P9-CJD-314

Handbook of Experimental Pharmacology

Continuation of Handbuch der experimentellen Pharmakologie

Vol. 62

Aminoglycoside Antibiotics

Contributors

I. R. Hooper · Y. Ito · T. Koeda · S. Kondo · S. Mitsuhashi
T. Okuda · N. Tanaka · T. Tsuchiya · K. Umemura
H. Umezawa · S. Umezawa · M. Yokota

Editors

H. Umezawa and I. R. Hooper

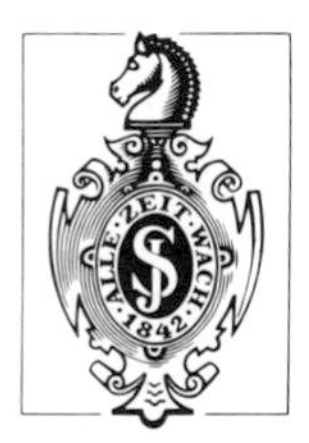

Springer-Verlag Berlin Heidelberg New York 1982

Professor Dr. HAMAO UMEZAWA

Institute of Microbial Chemistry, 14–23 Kamiosaki 3-Chome,
Shinagawa-ku, Tokyo, Japan

Dr. IRVING R. HOOPER

Research Associate, Duke University Marine Laboratory,
Pivers Island, Beaufort, NY 28516/USA

With 260 Figures

ISBN 3-540-11532-3 Springer-Verlag Berlin Heidelberg New York
ISBN 0-387-11532-3 Springer-Verlag New York Heidelberg Berlin

Library of Congress Cataloging in Publication Data. Main entry under title: Aminoglycoside Antibiotics (Handbook of experimental pharmacology; v. 62). Bibliography: p. Includes index. 1. Aminoglycosides–Therapeutic use. 2. Antibiotics. I. Umezawa, Hamao, 1914–. II. Hooper, Irving R., 1921–. III. Series. [DNLM: 1. Aminoglycosides. W1 HA51L v. 62/QU 75 A518] QP905.H3 vol. 62 [RM666.A456]. 615'.1s. 82-5638. ISBN 0-387-11532-3 (U.S.). [615'.329]. AACR2.

Printed in Germany.

Typesetting, printing, and bookbinding: Brühlsche Universitätsdruckerei, Giessen
2122/3130-543210

Preface

The first useful antibiotic found by screening was streptomycin. The late Prof. WAKSMAN started screening for antibacterial antibiotics in 1940 and, after finding actinomycin in 1941, he and his collaborators discovered streptomycin in 1944. This antibiotic made a great contribution in saving human lives from tuberculosis and acute serious infections. About 1957, after wide usage of such antibiotics as penicillin, streptomycin, chloramphenicol, tetracycline, and erythromycin, staphylococci and Gram negative organisms resistant to all or most antibiotic drugs appeared in hospital patients. The origin and treatment of such resistant strains became a major topic of investigation. At that time, kanamycin was discovered and used in the treatment of resistant infections. It may be said that the appearance of resistant strains stimulated a resurgence of research on new antibacterial antibiotics and their derivatives.

In 1965, kanamycin-resistant strains were found in hospital patients and, undertaking the study of the mechanisms of resistance, I found that resistant strains produce intracellular enzymes that can transfer either the terminal phosphate of ATP or the acetate of acetyl-CoA to the 3′-hydroxyl or the 6′-amino group of 2-deoxystreptamine-containing antibiotics. These results, reported in 1967, made it possible to design new synthetic derivatives that would inhibit the growth of kanamycin resistant strains of microorganisms. Thus, a new research area was opened: the development of aminoglycosides useful in the treatment of drug-resistant infections.

Developments in carbohydrate chemistry have made it possible to synthesize streptomycin, kanamycin and most other aminoglycoside antibiotics. From another ascpect, it can also be said that the successful total synthesis of these antibiotics has made great contributions to the progress of carbohydrate chemistry. Derivatives of aminoglycosides are now produced on an industrial scale.

Microorganisms have an almost unlimited ability to produce novel compounds. Even at present, new types of aminoglycosides are being found in microbial culture filtrates. The reasons so many varied secondary metabolites are found in microorganisms and the evolution and genetics of resistance are topics with great relevance to biological and medical science. Considering the biochemical characteristics of future resistant strains, microbiologists and chemists are studying new aminoglycosides and other structures that could inhibit the growth of present and future resistant strains. Up to now, most success has been obtained with β-lactam and aminoglycoside antibiotics.

As described, there have been many important accomplishments in the biochemistry and chemistry of aminoglycosides. In order to review these studies, this book was published. It is hoped that this book will contribute to the coming progress in studies of chemotherapy, antibiotics, and carbohydrate chemistry.

Dr. IRVING R. HOOPER, my friend who collaborated with me on the publication of this book, read carefully all manuscripts and corrected the English written by authors outside of English-speaking countries. In behalf of these authors I wish to thank Dr. HOOPER for his great effort in writing not only his manuscript but also for his careful review of the papers. I wish also to thank all contributors for their enthusiastic collaboration.

Tokyo HAMAO UMEZAWA

List of Contributors

Dr. Irving R. Hooper, Duke University Marine Laboratory, Pivers Island, Beaufort, NC 28516/USA

Dr. Yukio Ito, Microbial Research Laboratory, Tanabe Seiyaku Co., Ltd., 2-2-50 Kawagishi, Toda-Shi, Saitama-ken 335, Japan

Dr. Takemi Koeda, Research Laboratories, Meiji Seika Kaisha, Ltd., 760 Morooka-cho, Kohoku-ku, Yokohama-shi, Kanagawa-ken 222, Japan

Dr. Shinichi Kondo, Institute of Microbial Chemistry, 14-23 Kamiosaki 3-Chome, Shinagawa-ku, Tokyo 141, Japan

Dr. Susumu Mitsuhashi, Department of Microbiology, Laboratory of Bacterial Resistance, School of Medicine, Gunma University, Showa-machi, Maebashi-shi, Gunma-ken 371, Japan

Dr. Tomoharu Okuda, Microbial Research Laboratory, Tanabe Seiyaku Co., Ltd., 2-2-50 Kawagishi, Toda-shi, Saitama-ken 335, Japan

Dr. Nobuo Tanaka, Institute of Applied Microbiology, University of Tokyo, 1-1 Yayoi 1-Chome, Bunkyo-ku, Tokyo 113, Japan

Dr. Tsutomu Tsuchiya, Institute of Bioorganic Chemistry, 1416 Ida, Nakahara-ku, Kawasaki-shi, Kanagawa-ken 211, Japan

Dr. Koshiro Umemura, Research Laboratories, Meiji Seika Kaisha, Ltd., 760 Morooka-cho, Kohoku-ku, Yokohama-shi, Kanagawa-ken 222, Japan

Dr. Hamao Umezawa, Institute of Microbial Chemistry, 14–23 Kamiosaki 3-Chome, Shinagawa-ku, Tokyo 141, Japan

Dr. Sumio Umezawa, Institute of Bioorganic Chemistry, 1416 Ida, Nakahara-ku, Kawasaki-shi, Kanagawa-ken 211, Japan

Dr. Masayuki Yokota, Research Laboratories, Meiji Seika Kaisha, Ltd., 760 Morooka-cho, Kohoku-ku, Yokohama-shi, Kanagawa-ken 222, Japan

Contents

CHAPTER 1

The Naturally Occurring Aminoglycoside Antibiotics. I. R. HOOPER.

CHAPTER 2

Total Synthesis and Chemical Modification of the Aminoglycoside Antibiotics. S. UMEZAWA and T. TSUCHIYA. With 87 Figures

CHAPTER 3

Biosynthesis and Mutasynthesis of Aminoglycoside Antibiotics.
T. OKUDA and Y. ITO. With 42 Figures

CHAPTER 4

Antibacterial Activity of Aminoglycoside Antibiotics. S. MITSUHASHI. With 9 Figures

CHAPTER 5

Mechanism of Action of Aminoglycoside Antibiotics. N. TANAKA. With 21 Figures

CHAPTER 6

Mechanisms of Resistance to Aminoglycoside Antibiotics.
H. UMEZAWA and S. KONDO. With 16 Figures

CHAPTER 7

Toxicology and Pharmacology of Aminoglycoside Antibiotics.
T. KOEDA, K. UMEMURA, and M. YOKOTA. With 23 Figures

CHAPTER 1

The Naturally Occurring Aminoglycoside Antibiotics

I. R. HOOPER

A. Introduction

A large group of loosely related antibiotics containing aminosugars as their main components has traditionally been classed the aminoglycoside antibiotics. Since many of the most important members of this class of antibiotics contain an aminocyclitol moiety, the terms aminocyclitol antibiotics or aminoglycoside–aminocyclitol antibiotics have also been used to define the group. In this chapter we will include some simpler aminoglycoses and aminoglycosides which do not contain a cyclitol fragment because some of these compounds without a cyclitol closely resemble the typical aminoglycoside–aminocyclitol compounds in terms of biologic and chemical properties. Many other antibiotic groups contain aminoglycoside fragments, e.g., the macrolides, nuleosides, and anthracyclines. However, we will not discuss these types but only those compounds in which carbohydrate-like components make up the main structural units.

The aminoglycosides were among the earliest antibiotics to be studied. Streptomycin (SCHATZ et al. 1944) was one of the very earliest and the second antibiotic after penicillin, to reach widespread clinical usage. Many others of the group have attained widespread commercial usage and new aminoglycosides or new derivatives are still being vigorously investigated and marketed. The total world market for human clinical use of this class of compounds was estimated at approximately US-$ 525 million for 1978 at the manufacturers' level.

A majority of the aminoglycosides are produced by actinomycetes. The large, important group of gentamicin, sisomicin, and related compounds is produced by strains of *Micromonospora* and recently several new aminoglycosides have been isolated from bacterial fermentation.

Aminoglycosides are generally water-soluble basic compounds. Because of the general lack of solvent extractability, adsorption techniques have been most commonly used for the isolation and purification of these compounds. Probably the most widely applicable technique has been ion-exchange chromatography on weakly acidic cation-exchange resins such as Amberlite IRC-50. This material was developed for commercial use in the early days of streptomycin purification studies and has been indispensable for isolations in this field ever since. Besides its use for primary isolation of crude antibiotic it has been widely used in weakly basic buffer systems for the chromatographic purification and separation of closely related aminoglycosides. As with most other classes of antibiotics, usually a group of closely related compounds are produced by a single organism. In most cases the compounds are separated for clinical use but gentamicin, the largest selling aminoglycoside, is used as a defined, controlled mixture of the three closely related gentamicins, C_1, C_{1a}, and C_2.

The determination of the structure of new aminoglycosides usually depends upon hydrolysis of glycosidic, and in some cases amide, bonds to yield simpler fragments which often are sugars or aminosugars and a cyclitol. The polyhydroxylic, polyamino character of the compounds make it difficult to obtain good crystalline preparations and X-ray structural studies have played little part in aminoglycoside chemistry. However, modern spectroscopic techniques, especially nuclear magnetic resonance of protons and, more recently, ^{13}C nuclei, have made the structural assignment of fragments relatively simple. In some caes, the structure of intact molecules can be determined by these methods, especially when the new compound is a new member of a well-studied series.

The aminoglycosides are, in general, broad-spectrum antibiotics used primarily for treating infections with *Escherichia coli*, *Klebsiella*, *Proteus*, and *Enterobacter*. Their activity against *Pseudomonas* is variable, with some classes being among the most effective agents for treating these organisms. Recently, strains of normally sensitive bacteria have developed resistance to certain aminoglycoside antibiotics through inactivating enzymes. These resistance mechanisms are discussed in Chap. 6 of this handbook, and the steps taken to combat such resistance mechanisms by chemically modifying aminoglycosides are discussed in Chap. 2. The antimicrobial activity is discussed in detail in Chap. 4, so this chapter will make only a general assessment of antibacterial activity.

The arrangement of this chapter is somewhat arbitrary. The compounds are grouped according to the structural type and substitution pattern of the nonreducing moiety. This moiety is often a cyclitol and frequently is 2-deoxystreptamine (2-DOS). While this may seem to put undue emphasis on one portion of the molecule, it usually brings related compounds together and results in conveniently sized groups in most cases.

We have tried to include all the naturally occurring aminoglycosides but have not included compounds which, while active, have been reported only as degradation products of other active compounds. In general, we have not included compounds prepared by directed biosynthesis or mutasynthesis, since Chap. 3 deals with this subject. However, probably some of the naturally occurring compounds discussed in this chapter arise from the use of mutants or special media and many represent early examples of directed biosynthesis. Since the mechanism of their formation is unknown and since they were more or less chance observations, these early examples are included here.

B. Aminoglycoses and Noncyclitol Aminoglycosides

I. Aminoglycose Derivatives

Several simple glucosamines and their derivatives have been isolated from fermentation and shown to have weak antibacterial activity.

3-Amino-3-deoxy-D-glucose (1), a component of kanamycin, was isolated from *Bacillus aminoglucosidicus* ATCC 21143 (S. UMEZAWA et al. 1967a) and shown to have weak antibacterial activity. Fermentations yield up to 4 mg/ml of the

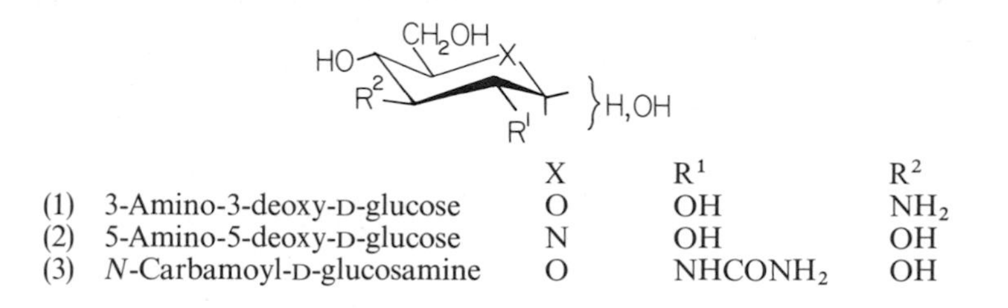

	X	R^1	R^2
(1) 3-Amino-3-deoxy-D-glucose	O	OH	NH_2
(2) 5-Amino-5-deoxy-D-glucose	N	OH	OH
(3) *N*-Carbamoyl-D-glucosamine	O	$NHCONH_2$	OH

aminosugar which is isolated by adsorption on Amberlite IRC-50. Nojirimycin (2), R-468, SF-425, 5-amino-5-deoxy-D-glucose has weak antibacterial and antifungal activity (NISHIKAWA and ISHIDA 1965). The unique piperidinose structure was reported by INOUYE et al. (1966). Nojirimycin has been shown to be a potent glucosidase inhibitor (NIWA et al. 1970).

N-Carbamoyl-D-glucosamine (3), SF 1993, has been isolated from *Streptomyces halstedii* cultures grown on the surface of agar (SHOMURA et al. 1979; OMOTO et al. 1979). It can be produced in submerged fermentations by the use of conditions or strains which prevent fragmentation of the mycelium. The active material was isolated by carbon adsorption and purified with Sephadex LH-20. It is weakly active against some gram-negative bacteria and some fungi.

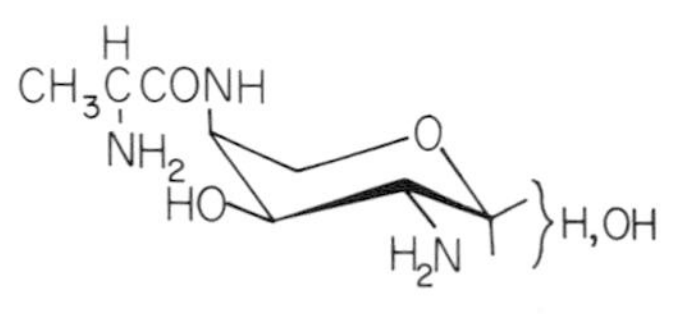

(4) Prumycin

Prumycin (4), 4-D-alanyl-2,4-diamino-2,4-dideoxy-L-arabinose, was isolated from fermentations of a *Streptomyces* sp. by Amberlite IRC-50 adsorption and shown to have activity against some phytopathogenic fungi (HATA et al. 1971; OMURA et al. 1973). The structure determination was reported in 1974 (OMURA et al.). Prumycin is inactive against most bacteria and yeasts. Recently it was reported (OKUBO et al. 1979) to have potent antitumor activity in several experimental mouse tumor systems.

II. Disaccharides and Pseudodisaccharides

Several nonreducing disaccharides have been isolated from fermentations and shown to have weak antibacterial activity. In many cases the activity is media dependent and is of little practical interest.

α,α-Trehalosamine (5) was first isolated from a streptomyces (ARCAMONE and BIZIOLI 1957) and later synthesized (S. UMEZAWA et al. 1967b). It is active against *Mycobacterium tuberculosis* at 2 μg/ml but is blocked by trehalose. The 2-epimer of trehalosamine, α-D-mannosyl-2-amino-2-deoxy-α-D-glucoside (6) was isolated by URAMOTO et al. (1967). It is coproduced with trehalosamine by *Streptomyces virginiae* and is active against *Mycobacterium smegmatis*.

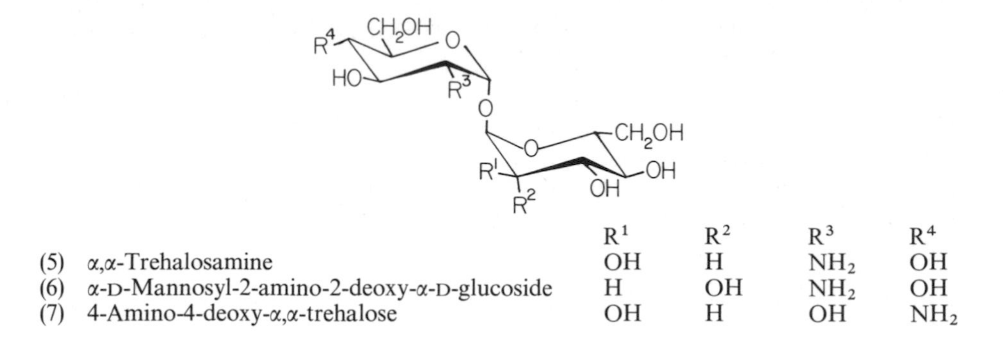

		R¹	R²	R³	R⁴
(5)	α,α-Trehalosamine	OH	H	NH_2	OH
(6)	α-D-Mannosyl-2-amino-2-deoxy-α-D-glucoside	H	OH	NH_2	OH
(7)	4-Amino-4-deoxy-α,α-trehalose	OH	H	OH	NH_2

The 4-amino derivative of α,α-trehalose (7) was isolated from a *Streptomyces* strain by NAGANAWA et al. (1974). It is weakly active against *E. coli* and *Bacillus subtilis* but is inactive against *M. smegmatis* ATCC 607, while trehalosamine is active against this organism. Although the 2-amino and 4-amino compounds are active, synthetic 6-amino-6-deoxy-α,α-trehalose (HANESSIAN and LAVALLEE 1972) has no appreciable antibacterial activity.

The sorbistins are a new group of aminoglycoside antibiotics in which an aminoglucose is glycosidically linked to a diamino polyalcohol. However, the aglycone is an open chain diaminohexitol. The antibacterial spectrum is typical of aminoglycosides but with considerably less activity, although the sorbistins do show activity against many of the aminoglycoside-resistant strains. The sorbistins were studied independently by three groups, each of which reported the isolation and structural identification of this new class of aminoglycoside antibiotics.

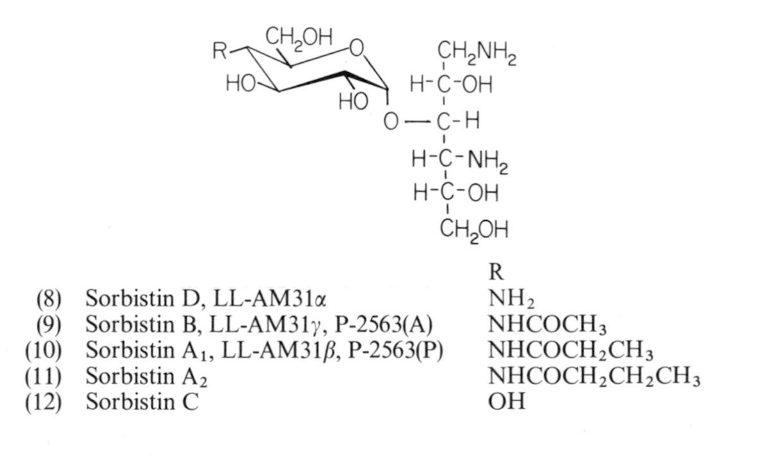

		R
(8)	Sorbistin D, LL-AM31α	NH_2
(9)	Sorbistin B, LL-AM31γ, P-2563(A)	$NHCOCH_3$
(10)	Sorbistin A_1, LL-AM31β, P-2563(P)	$NHCOCH_2CH_3$
(11)	Sorbistin A_2	$NHCOCH_2CH_2CH_3$
(12)	Sorbistin C	OH

The compounds were isolated by Amberlite IRC-50 adsorption (TSUKIURA et al. 1976; KIRBY et al. 1977a; NARA et al. 1978a). Structural determination (KONISHI et al. 1976; KIRBY et al. 1977b; NARA et al. 1978b, c) was largely carried out by hydrolysis and isolation of fragments with structural assignment carried out mainly by spectroscopic methods. The structure of sorbistin A_1 was confirmed by X-ray analysis of the hydrobromide (KAMIYA et al. 1978). One structure proof of the aglycone involved the reduction of the oxime of 4-amino-4-deoxy-D-glucose, obtained from the sugar portion of sorbistin, to a 1,4-diamino-1,4-dideoxyhexitol identical to the aglycone of sorbistin (KONISHI et al. 1976).

The antibiotics are produced by *Pseudomonas sorbicinii* (TOMITA et al. 1976), *P. fluorescens* (NARA et al. 1978a), and *Streptoverticillium* sp. (KIRBY et al. 1977a). Sorbistin A_1 (10), with the propionyl side chain on the 4-amino group of the aminoglucose, is the most active of the group, being approximately two to four times as active as the acetyl derivative, sorbistin B (9), or the butyryl derivative, sorbistin A_2 (11). Sobistin A_1 is approximately $^1/_{50}$ as active as kanamycin against a standard *E. coli* strain but is active against several aminoglycoside-resistant strains. The free amino compound, sorbistin D (8), and the hydroxy analog, sorbistin C (12), are biologically inactive.

III. Trisaccharides

A unique group of aminoglycosides, the glycocinnamoylspermidines, has recently been reported by MARTIN et al. (1978). These compounds are produced by an un-

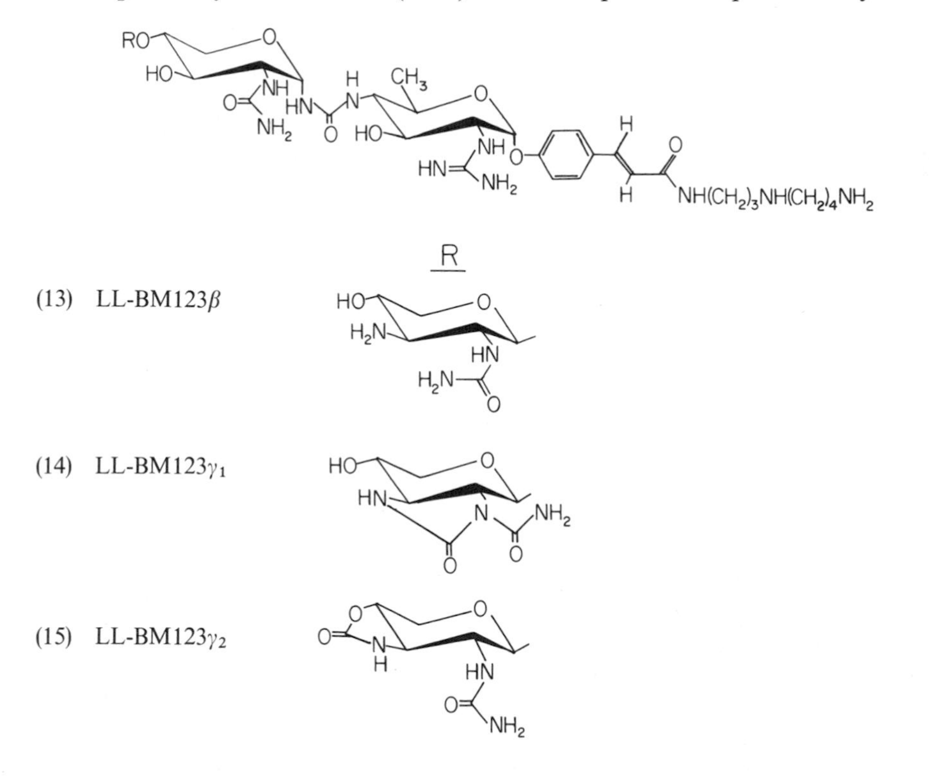

identified species of *Nocardia* (TRESNER et al. 1978), together with LL-BM123 α, a myoinosamine-containing antibiotic (ELLESTAD et al. 1977) which will be discussed in Sect. D.II. The compounds were isolated and purified by ion-exchange chromatography on CM-Sephadex. Structures were determined by hydrolysis and spectral studies (ELLESTAD et al. 1978). LL-BM123 γ, a mixture of γ_1 (14) and γ_2 (15), is two to four times more potent than LL-BM123 β (13) and is one-half to one-fourth as potent as gentamicin against most organisms tested, with a spectrum typical of the aminoglycoside antibiotics.

It is, however, much less active than gentamicin against *Pseudomonas* and is more toxic. Modification studies have given derivatives with improvements in both activity and toxicity (HLAVKA et al. 1978; KUCK and REDIN 1978). The isopropyl derivative obtained by alkylation of the terminal amine of the spermidine moiety compares favorably in activity to gentamicin and has activity against some aminoglycoside-resistant strains.

C. Aminocyclitol Aminoglycosides Containing Streptamine, 2-Deoxystreptamine, or Their Derivatives

The largest group of aminoglycosides consists of those in which the aglycone is 2-deoxystreptamine (2-DOS) (16), streptamine (17), or streptidine (18).

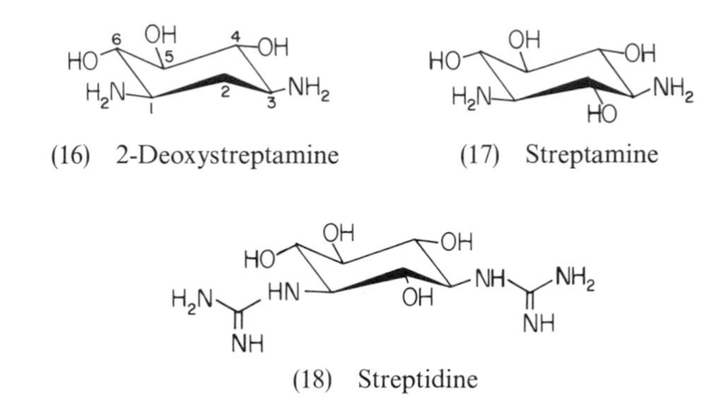

(16) 2-Deoxystreptamine (17) Streptamine

(18) Streptidine

These aminocyclitols are interesting in that the free cyclitol is optically inactive, but substitution on one side of the plane of symmetry produces optically active compounds. The numbering of the ring atoms is as shown for 2-DOS in which numbering begins with the nitrogen-bearing carbon atom having the *R* configuration. Although many 2-DOS compounds are found with a monosubstituted aglycone, the most active generally have 4,5 or 4,6 substitution patterns and are pseudotri- or tetrasaccharides. Monosubstituted 2-DOS compounds with high activity are known, e.g., streptomycin or apramycin, but these are also pseudotrisaccharides. In disubstituted compounds the sugar attached to the 4 position of 2-DOS or another aglycone is given primed numbers and that at the 5 or 6 position is given double primed numbers.

The first compound of this class to be investigated was streptomycin (32) (SCHATZ et al. 1944), containing the cyclitol streptidine (18). Of the very important 2-DOS-containing group, the first to be studied was neomycin (48) (WAKSMAN and LECHEVALIER 1949; H. UMEZAWA et al. 1949).

The structure and biologic activity relationships of the 2-DOS-containing aminoglycosides have been intensively reviewed by PRICE et al. (1974, 1977). Chemical modification of this class of antibiotic continues at a rapid pace with new interesting derivatives announced each year.

I. Monosubstituted Streptamine and 2-Deoxystreptamine Aminoglycosides

Accompanying some of the common 4,5- or 4,6-disubstituted pseudotri- and pseudotetrasaccharides, such as neomycin, are the corresponding 4-substituted disaccharides which generally have appreciable antibacterial activity but less than that of the disubstituted compounds. Often these disaccharides have been isolated first as degradation products of the disubstituted compounds and have later been found as primary fermentation products. Other unique compounds with monosubstituted 2-DOS are also found as primary fermentation products with no disubstituted counterparts.

1. 4- or 6-Substituted Cyclitol

One of the most interesting monosubstituted compounds is apramycin (19), or nebramycin factor 2, as it was known in the early literature. It is produced by *Streptomyces tenebrarius* (HIGGENS and KASTNER 1968), together with several 2-DOS-disubstituted compounds of the nebramycin complex (STARK et al. 1968). It is surprisingly active compared with other 4-monosubstituted 2-DOS compounds such as neamine which is $^1/_8$ to $^1/_{16}$ as active as apramycin against typical organisms. In addition it is resistant to many of the aminoglycoside inactivating enzymes and so is active against many resistant strains. The activity of apramycin is approximately one-fourth that of gentamicin. The nebramycin complex is isolated from the fermentation by Amberlite IRC-50 adsorption and is separated into components by chromatography on cation-exchange resins (THOMPSON and PRESTI 1968; KOCH et al. 1973). The octadiose sugar which exists as a rigid bicyclic system is a unique feature of this interesting antibiotic. The structure was determined from hydrolytic and spectral data and was confirmed by X-ray crystallography (O'CONNOR et al. 1976).

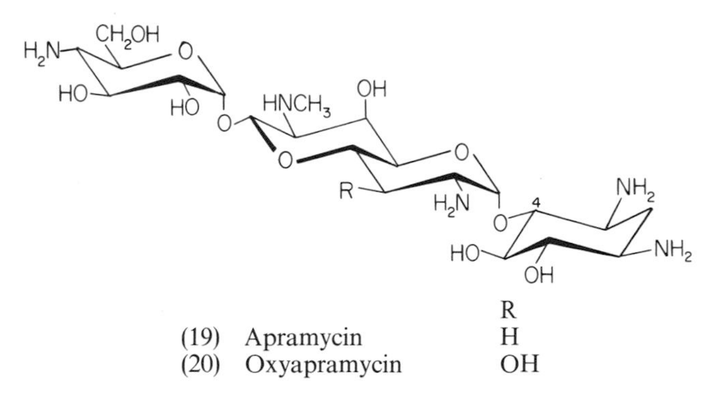

		R
(19)	Apramycin	H
(20)	Oxyapramycin	OH

Oxyapramycin (20) (nebramycin factor 7) is produced as a minor component accompanying apramycin in fermentations of a mutant of *S. tenebrarius* which produces mainly apramycin (DORMAN et al. 1976).

Among the pseudodisaccharides which can be considered as incomplete tri- or tetrasaccharides are several aminoglucosyl derivatives of 2-DOS.

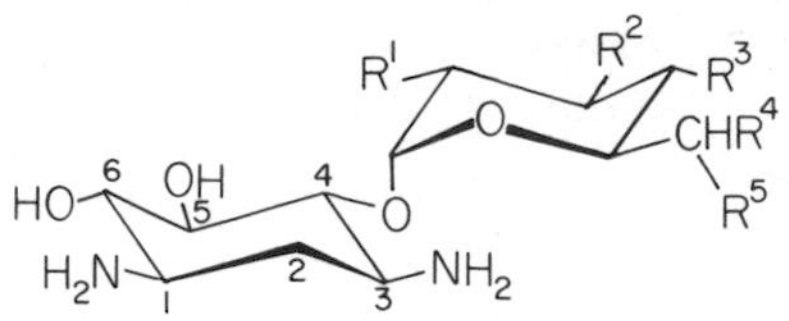

		R^1	R^2	R^3	R^4	R^5
(21)	Neamine	NH_2	OH	OH	NH_2	H
(22)	Nebramine	NH_2	H	OH	NH_2	H
(23)	Paromamine	NH_2	OH	OH	OH	H
(24)	Lividamine	NH_2	H	OH	OH	H
(25)	NK-1003	OH	OH	OH	NH_2	H
(26)	4-Deoxyneamine	NH_2	OH	H	NH_2	H
(27)	Gentamine C_1	NH_2	H	H	$NHCH_3$	CH_3
(28)	Gentamine C_2	HN_2	H	H	NH_2	CH_3
(29)	Gentamine C_{1a}	NH_2	H	H	NH_2	H

Neamine (21), originally designated neomycin A, was isolated by PECK et al. (1949) from the neomycin complex and was later shown to be identical to the principal acid degradation product of the neomycins (LEACH and TEETERS 1951). It has about one-tenth the activity of the neomycin complex. It is used as the basis of comparison for 4- or 6-substituted 2-DOS derivatives in the review by PRICE et al. (1974, 1977). Although it is more potent than most of the 4- or 6-monosubstituted derivatives in this group, it is approximately 50-fold less active than gentamicin. The chemistry of the entire neomycin complex is discussed by RINEHART (1961). Paromamine (23), a 2-amino-2-deoxy-α-D-glucosyl derivative of 2-DOS, is a member of the paromomycin complex (HASKELL et al. 1959; RINEHART 1961). It is much less active than neamine, just as paromomycin is less active than neomycin.

Recently two additional disaccharides have been characterized from a study of the minor components of the *S. tenebrarius* fermentation which yields tobramycin (66) and apramycin (19) (KOCH et al. 1978).

Nebramycin factor 8 is nebramine (22), or 3′-deoxyneamine, while nebramicyn factor 9 has been shown to be lividamine (24), or 3′-deoxyparomamine. NK-1003 (25), 4-O-(6-amino-6-deoxy-α-D-glucopyranosyl)-2-deoxystreptamine, may be produced by the mild acid hydrolysis of kanamycin but has also been isolated by ion-exchange chromatography from fermentation of a mutant *S. kanamyceticus* culture (MURASE et al. 1970). It was weak antibacterial activity.

Seldomycin factor 2 (26), or 4′-deoxyneamine, was isolated from fermentations of *S. hofunensis* by cation-exchange resin and silica gel chromatography (SATO et al. 1977) as a member of the seldomycin complex. The structure was determined to be as shown by spectral analyses (EGAN et al. 1977 a) and confirmed by comparison with 4′-deoxyneamine obtained from degradation of 4′-deoxybutirosin (KONISHI et al. 1974). It appears to be somewhat more active than neamine.

BERDY et al. (1977), in an extensive study of minor components, showed that three 4-substituted 2-DOS pseudodisaccharides corresponding to the three main gentamicin fractions occur in the fermentation of a gentamicin-producing *Micromonospora* culture. These compounds, designated gentamine C_1 (27), C_2 (28), and C_{1a} (29), were described earlier as degradation products of the gentamicins. BERDY et al. reported that these compounds all showed broad antibacterial activity.

There are two examples of a pseudodisaccharide of 2-DOS substituted at the 6 rather than the 4 position. NK-1012-2 (30), 6-O-(3-amino-3-deoxy-α-D-gluco-

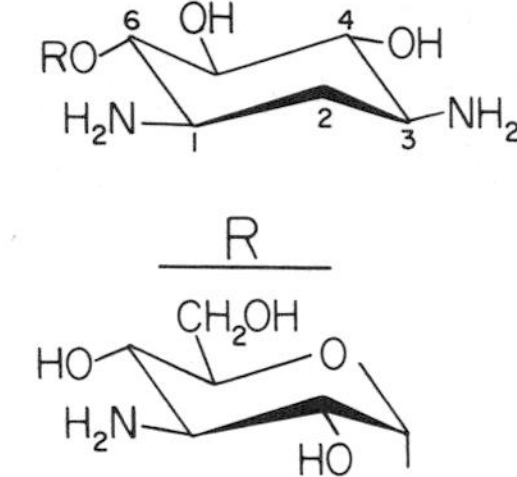

(30) NK-1012-2

(31) Garamine

pyranosyl)-2-deoxystreptamine, is obtainable from kanamycin and has been reported (MURASE et al. 1970) to be present in fermentation broths of a mutant strain of *S. kanamyceticus*. It is very weakly active, and is even less active than NK-1003. The pseudodisaccharide from the gentamicin C complex containing 2-DOS and its 6-O substituent, garamine (31), was isolated by BERDY et al. (1977) in their work on minor components in the gentamicin fermentation.

Streptomycin (32) and its relatives constitute an important group of monosubstituted aminocyclitol antibiotics. Most of the structure work on streptomycin was carried out before the advent of modern spectroscopic techniques. This early work was reviewed by LEMIEUX and WOLFROM (1948) and later studies are included in the review by S. UMEZAWA (1974). The early isolation work involved carbon adsorption and elution with alumina chromatography for purification. The weak cation-exchange resins with CO_2H groups soon replaced carbon as the preferred adsorbent for purification of the antibiotic on both the laboratory and commercial scale.

Streptomycin has a broad spectrum of activity against most of the gram-negative organisms except *Pseudomonas*, many gram-positive organisms, and *M. tuberculosis*.

Mannosidostreptomycin (33), or streptomycin B as it was formerly called, occurred together with streptomycin in the early fermentations of *S. griseus*. It was first reported by FRIED and TITUS (1947, 1948). It is about one-fourth to one-eight as active as streptomycin with a similar spectrum. The mannosyl moiety attached to the *N*-methyl-L-glucosamine fragment (C) can be enzymatically removed by a mannosidostrepomycinase found in streptomycin-producing cultures of *S. griseus* (PERLMAN and LANGLYKE 1948).

Most of the other variants on the streptomycin structure involve changes in the unusual branched chain sugar, streptose, the central moiety (B). The B+C disaccharide is termed streptobiosamine and is linked to streptidine by an α-L linkage while the *N*-methyl-L-glucosamine is also linked by an α-L linkage to the streptose.

		R^1	R^2	R^3	R^4	R^5
(32)	Streptomycin	NH–C(=NH)–NH_2	CHO	CH_3	H	CH_3
(33)	Mannosidostreptomycin	NH–C(=NH)–NH_2	CHO	CH_3	D-Manno-pyranosyl	CH_3
(34)	Dihydrostreptomycin	NH–C(=NH)–NH_2	CH_2OH	CH_3	H	CH_3
(35)	Hydroxystreptomycin	NH–C(=NH)–NH_2	CHO	CH_2OH	H	CH_3
(36)	*N*-Demethylstreptomycin	NH–C(=NH)–NH_2	CHO	CH_3	H	H
(37)	Glebomycin	$OCONH_2$	CH_2OH	CH_3	H	CH_3

Dihydrostreptomycin (34) was produced in early structural studies by catalytic hydrogenation of streptomycin but may also be prepared by direct fermentation (TATSUOKA et al. 1957). It is very similar in activity to streptomycin. Hydroxystreptomycin (35) was first reported by HOSOYA et al. (1950) under the name reticulin, as a product of *S. reticuli*. It was recognized that it was related to streptomycin but the relationship was unknown until BENEDICT et al. (1950) reported on hydroxystreptomycin. *N*-Demethylstreptomycin (36) is produced from *S. griseus* grown in the presence of DL-ethionine (HEDING 1968), an inhibitor of methylation.

Glebomycin (37), or bluensomycin, was reported independently by two groups of workers (MIYAKI et al. 1962; BANNISTER and ARGOUDELIS 1963). One of the guanidino groups of the streptidine is replaced by the O-carbamoyl group (NAITO 1962). The absolute configuration was determined by BARLOW and ANDERSON (1972) to be as shown. Glebomycin is produced by a *Streptomyces* strain (OHMORI et al. 1962) and is about one-fifth to one-tenth as active as streptomycin (OKANISHI et al. 1962).

2. 5-Substituted Cyclitol

An interesting group of compounds with an unusual orthoester structure has been studied by several groups of investigators and reported under various names over the past few years.

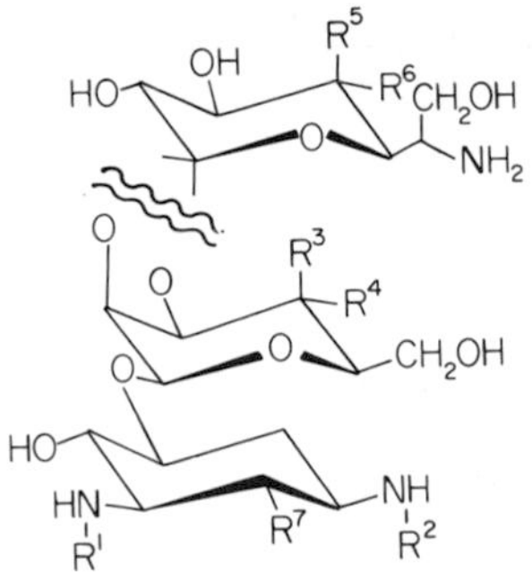

		R^1	R^2	R^3	R^4	R^5	R^6	R^7
(38)	Hygromycin B	H	CH_3	OH	H	OH	H	H
(39)	Destomycin A	CH_3	H	OH	H	OH	H	H
(40)	Destomycin B	CH_3	CH_3	H	OH	H	OH	H
(41)	Destomycin C	CH_3	CH_3	OH	H	OH	H	H
(42)	A-396-I	H	H	OH	H	OH	H	H
(43)	SS-56-C	H	H	OH	H	OH	H	OH
(44)	A-16316-C	CH_3	CH_3	H	OH	OH	H	H

Hygromycin B (38) was first isolated by MANN and BROMER (1958) from *S. hygroscopicus*, which also produces hygromycin A. It was found to have the structure shown by WILEY et al. (1962) and NEUSS et al. (1970). The aminocyclitol (moiety C) is (+)-*N*-methyl-2-deoxystreptamine and linked to it by a β-glycosidic bond is a talose or mannose fragment (B). A unique amino acid (A), termed destomic acid (KONDO et al. 1966 b) and shown to be 6-amino-6-deoxy-L-*glycero*-D-*galacto*-heptonic acid, or its 4 epimer, *epi*-destomic acid, is bound by orthoester formation to the 1- and 2-hydroxyls of the talose or mannose moiety. The configuration of the orthoester carbon is unknown.

Destomycin A (39) and B (40) were isolated by KONDO et al. (1965 a) from *S. rimofaciens* and the structures were reported in several papers from the same group (KONDO et al. 1965 b, 1966 a, b, 1975). Destomycin C (41) was found as a minor component of the crude destomycin preparation (SHIMURA et al. 1975). The aminocyclitol (C) is (−)-*N*-methyl-2-deoxystreptamine in destomycin A and *N*,*N'*-dimethyl-2-deoxystreptamine in destomycin B and C. The central neutral sugar moiety (B) is mannose in destomycin B and talose in destomycin A and C. While destomycin A and C contain destomic acid as the amino acid moiety (A), destomycin B has the 4 epimer, *epi*-destomic acid, or 6-amino-6-deoxy-L-*glycero*-D-*gluco*-heptonic acid.

Antibiotic A-396-I (42) was isolated from *Streptoverticillium eurocidicus* by SHOJI et al. (1970), together with hygromycin B (A-396-II) (38). It is made up of 2-DOS, talose, and destomic acid (SHOJI and NAKAGAWA 1970).

Another new member of this family, SS-56-C (43), was found in fermentations of *Streptomyces eurocidicus* by INOUYE et al. (1973). The aminocyclitol here is streptamine, to which is linked talose and destomic acid. Also present in the fermentation were A-396-I (42) (SS-56-D), the deoxystreptamine analog of SS-56-C, and two bioinactive products, SS-56-A and B, the 5-β-mannoside and 5-β-taloside respectively of 2-DOS.

Antibiotic A-16316-C (44) was studied by TAMURA et al. (1975) and shown to be an analog containing *N,N′*-dimethyl-2-deoxystreptamine, mannose, and destomic acid. It is produced by *Streptoverticillium eurocidicus* which also produces A-396-I (A 16316-A) (42) and hygromycin B (A-396-II) (A 16316-B) (38).

A possible new member of this group is AB-74 (TAMURA et al. 1976a, b). It is produced by *Streptomyces aquacanus*, together with hygromycin B (38) and neomycin A (21), B (48), and C (49). It yields the same components as destomycin C (41), i.e., destomic acid, D-talose, and *N,N′*-dimethyl-2-deoxystreptamine. However, there are differences in the optical rotation and ^{1}H- and ^{13}C-NMR spectra. It remains to be determined whether this is yet another member of this extensive family. The members of the hygromycin B family are all isolated by cation-exchange resin chromatography. They have a broad range of activity against gram-positive and gram-negative bacteria, fungi, and helminths.

II. Disubstituted 2-Deoxystreptamine Aminoglycosides

1. 4,5-Disubstituted Cyclitol

a) Pseudotrisaccharides

Several pseudotrisaccharides have been found recently as primary fermentation products, although in many cases they represent fragments of the more complex neomycin-type antibiotics.

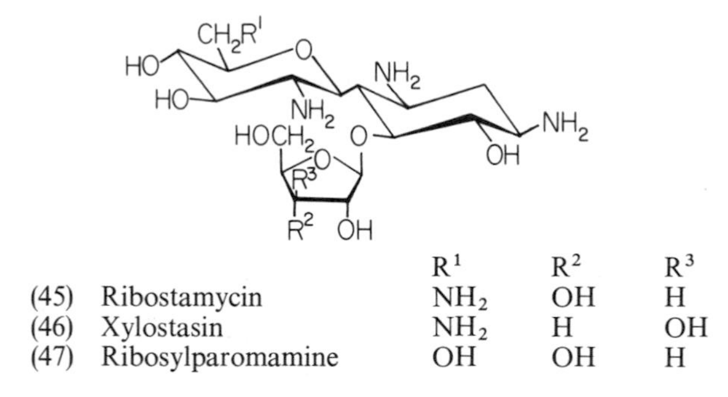

		R^1	R^2	R^3
(45)	Ribostamycin	NH_2	OH	H
(46)	Xylostasin	NH_2	H	OH
(47)	Ribosylparomamine	OH	OH	H

Ribostamycin (45), SF-733, was isolated from cultures of *Streptomyces ribosidificus* (SHOMURA et al. 1970) and shown to be 5-O-β-D-ribofuranosyl neamine (AKITA et al. 1970). After purification with Amberlite IRC-50 and CG-50 it can be crystallized. It is 5–10 times more active than neamine and is roughly comparable in activity to kanamycin. It is widely used clinically in Japan.

The *xylo* epimer, xylostasin (46), was isolated by degradation of the antibiotic butirosin and shown to have approximately the same antibacterial activity as ribostamycin (TSUKIURA et al. 1973a). It was also reported as a primary fermentation product produced by two *Bacillus subtilis* strains (HORII et al. 1974).

A third member of this family, 5-β-D-ribosylparomamine (47), was first prepared by degradation of Bu-1709 E_2 (TSUKIURA et al. 1973b) and of paromomycin (TAKAMOTO and HANESSIAN 1974) and was later found in fermentations of a *Streptomyces*, which also produced paromomycin (52) (KIRBY et al. 1977b). It is $^{1}/_{10}$

to $^{1}/_{20}$ as active as ribostamycin, just as paromomycin is weaker in biologic activity than neomycin.

b) Pseudotetra- and Pseudopentasaccharides

The neomycin group of antibiotics is similar to the group discussed in Sect. C.II.1.a but the pentose moiety, which in neomycin-type compounds is always ribose, is substituted by another aminosugar residue giving compounds which are generally more bioactive than the pseudotrisaccharides.

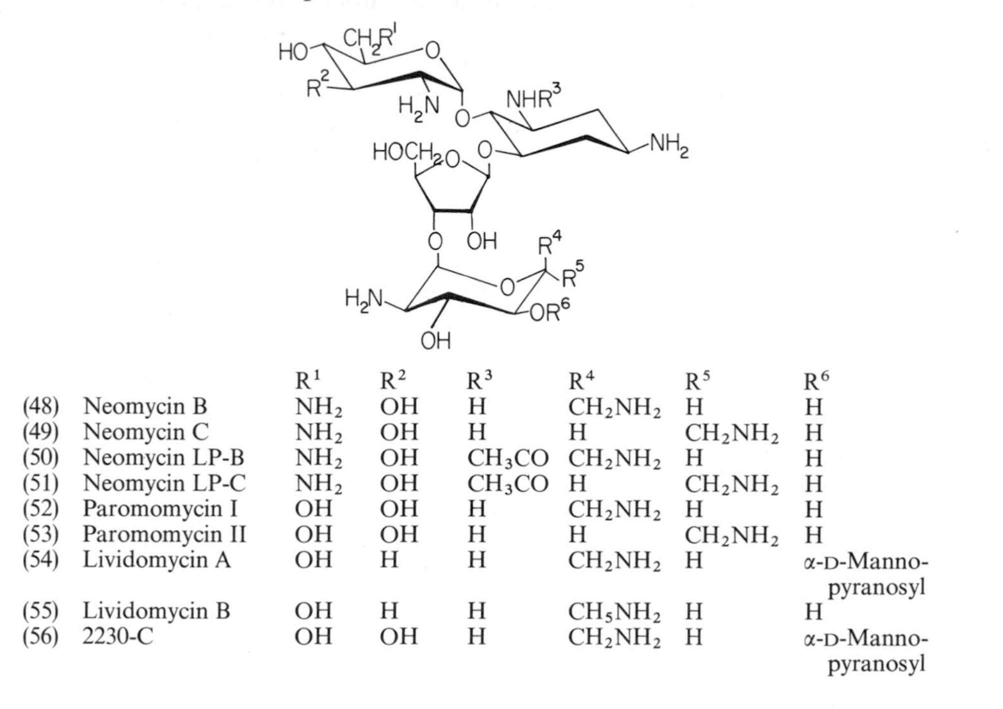

		R^1	R^2	R^3	R^4	R^5	R^6
(48)	Neomycin B	NH_2	OH	H	CH_2NH_2	H	H
(49)	Neomycin C	NH_2	OH	H	H	CH_2NH_2	H
(50)	Neomycin LP-B	NH_2	OH	CH_3CO	CH_2NH_2	H	H
(51)	Neomycin LP-C	NH_2	OH	CH_3CO	H	CH_2NH_2	H
(52)	Paromomycin I	OH	OH	H	CH_2NH_2	H	H
(53)	Paromomycin II	OH	OH	H	H	CH_2NH_2	H
(54)	Lividomycin A	OH	H	H	CH_2NH_2	H	α-D-Mannopyranosyl
(55)	Lividomycin B	OH	H	H	CH_5NH_2	H	H
(56)	2230-C	OH	OH	H	CH_2NH_2	H	α-D-Mannopyranosyl

Pseudotetra- and pentasaccharides may be grouped into four groups. The neomycins have a 2,6-diamino-2,6-dideoxy-*β*-D-glucopyranosyl residue attached to the 4 position of the 2-DOS moiety. In the paromomycins this group is 2-amino-2-deoxy-glucosyl and in the lividomycins it is 2-amino-2,3-dideoxy-α-D-glucopyranosyl. Compound 2230-C is a mannosylparomomycin. The neomycins were first reported by WAKSMAN and LECHEVALIER (1949). The early work on the neomycins has been reviewed by RINEHART (1961) who contributed to their structural elucidation. Neomycin B (48) and neomycin C (49) differ in the configuration of the diaminosugar attached to the ribose moiety. The two sugars, 2,6-diamino-2,6-dideoxy-L-idose (neosamine B from neomycin B) and 2,6-diamino-2,6-dideoxy-D-glucose (neosamine C) are epimers at the 5 position. They have comparable activity.

The fourth group, the 3-*N*-acetyl derivatives of neomycin, LP-B (50) and LP-C (51), occur as minor components of the neomycin mixture prepared from *Streptomyces fradiae* cultures (CHILTON 1963; CLAES et al. 1974). They are much less active than the parent compounds. CLAES et al. (1974) also showed that mono-*N*-acetyl neamine is also present in the mixture together with small amounts of the paromomycins, ribostamycin, and a disaccharide containing neosamine C linked to *myo*-inositol. HESSLER et al. (1970) had previously shown that paromomycins could be found in neomycin.

The paromomycins, with a glucosamine residue at the 4 position of 2-DOS and either neosamine B in paromomycin I (52) or neosamine C in paromomycin II (53), have been reported under many names: catenulin (DAVISSON et al. 1952), hydroxymycin (VAISMAN and HAMELIN 1958), amminosidin (CANEVAZZI and SCOTTI 1959), and zygomycin A (HORII et al. 1963). The name paromomycin is used because the structural elucidation of these compounds was carried out with material designated paromomycin (HASKELL et al. 1959; RINEHART 1961) and the identity of these materials was established later (SCHILLINGS and SCHAFFNER 1962).

Lividomycin A (54), B (55), and 2230-C, or mannosylparomomycin (56), are produced by *Streptomyces lividus* (ODA et al. 1971a). Lividomycin A and B are distinguished from paromomycin I by the presence of a 2,3-dideoxy-2-amino-glucose residue linked to the 4 position of 2-DOS. The lack of the 3′-OH group affects the activity against resistant strains which are resistant by virtue of the ability to phosphorylate the 3′-OH of similar antibiotics. Lividomycin A and 2230-C have an α-D-mannopyranosyl residue attached to the neosamine B moiety on the ribose. The complex was isolated by cation-exchange adsorption (MORI et al. 1971). Lividomycin B has activity similar to paromomycin which was also isolated from the fermentations (2230-D), while lividomycin A and 2230-C are approximately one-half as active against sensitive strains. Structural studies leading to the assignment of the structures shown were carried out by ODA et al. (1971b, c) and MORI et al. (1972a, b).

2. 4,6-Disubstituted Cyclitol

This is the largest group of antibiotics to be discussed and includes those that are clinically most important, i.e., gentamicin, tobramycin, and kanamycin.

a) Kanamycin, Tobramycin, and Related Compounds

Kanamycin A (57) was discovered by H. UMEZAWA et al. (1957) (TAKEUCHI et al. 1957) in fermentations of *S. kanamyceticus*. Two minor components were also produced, kanamycin B (58) (SCHMITZ et al. 1958) and kanamycin C (59) (MURASE et al. 1961). Kanamycin A, with a good broad spectrum of antibacterial activity, including activity against *M. tuberculosis*, soon gained widespread clinical usage. The structure of kanamycin, except for the configuration of the 2-DOS moiety, was solved almost simultaneously by three groups (CRON et al. 1958; S. UMEZAWA et al. 1959; OGAWA et al. 1959). The remaining structural point, the position of attachment to the 2-DOS fragment, was reported by HICHENS and RINEHART (1963) and by TATSUOKA et al. (1964). The structure of kanamycin was confirmed by X-ray analysis of kanamycin sulfate (KOYAMA et al. 1968). The structure of kanamycin B was reported by ITO et al. (1964) and that of kanamycin C by MURASE (1961). Paromamine (23) and 6-*0*-(3-amino-3-deoxy-α-D-glucopyranosyl)-2-deoxystreptamine have been isolated as minor components of a commercial kanamycin mixture (CLAES et al. 1973).

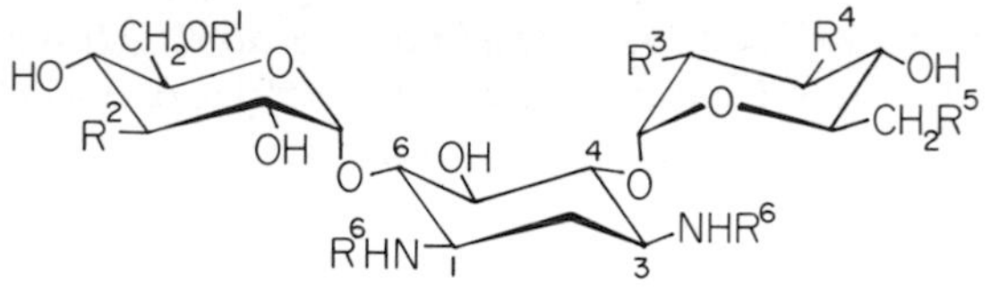

		R^1	R^2	R^3	R^4	R^5	R^6
(57)	Kanamycin A	H	NH_2	OH	OH	NH_2	H
(58)	Kanamycin B	H	NH_2	NH_2	OH	NH_2	H
(59)	Kanamycin C	H	NH_2	NH_2	OH	OH	H
(60)	NK-1001	H	OH	OH	OH	NH_2	H
(61)	NK-1012-1	H	OH	NH_2	OH	NH_2	H
(62)	NK-1013-1	H	$NHCOCH_3$	NH_2	OH	NH_2	H, $COCH_3$
(63)	NK-1013-2	H	NH_2	NH_2	OH	NH_2	H, $COCH_3$
(64)	Nebramycin factor 4	$CONH_2$	NH_2	NH_2	OH	NH_2	H
(65)	Nebramycin factor 5′	$CONH_2$	NH_2	NH_2	H	NH_2	H
(66)	Tobramycin	H	NH_2	NH_2	H	NH_2	H
(67)	Nebramycin factor 11	H	NH_2	$NHCONH_2$	H	NH_2	H
(68)	Nebramycin factor 12	H	OH	NH_2	H	NH_2	H
(69)	Nebramycin factor 13	H	NH_2	NH_2	H	$NHCONH_2$	H

The NK compounds are all minor components found in the fermentation of a mutant strain of *S. kanamyceticus* (MURASE et al. 1970). NK-1001 (60) and NK-1012-1 (61) have α-D-glucosyl residues at the 6 position of 2-DOS in place of a 3-amino-3-deoxy-α-D-glucosyl moiety. NK-1013-1 (62) and NK-1013-2 (63) are *N*-acetylated derivatives of kanamycin B. They all have some bioactivity, although less than kanamycin.

Among the major kanamycins, kanamycin B is approximately twice as active as kanamycin A, while kanamycin C is one-fourth as active as kanamycin A.

Tobramycin (66) is the most important member of the nebramycin complex (STARK et al. 1968; HIGGENS and KASTNER 1968; THOMPSON and PRESTI 1968). It was first designated nebramycin factor 6 and the structure was reported by KOCH and RHOADES (1971) to be 3′-deoxykanamycin B. The structure of some other components was clarified by KOCH et al. (1973). Factor 5 was shown to be kanamycin B. Factor 4 (64) is 6″-O-carbamoylkanamycin B and factor 5′ (65) is 6″-O-carbamoyltobramycin. STARK et al. (1971) showed that the parent strain produces mainly apramycin (19) and factors 4 and 5′ which yield kanamycin B and tobramycin during isolation. Factors 4 and 5′ are about as active as kanamycin B against sensitive strains. Tobramycin is approximately twice as active and is also active against *Pseudomonas* strains.

KOCH et al. (1978) reported on the isolation and characterization of additional nebramycin complex components. Nebramycin factor 11 (67) is 2′-*N*-carbamoyltobramycin. Factor 12 (68), like NK-1012-1, is a 6-O-α-D-glucopyranosyl-2-deoxystreptamine derivative but in factor 12 the 4 substituent is 2,6-diamino-2,3,6-trideoxy-α-D-glucopyranosyl, the moiety found in tobramycin. NK-1012-1 has also been identified in this study of the *S. tenebrarius* products. It was earlier referred to as nebramycin factor 3. Nebramycin factor 13 (69) is 6′-*N*-carbamoyltobramycin. All three of the newly described factors are significantly less active than tobramycin or apramycin.

b) Gentamicins Containing Garosamine

One of the most important groups of aminoglycosides includes the gentamicins and related compounds. The group discussed here includes those with the branched chain sugar garosamine at the 6 position of 2-DOS.

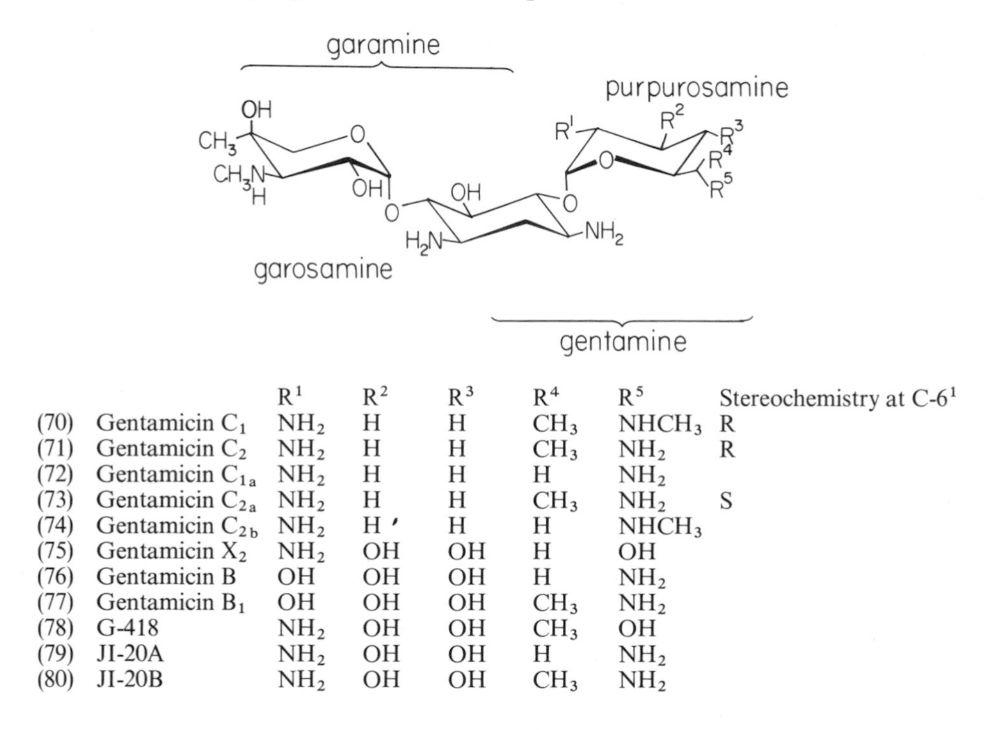

		R^1	R^2	R^3	R^4	R^5	Stereochemistry at C-6[1]
(70)	Gentamicin C_1	NH_2	H	H	CH_3	$NHCH_3$	R
(71)	Gentamicin C_2	NH_2	H	H	CH_3	NH_2	R
(72)	Gentamicin C_{1a}	NH_2	H	H	H	NH_2	
(73)	Gentamicin C_{2a}	NH_2	H	H	CH_3	NH_2	S
(74)	Gentamicin C_{2b}	NH_2	H	H	H	$NHCH_3$	
(75)	Gentamicin X_2	NH_2	OH	OH	H	OH	
(76)	Gentamicin B	OH	OH	OH	H	NH_2	
(77)	Gentamicin B_1	OH	OH	OH	CH_3	NH_2	
(78)	G-418	NH_2	OH	OH	CH_3	OH	
(79)	JI-20A	NH_2	OH	OH	H	NH_2	
(80)	JI-20B	NH_2	OH	OH	CH_3	NH_2	

The commercial material gentamicin consists primarily of gentamicin C_1 (70), C_2 (71), and C_{1a} (72), which were first reported by WEINSTEIN et al. (1964) to be produced by *Micromonospora purpurea*. Since then several other members of the group have been isolated from *Micromonospora* fermentations and recently some closely related compounds from *Streptomyces* sp. The designation -micin in the name has been used to distinguish the *Micromonospora*-derived materials from those produced by *Streptomyces* strains which are often given the suffix -mycin.

Gentamicin has become the largest selling aminoglycoside on the world market, excluding the USSR and other Comecon Countries, accounting for approximately one-half the total aminoglycoside sales. The structure was elucidated by Schering workers (COOPER 1971; COOPER et al. 1971; DANIELS et al. 1971; DANIELS 1975).

The gentamicins first discovered, the gentamicin C complex, were characterized by the presence of the branched chain sugar garosamine linked to the 6 position of 2-DOS in place of the 3-amino-3-deoxyglucose found in kanamycin. Also the 4 substituent was an α-2,6-diaminoglucosyl derivative with deoxygenation at C-3 and C-4 and varying substitution of methyl at C-6 or the 6-amino group. They are two to four times as potent as kanamycin with good activity against *Pseudomonas* (WEINSTEIN et al. 1967).

Of the minor components of the gentamicin C complex, gentamicin C_{2a} (73) is the epimer at C-6′ of gentamicin C_2 (DANIELS et al. 1975). BERDY et al. (1977) have given a good description of the isolation and identification of many of the gentamicin-related compounds found in a *Micromonospora* fermentation. Gentamicin C_{2b} (74) has also been reported as XK-62-2 or sagamicin (DANIELS et al. 1976; OKACHI et al. 1974; NARA et al. 1975; EGAN et al. 1975). It appears as a major component, together with gentamicin C_{1a}, in fermentations of a *Micromonospora* strain.

It would seem that substitution of CH_3 for H at C-6′ and on the 6′-NH_2 should lead to four compounds. However, substitution on the methylene at C-6′ can give rise to two epimers, which have been found in the case of the amino compounds. The missing compound is the dimethyl-substituted compound with *S* stereochemistry at C-6′.

Besides the gentamicin C group of garosamine-containing aminoglycosides, there are several compounds with oxygenation at C-3′ and C-4′ of the 4 substituent on 2-DOS occurring as minor components of the fermentation of *M. purpurea* or related cultures (WAGMAN et al. 1972; BERDY et al. 1977).

Gentamicin X_2 (75) is the 6-garosaminyl derivative of paromamine containing 2-amino-2-deoxyglucose, while in gentamicin B (76) the 4 substituent is 6-amino-6-deoxyglucose and JI-20A (79) contains 2,6-diamino-2,6-dideoxyglucose,that is, JI-20A in 6-garosaminyl neamine. Gentamicin B_1 (77) is the 6′-*C*-methyl derivative of gentamicin B, G-418 (78) is the corresponding derivative of gentamicin X_2, and JI-20B (80) is the 6′-*C*-methyl derivative of JI-20A.

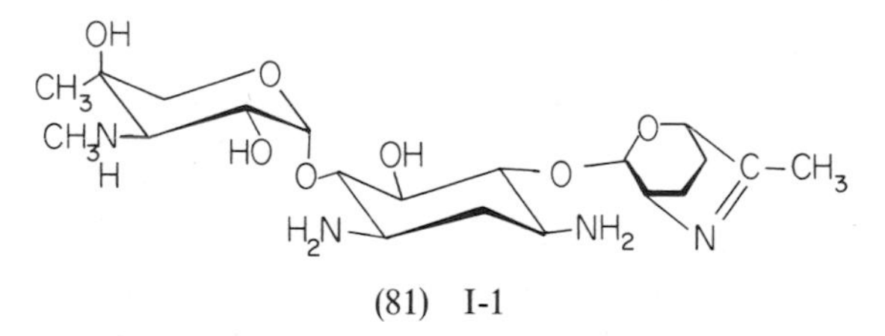

(81) I-1

BERDY et al. (1977) have reported a unique compound of the garosamine-containing class (81) with the structure shown (compound I-1). The structure was determined by mass spectrometry and ^{13}C-NMR studies. Another minor product from the work of BERDY et al. was compound V-2, 3″-*N*-demethyl gentamicin C_2, in which the garosamine moiety is lacking the *N*-methyl substituent.

c) Gentamicins and Seldomycins Containing an Aminopentose

Several minor gentamicin components containing a pentose moiety at C-6 of 2-DOS have been isolated and characterized (MAEHR and SCHAFFNER 1967) and shown to have the structures depicted in (82)–(91) (NAGABUSHAN et al. 1975a, b).

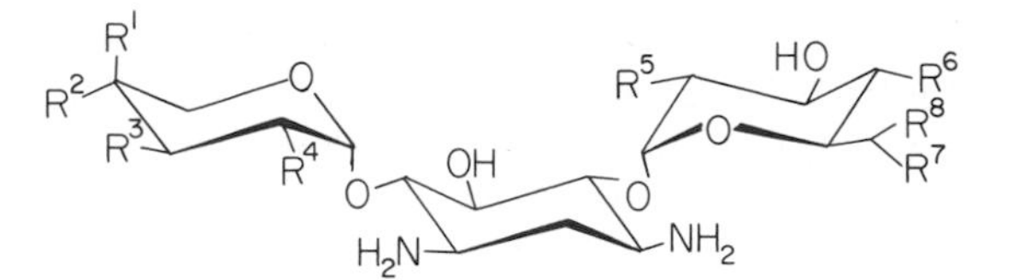

		R^1	R^2	R^3	R^4	R^5	R^6	R^7	R^8
(82)	Gentamicin A	H	OH	$NHCH_3$	OH	NH_2	OH	OH	H
(83)	Gentamicin A_1	OH	H	$NHCH_3$	OH	NH_2	OH	OH	H
(84)	Gentamicin A_2	H	OH	OH	OH	NH_2	OH	OH	H
(85)	Gentamicin A_3	OH	H	$NHCH_3$	OH	OH	OH	NH_2	H
(86)	Gentamicin A_4	H	OH	NCH_3 (N–CHO)	OH	NH_2	OH	OH	H
(87)	Seldomycin factor 1	H	OH	OH	NH_2	NH_2	OH	OH	H
(88)	Seldomycin factor 3	H	OH	OH	NH_2	NH_2	OH	NH_2	H
(89)	Seldomycin factor 5	H	OCH_3	NH_2	NH_2	NH_2	H	NH_2	H
(90)	II-2	H	OH	$NHCH_3$	OH	NH_2	OH	OH	CH_3
(91)	III-1	OH	H	$NHCH_3$	OH	NH_2	OH	OH	CH_3

The gentamicin A complex (Maehr and Schaffner 1967) contains a simple pentose or aminopentose related to garosamine but missing the C–CH_3 group at the 4″ position. Epimers are found at the 4″ position.

Gentamicin A_2 (84) (Nagabushan et al. 1975b) is unique in having a nonbasic sugar at the 6 position of 2-DOS in place of garosamine. Thus gentamicin A_2 is the 6-O-xyloside of paromamine. Gentamicin A (82) and A_1 (83) contain a methylaminopentose, designated gentosamine for gentamicin A (Maehr and Schaffner 1970). The pentose in gentamicin A_1 is epimeric at C-4″ with that in gentamicin A. Both compounds are the 6-O-glycosides of paromamine. Gentamicin A_3 (85) is the *epi*-gentosaminide of the disaccharide derived from substitution of 6-amino-6-deoxy-D-glucose on 2-DOS while gentamcin A_4 (86) is gentamicin A *N*-formylated at the methylamino group of the gentosamine moiety.

While the gentamicins with the 3′,4′ deoxygenation are generally more potent than the corresponding kanamycins, the oxygenated compounds discussed above are generally comparable in activity to the corresponding kanamycins.

Two other minor compounds related to the gentamicin A complex have been isolated by Berdy et al. (1977). Compound II-2 (90) is the C-6′-methyl derivative of gentamicin A and compound III-I (91) is the corresponding derivative of gentamicin A_1, the 4″-epimer of gentamicin A.

A group of aminoglycosides containing an aminopentose moiety at the 6 position of 2-DOS was isolated from *Streptomyces hofunensis* in contrast to all the compounds of this class previously discussed which have been produced by *Micromonospora* (Nara et al. 1977a). The complex was isolated by cation-exchange resin adsorption and purified by silica gel chromatography (Sato et al. 1977).

Seldomycin factor 2 (26) has been discussed in Sect. C.I.1. It was the pseudodisaccharide formed by the α-glycosidic attachment of 2,6-diamino-2-4,6-trideoxy-D-glucose to the 4 position of 2-DOS (Egan et al. 1977a) or 4′-deoxyneamine. In seldomycin factor 5 (89) this pseudodisaccharide is substituted at the 6 position of

2-DOS with an O-methyl diaminopentose, designated seldose (McALPINE et al. 1977). Thus seldomycin factor 5 is 6-O-(2,3-diamino-2,3-dideoxy-4-O-methyl-α-D-*xylo*-pyranosyl)-4′-deoxyneamine. This is the first example of a naturally occurring diaminosugar substituted at the 6 position of 2-DOS.

Seldomycin factor 1 (87) is 6-O-(2-amino-2-deoxy-α-D-xylopyranosyl) paromamine and seldomycin factor 3 (88) consists of the same aminopentose substituted at the 6-O position of neamine. Seldomycin factor 5 shows the highest biologic activity of the group, being roughly similar to, or slightly weaker than, kanamycin. Factor 1 is quite weak and factor 2 is about one-half as active as factor 5 (NARA et al. 1977a).

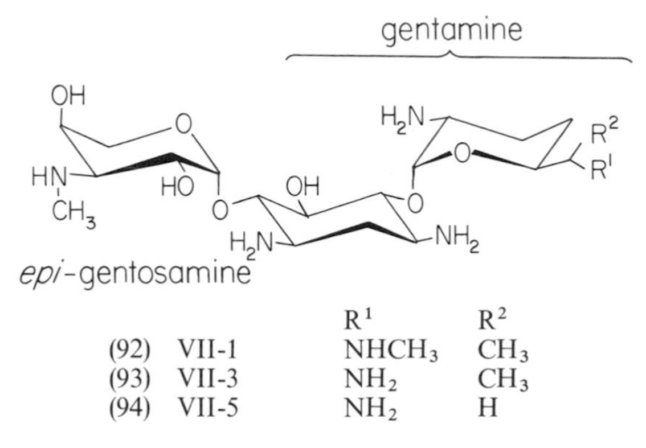

		R^1	R^2
(92)	VII-1	$NHCH_3$	CH_3
(93)	VII-3	NH_2	CH_3
(94)	VII-5	NH_2	H

Three other compounds of this general class isolated by BERDY et al. (1977) are shown in (92)–(94). In these compounds *epi*-gentosamine is linked to pseudodisaccharides (gentamines) of the gentamicin C type. Compound VII-1 (92) contains gentamine C_1, compound VII-3 (93) contains gentamine C_2 or C_{2a} (stereochemistry at C-6′ unknown), and compound VII-5 (94) contains the gentamine derived from gentamicin C_{1a}.

d) Sisomicins

WEINSTEIN et al. (1970) reported the discovery of a second novel family of *Micromonospora*-produced aminoglycosides. Additional studies were reported by WAGMAN et al. (1970) and WAITZ et al. (1970).

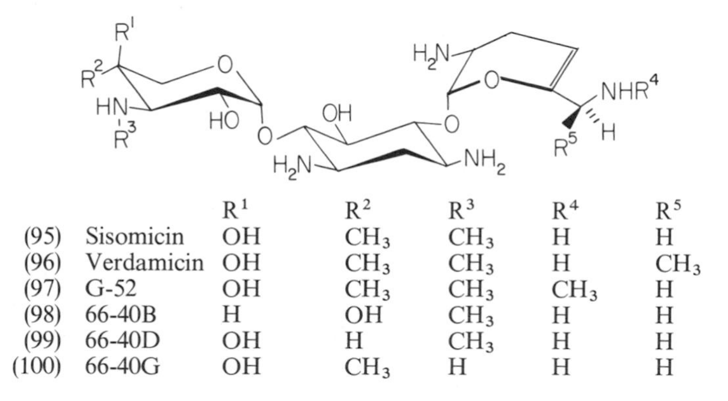

		R^1	R^2	R^3	R^4	R^5
(95)	Sisomicin	OH	CH_3	CH_3	H	H
(96)	Verdamicin	OH	CH_3	CH_3	H	CH_3
(97)	G-52	OH	CH_3	CH_3	CH_3	H
(98)	66-40B	H	OH	CH_3	H	H
(99)	66-40D	OH	H	CH_3	H	H
(100)	66-40G	OH	CH_3	H	H	H

The first of this group to be evaluated was sisomicin (95), formerly designated 66-40. The members of this class are characterized by the presence of an unsaturated ($\Delta^{4,5}$) derivative of purpurosamine at the 4 position of 2-DOS. Sisomicin has garosamine as the 6 substituent and an unsaturated aminosugar related to gentamicin C_{1a} as the 4 substituent on 2-DOS. The structure was reported by REIMANN et al. (1974). It was first found in fermentations of *M. inyoensis* (WEINSTEIN et al. 1970).

Verdamicin (96) was isolated from fermentations of *M. grisea* (WEINSTEIN et al. 1975) where it occurs together with sisomicin. Verdamicin is 6′-C-methylsisomicin. The unsaturated moiety can be considered as deriving from gentamine C_2. Antibiotic G-52 (97) (MARQUEZ et al. 1976; DANIELS et al. 1976) is produced by *M. zionensis* together with sisomicin. It is 6′-*N*-methylsisomicin, or the 4′-unsaturated derivative of gentamicin C_{2b}.

Several minor components have been found in the original sisomicin fermentation. 66-40B (98) and 66-40D (99) have the same gentamine-like pseudodisaccharide as sisomicin (DAVIES et al. 1975; LEE et al. 1976), but the 6-substituent is *epi*-gentosamine in 66-40B and gentosamine in 66-40D. These compounds thus are the 4″-epimers of 4″-demethylsisomicin. A third component of the mixture, 66-40G (100), was recently reported (KUGELMAN et al. 1978) to be 3″-*N*-demethylsisomicin.

Another minor component of the *M. inyoensis* fermentation is 66-40C (101) in which two molecules of sisomicin are linked together by imine bridges (DAVIES et al. 1977).

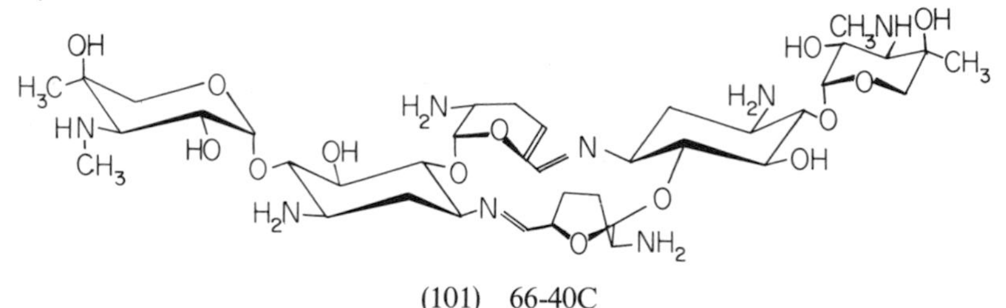

(101) 66-40C

Sisomicin is approximately twice as active as gentamicin while the minor components generally have activity similar to that of sisomicin.

III. 1-*N*-Acyl Substituted Cyclitol

The butirosins and related compounds are an interesting group of agents from *Bacillus* fermentations.

Their most unusual feature is the presence of a hydroxyamino acid side chain linked by an amide bond to the amino group of C-1 of the 2-DOS moiety. Otherwise the butirosins resemble the 4,5-substituted pseudotrisaccharides, ribostamycin and xylostasin, discussed in Sect. C.II.1.a. Butirosin A (102) and B (103) are derived from *B. circulans* fermentations (DION et al. 1972). Butirosin A is the amino acid derivative of xylostasin (46). The amino acid moiety is L(−)-γ-amino-α-hydroxybutyric acid (WOO et al. 1971). Butirosin B is the similar derivative of the ribose-containing compound ribostamycin (45).

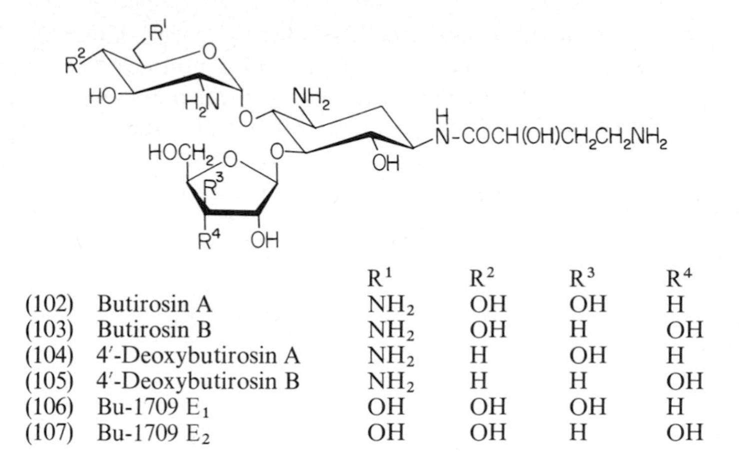

		R^1	R^2	R^3	R^4
(102)	Butirosin A	NH_2	OH	OH	H
(103)	Butirosin B	NH_2	OH	H	OH
(104)	4′-Deoxybutirosin A	NH_2	H	OH	H
(105)	4′-Deoxybutirosin B	NH_2	H	H	OH
(106)	Bu-1709 E_1	OH	OH	OH	H
(107)	Bu-1709 E_2	OH	OH	H	OH

The butirosins are about as active as kanamycin or ribostamycin but show good activity against *Pseudomonas* which is lacking in the nonacylated compounds.

The 4′-deoxybutirosins A (104) and B (105), earlier termed Bu-1975 C_1 and C_2, occur together with the butirosins in a *B. circulans* fermentation (KAWAGUCHI et al. 1974; KONISHI et al. 1974). Their activity is similar to that of the butirosins but with a somewhat broader spectrum.

Another pair of related compounds also occurs in the butirosin fermentation: Bu-1709 E_1 (106), the xylose-containing compound, and Bu-1709 E_2 (107), the ribose-containing epimer, both have paromamine rather than neamine moieties (TSUKIURA et al. 1973b). As would be expected, they are somewhat less active than the neamine analogs.

D. Aminoglycosides with Cyclitol Aglycones Other than Streptamine or 2-Deoxystreptamine

I. Nonbasic Cyclitol

Kasugamycin (108) (H. UMEZAWA et al. 1965) is produced by *Streptomyces kasugaensis*.

It has activity primarily against gram-negative organisms, including *Pseudomonas*, but is has found widespread commercial use as an inhibitor of *Piricularia*

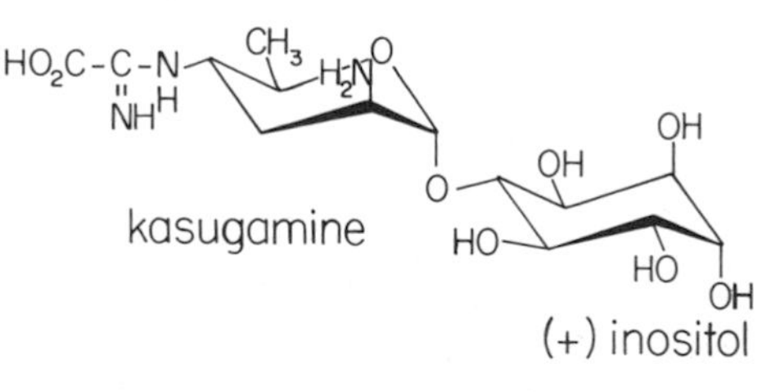

(108) Kasugamycin

oryzae, the organism which causes rice blast disease. Degradation yields oxalic acid, (+)-inositol, and the unusual aminosugar 2,4-diamino-2,3,4,6-tetradeoxy-D-*arabino*-hexose. The structure determined by chemical methods (SUHARA et al. 1966) was confirmed by X-ray analyses (IKEKAWA et al. 1966).

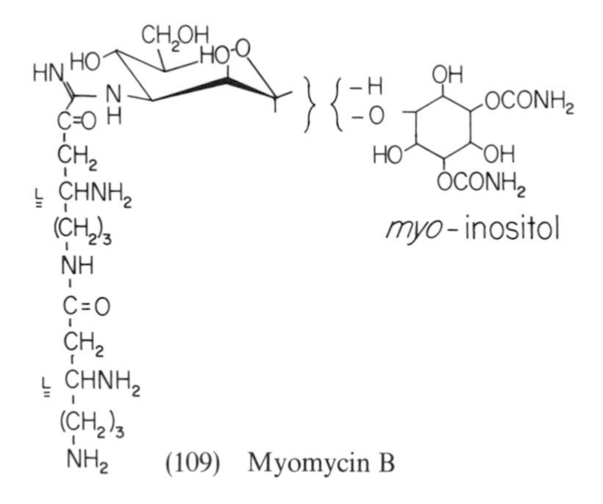

(109) Myomycin B

The cyclitol *myo*-inositol is a component of myomycin B (109), the major component of the myomycin complex (FRENCH et al. 1973). Myomycin is produced by a *Nocardia* sp. and is isolated by the usual ion-exchange procedure or by carbon adsorption. It has weak activity against gram-positive and gram-negative organisms. Structural studies showed that myomycin B contains L-β-lysine, *myo*-inositol, and 3-guanidino-3-deoxy-D-mannose. The structure shown was derived from degradative data and leaves uncertain the glycosidic configuration and the point of attachment to the inositol moiety; the attachment of the peptide to the mannose moiety is also uncertain. Myomycin A and C resemble myomycin B structurally.

II. Monoaminocyclitol

The compound minosaminomycin (110) is related to kasugamycin. It was isolated from a *Streptomyces* (HAMADA et al. 1974). It is very weakly active against some gram-positive and gram-negative bacteria but has considerable activity against *Mycobacterium* strains. The structure was determined by IINUMA et al. (1975). It was found that kasugamine was one moiety and the new aminocyclitol, 1-D-1-amino-1-deoxy-*myo*-inositol, is related to the cyclitol found in kasugamycin.

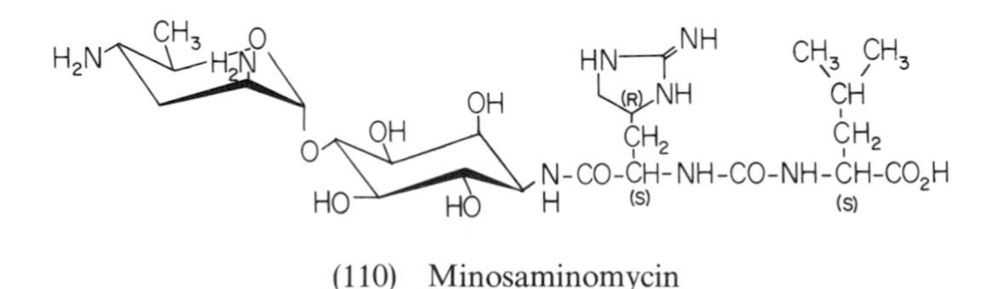

(110) Minosaminomycin

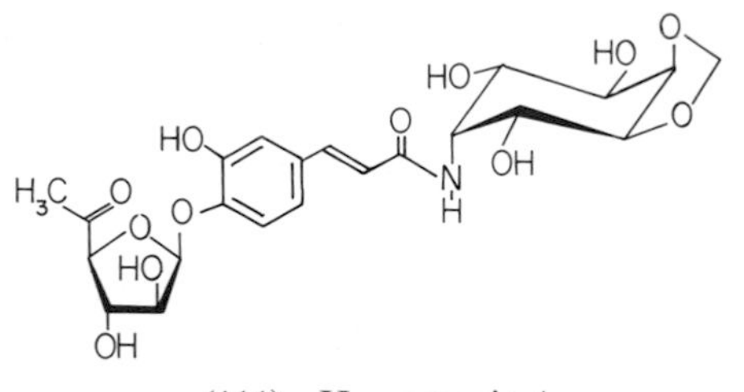

(111) Hygromycin A

Hygromycin A (111) was first isolated from *S. hygroscopicus* which also produces hygromycin B (38) which has been discussed in Sect. C.I.2 (PITTENGER et al. 1953; MANN et al. 1953). The antibiotic has also been reported from other sources and extensive structural studies were finally completed by KAKINUMA et al. (1976) who solved the remaining structural problems. One of the final points to be determined was the location of the methylene bridge on the neoinosamine-2 moiety.

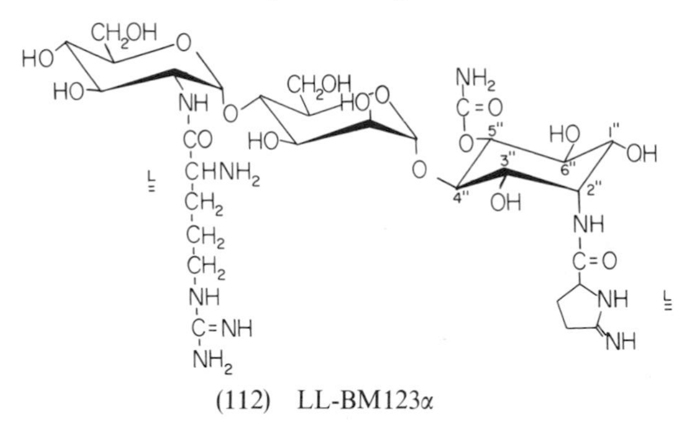

(112) LL-BM123α

The compound LL-BM123α (112) (ELLESTAD et al. 1977) is produced by the same *Nocardia* sp. which produces the LL-BM123β, γ_1, and γ_2 compounds discussed in Sect. B.III. The latter compounds do not include a cyclitol moiety but contain a basic trisaccharide linked to cinnamoylspermidine. LL-BM123α is a substituted disaccharide, glucosaminylmannose, linked to *myo*-inosamine-2. The position of the attachment to the cyclitol, either at 4″ or 6″, is still uncertain. LL-BM123α has moderate activity against gram-negative organisms.

The validamycins contain the unusual cyclitol validoxylamine. In the validamycins this cyclitol is glycosylated at varying positions and to varying degrees. The complex is produced by a variant strain of *S. hygroscopicus* (IWASA et al. 1970). Validamycin A (115) is the main component. The validamycins are inactive against the usual bacteria and fungi but show good in vivo activity against the sheath blight of rice plants and are used commercially for this purpose (IWASA et al. 1971 a, b). Validoxylamine A (113) and B (114) are also components of the fermentation mixture and are weakly active in the sheath blight test. The minor validamycins C (117), D (118), E (119), and F (120) differ in the location and number of glycosyl groups. Validamycin B (116) is hydroxyvalidamycin A containing the validoxylamine B cyclitol instead of the more common validoxylamine A (HORII et al. 1972).

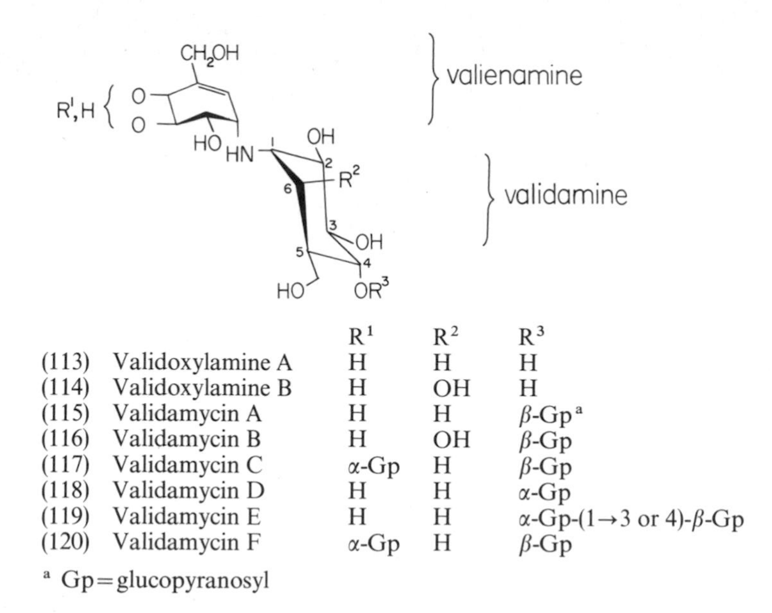

		R^1	R^2	R^3
(113)	Validoxylamine A	H	H	H
(114)	Validoxylamine B	H	OH	H
(115)	Validamycin A	H	H	β-Gp[a]
(116)	Validamycin B	H	OH	β-Gp
(117)	Validamycin C	α-Gp	H	β-Gp
(118)	Validamycin D	H	H	α-Gp
(119)	Validamycin E	H	H	α-Gp-(1→3 or 4)-β-Gp
(120)	Validamycin F	α-Gp	H	β-Gp

[a] Gp = glucopyranosyl

The structural studies reported (HORII et al. 1971 a, b; KAMIYA et al. 1971; KAMEDA and HORII 1972; HORII and KAMEDA 1972) did not lead to a definite assignment for the substitution of the sugar residue on the valienamine moiety in validamycins C and F. The glucoyl substitution in validamycin A was assigned to the hydroxyl at C-3 of validamine by periodate studies. Recently, however, SUAMI et al. (1980) unequivocally showed by synthetic studies that validamycin A has the structure shown with the glucosyl substituent at C-4 of validamine. We have assumed that the position of attachment of the R^3 sugar is the same in all the validamycins since the proof of their structure usually involves isolation of validamycin A. This point will probably be clarified in the near future.

III. Diaminocyclitol

Spectinomycin (121), formerly called actinospectacin, was first reported by MASON et al. (1961) and BERGY et al. (1961). It is produced by *Streptomyces spectabilis* fer-

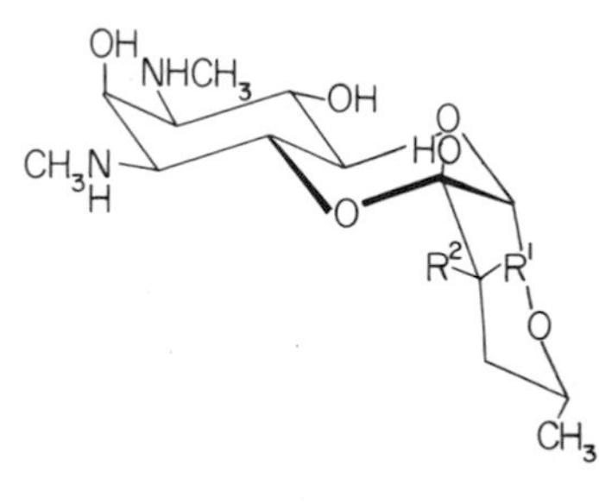

(121) Spectinomycin hydrate $R^1 = R^2 = OH$
(122) Dihydrospectinomycin $R^1 = OH, R^2 = H$

mentation. It is active against gram-positive and gram-negative bacteria and was recently released for clinical use in resistant gonorrhea. Dihydrospectinomycin (122) is also found in the fermentation (HOEKSEMA and KNIGHT 1975). Chemical degradation established the structure of the molecule (WILEY et al. 1963) and it was shown that the cyclitol was *N,N′*-dimethyl-2-*epi*-streptamine. The final stereochemical points were determined by X-ray analyses (COCHRAN and ABRAHAM 1972).

Recently several closely related compounds in which the cyclitol moiety is a 1,4-diaminocyclitol have been reported by several groups of workers.

		R^1	R^2	R^3	R^4	R^5
(123)	Fortimicin B	NH_2	H	OH	CH_3	H
(124)	Fortimicin KE	NH_2	H	OH	H	H
(125)	Sporaricin B	H	NH_2	H	CH_3	H
(126)	Sannamycin B	NH_2	H	H	H	CH_3

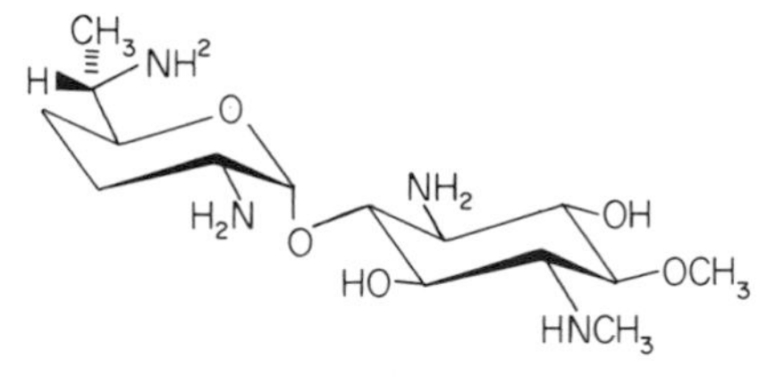

(127) Fortimicin E

Fortimicin A (128) and B (123) were the first of this group to be described (NARA et al. 1977b; OKACHI et al. 1977, EGAN et al. 1977b; GIROLAMI and STAMM 1977). Fortimicin B has only weak antibacterial activity while fortimicin A has typical aminoglycoside antibacterial activity which is roughly comparable to that of kanamycin. However, it has considerable activity against common aminoglycoside-resistant strains but not against *Pseudomonas*. The main structural difference between the fortimicin A and B group is the presence of glycine or similar substitution on the methylamino group at C-4 of fortamine. The structural studies (EGAN et al. 1977b) indicated that the cyclitol moiety exists in a different conformation in fortimicin B than in fortimicin A. The structure of fortimicin B was independently confirmed by X-ray crystallography (HIRAYAMA et al. 1978). Although detailed conformational studies have not been reported for other compounds of this group, it is assumed that the differing conformation of the substituted and unsubstituted compounds is a common feature of these compounds. The fortimicins were isolated from *Micromonospora olivoasterospora*. Other minor products in the fermentation include fortimicin C (129), D (130), and KE (124) reported by SUGIMOTO et al. (1979) with structures as shown (IIDA et al. 1979). Fortimicin C has hydantoic acid substituted for glycine of fortimicin A, while fortimicin D and KE are 6′-demethyl-fortimicin A and B respectively. As would be expected fortimicin KE is weakly active. Fortimicin C is somewhat less active than fortimicin A while the activity of fortimicin D is equal to that of fortimicin A.

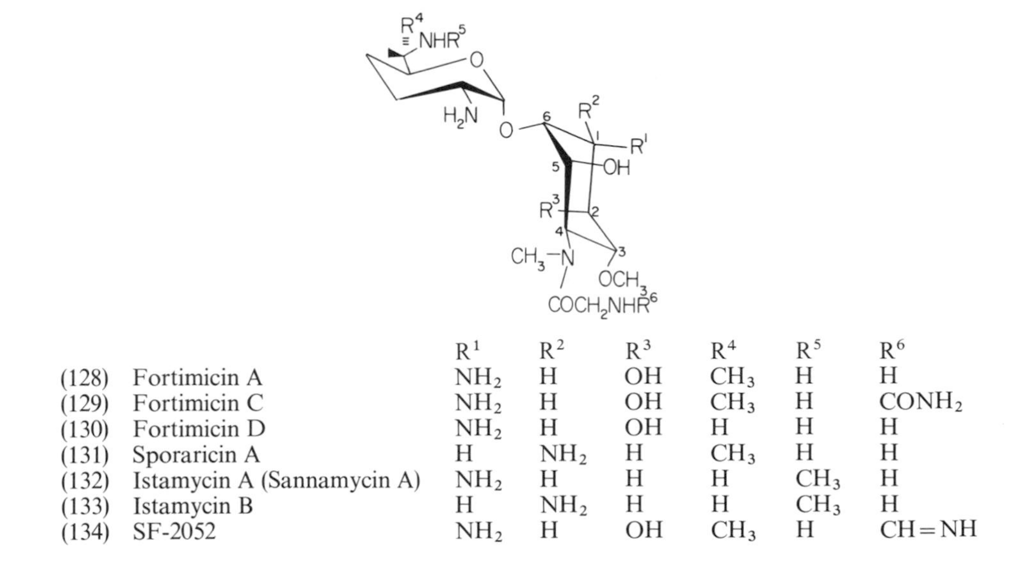

		R^1	R^2	R^3	R^4	R^5	R^6
(128)	Fortimicin A	NH_2	H	OH	CH_3	H	H
(129)	Fortimicin C	NH_2	H	OH	CH_3	H	$CONH_2$
(130)	Fortimicin D	NH_2	H	OH	H	H	H
(131)	Sporaricin A	H	NH_2	H	CH_3	H	H
(132)	Istamycin A (Sannamycin A)	NH_2	H	H	H	CH_3	H
(133)	Istamycin B	H	NH_2	H	H	CH_3	H
(134)	SF-2052	NH_2	H	OH	CH_3	H	CH=NH

Recently fortimicin E (127) was reported (KURATH et al. 1979). It is only weakly active. It is epimeric with fortimicin B at C-3 and C-4, with an all-equatorial conformation for the cyclitol moiety.

The isolation and properties of the sporaricins were reported by DEUSHI et al. (1979a). The producing organism is a nocardioform actinomycete, *Saccharopolyspora hirsuta* subsp. *kobensis* (IWASAKI et al. 1979). Sporaricin A (131) and sporaricin B (125) are epimeric at C-1 and lack the -OH at C-2 which is present in the corresponding fortimicin A and B (DEUSHI et al. 1979b). The activity of the sporaricins is comparable to that of the fortimicins.

The istamycins A (132) and B (133) were isolated from *Streptomyces tenjimariensis* (OKAMI et al. 1979). Both compounds have an N-CH_3 group at C-6′ but lack the 6′-C-methyl of the sporaricins and fortimicins. The cyclitol of istamycin B is the same as that of sporaricin A while istamycin A is the 2-epimer.

Sannamycin A (132) and B (126) were reported from the same laboratory that discovered the sporaricins (DEUSHI et al. 1979c). They are isolated from fermentations of a *Streptomyces* sp. Sannamycin A is somewhat weaker in activity than the previously reported members of the glycine-containing group. It is identical to istamycin A (WATANABE et al. 1979). Sannamycin B contains 2-deoxyfortamine as the cyclitol residue.

Another member of the group reported recently is SF-2052 (134) (INOUYE et al. 1979) which is produced by an actinomycete, *Dactylosporangium matsuzakiense*. It is identical to fortimicin A except for a formimino substitution on the amino group of the glycine moiety of fortimicin A. It appears to be somewhat less active biologically than fortimicin A, although it may have relatively more anti-*Pseudomonas* activity.

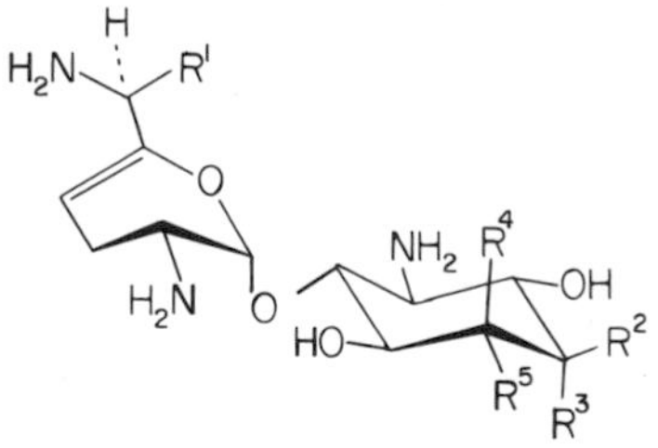

		R^1	R^2	R^3	R^4	R^5
(135)	Fortimicin KF	H	H	OCH_3	H	$NHCH_3$
(136)	Fortimicin G	CH_3	H	OCH_3	H	$NHCH_3$
(137)	Fortimicin G_1	CH_3	OCH_3	H	H	$NHCH_3$
(138)	Fortimicin G_2	CH_3	H	OCH_3	$NHCH_3$	H
(139)	Fortimicin G_3	CH_3	H	OCH_3	NCH_3 $COCH_2NH_2$	H

Some new members of the fortimicin series have been reported in a preliminary communication (TAKAHASHI et al. 1979). They are minor components of the fortimicin A fermentation and contain an unsaturated purpurosamine moiety, such as is found in the sisomicins. The structures are shown in (135)–(139) although the conformation was not reported. Presumably fortimicin G_3 would have the inverted conformation of the other glycine-substituted fortimicins.

References

Akita E, Tsuruoka T, Ezaki N, Niida T (1970) Studies on antibiotic SF-733, a new antibiotic. II. Chemical structure of antibiotic SF-733. J Antibiot (Tokyo) 23:173–183

Arcamone F, Bizioli F (1957) Isolation and constitution of trehalosamine, a new aminosugar from a streptomyces. Gazz Chim Ital 87:896–902

Bannister B, Argoudelis AD (1963) The chemistry of bluensomycin. I. The structure of bluensidine. II. The structure of bluensomycin. J Am Chem Soc 85:119–120, 234–235

Barlow CB, Anderson L (1972) A study of the structure of bluensomycin with the tetramminecopper reagent. J Antibiot (Tokyo) 25:281–286

Benedict RG, Stodola FH, Shotwell OL, Borud AM, Lindenfelser LA (1950) A new streptomycin. Science 112:77–78

Berdy J, Pauncz HK, Vajna ZM, Horvath G, Gyimesi J, Koczka I (1977) Metabolites of gentamicin-producing *Micromonospora* species. I. Isolation and identification of metabolites. J Antibiot (Tokyo) 30:945–954

Bergy ME, Eble TE, Herr RR (1961) Actinospectacin, a new antibiotic. IV. Isolation, purification and chemical properties. Antibiot Chemother 11:661–664

Canevazzi G, Scotti T (1959) Description of a new species of streptomycetes producing a new antibiotic, amminosidin. Giorn Microbiol 7:242–250

Chilton WS (1963) The structure of neomycins LP-B and LP-C. PhD thesis, University of Illinois

Claes PJ, Vanderhaeghe H, Compernolle F (1973) Isolation and identification of minor components of commercial kanamycin. Antimicrob Agents Chemother 4:560–563

Claes PJ, Compernolle F, Vanderhaeghe H (1974) Chromatographic analyses of neomycin. Isolation and determination of minor components. J Antibiot (Tokyo) 27:931–942
Cochran TG, Abraham DJ (1972) Sterochemistry and absolute configuration of the antibiotic spectinomycin: an X-ray diffraction study. J Chem Soc Chem Comm 1972:4944–4945
Cooper DJ (1971) Comparative chemistry of some aminoglycoside antibiotics. Pure Appl Chem 28:455–567
Cooper DJ, Daniels PJL, Yudis MD, Marigliano HM, Guthrie RD, Bukhari STK (1971) The gentamicin antibiotics. 3. The gross structures of gentamicin C components. J Chem Soc (C) 1971:3126–3129
Cron MJ, Evans DK, Palermiti FM, Whitehead DF, Hooper IR, Chu P, Lemieux RU (1958) Kanamycin. V. The structure of kanosamine. J Am Chem Soc 80:4741
Daniels PJL (1975) The elucidation of the structures of gentamicin and sisomicin and the current status of clinical resistance to these antibiotics. In: Mitsuhashi S (ed) Aminoglycoside antibiotics. University Park Press, Tokyo (Drug action and drug resistance in bacteria, vol 2, pp 77–111)
Daniels PJL, Tkach R, Kugelman M, Mallams AK, Vernay HF, Weinstein MJ, Jehaskel A (1971) Mass spectral studies on aminocyclitol antibiotics. Chem Commun (J Chem Soc Sect D) 1971:1629–1631
Daniels PJL, Luce C, Nagabushan TL, Jaret RS, Schumacher D, Reimann H, Ilavsky J (1975) The gentamicin antibiotics. 6. Gentamcin C_{2b}, an aminoglycoside antibiotic produced by *Micromonospora purpurea* mutant J1-33. J Antibiot (Tokyo) 28:35–41
Daniels PJL, Jaret RS, Nagabushan TL, Turner WN (1976) The structure of G-52, a new aminocyclitol-aminoglycoside antibiotic produced by *Micromonospora zionensis*. J Antibiot (Tokyo) 29:488–491
Davies DH, Greeves D, Mallams AK, Morton JB, Tkach RT (1975) Structures of the aminoglycoside antibiotics 66-40B and 66-40D produced by *Micromonospora inyoensis*. J Chem Soc Perkin I 1975:814–818
Davies DH, Greeves D, Mallams AK, Morton JB, Tkach RW (1977) Structure of aminoglycoside 66-40C, a novel unsaturated imine produced by *Micromonospora inyoensis*. J Chem Soc Perkin I 1977:1407–1411
Davisson JW, Solomons JA, Lees TM (1952) Catenulin, a new antibiotic. Antibiot Chemother 2:460–462
Deushi T, Iwasaki A, Kamiya K, Kunieda T, Mizoguchi T, Nakayama M, Itoh H, Mori T, Oda T (1979a) A new broad-spectrum aminoglycoside antibiotic complex, sporaricin. I. Fermentation, isolation and characterization. J Antibiot (Tokyo) 32:174–180
Deushi T, Nakayama M, Watanabe I, Mori T, Naganawa H, Umezawa H (1979b) A new broad-spectrum aminoglycoside antibiotic complex, sporaricin. III. The structures of sporaricins A and B. J Antibiot (Tokyo) 32:187–193
Deushi T, Iwasaki A, Kamiya K, Mizoguchi T, Nakayama M, Itoh H, Mori T (1979c) New aminoglycoside antibiotics, sannamycin. J Antibiot (Tokyo) 32:1061–1065
Dion HW, Woo PWK, Willmer NE, Keru DL, Onaga J, Fusari SA (1972) Butirosin a new aminoglycoside antibiotic complex. Isolation and characterization. Antimicrob Agents Chemother 2:84–88
Dorman DE, Paschal JW, Merkel KE (1976) ^{15}N Nuclear magnetic resonance spectroscopy. The nebramycin aminoglycosides. J Am Chem Soc 98:6885–6888
Egan RS, DeVault RL, Mueller SL, Levenberg MI, Sinclair AC, Stanaszek RS (1975) A new antibiotic XK-62-2. III. The structure of XK-62-2, a new gentamicin C complex antibiotic. J Antibiot (Tokyo) 29:29–34
Egan RS, Sinclair AC, DeVault RL, McAlpine JB, Mueller SL, Goodley PC, Stanaszek RS, Cirovic M, Mauritz RJ, Mitscher LA, Shirakata K, Sato S, Iida T (1977a) A new aminoglycoside antibiotic complex – the seldomycins. III. The structures of seldomycin factors 1 and 2. J Antibiot (Tokyo) 30:31–38
Egan RS, Stanaszek RS, Cirovic M, Mueller SL, Tadanier J, Martin JR, Collum P, Goldstein AW, DeVault RL, Sinclair AC, Fager EE, Mitscher LA (1977b) Fortimicins A and B, new aminoglycoside antibiotics. III. Structural identification. J Antibiot (Tokyo) 30:552–563

Ellestad GA, Martin JH, Morton GO, Sassiver ML, Lancaster JE (1977) Structure of LL-BM123α, a new myoinosamine-2 containing antibiotic. J Antibiot (Tokyo) 30:678–680
Ellestad GA, Cosulich DB, Broshard RW, Martin JH, Kunstmann MP, Morton GO, Lancaster JE, Fulmor W, Lovell FM (1978) Glycocinnamoylspermidines, a new class of antibiotics. III. Structures of LL-BM123β, γ_1 and γ_2. J Am Chem Soc 100:2515–2524
French J, Bartz Q, Dion H (1973) Myomycin, a new antibiotic. J Antibiot (Tokyo) 26:272–283
Fried J, Titus E (1947) Streptomycin B, an antibiotically active constituent of streptomycin concentrates. J Biol Chem 168:391–392
Fried J, Titus E (1948) Streptomycin. VIII. Isolation of mannosidostreptomycin (streptomycin B). J. Am Chem Soc 70:3615–3618
Girolami RL, Stamm JM (1977) Fortimicins A and B, new aminoglycoside antibiotics. IV. In vitro study of fortimicin A compared with other aminoglycosides. J Antibiot (Tokyo) 30:564–570
Hamada M, Kondo S, Yokoyama T, Miura K, Iinuma K, Yamamoto H, Maeda K, Takeuchi T, Umezawa H (1974) Minosaminomycin, a new antibiotic containing *myo*-inosamine. J Antibiot (Tokyo) 27:81–83
Hanessian S, Lavallee P (1972) Synthesis of 6-amino-6-deoxy-α, α-trehalose: a positional isomer of trehalosamine. J Antibiot (Tokyo) 25:683–684
Haskell TH, French JC, Bartz QR (1959) Paromomycin. IV. Structural studies. J Am Chem Soc 81:3482–3483
Hata T, Omura S, Katagiri M, Atsumi K, Awaya J, Higashikawa S, Yasui K, Terada H, Kuyama S (1971) A new antifungal antibiotic, prumycin. J Antibiot (Tokyo) 24:900–901
Heding H (1968) N-Demethylstreptomycin. I. Microbiological formation and isolation. Acta Chem Scand 22:1649–1654
Hessler EJ, Jahnke HK, Robertson JH, Tsuji K, Rinehart KL Jr, Shier WT (1970) Neomycins D, E and F: identity with paromamine, paromomycin I and paromomycin II. J Antibiot (Tokyo) 23:464–466
Hichens M, Rinehart KL Jr (1963) Chemistry of the neomycins. XII. The absolute configuration of deoxystreptamine in the neomycins, paromomycins and kanamycins. J Am Chem Soc 85:1547–1548
Higgens CE, Kastner RE (1968) Nebramycin, a new broad spectrum antibiotic complex. II. Description of *Streptomyces tenebrarius*. Antimicrob Agents Chemother 1967:324–331
Hirayama N, Shirahata K, Ohashi Y, Sasada Y, Martin JR (1978) Structure of fortimicin B. Acta Crystallogr Sect B Struct Crystallogr Cryst Chem B34:2648–2650
Hlavka JJ, Bitha P, Boothe J, Fields T (1978) Glycocinnamoylspermidines, a new class of antibiotics. IV. Chemical modification of LL-BM123γ. J Antibiot (Tokyo) 31:477–479
Hoeksema H, Knight JC (1975) The production of dihydrospectinomycin by *Streptomyces spectabilis*. J Antibiot (Tokyo) 28:240–241
Horii S, Kameda Y (1972) Structure of the antibiotic validamycin A. J Chem Soc Chem Comm 1972:747–748
Horii S, Hitomi H, Miyake A (1963) Chemistry of zygomycin A: separation of zygomycin A_1 and zygomycin A_2 and their characterization. J Antibiot (Tokyo) A16:144–145
Horii S, Iwasa T, Kameda Y (1971 a) Studies on validamycins, new antibiotics. V. Degradation studies. J Antibiot (Tokyo) 24:57–58
Horii S, Iwasa T, Mizuta E, Kameda Y (1971 b) Studies on validamycins, new antibiotics. VI. Validamine, hydroxyvalidamine and validatol, new cyclitols. J Antibiot (Tokyo) 24:59–63
Horii S, Kameda Y, Kawahara K (1972) Studies on validamycins, new antibiotics. VIII. Isolation and characterization of validamycins C, D, E and F. J Antibiot (Tokyo) 25:48–53
Horii S, Nogami I, Mizokami N, Arai Y, Yoneda M (1974) New antibiotic produced by bacteria, 5-β-D-xylofuranosylneamine. Antimicrob Agents Chemother 5:578–581
Hosoya S, Soeda M, Kamatsu N, Sonoda Y (1950) A new antibiotic, reticulin, produced by *Streptomyces reticuli*. J Antibiot (Tokyo) [Suppl A] 3:66–71
Iida T, Sato M, Matsubara I, Mori Y, Shirahata K (1979) The structures of fortimycins C, D and KE. J Antibiot (Tokyo) 32:1273–1279

Iinuma K, Kondo S, Maeda K, Umezawa H (1975) Structure of minosaminomycin. J Antibiot (Tokyo) 28:613–615
Ikekawa T, Umezawa H, Iitaka Y (1966) The structure of kasugamycin hydrobromide by X-ray crystallographic analysis. J Antibiot (Tokyo) A19:49–50
Inouye S, Tsuruoka T, Niida T (1966) The structure of nojirimycin, a piperidinose sugar antibiotic. J Antibiot (Tokyo) A19:288–292
Inouye S, Shomura T, Watanabe H, Totsugawa K, Niida T (1973) Isolation and gross structure of a new antibiotic SS-56 C and related compounds. J Antibiot (Tokyo) 26:374–385
Inouye S, Ohba K, Shomura T, Kojima M, Tsuruoka T, Yoshida J, Kato N, Ito M, Amano S, Omoto S, Ezaki N, Ito T, Niida T, Watanabe K (1979) A novel aminoglycoside antibiotic substance SF-2052. J Antibiot (Tokyo) 32:1354–1356
Ito T, Nishio M, Ogawa H (1964) The structure of kanamycin B. J Antibiot (Tokyo) A17:189–193
Iwasa T, Yamamoto H, Shibata M (1970) Studies on validamycins, new antibiotics. I. *Streptomyces hygroscopicus* var. *limoneus* nov. var., validamycin producing organism. J Antibiot (Tokyo) 23:595–602
Iwasa T, Higashide E, Yamamoto H, Shibata M (1971 a) Studies on validamycins, new antibiotics. II. Production and biological properties of validamycins A and B. J Antibiot (Tokyo) 24:107–113
Iwasa T, Kameda Y, Asai M, Horii S, Mizuno K (1971 b) Studies on validamycins, new antibiotics. IV. Isolation and characterization of validamycins A and B. J Antibiot (Tokyo) 24:119–123
Iwasaki A, Itoh H, Mori T (1979) A new broad spectrum aminoglycoside antibiotic complex, sporaricin. II. Taxonomic studies on the sporaricin producing strain *Saccharopolyspora hirsuta* subsp. *kobensis* nov. subsp. J Antibiot (Tokyo) 32:180–186
Kakinuma K, Kitahara S, Watanabe K, Sakagami Y, Fukuyasu T, Shimura M, Ueda M, Sekizawa Y (1976) On the structure of hygromycin. The location of a methylene substituent and the anomeric configuration of the *arabino*-hexidose moiety. J Antibiot (Tokyo) 29:771–773
Kameda Y, Horii S (1972) The unsaturated cyclitol part of the new antibiotics, the validamycins. J Chem Soc Chem Comm 1972:746–747
Kamiya K, Wada Y, Horii S, Nishikawa M (1971) Studies on validamycins, new antibiotics. VII. The X-ray analysis of validamine hydrobromide. J Antibiot (Tokyo) 24:317–318
Kamiya K, Wada Y, Nara K (1978) X-ray analysis of an aminoglycoside antibiotic P-2563(P) monohydrobromide. Chem Pharm Bull 26:2040–2045
Kawaguchi H, Tomita K, Hoshiya T, Miyaki T, Fujisawa K, Kimeda M, Numata K, Konishi M, Tsukiura H, Hatori M, Koshiyama H (1974) Aminoglycoside antibiotics. V. The 4′-deoxybutirosins (BU-1975 C_1 and C_2). New aminoglycoside antibiotics of bacterial origin. J Antibiot (Tokyo) 27:460–470
Kirby JP, van Lear GE, Morton GO, Gore WE, Curran WV, Borders DB (1977 a) LL-AM31 antibiotic complex: aminoalditol antibiotics from a *Streptoverticillium*. J Antibiot (Tokyo) 30:344–347
Kirby JP, Borders DB, Van Lear GE (1977 b) Structure of LL-BM408, an aminocyclitol antibiotic. J Antibiot (Tokyo) 30:175–177
Koch KF, Rhoades JA (1971) Structure of nebramycin factor 6. Antimicrob Agents Chemother 1970:309–313
Koch KF, Davis FA, Rhoades JA (1973) Nebramycin: Separation of the complex and identification of factors 4, 5 and 5′. J Antibiot (Tokyo) 26:745–751
Koch KF, Merkel KE, O'Connor SC, Occolowitz JL, Paschal JW, Dorman DE (1978) Structures of some of the minor aminoglycoside factors of the nebramycin fermentation. J Org Chem 43:1430–1434
Kondo S, Sezaki M, Koike M, Shimura M, Akita E, Satoh K, Hara T (1965 a) Destomycins A and B, two new antibiotics produced by a *Streptomyces*. J Antibiot (Tokyo) A18:38–42
Kondo S, Sezaki M, Koike M, Akita E (1965 b) Destomycin A. The acid hydrolysis and the partial structure. J Antibiot (Tokyo) A18:192–194

Kondo S, Akita E, Koike M (1966a) The structure of destomycin A. J Antibiot (Tokyo) A19:139–140
Kondo S, Akita E, Sezaki M (1966b) A new polyhydroxy amino acid, destomic acid, the hydrolysis product of destomycin A. J Antibiot (Tokyo) A19:137–138
Kondo S, Iinuma K, Naganawa H, Shimura M, Sekizawa Y (1975) Structural studies on destomycins A and B. J Antibiot (Tokyo) 28:79–82
Konishi M, Numata K, Shimoda K, Tsukiura H, Kawaguchi H (1974) Aminoglycoside antibiotics. VI. Structure determination of 4′-deoxybutirosins (BU-1975 C_1 and C_2). J Antibiot (Tokyo) 27:471–483
Konishi M, Kamata S, Tsuno T, Numata K, Tsukiura H, Naito T, Kawaguchi H (1976) Sorbistin, a new aminoglycoside antibiotic complex of bacterial origin. III. Structure determination. J Antibiot (Tokyo) 29:1152–1162
Koyama G, Iitaka Y, Maeda K, Umezawa H (1968) The crystal structure of kanamycin. Tetrahedron Lett 15:1875–1879
Kuck NA, Redin GS (1978) Glycocinnamoylspermidines, a new class of antibiotics. V. Antibacterial evaluation of the isopropyl derivative of LL-BM123γ. J Antibiot (Tokyo) 31:405–409
Kugelman M, Jaret RS, Mittelman S, Gau W (1978) The structure of aminoglycoside antibiotic 66-40G produced by *Micromonospora inyoensis*. J Antibiot (Tokyo) 31:643–645
Kurath P, Grampovnik D, Tadanier J, Martin JR, Egan RS, Stanaszek RS, Cirovic M, Washburn WH, Hill P, Dunnigan DA, Leonard JE, Johnson P, Goldstein AW (1979) 4-N-Acylfortimicins E. J Antibiot (Tokyo) 32:884–890
Leach BE, Teeters CM (1951) Neamine, an antibacterial degradation product of neomycin. J Am Chem Soc 73:2794–2797
Lee BK, Condon RG, Wagman GH, Weinstein MJ, Katz E (1976) *Micromonospora*-produced sisomicin components. J Antibiot (Tokyo) 29:677–684
Lemieux RU, Wolfrom ML (1948) The chemistry of streptomycin. Adv Carbohydr Chem 3:337–384
Maehr H, Schaffner CP (1967) The chemistry of the gentamicins. I. Characterization and gross structure of gentamicin A. J Am Chem Soc 89:6787–6788
Maehr H, Schaffner CP (1970) Chemistry of gentamicins. II. Stereochemistry and synthesis of gentosamine. Total structure of gentamicin A. J Am Chem Soc 92:1697–1700
Mann RL, Gale RM, Van Abeele FR (1953) Hygromycin. II. Isolation and properties. Antibiot Chemother 3:1279–1282
Mann RL, Bromer WW (1958) The isolation of a second antibiotic from *Streptomyces hygroscopicus*. J Am Chem Soc 80:2714–2716
Marquez JA, Wagman GH, Testa RT, Waitz JA, Weinstein MJ (1976) A new broad spectrum aminoglycoside antibiotic, G-52, produced by *Micromonospora zionensis*. J Antibiot (Tokyo) 29:483–487
Martin JH, Kunstmann MP, Barbatschi F, Hertz M, Ellestad GA, Dann M, Redin GS, Dornbush AC, Kuck NA (1978) Glycocinnamoylspermidines, a new class of antibiotics. II. Isolation, physicochemical and biological properties of LL-BM123β, γ_1 and γ_2. J Antibiot (Tokyo) 31:398–404
Mason DJ, Dietz A, Smith R (1961) Actinospectacin, a new antibiotic. I. Discovery and biological properties. Antibiot Chemother 11:118–122
McAlpine JB, Sinclair AC, Egan RS, DeVault RL, Stanaszek RS, Cirovic M, Mueller SL, Goodley PC, Mauritz RJ, Wideburg NE, Mitscher LA, Shirahata K, Matsushima H, Sato S, Iida (1977) A new aminoglycoside antibiotic complex – the seldomycins. IV. The structure of seldomycin factor 5. J Antibiot (Tokyo) 30:39–49
Miyaki T, Tsukiura H, Wakae M, Kawaguchi H (1962) Glebomycin, a new member of the streptomycin class. II. Isolation and physicochemical properties. J Antibiot (Tokyo) A15:15–19
Mori T, Ichiyanagi T, Kondo H, Tokunaga K, Oda T, Munakata K (1971) Studies on new antibiotic lividomycins. II. Isolation and characterization of lividomycins A, B and other aminoglycosidic antibiotics produced by *Streptomyces lividus*. J Antibiot (Tokyo) 24:339–346

Mori T, Kyotani Y, Watanabe I, Oda T (1972a) Chemical conversion of lividomycin A into lividomycin B. J Antibiot (Tokyo) 25:149–150
Mori T, Kyotani Y, Watanabe I, Oda T (1972b) The structure of mannosylparomomycin (No 2230-C). J Antibiot (Tokyo) 25:317–319
Murase M (1961) Structural studies on kanamycin C. J Antibiot (Tokyo) A14:367–368
Murase M, Wakazawa T, Abe M, Kawaji S (1961) Studies on kanamycin C. J. Antibiot (Tokyo) A14:156–157
Murase M, Ito T, Fukatsu S, Umezawa H (1970) Studies on kanamycin related compounds produced during fermentation by mutants of *Streptomyces kanamyceticus*. Isolation and properties. In: Umezawa H (ed) Progress in antimicrobial and cancer chemotherapy. Proceedings of the 6th International Congress on Chemotherapy, vol II. University Park Press, Baltimore, pp 1098–1110
Nagabushan TL, Daniels PJL, Turner WN, Morton JB (1975a) The gentamicin antibiotics. 7. Structure of the gentamicin antibiotics A_1, A_3 and A_4. J Org Chem 40:2830–2834
Nagabushan TL, Daniels PJL, Jaret RS, Morton JB (1975b) The gentamicin antibiotics. 8. Structure of gentamicin A_2. J Org Chem 40:2835–2836
Naganawa H, Usui N, Takita T, Hamada M, Maeda K, Umezawa H (1974) 4-Amino-4-deoxy-α,α-trehalose, a new metabolite of a streptomyces. J Antibiot (Tokyo) 27:145–146
Naito T (1962) Glebomycin, a new member of the streptomycin class. IV. Structure of glebomycin (in Japanese). J Antibiot (Tokyo) B15:373–379
Nara T, Kawamoto I, Okachi R, Takasawa S, Yamamoto M, Sato S, Sato T, Morikawa A (1975) New antibiotics XK-62-2 (sagamicin). II. Taxonomy of the producing organism, fermentative production and characterization of sagamicin. J Antibiot (Tokyo) 28:21–28
Nara T, Yamamoto M, Takasawa S, Sato S, Sato T, Kawamoto I, Okachi R, Takahashi I, Morikawa A (1977a) An new aminoglycoside antibiotic complex – the seldomycins. I. Taxonomy, fermentation and antibacterial properties. J Antibiot (Tokyo) 30:17–24
Nara T, Yamamoto M, Kawamoto I, Takayama K, Okachi R, Takasawa S, Sato T, Sato S (1977b) Fortimicins A and B, new aminoglycoside antibiotics. I. Producing organism, fermentation and biological properties of fortimicins. J Antibiot (Tokyo) 30:533–540
Nara K, Sumino Y, Katamoto K, Akiyama S, Asai M (1978a) The chemistry of aminoglycoside antibiotics from *Pseudomonas fluorescens*. I. Isolation, characterization and partial structure of P-2563(P) (sorbistin A_1) and P-2563(A) (sorbistin B). Chem Pharm Bull 26:1075–1082
Nara K, Katamoto K, Suzuki S, Akiyama S, Mizuta E (1978b) The chemistry of aminoglycoside antibiotics from *Pseudomonas fluorescens*. II. Absolute configuration of the diaminopolyol, the aglycone of P-2563(P) (sorbistin A_1) and P-2563(A) (sorbistin B). Chem Pharm Bull 26:1083–1090.
Nara K, Katamoto K, Suzuki S, Mizuta E (1978c) The chemistry of aminoglycoside antibiotics from *Pseudomonas fluorescens*. III. Absolute configuratation of P-2563(P) (sorbistin A_1) and P-2563(A) (sorbistin B). Chem Pharm Bull 26:1091–1099
Neuss N, Koch KF, Molloy BB, Day W, Huckstep LL, Dorman DE, Roberts JD (1970) Structure of hygromycin B, an antibiotic from *Streptomyces hygroscopicus;* the use of CMR spectra in structure determination, I. Helv Chem Acta 53:2314–2319
Nishikawa T, Ishida N (1965) A new antibiotic R-468 active against drug-resistant *Shigella*. J Antibiot (Tokyo) A18:132–133
Niwa T, Inouye S, Tsuruoka T, Koaze Y, Niida T (1970) Nojirimycin as a potent inhibitor of glucosidase. Agric Biol Chem 34:966–968
O'Connor S, Lam LKT, Jones ND, Chaney MO (1976) Apramycin, a unique aminocyclitol antibiotic. J Org Chem 41:2087–2092
Oda T, Mori T, Ito H, Kunieda T (1971a) Studies on new antibiotic lividomycins. I. Taxonomic studies on the lividomycin-producing strain *Streptomyces lividus* nov. sp. J Antibiot (Tokyo) 24:333–338
Oda T, Mori T, Kyotani Y (1971b) III. Partial structure or lividomycin A. J Antibiot (Tokyo) 24:503–510
Oda T, Mori T, Kyotani Y, Nakayama M (1971c) Structure of lividomycin A. J Antibiot (Tokyo) 24:511–518

Ogawa H, Ito S, Kondo S, Inoue S (1959) The structure of an antibiotic kanamycin. Bull Agric Chem Soc Jpn 23:289–310

Ohmori T, Okanishi M, Kawaguchi H (1962) Glebomycin, a new member of the streptomycin class. III. Taxonomic studies on strain no 12096 producer of glebomycin. J Antibiot (Tokyo) A15:21–27

Okachi R, Kawamoto I, Takasawa S, Yamamoto M, Sato S, Sato T, Nara T (1974) A new antibiotic XK-62-2 (sagamicin) I. Isolation, physicochemical and antibacterial properties. J Antibiot (Tokyo) 27:793–800

Okachi R, Takasawa S, Sato T, Sato S, Yamamoto M, Kawamoto I, Nara T (1977) Fortimicins A and B, new aminoglycoside antibiotics. II. Isolation, physicochemical and chromatographic properties. J Antibiot (Tokyo) 30:541–551

Okami Y, Hotta K, Yoshida M, Ikeda D, Kondo S, Umezawa H (1979) New aminoglycoside antibiotics, istamycins A and B. J Antibiot (Tokyo) 32:964–966

Okanishi M, Koshiyama H, Ohmori T, Matsuzaki M, Ohashi S, Kawaguchi K (1962) Glebomycin, a new member of the streptomycin class. I. Biological studies. J Antibiot (Tokyo) A15:7–14

Okubo S, Nakamura N, Ito K, Marumo H, Tanaka M, Omura S (1979) Antitumor activity of prumycin. J Antibiot (Tokyo) 32:347–354

Omoto S, Shomura T, Suzuki H, Inouye S (1979) Studies on *Actinomycetales* producing antibiotics only on agar culture. II. Isolation, structure and biological properties of N-carbamoyl-D-glucosamine (substance SF-1993). J Antibiot (Tokyo) 32:436–441

Omura S, Katagiri M, Awaya J, Atsumi K, Oiwa R, Hata T, Higashikawa K, Yasui K, Terada H, Kuyama S (1973) Production and isolation of a new antifungal antibiotic, prumycin, and taxonomic studies of *Streptomyces* sp., strain no. F-1028. Agric Biol Chem 37:2805–2812

Omura S, Katagiri M, Atsumi K, Hata T, Jakubowski AA, Springs EB, Tishler M (1974) Structure of prumycin. J Chem Soc Perkin I 1974:1627–1631

Peck RL, Hoffhine CE Jr, Gale P, Folkers K (1949) *Streptomyces* antibiotics. XXIII. Isolation of neomycin A. J Am Chem Soc 71:2590-2591

Perlman D, Langlyke AF (1948) The occurrence of mannosidostreptomycinase. J Am Chem Soc 70:3968

Pittenger RC, Wolfe RN, Hoehn MM, Marks PN, Daily WA, McGuire JM (1953) Hygromycin. I. Preliminary studies on the production and biologic activity of a new antibiotic. Antibiot Chemother 3:1268–1278

Price KE, Godfrey JC, Kawaguchi H (1974) Effect of structural modifications on the biological properties of aminoglycoside antibiotics containing 2-deoxystreptamine. Adv Appl Microbiol 18:191–307. Reprinted in: Perlman D (ed) (1977) Structure-activity relationships among the semisynthetic antibiotics. Academic Press, New York San Francisco London, pp 239–355, 357–395 [Suppl]

Reimann H, Cooper DJ, Mallams AK, Jaret RS, Yehaskel A, Kugelman M, Vernay HF, Schumacher D (1973) The structure of sisomicin, a novel unsaturated aminocyclitol antibiotic from *Micromonospora inyoensis*. J Org Chem 39:1451–1459

Rinehart KL Jr (1961) The neomycins and related antibiotics. Wiley and Sons, New York

Sato S, Takasawa S, Sato T, Yamamoto M, Okachi R, Kawamoto I, Iida T, Morikawa A, Nara T (1977) A new aminoglycoside antibiotic complex – the seldomycins. II. Isolation, physicochemical and chromatographic properties. J Antibiot (Tokyo) 30:25–30

Schatz A, Bugie E, Waksman SA (1944) Streptomycin, a substance exhibiting antibiotic activity against Gram-positive and Gram-negative bacteria. Proc Soc Exp Biol Med 55:66–69

Schillings RT, Schaffner CP (1962) Differentiation of catenulin-neomycin antibiotics; identity of catenulin, paromomycin, hydroxymycin and aminosidin. Antimicrob Agents Chemother 1961:274–285

Schmitz H, Fardig OB, O'Herron FA, Rousche MA, Hooper IR (1958) Kanamycin. III. Kanamycin B. J Am Chem Soc 80:2911

Shimura M, Sekizawa Y, Iinuma K, Naganawa H, Kondo S (1975) Destomycin C, a new member of destomycin family antibiotics. J Antibiot (Tokyo) 28:83–84

Shoji J, Nakagawa Y (1970) Structural features of antibiotic A-396-I. J Antibiot (Tokyo) 23:569–571

Shoji J, Kozuki S, Mayama M, Kawamura Y, Matsumoto K (1970) Isolation of a new water soluble basic antibiotic A-396-I. J Antibiot (Tokyo) 23:291–294

Shomura T, Ezaki N, Tsuruoka T, Niwa T, Akita E, Niida T (1970) Studies on antibiotic SF-733, a new antibiotic. I. Taxonomy, isolation and characterization. J Antibiot (Tokyo) 23:155–161

Shomura T, Yoshida J, Amano S, Kojima M, Inouye S, Niida T (1979) Studies on *Actinomycetales* producing antibiotics only on agar culture. I. Screening, taxonomy and morphology-productivity relationship of *Streptomyces halstedii*, strain SF-1993. J Antibiot (Tokyo) 32:427–435

Stark WM, Hoehn MM, Knox NG (1968) Nebramycin, a new broad spectrum antibiotic complex. I. Detection and biosynthesis. Antimicrob Agents Chemother 1967:314–323

Stark WM, Knox NG, Wilgus RM (1971) Strains of *Streptomyces tenebrarius* and biosynthesis of nebramycin. Folia Microbiol (Praha) 16:205–217

Suami T, Ogawa S, Chida N (1980) The revised structure of validamycin A. J Antibiot (Tokyo) 33:98–99

Sugimoto M, Ishii S, Okachi R, Nara T (1979) Fortimicins C, D, and KE, new aminoglycoside antibiotics. J Antibiot (Tokyo) 32:868–873

Suhara Y, Maeda K, Umezawa H, Ohno M (1966) Chemical studies on kasugamycin. V. The structure of kasugamycin. Tetrahedron Lett 1966:1239–1244

Takahashi K, Iida T, Takazawa S, Shimura G, Shirakata K (1979) The structures of fortimicins. Abstr Meet Am Chem Soc 177 Pt 1 CARB 22

Takamoto T, Hanessian S (1974) Aminoglycoside antibiotics: chemical transformation of paromomycin into a bioactive pseudotrisaccharide. Tetrahedron Lett 1974:4009–4012

Takeuchi T, Hikiji T, Nitta K, Yamazaki S, Abe S, Takayama H, Umezawa H (1957) Biological studies on kanamycin. J Antibiot (Tokyo) A10:107–114

Tamura A, Furuta R, Kotani H (1975) Antibiotic A-16316-C, a new water-soluble basic antibiotic. J Antibiot (Tokyo) 28:260–265

Tamura A, Furuta R, Naruto S (1976a) Isolation of an antibiotic AB-74, related to destomycin C. J Antibiot (Tokyo) 29:590–591

Tamura A, Furuta R, Kotani H (1976b) Taxonomic studies on *Streptomyces aquacanus*, antibiotic AB-74 producing organism. J Antibiot (Tokyo) 29:592–594

Tatsuoka S, Kusaka T, Miyake A, Inoue M, HItomi H, Shiraishi Y, Iwasaki H, Imanishi M (1957) Antibiotics. XVI. Isolation and identification of dihydrostreptomycin produced by a new streptomyces: *Streptomyces humidus nov. sp.* Pharm Bull 5:343

Tatsuoka S, Horii S, Rinehart KL Jr, Nakabayashi T (1964) The absolute configuration of streptidine in dihyrostreptomycin and of deoxystreptamine in kanamycin A. J Antibiot (Tokyo) A17:88–89

Thompson RG, Presti EA (1968) Nebramycin, a new broad spectrum antibiotic complex. III. Isolation and chemical-physical properties. Antimicrob Agents Chemother 1967:332–340

Tomita K, Hoshino Y, Venoyama Y, Fujisawa K, Tsukiura H, Kawaguchi H (1976) Sorbistin, a new aminoglycoside antibiotic complex of bacterial origin. II. Isolation and taxonomy of sorbistin-producing organism. J Antibiot (Tokyo) 29:1147–1151

Tresner HD, Korshalla JH, Fantini AA, Korshalla JD, Kirby JP, Goodman JJ, Kele RA, Shay AJ, Borders DB (1978) Glycocinnamoylspermidines, a new class of antibiotics. I. Description and fermentation of the organism producing the LL-BM123 antibiotics. J Antibiot (Tokyo) 31:394–397

Tsukiura H, Fujisawa K, Konishi M, Saito K, Numata K, Ishikawa H, Miyaki T, Tomita K, Kawaguchi H (1973a) Aminoglycoside antibiotics. III. Bio-active degradation products from butirosins and semi-synthesis of butirosin analogs. J Antibiot (Tokyo) 26:351–357

Tsukiura H, Saito K, Kobaru S, Konishi M, Kawaguchi H (1973b) Aminoglycoside antibiotics. IV: BU-1709 E_1 and E_2, new aminoglycoside antibiotics related to the butirosins. J Antibiot (Tokyo) 26:386–388

Tsukiura H, Hanada M, Saito K, Fujisawa K, Miyaki T, Koshiyama H, Kawaguchi H (1976) Sorbistin, a new aminoglycoside antibiotic complex of bacterial origin. I. Production, isolation and properties. J Antibiot (Tokyo) 29:1137–1146
Umezawa H, Tazaki T, Okami Y, Fukuyama S (1949) Studies on the streptothricin group substances. On streptothricin A and streptothricin B (in Japanese). J Antibiot (Tokyo) 3:232–235
Umezawa H, Ueda K, Maeda K, Yagishita K, Kondo S, Okami Y, Utahara R, Osata Y, Nitta K, Takeuchi T (1957) Production and isolation of a new antibiotic, kanamycin. J Antibiot (Tokyo) A10:181–189
Umezawa H, Okami Y, Hashimoto T, Suhara Y, Hamada M, Takeuchi T (1965) A new antibiotic, kasugamycin. J Antibiot (Tokyo) A18:101–103
Umezawa S (1974) Structures and syntheses of aminoglycoside antibiotics. Adv Carbohydr Chem 30:111–182
Umezawa S, Ito Y, Fukatsu S (1959) Studies on antibiotics and related substances VII. The structure of kanamycin. Bull Chem Soc Jpn 32:81–84
Umezawa S, Umino K, Shibahara S, Hamada M, Omoto S (1967a) Fermentation of 3-amino-3-deoxy-D-glucose. J Antibiot (Tokyo) A20:355–360
Umezawa S, Tatsuta K, Muto R (1967b) Synthesis of trehalosamine. J Antibiot (Tokyo) A20:388–389
Uramoto M, Otake N, Yonehara H (1967) Mannosyl glucosaminide, a new antibiotic. J Antibiot (Tokyo) A20:236–237
Vaisman A, Hamelin A (1958) Hydroxymycin, a new antibiotic active against *Trichomonas vaginalis*. C R Acad Sci [D] (Paris) 247:163–165
Wagman GH, Testa RT, Marquez JA (1970) Antibiotic 6640. II. Fermentation, isolation and properties. J Antibiot (Tokyo) 23:555–558
Wagman GH, Marquez JA, Bailey JV, Cooper D, Weinstein J, Tkach R, Daniels PJL (1972) Chromatographic separation of some minor components of the gentamicin complex. J Chromatogr 70:171–173
Waitz JA, Moss EL, Oden EM, Weinstein MJ (1970) Antibiotic 6640. III. Biological studies with antibiotic 6640, a new broad-spectrum aminoglycoside antibiotic. J Antibiot (Tokyo) 23:559–565
Waksman SA, Lechevalier HA (1949) Neomycin, a new antibiotic active against streptomycin-resistant bacteria, including tuberculosis organisms. Science 109:305–307
Watanabe I, Deushi T, Yamaguchi T, Kamiya K, Nakayama M, Mori T (1979) The structural elucidation of aminoglycoside antibiotics, sannamycins A and B. J Antibiot (Tokyo) 32:1066–1068
Weinstein MJ, Leudemann GM, Oden EM, Wagman H (1964) Gentamicin, a new broad-spectrum antibiotic complex. Antimicrob Agents Chemother 1963:1–7
Weinstein MJ, Wagman GH, Oden EM, Marquez JA (1967) Biological activity of the antibiotic components of the gentamicin complex. J Bacteriol 94:789–790
Weinstein MJ, Marquez JA, Testa RT, Wagman GH, Oden EM, Waitz JA (1970) Antibiotic 6640, a new *Micromonospora*-produced aminoglycoside antibiotic. J Antibiot (Tokyo) 23:551–554
Weinstein MJ, Wagman GH, Marquez JA, Testa RT, Waitz JA (1975) Verdamicin, a new broad spectrum aminoglycoside antibiotic. Antimicrob Agents Chemother 7:246–249
Wiley PF, Sigal MV Jr, Weaver O (1962) Degradation products of hygromycin B. J Org Chem 27:2793-2796
Wiley PF, Argoudelis AD, Hoeksema H (1963) The chemistry of actinospectacin. IV: The determination of the structure of actinospectacin. J Am Chem Soc 85:2652
Woo PWK, Dion HW, Bartz QR (1971) Butirosins A and B, aminoglycoside antibiotics. III. Structures. Tetrahedron Lett 1971:2625–2628

CHAPTER 2

Total Synthesis and Chemical Modification of the Aminoglycoside Antibiotics

S. UMEZAWA and T. TSUCHIYA

A. Introduction

The number of structurally elucidated aminoglycoside antibiotics of microbial origin is now about one hundred. Various aminoglycoside antibiotics have been introduced into, and have become established in, chemotherapy. The study of this group of antibiotics has provided some fascinating and challenging problems in the field of carbohydrate chemistry. After several decades of work on the determination of chemical structures of naturally occurring aminoglycoside antibiotics, it was inevitable that organic chemists would turn their attention toward total synthesis; however, the synthetic chemistry of this important group of antibiotics was rather slow in developing until the end of the 1960s.

During the past ten years or so, remarkable progress has been made in the synthetic chemistry of this field. Total syntheses of a number of aminoglycoside antibiotics, including streptomycin, dihydrostreptomycin, neomycin C, kanamycin A, B, and C, kasugamycin, ribostamycin, tobramycin, butirosin B, minosaminomycin, spectinomycin, and istamycin A, have been accomplished.

Furthermore, extension of the procedures of the total synthesis combined with the knowledge of the mechanisms of resistance of resistant organisms opened the way to planned chemical modification of aminoglycoside antibiotics to overcome inactivating enzymes, and a great number of synthetic aminoglycoside antibiotics which are remarkably active against resistant bacteria have been successfully prepared.

This chapter is concerned with the synthetic aspects. Since several excellent reviews (HANESSIAN and HASKELL 1970; S. UMEZAWA 1974; COX et al. 1977) of the chemistry of aminoglycoside antibiotics have appeared, the present chapter will cover, in outline, the key literatures, placing major emphasis on recent advances.

The classification of aminoglycoside antibiotics in this chapter is based on overall common structural relationships, being divided into the following six groups:

1. Streptomycin group.
2. Pseudodisaccharides which contain 4-substituted 2-deoxystreptamine – paromamine, neamine, and related compounds.
3. Pseudotrisaccharides which contain 4,5-disubstituted 2-deoxystreptamine – ribostamycin, butirosins, and related compounds.
4. Pseudotetra- and pseudopentasaccharides which contain 4,5-disubstituted 2-deoxystreptamine – neomycins, paromomycins, lividomycins, and related compounds.

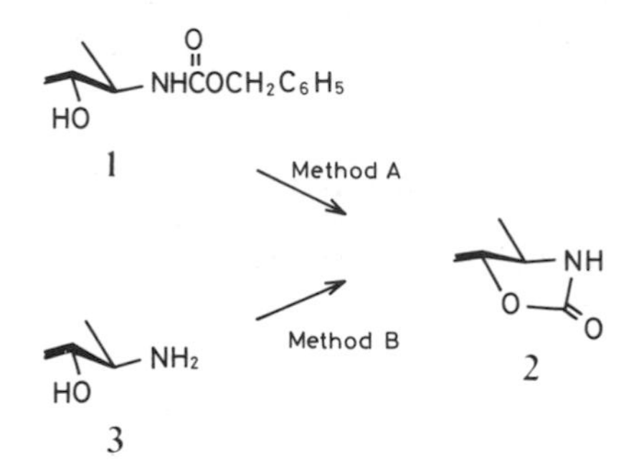

Fig. 1. Protection of *vicinal trans*-diequatorial NH_2 and OH

5. Pseudotrisaccharides which contain 4,6-disubstituted 2-deoxystreptamine – kanamycins, tobramycin, gentamicins, and related compounds.
6. Others including kasugamycin, spectinomycin, fortimicins, sorbistins, minosaminomycin, trehalosamine, and related compounds.

B. Several Reactions and Methods Generally Useful for the Synthesis of Aminoglycoside Antibiotics

I. Simultaneous Protection of Vicinal Trans-Equatorial Amino and Hydroxyl Groups

The simultaneous protection of *trans*-equatorial amino and hydroxyl groups has great advantages in aminoglycoside synthesis. For this purpose, efficient, facile procedures have been developed (Fig. 1).

When a benzyloxycarbonylamino derivative (1) of pyranosides or aminocyclitols having vicinal *trans*-diequatorial amino and hydroxyl groups is treated with sodium hydride or potassium butoxide in *N*,*N*-dimethylformamide (DMF) under nitrogen, a cyclic carbamate derivative (2) is formed in excellent yield (method A) (D. IKEDA et al. 1972). As an alternative procedure (method B), treatment of an aminosugar or aminocyclitol (3) with either phenoxycarbonyl chloride or *p*-nitrophenoxycarbonyl chloride in the presence of a basic resin or alkali in aqueous media affords a cyclic carbamate derivative (S. UMEZAWA et al. 1971c). The great value of these reagents lies in the fact that they are specific for amino alcohols and do not react with diols. The carbamate group is readily removed by mild alkali, such as barium hydroxide. Another advantage of the cyclic carbamate group is that it can withstand acidic treatment, whereas cyclic acetals and ketals are readily hydrolyzed by acid. Cyclic carbamate formation combined with cyclic acetal formation has been useful for a number of aminoglycoside syntheses.

II. Selective Cyclic Acetalation

The value of cyclic acetals for the protection of hydroxyl groups in carbohydrate chemistry is well known. Among acetalation reactions, the ketal-exchange reaction

(EVANS et al. 1967) has been extremely useful in aminoglycoside syntheses. The method involving the use of cyclohexanone dimethyl ketal or 2,2-dimethoxypropane in DMF in the presence of a catalytic amount of *p*-toluenesulfonic acid made it possible to form a ketal ring between adjacent *trans*-hydroxyls. Furthermore, different cyclic acetals often show different stability toward acid and selective acetalation is possible, often affording key intermediates; many examples will be found in subsequent sections.

III. 1,2-cis-Glycosylation of Aminosugars

The synthesis of aminoglycoside antibiotics often involves the formation of a 1,2-*cis*-pyranoside. Among several glycosylation reactions, the Koenigs–Knorr condensation is still the most widely applicable to glycoside synthesis. Stereochemical control of the Koenigs–Knorr condensation is unreliable, depending on the structures of the sugar component and aglycon; however, the use of nonparticipating groups as the substituent at C-2 of the sugar component was found to selectively produce 1,2-*cis*-pyranosides. Thus, for 2-amino-2-deoxysugars, the use of Schiff base derivatives and 2,4-dinitrophenyl derivatives (S. UMEZAWA and KOTO 1966) successfully gives the 1,2-*cis*-pyranosides. Schiff base derivatives are especially useful in giving stereospecific 1,2-*cis*-glycoside synthesis (S. UMEZAWA et al. 1972a), as exemplified by the syntheses of paromamine, dihydrostreptomycin, and neomycin C. For 2-hydroxy aminosugars, the use of the benzyl group selectively gives the 1,2-*cis*-pyranosides, as exemplified by the synthesis of kanamycin A and others. The above-modified Koenigs–Knorr condensation requires strictly anhydrous conditions, therefore, carefully dried solvents should be used.

It should be noted that 2-azidosugars (PAULSEN et al. 1979) and 1-*O*-imidyl-β-D-sugars (SINAŸ 1978) are reported to be useful precursors of α-D-glycosides.

Another useful 1,2-*cis*-glycosylation reaction involves addition reactions to glucals. The addition of nitrosyl chloride to a protected D-glucal gives a dimeric product with α-D-*gluco*-configuration. The glycosylating agent reacts with molar portions of alcohols in DMF to give the corresponding 2-oximino-α-D-glycosides by an elimination–addition mechanism. Hydrogenation then gives glucosaminides and, more particularly, deoximination can be effected to give the keto analogs which on reduction with sodium borohydride give α-D-glucopyranosides. (For examples see LEMIEUX et al. 1973; KUGELMAN et al. 1976b–d).

CLEOPHAX et al. (1978a, b) have reported that α-linked aminocyclitol glycosides can be prepared from a protected 2-*O*-acyl glucal and an appropriately functionalized cyclitol derivative by a boron trifluoride–ether catalyzed addition reaction followed by hydrogenation of the resulting double bond. CANAS-RODRIGUEZ and MARTINEZ-TOBED (1979) also reported the syntheses of pseudotrisaccharides derived from 2,5-dideoxystreptamine by the boron trifluoride catalyzed addition of alcohols to glycals.

IV. Selective Deoxygenation Reactions

Selective deoxygenation reactions are required for the modification of aminoglycoside antibiotics, as described in Sect. C.

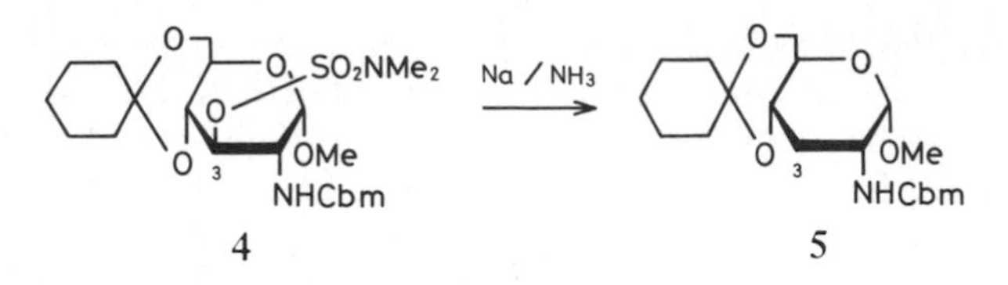

Fig. 2. 3-Deoxygenation. (Cbm = CO_2Me)

1. 3-Deoxygenation

In α-D-glucopyranosides, the difficulty lies in the deoxygenation of a secondary hydroxyl group attached to a carbon atom at which an S_N2 process is hindered. As an approach to this problem, radical-type deoxygenation reactions have recently been developed (BARTON and MCCOMBIE 1975; BARTON and SUBRAMANIAN 1977; IRELAND et al. 1972; OIDA et al. 1975; DESHAYES et al. 1975; PETE et al. 1977; COLLINS and MUNASINGHE 1977; BILLINGHAM et al. 1977; BELL et al. 1977; KISHI et al. 1979). TSUCHIYA et al. (1978b) reported a method involving treatment of a 3-*O*-(*N*,*N*-dimethylsulfamoyl) derivative (4) with sodium metal in liquid ammonia, as exemplified in Fig. 2.

This method was successfully applied to the transformation of dihydrostreptomycin into its 3″-deoxy derivative, namely 3″-deoxydihydrostreptomycin, which is remarkably active against resistant bacteria (S. UMEZAWA to be published).

HASKELL et al. (1977) described a 3-deoxygenation which includes nucleophilic displacement of the 3-*O*-trifluoromethylsulfonyl function by benzenethiolate under mild conditions and subsequent desulfurization with sodium in liquid ammonia.

BARTON and MCCOMBIE (1975) reported that *S*-methyl dithiocarbonates or thiobenzoates derived from secondary alcohols are reduced to the corresponding hydrocarbons on treatment with tributylstannane and suggested the particular applicability of this method in aminoglycoside chemistry. This method has been extended to the modification of aminoglycoside antibiotics, and 5-deoxykanamycin B, 3′,4′,5-trideoxykanamycin B, 3′,4′,5-trideoxy-3′-enokanamycin B, 6-deoxybutirosin A, and 3′-deoxybutirosin A have been prepared from kanamycin B or butirosin A (HAYASHI et al. 1978) (see Sect. C.III.3.c).

A useful 3-deoxygenation involves a sequence of reactions including selective tosylation. Whereas mesylation of 2,6-di-*N*-protected 2,6-diamino-2,6-dideoxy-α-D-glucopyranosides gives 3,4-di-*O*-mesyl derivatives, toslyation is selective for the 3-hydroxyl group and allows, by iodination followed by hydrogenolysis, a convenient synthesis of 3-deoxy derivatives. For example, 3′-deoxykanamycin B (tobramycin) (TAKAGI et al. 1973, 1976), 3′-deoxyribostamycin (D. IKEDA et al. 1973b), and 3′-deoxybutirosin B (D. IKEDA et al. 1975, 1976) were synthesized by this method.

Another useful 3′-deoxygenation involves the use of inactivating enzymes. For example, kanamycin B 3′-phosphate was prepared by use of a phosphotransferase enzyme and the inactivated derivative was converted into the 3′-chloro derivative by treatment with trimethylsilylchloride, which by subsequent catalytic dechlorination led to 3′-deoxykanamycin B (OKUTANI et al. 1977) (see Sect. C.V.1.b).

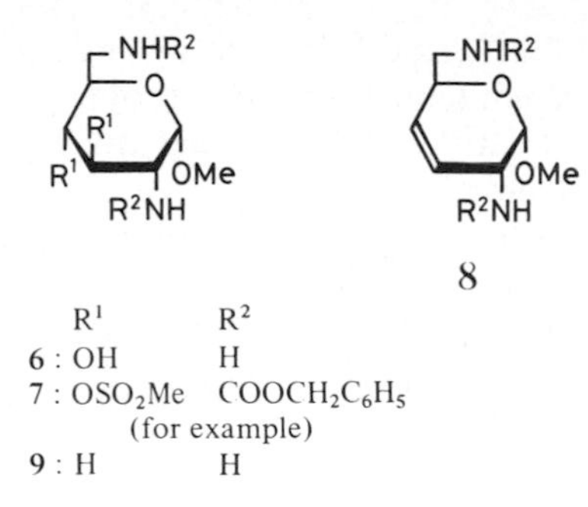

Fig. 3. 3,4-Dideoxygenation

2. 3,4-Dideoxygenation

2,6-Diamino-2,6-dideoxy-D-glucose (6), a component of a number of aminoglycoside antibiotics such as kanamycin B, neomycins, ribostamycin, butirosins, and others, was transformed into its 3,4-dideoxy derivative (9) as outlined in Fig. 3 (S. UMEZAWA et al. 1972d). The two amino groups of the glycoside were protected with methoxycarbonyl, ethoxycarbonyl, or benzyloxycarbonyl groups, and the two hydroxyl groups were mesylated or benzylsulfonylated to give the 3,4-disulfonate (7). Tosylation gave an almost completely selective reaction at the 3-OH. Treatment of the disulfonate with sodium iodide and an excess of zinc dust in hot DMF afforded the 3,4-unsaturated sugar (8) in excellent yield. Catalytic hydrogenation of (8) and deprotection gave the 3,4-dideoxyaminoglycoside (9). This deoxygenation opened the way to the transformation of neamine, kanamycin B, ribostamycin, and butirosin B into their 3′,4′-dideoxy derivatives, which are active against resistant bacteria.

HAYASHI et al. (1977) described the removal of vicinal mesyloxy groups with naphthalene-sodium. YONETA et al. (1979) recently reported another method for the above 3′-ene formation which involved the cleavage of an epoxide ring to iodohydrin followed by treatment with p-toluenesulfonyl chloride in pyridine. BARRETT et al. (1979) reported the preparation of olefins from vicinal diols by reaction of the derived bisdithiocarbonates with tributylstannane in toluene and suggested its application to the modification of aminoglycoside antibiotics.

V. Selective *N*-Protection via Temporary Metal Chelation of Vicinal and Nonvicinal Amino–Hydroxy or Amino–Amino Groups

In the area of semisynthesis and modification of aminoglycoside antibiotics, methods for selective *N*-acylation and *N*-alkylation are in demand. Metal chelation has recently been introduced as an efficient means of meeting this need. The method is based on the temporary protection of suitably disposed amino–hydroxy or amino–amino functions as metal chelates and subsequent acylation or alkylation of the unbound amino group(s). HANESSIAN and PATIL (1978) described the selective *N*-acylation of kanamycin A via chelation of the vicinal amino–hydroxy group with Cu^{2+}. NAGABHUSHAN et al. (1978c) described the *N*-acylation of sisomicin, gentamicins, and kanamycin A via chelation of the nonvicinal amino–hydroxy group (with Co^{2+}, Ni^{2+}, and Cu^{2+}) between the 1 and 2″ positions as well as the chelation of the vicinal amino–hydroxy group (see Fig. 71). CARNEY et al. (1978) utilized chelation of Cu^{2+} between vicinal amino groups in the selective *N*-acylation of seldomycin factor 5.

CRON et al. (1979) reported that the *N*-acylation of partially trimethylsilylated kanamycin A in acetone proceeded selectively at the 1-*N* position rather than the usual 6′-*N* position. TSUCHIYA et al. (1979 b) reported an efficient method for the regiospecific 1-*N*-acylation of kanamycin-related antibiotics which involves zinc chelation followed by regiospecific *N*-trifluoroacetylation (see Fig. 53).

VI. Determination of the Configurations of Aminopyranosides and Aminocyclitols by the Shift in Optical Rotation Due to Copper (II) Chelate Formation

The Reeves method (REEVES 1951) for determination of the configuration of pyranosides is well known and has greatly contributed to the structural determination of aminoglycoside antibiotics. However, the Reeves method is limited to the vicinal diol system. S. UMEZAWA et al. (1966 b) found a useful method for the vicinal amino–hydroxy systems using tetrammine-copper (II) sulfate (TACu) as a chelating agent.

This reagent has found widespread application. The most striking characteristic of TACu is that it forms, in an aqueous solution, a copper complex only with vicinal amino and hydroxyl groups, but not with vicinal hydroxyl groups, whereas the Cupra B reagent of the Reeves method forms a complex with vicinal hydroxyl groups. In the six-membered chair form, a pair of contiguous *trans*-diequatorial amino and hydroxyl groups gives roughly $\Delta[M]_{TACu}$ of $\pm 900°$ according to the 60° dihedral angle between the amino and hydroxyl groups which may be clockwise (negative) or anticlockwise (positive). On the other hand, the $\Delta[M]_{Cupra\,B}$ gives roughly $\pm 2{,}000°$ for a hydroxy–hydroxy system, according to the direction of dihedral angle. A solution of cuprous chloride in concentrated ammonia also give the same results as the Cupra B reagent. This reagent, called CuAm, is easy and simple to prepare (S. UMEZAWA et al. 1966 b).

For example, D-glucosamine glycoside provides an important observation. There are two combinations, namely, hydroxy–hydroxy and amino–hydroxy systems. TACu forms a complex with the amino–hydroxy system, while Cupra B or CuAm forms a complex with the hydroxy–hydroxy system, giving reasonable $\Delta[M]$ values (Fig. 4).

The TACu method has found further application in the structural determination of pseudodisaccharides; for example, paromamine was differentiated from its positional isomer (S. UMEZAWA et al. 1972 a). An interesting example is the structural determination of the diastereomers of protected streptosyldeoxystreptamine (PAULSEN et al. 1977).

BARLOW and GUTHRIE (1967) described a study of the optical rotatory shift and conductance changes in cuprammonium solutions of eight isomeric aminoglycosides.

$$\Delta[M]_{TACu} = ([\alpha]_{436}\mathrm{TACu} - [\alpha]_{436}\mathrm{H_2O}) \cdot \frac{\mathrm{Mol.\ wt}}{100} \quad \ldots\ldots (1)$$

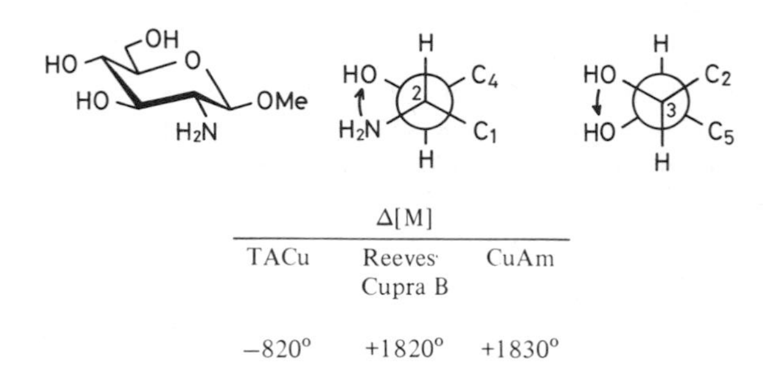

Δ[M]		
TACu	Reeves-Cupra B	CuAm
−820°	+1820°	+1830°

Fig. 4

Several applications of circular dichroism to aminoglycosides have been described (KUGELMAN et al. 1976b, c; HANESSIAN and PATIL 1978; BARLOW et al. 1979; BYSTRICKY et al. 1979).

C. Total Synthesis and Modification of Aminoglycoside Antibiotics

The first total synthesis of this group of antibiotics was reported by S. UMEZAWA and KOTO (1966) with the synthesis of paromamine, followed by the synthesis of neamine (neomycin A) (S. UMEZAWA et al. 1967c). Paromamine is a constituent of kanamycin C, paromomycins, and others. Neamine is a constituent of neomycin, kanamycin B, ribostamycin, butirosins, and others. Both antibiotics were isolated from *Streptomyces* cultures. These syntheses of pseudodisaccharides provided useful intermediates for further syntheses of more complex aminoglycoside antibiotics. Kanamycin A (S. UMEZAWA et al. 1968b; NAKAJIMA et al. 1968a), Kanamycin B (S. UMEZAWA et al. 1968c), and kanamycin C (S. UMEZAWA et al. 1968a) were synthesized. The total synthesis of dihydrostreptomycin and streptomycin was accomplished by S. UMEZAWA et al. (1974a, c, 1975).

A difficulty associated with the synthesis of these antibiotics was the formation of the 1,2-*cis*-glycosidic linkages in a regiospecific manner, for which early syntheses were particularly deficient. Another unavoidable difficulty lay in the selective or specific protection of many functional groups. Needless to say, modern instrumental techniques, particularly nuclear magnetic resonance (NMR) spectroscopy, mass spectroscopy, Reeves' copper complexing method and its modification for configurational studies (see Sect. B.VI), thin-layer chromatography, and gas-liquid chromatography have greatly contributed to the advances in this area. [For examples see the report by DORMAN et al. (1976) for ^{15}N NMR spectroscopy and that by DANIELS et al. (1976b) for mass spectroscopy].

On the other hand, the mechanisms of inactivation (H. UMEZAWA 1970, 1974, 1979) of aminoglycoside antibiotics by resistant organisms have been elucidated. The mechanisms gave clues which led to the remarkable improvement of the antibacterial activity of aminoglycoside antibiotics. There were two approaches to new derivatives: (1) total synthesis, or (2) partial synthesis from natural antibiotics. The initial approach involved the total synthesis of 3′-deoxykanamycin A (S. UMEZAWA et al. 1971 a) and 3′-*O*-methylkanamycin A (H. UMEZAWA et al. 1972 b) by a sequence of reactions similar to the total synthesis of kanamycins. Thus, it was found that the synthetic 3′-deoxykanamycin A exhibited remarkable antibacterial activity against resistant bacteria, including resistant *Escherichia coli* and *Pseudomonas*, as well as against common bacteria, whereas the 3′-*O*-methylkanamycin A was almost devoid of activity. These results allowed the rational modification of aminoglycoside antibiotics to improve antibacterial activity against resistant bacteria. Subsequently, regioselective deoxygenation of natural aminoglycoside antibiotics has been studied extensively, and furthermore deoxygenation, not only at C-3′ but also at other positions, has been studied. The semisynthetic antibiotic 3′,4′-dideoxykanamycin B (dibekacin) (H. UMEZAWA et al. 1971; S. UMEZAWA et al. 1972 e) has been developed commercially as a drug for resistant infections.

On the other hand, it was suggested that the amino group at C-1 or C-3 of the deoxystreptamine moiety is involved in the binding of antibiotics with the 3′-*O*-phosphotransferase (H. UMEZAWA 1970; DOI et al. 1968) and, in fact, butirosin (WOO et al. 1971), which has an (*S*)-4-amino-2-hydroxybutyryl residue at the C-1 amino group, inhibits the growth of resistant strains. Furthermore, amikacin, which has the same aminoacyl residue at the C-1 amino group of kanamycin A, was prepared and proved to have a broad antibacterial spectrum against resistant and sensitive bacteria (KAWAGUCHI et al. 1972). Amikacin has recently been developed commercially. Modification of aminoglycoside antibiotics by acylation of the amino group at C-1 is of current interest as is the above-mentioned deoxygenation. Selective 1-*N*-acylation has been hampered by the difficulty in differentiating the reactivity of the many functional groups. However, efficient methods have been developed, including selective protection via temporary metal chelation (see Sect. B.V).

Furthermore, modification of aminoglycoside antibiotics by the combination of deoxygenation with *N*-acylation has provided compounds with significant activity against a wide range of resistant organisms.

I. Streptomycin Group

1. Total Synthesis of Streptomycin and Dihydrostreptomycin

The synthesis of the individual components, streptidine (WOLFROM and POLGLASE 1948; WOLFROM et al. 1950), streptose and dihydrostreptose (DYER et al. 1965), and *N*-methyl-L-glucosamine (KUEHL et al. 1947) had been reported by 1965. The total synthesis of dihydrostreptomycin (16) was accomplished by S. UMEZAWA et al. (1974 a) (Fig. 5).

The key intermediates for the first stage were the isopropylidene derivative (10) of benzyl dihydrostreptoside and the Schiff base of L-acetobromoglucosamine (11). Condensation of (10) and (11) by a modified Koenigs–Knorr reaction, followed by a sequence of reactions including *N*-methylation, led to benzyl dihydrostreptobiosaminide (12). In the second phase, the dihydrostreptobiosaminide was transformed into a blocked glycosyl chloride (13) through steps which included blocking

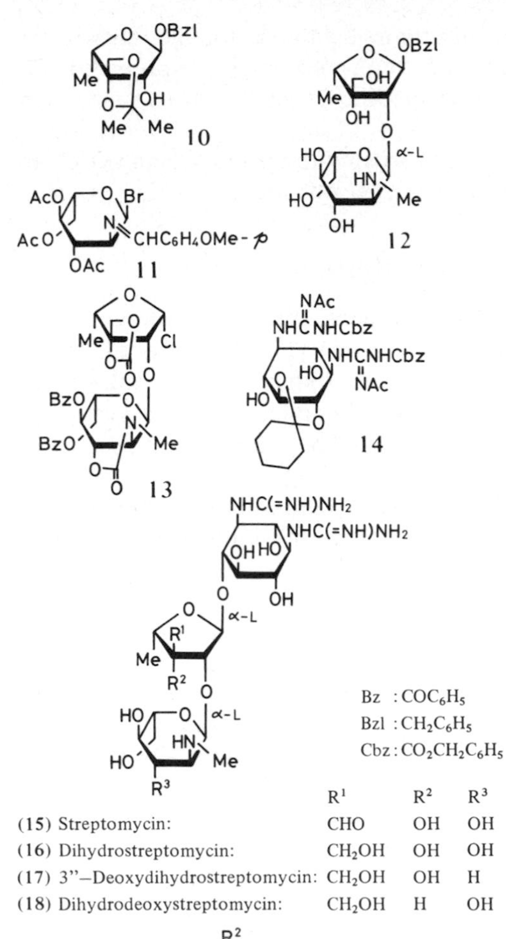

Bz : COC_6H_5
Bzl : $CH_2C_6H_5$
Cbz : $CO_2CH_2C_6H_5$

	R^1	R^2	R^3
(15) Streptomycin:	CHO	OH	OH
(16) Dihydrostreptomycin:	CH_2OH	OH	OH
(17) 3"–Deoxydihydrostreptomycin:	CH_2OH	OH	H
(18) Dihydrodeoxystreptomycin:	CH_2OH	H	OH

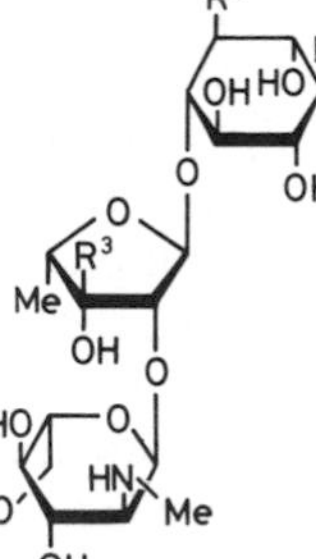

	R^1	R^2	R^3
(19) Deamidinodihydrostreptomycin:	NH_2	NH_2	CH_2OH
(20) Dideamidinostreptomycylamine:	NH_2	NH_2	CH_2NH_2
(21) 1–Deamidinodihydrostreptomycin:	NH_2	$NHC(=NH)NH_2$	CH_2OH
(22) 3–Deamidinodihydrostreptomycin:	$NHC(=NH)NH_2$	NH_2	CH_2OH
(23) 1–*N*–[(*S*)–4–Amino–2–hydroxybutyryl]–1–deamidinodihydrostreptomycin:	(*S*) $NHCOCH(OH)CH_2CH_2NH_2$	$NHC(=NH)NH_2$	CH_2OH
(24) 1–Deamidino–1–*N*–[(*S*)–4–guanidino–2–hydroxybutyryl]dihydrostreptomycin:	(*S*) $NHCOCH(OH)CH_2CH_2$–$NHC(=NH)NH_2$	$NH(C=NH)NH_2$	CH_2OH

Fig. 5

with cyclic carbamate and chlorination with thionyl chloride. On the other hand, the suitably blocked derivative of streptidine [(14), racemate] was prepared. Finally, (13) was condensed with (14), and deblocking afforded dihydrostreptomycin (16).

In another regiospecific synthesis of dihydrostreptomycin (YAMASAKI et al. 1978), an optically active streptidine derivative (14) was used.

2. Chemical Modification of Streptomycin and Diyhdrostreptomycin

Dihydrostreptomycin (16) was the first semisynthetic aminoglycoside antibiotic produced by catalytic hydrogenation of streptomycin (15) (BARTZ et al. 1946), though dihydrostreptomycin was later found to be produced by fermentation of a *Streptomyces* sp. Reduction of streptomycin with aluminum amalgam gives dihydrodeoxystreptomycin (18) (H. IKEDA et al. 1956). The antibacterial spectra of these modifications are similar.

The reactivity of the aldehyde group in streptomycin has been utilized to prepare a number of derivatives; however, except for the above dihydro derivatives, all of them show diminished activity. Condensation of streptomycin with nitromethane changed the CHO into $CH(OH)CH_2NO_2$, which was further reduced to $CH(OH)CH_2NH_2$ (HEDING et al. 1972). Reductive amination gave a series of compounds having CH_2NHR (HEDING and DIEDRICHSEN 1975). Reduction to a methyl group and oxidation to a carboxyl group gave poor activities (HEDING 1969; HEDING et al. 1972). The streptomycin hydrazone (streptonicozid) formed with isonicotinylhydrazine was reported to exert the therapeutic effect of both components (PENNINGTON et al. 1953).

Deamidinodihydrostreptomycin (19) (BODANSZKY 1954; POLGLASE 1962) had almost no antibacterial activity. *N,N'*-(dialkoxyphenylthio)carbamoyldideamidinodihydrostreptomycin was weakly active (LAZAREVA et al. 1968). Undecabenzoylstreptomycin was reported to have antiviral activity (GOLUBEV et al. 1970). Dideamidinostreptomycylamine (20) was prepared by alkaline degradation of streptomycylamine obtained by reduction of streptomycin oxime (CLAES et al. 1971). 1-Deamidino- and 3-deamidinodihydrostreptomycin (21) and (22) were prepared and comparison of their antibacterial spectra showed that the 3-guanidino group of dihydrostreptomycin is more important than the 1-guanidino group for antibacterial activity. 1-*N*-[(*S*)-4-Amino-2-hydroxybutyryl]-1-deamidinodihydrostreptomycin (23) and 1-deamidino-1-*N*-[(*S*)-4-guanidino-2-hydroxybutyryl]-dihydrostreptomycin (24) were prepared but showed poor activity (USUI et al. 1978), indicating that the introduction of the peculiar aminoacyl residue, which is remarkably effective for the improvement of the antibacterial spectra of the ribostamycin and kanamycin groups of antibiotics, is not effective in the streptomycin group.

Studies of the biochemical mechanism of resistance suggested that 3″-deoxydihydrostreptomycin (17) should be active against resistant strains, and SANO et al. (1976, 1977) synthesized this compound by a total synthesis similar to that of dihydrostreptomycin. The deoxy derivative inhibited both sensitive and resistant strains, as expected, except for *Pseudomonas aeruginosa* which produces 6-adenylyltransferase. This derivative was also prepared by transformation of natural dihydrostreptomycin (S. UMEZAWA, to be published).

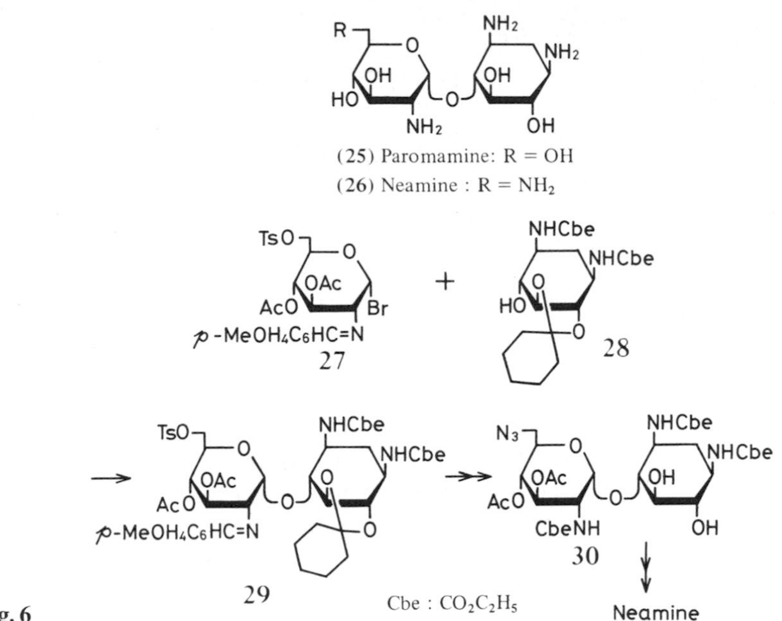

Fig. 6

II. Pseudodisaccharides Containing 4-Substituted 2-Deoxystreptamine – Paromamine, Neamine, and Related Compounds

1. Synthesis of Paromamine and Neamine

The synthesis of pseudodisaccharides has provided useful intermediates for further synthesis of more complex aminoglycosides. S. UMEZAWA and KOTO (1966) synthesized paromamine, and subsequently neamine (PECK et al. 1949) was derived (S. UMEZAWA et al. 1967c) from paromamine. An improved synthesis of paromamine was effected (S. UMEZAWA et al. 1972a) with a Schiff base derivative of the sugar component and a more protected 2-deoxystreptamine. Another synthesis of tetra-*N*-acetyl neamine was reported by KOHNO et al. (1975). A recent synthesis by HARAYAMA et al. (1979) involved condensation of (27) and (28) as shown in Fig. 6.

Several position isomers of paromamine and neamine, including 6-*O*-(2-amino-2-deoxy-α-D-glucopyranosyl)-2-deoxystreptamine (S. UMEZAWA et al. 1972a), 5-*O*-isomer of paromamine (S. UMEZAWA et al. 1966a), and that of neamine (FUKAMI et al. 1975), have been prepared.

2. Deoxygenated Derivatives

3′,4′-Dideoxyneamine, which is active against resistant bacteria, was synthesized (JIKIHARA et al. 1973) by the method developed by UMEZAWA's group (see Sect. B.IV.2).

5-Deoxy-, 6-deoxy-, and 5,6-dideoxyneamines were prepared (SUAMI et al. 1977a) from neamine and the first compound was found to be one and a half times more active than neamine. 3′,4′,5,6-Tetradeoxyneamine was prepared (CANAS-

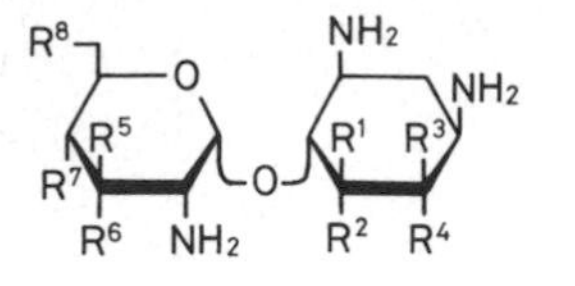

	R_1	R_2	R_3	R_4	R_5	R_6	R_7	R_8
(31) 3'–Epiparomamine	: OH	H	H	OH	H	OH	OH	OH
(32) 3'–Epineamine	: OH	H	H	OH	H	OH	OH	NH_2
(33) 5–Epineamine	: H	OH	H	OH	OH	H	OH	NH_2
(34) 6–Epineamine	: OH	H	OH	H	OH	H	OH	NH_2
(35) 5, 6–Diepineamine	: H	OH	OH	H	OH	H	OH	NH_2
(36) 4'–Deoxy–3'–epineamine	: OH	H	H	OH	H	OH	H	NH_2

Fig. 7

RODRIGUEZ and RUIZ-POVEDA 1977), as well as the 5,6-dideoxyneamine, and both compounds had antibacterial activity similar to neamine. Tetrakis(*N*-methoxycarbonyl) derivatives of 3′-deoxyneamine (KOCH and RHOADES 1971) and 4′-deoxyneamine (KONISHI et al. 1974) were prepared (PFEIFFER et al. 1979) via the 3′,4′-epoxy of 4′-oxo-3′-*O*-tosyl derivatives, respectively.

3. Epimerized Derivatives

3′-Epiparomamine (31) was prepared (HANESSIAN et al. 1973) by oxidation at C-3′ of a protected paromamine derivative followed by reduction of the 3-ulose with sodium borohydride. 3′-Epineamine (32) (HANESSIAN et al. 1978d) was similarly prepared. The compound was not a substrate for the phosphotransferases and showed only weak antibacterial activity for common strains. 4′-Deoxy-3′-epineamine (36) (AKITA et al. 1979a) was also reported. 5- and 6-Epineamines (33) and (34) were similarly prepared from neamine (SUAMI et al. 1978a) and 5,6-diepineamine (35) was prepared via the corresponding 5,6-epoxy compound (Fig. 7). Compounds (34) and (35) were less active than neamine, while (33) had activity comparable to that of neamine, but slight activity against some kanamycin-resistant strains.

4. Amino-Deoxy Derivatives

5-Amino-5-deoxy- (37), 6-amino-6-deoxy- (38), and 5-amino-5-deoxy-5,6-diepineamine (39) have been prepared (NISHIYAMA et al. 1978) through the 5-epichloro-, 6-epichloro-, and 5,6-epoxy compounds, respectively, by way of azidolysis or, in the case of (39), by the action of boron trifluoride in acetonitrile. These compounds were less active than neamine. PFEIFFER et al. (1979) prepared the 3′- or 4′-amino derivatives (40)–(43), which were less active than neamine (Fig. 8). The synthetic route to (40) is shown as a typical example in Fig. 9.

5. Derivatives Having a Side Chain or Longer Chain

6′-*C*-Aminomethyl-3′-deoxyparomamine (55) was prepared (YAMAGUCHI et al. 1977a) starting from 3′-deoxyparomamine (ODA et al. 1971) via the 6′-aldehyde de-

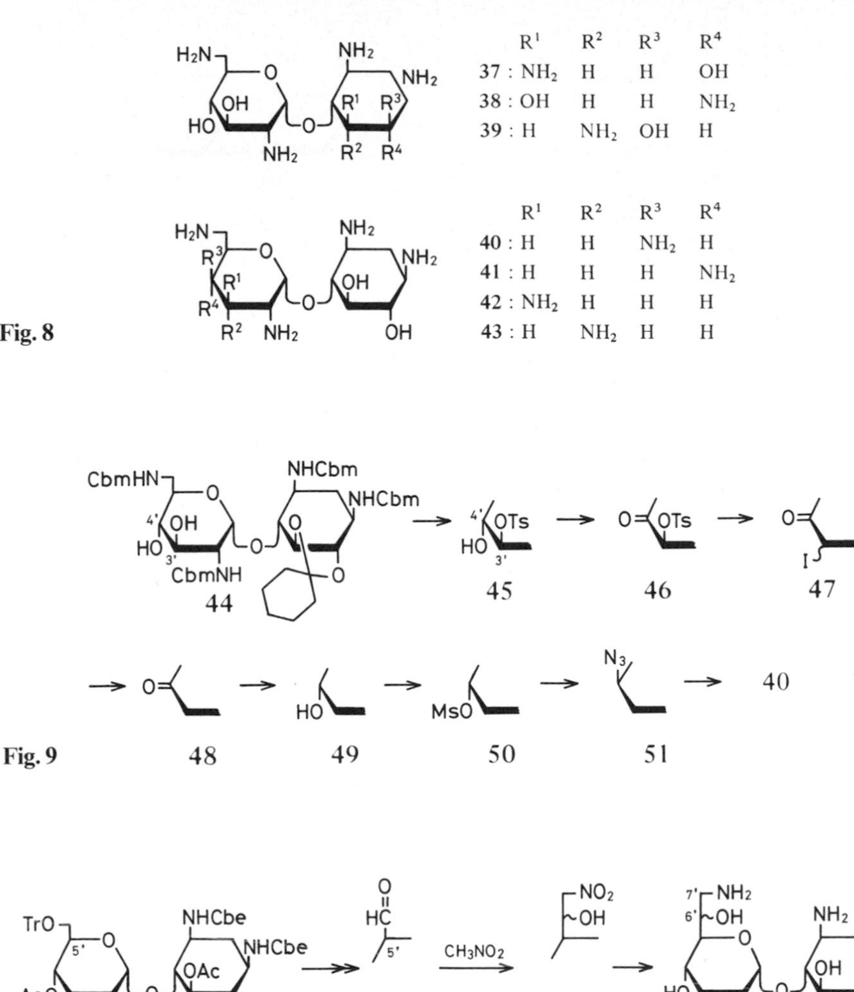

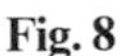

Fig. 8

Fig. 9

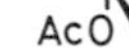

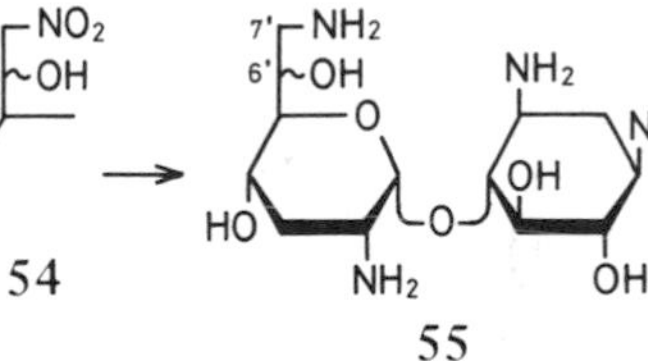

Fig. 10

Tr : $C(C_6H_5)_3$

rivative (53). This modification had decreased activity compared with neamine, suggesting that the 6′-amino group (not the 7′-amino) may be important for the antibacterial activity of neamine-related compounds (Fig. 10). The 6′-*C*-methyl derivative (57) and (58) with weak activity was prepared (D. IKEDA et al. 1979a) from 3′,4′-dideoxyneamine (S. UMEZAWA et al. 1971b) via the 6′-aldehyde derivative (56), which was treated with diazomethane followed by reductive amination (Fig. 11). PFEIFFER et al. (1979) prepared derivatives having a side chain at C-3 (59) or at C-4 (60), which were less active than neamine (Fig. 12). 6-Deoxy-5-methylneamine (MAGERLEIN 1979) was prepared by a route involving treatment of the corresponding 5-oxo derivative with methyl magnesium bromide.

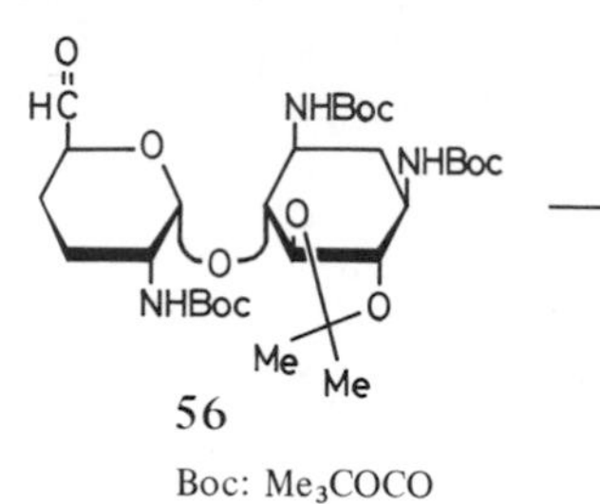

56

Boc: Me_3COCO

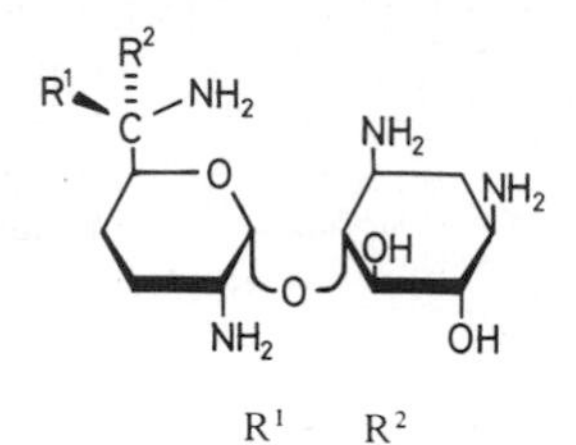

	R^1	R^2
57 :	H	CH_3
58 :	CH_3	H

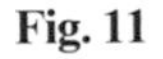

Fig. 11

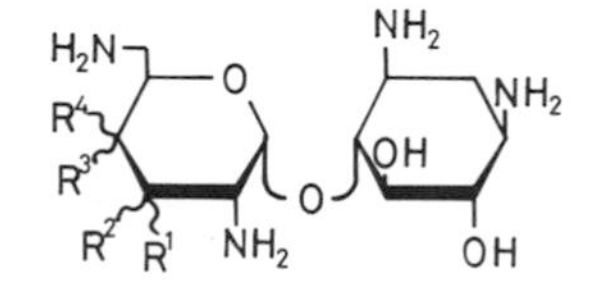

	R^1, R^2	R^3, R^4
59 :	H, CH_2OH	H, H
60 :	H, H	H, CH_3 or CH_2OH

Fig. 12

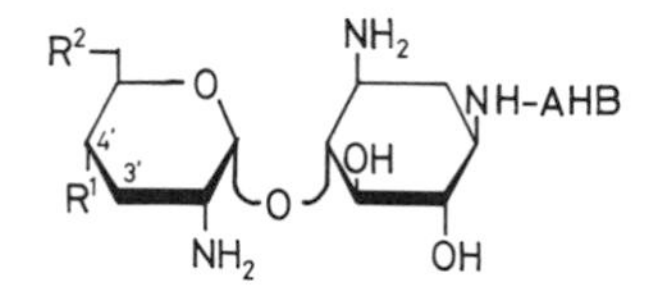

	R^1	R^2
61 :	H	NH_2
62 :	OH	OH

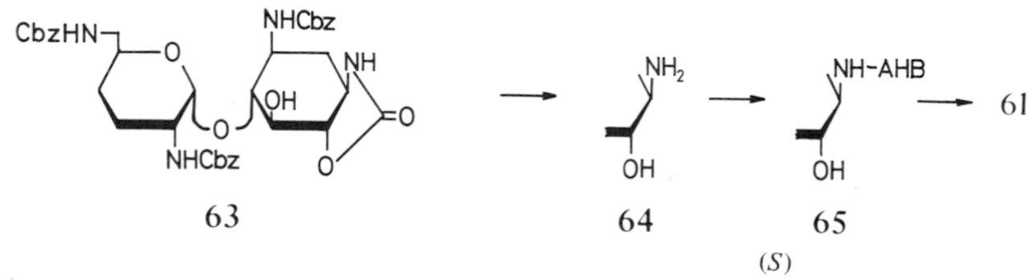

63 64 65

Fig. 13

AHB: $\overset{(S)}{COCH(OH)}CH_2CH_2NH_2$

6. 1-*N*-Acyl Derivatives

1-*N*-[(*S*)-4-Amino-2-hydroxybutyryl]-3′,4′-dideoxyneamine (61) was prepared (S. UMEZAWA et al. 1973) via the route outlined in Fig. 13 and showed higher antibacterial activity than 3′,4′-dideoxyneamine (see Sect. C.II.2) against both sensitive and resistant bacteria. 1-*N*-[(*S*)-4-Amino-2-hydroxybutyryl]-3′-deoxyparomamine (62) (WATANABE et al. 1975a) was weakly antibacterial.

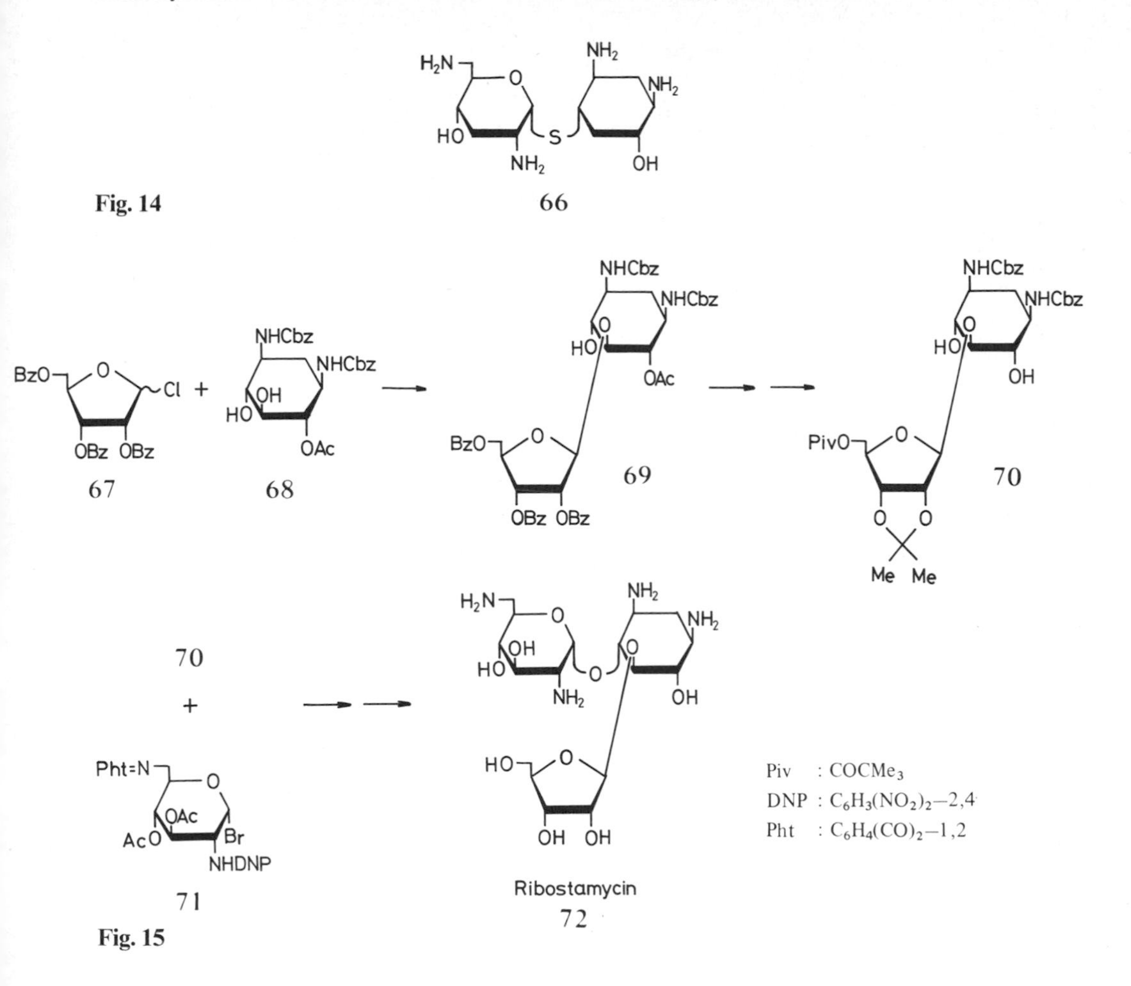

Fig. 14

Fig. 15

7. Other Derivatives

The 2′-fluoro derivatives, 4-*O*- and 5-*O*-(2′,3′-dideoxy-2′-fluoro-α-D-ribohexopyranosyl)-2,6-dideoxystreptamine (Vass et al. 1979) have been reported. A thio analog of neamine, (1*S*, 2*S*, 4*R*, 5*R*)-2,4-diamino-5-hydroxycyclohexyl-2,6-diamino-2,3,6-trideoxy-1-thio-α-D-*ribo*-hexopyranoside (66), was prepared (Kavadias et al. 1979) and showed no inhibition in the growth of *Staphylococcus aureus*. 4-*O*-(3′-Deoxy-α-D-*ribo*-hexopyranosyl-2,6-dideoxystreptamine (Cleophax et al. 1978a, b) was synthesized.

III. Pseudotrisaccharides Containing 4,5-Disubstituted 2-Deoxystreptamine – Ribostamycin, Butirosins, and Related Compounds

1. Synthesis of Ribostamycin and Related Pseudotrisaccharides

Ribostamycin (72) was first synthesized (Ito et al. 1970) from neamine. A synthesis of ribostamycin by Fukami et al. (1976, 1977a, b) is outlined in Fig. 15. Suami et

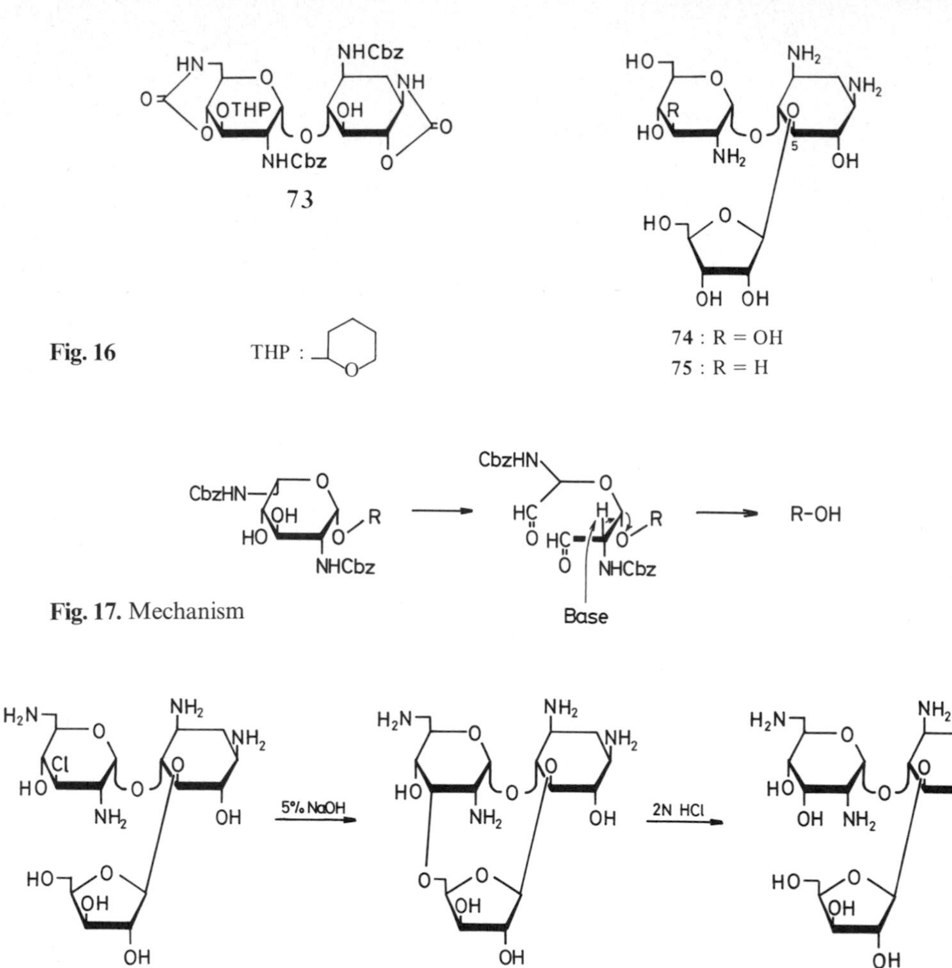

Fig. 16

Fig. 17. Mechanism

Fig. 18

al. (1977b) synthesized ribostamycin from 6,3′,4′-tri-*O*-acetyl-1,3,2′,6′-tetrakis(*N*-ethoxycarbonyl)neamine (SUAMI et al. 1976) and (67). Another synthesis utilized a cyclic carbamate (73), which was condensed with (67) (KUMAR and REMERS 1978).

5-*O*-Ribosylparomamine (74) was prepared (TAKAMOTO and HANESSIAN 1974; HANESSIAN et al. 1978a) from 4′,6′-*O*-benzylidene-pentakis(*N*-benzyloxycarbonyl)paromomycin by cleaving the 2,6-diamino-2,6-dideoxyidopyranose portion by periodate oxidation followed by treatment with triethylamine, as shown briefly in Fig. 17. The compound was later obtained by fermentation and has slight antibacterial activity (KIRBY et al. 1977).

Deneosaminyllividomycin B, namely, 3′-deoxy-5-*O*-ribosylparomamine (75) (YAMAGUCHI et al. 1977b), was prepared from lividomycin B by periodate oxidation in a similar manner as above.

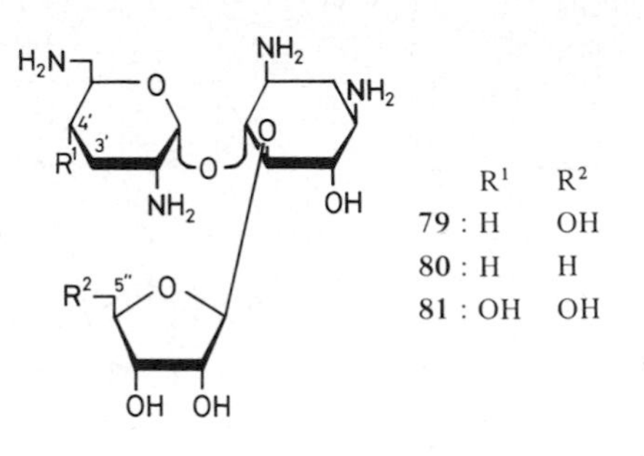

	R^1	R^2
79 :	H	OH
80 :	H	H
81 :	OH	OH

Fig. 19

SUAMI et al. (1977b) prepared 5-*O*-β-D-glucopyranosylneamine which showed decreased activity compared to neamine, suggesting that the attachment of a β-D-ribo- or β-xylo-furanosyl unit at C-5 is important to enhance the activity of neamine. However, biologically prepared 5-*O*-α-D-glucopyranosylneamine (ENDO and PERLMAN 1972) was reported to be more active than neamine.

CLEOPHAX et al. (1978b) prepared 2,6-dideoxy-4-*O*-(3-deoxy-α-D-*ribo*hexopyranosyl)-5-*O*-ribosylstreptamine. 3′-Epixylostasin (78) was prepared (ASAKO et al. 1978) from 3′-chloro-3′-deoxyxylostasin (76) (OKUTANI et al. 1977) by alkaline treatment, followed by acidic cleavage of the intermediate cyclic compound (77). This compound (78) was devoid of antibacterial activity (Fig. 18).

2. Deoxy Derivatives

3′,4′-Dideoxy and 3′,4′,5″-trideoxyribostamycin (79) and (80) were synthesized by S. UMEZAWA et al. (1972b) and showed activity against ribostamycin- and kanamycin-resistant bacteria. 3′-Deoxyribostamycin (81) (D. IKEDA et al. 1973b) was found to have higher activity than 3′,4′-dideoxyribostamycin (Fig. 19).

3. 1-*N*-Acyl and 1-*N*-Alkyl Derivatives of 4,5-Disubstituted Pseudotrisaccharides

a) Synthesis of Butirosins

Butirosins A and B (82) and (83) (WOO et al. 1971) have been found to exhibit broad antibacterial activity against gram-positive and gram-negative bacteria, including *Pseudomonas aeruginosa* and kanamycin- and gentamicin-resistant clinical strains (Fig. 20). The first total synthesis of an antibiotic of this group was accomplished by D. IKEDA et al. (1972, 1974) with the synthesis of butirosin B. This synthesis involved a regiospecific 1-*N*-acylation of protected ribostamycin (88) with an active ester of the *N*-protected (*S*)-4-amino-2-hydroxybutyric acid as outlined in Fig. 21. Another regiospecific synthesis (KUMAR and REMERS 1978) involved condensation of 2,3,5-tri-*O*-acetylribosyl chloride with a protected *N*-acylneamine derivative (91) as shown in Fig. 22. The structurally related antibiotics Bu-1709E_1 (84) and E_2 (85) were isolated from fermentation broths (TSUKIURA et al. 1973). Both compounds are less active than butirosins.

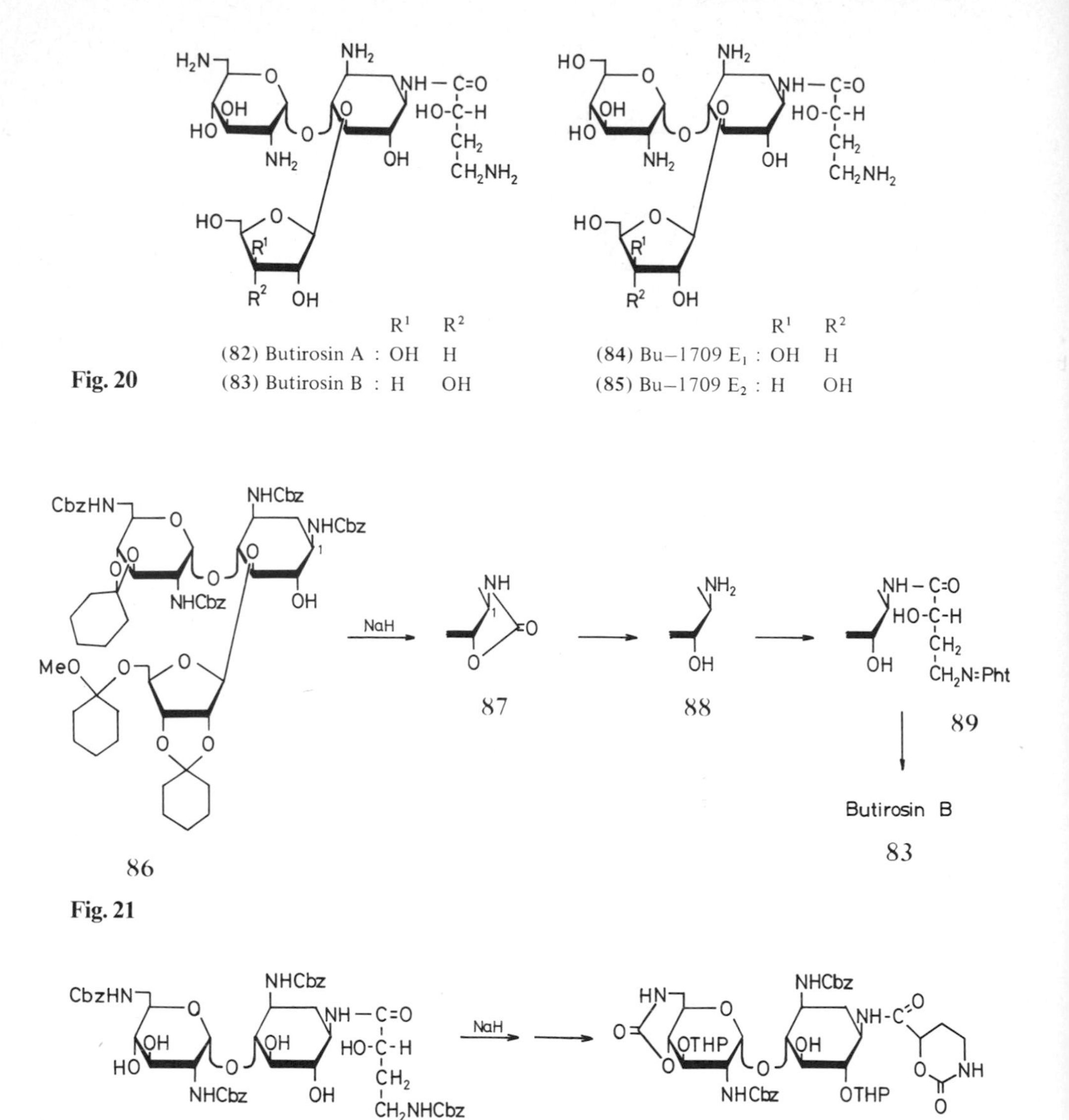

Fig. 20

Fig. 21

Fig. 22

b) Synthesis of 3′,4′-Dideoxybutirosins

The synthesis of 3′,4′-dideoxybutirosin B (93) was accomplished by D. IKEDA et al. (1973a, 1974) by a sequence of reactions involving treatment of the 3′,4′-di-*O*-mesyl derivative (94) of a protected butirosin B derivative (D. IKEDA et al. 1972) with sodium iodide–zinc dust in DMF (TIPSON and COHEN 1965; ALBANO et al. 1966) to give unsaturation (95) as shown in Fig. 23. The 3′,4′-dideoxybutirosin B was found to be more effective against resistant bacteria than butirosin B. This finding stimulated the synthesis of other deoxy derivatives of butirosins. 3′,4′-Dideoxy-

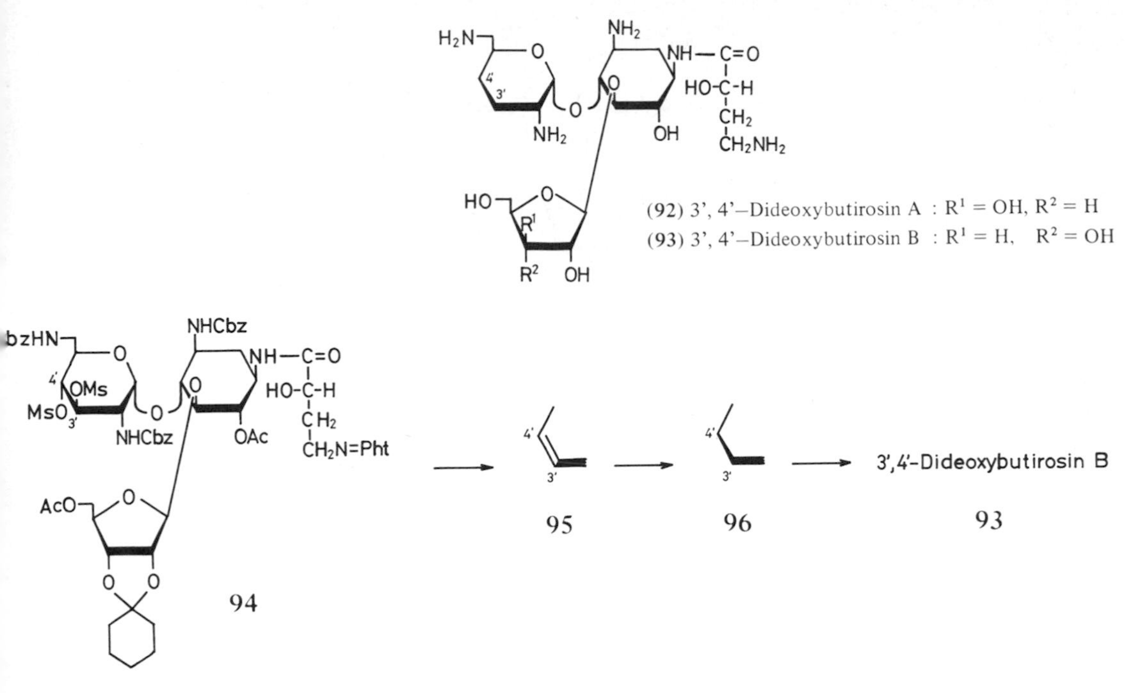

Fig. 23

butirosin A (92) was similarly synthesized (SAEKI et al. 1974) and also showed an excellent antibacterial spectrum. 3′,4′-Dideoxybutirosin A (92) was further prepared (SAEKI et al. 1977) starting from butirosin A, utilizing selective *O*-benzoylation followed by 3′,4′-di-*O*-mesylation and 3′,4′-unsaturation. The 3′,4′-unsaturation of the 3′,4′-di-*O*-mesyl derivative was also effected with naphthalene-sodium (HAYASHI et al. 1977).

c) Synthesis of 3′-Deoxybutirosins

3′-Deoxybutirosin B (98) was first prepared from a ribostamycin derivative (99) by the route shown in Fig. 24 (D. IKEDA et al. 1975, 1976) and was found to be more active than butirosin B and 3′,4′-dideoxybutirosin B (93). Improved syntheses of 3′-deoxybutirosin B and 3′-deoxybutirosin A involved condensation of a protected 3′-deoxyparomamine derivative with a protected ribosyl or xylosyl halide followed by 1-*N*-acylation and 6′-amination (WATANABE et al. 1977a, b).

3′-Deoxybutirosin A (97) was obtained (OKUTANI et al. 1977) by a unique method utilizing butirosin A 3′-phosphate (YAGISAWA et al. 1972) obtained by inactivation of butirosin A by enzymatic action (Fig. 25). When the 3′-phosphate (104) was treated with bis(trimethylsilyl)acetamide–trimethylchlorosilane in pyridine and then hydrolyzed, 2′,3′-epimino-2′-deamino-3′-deoxybutirosin A (105) was obtained. Catalytic hydrogenation of the epimine followed by separation by ligand-exchange chromatography gave 3′-deoxybutirosin A (97). Another 3′-deoxygenation via the 2′,3′-epimine was also reported (FUKASE et al. 1978). *N*-Pro-

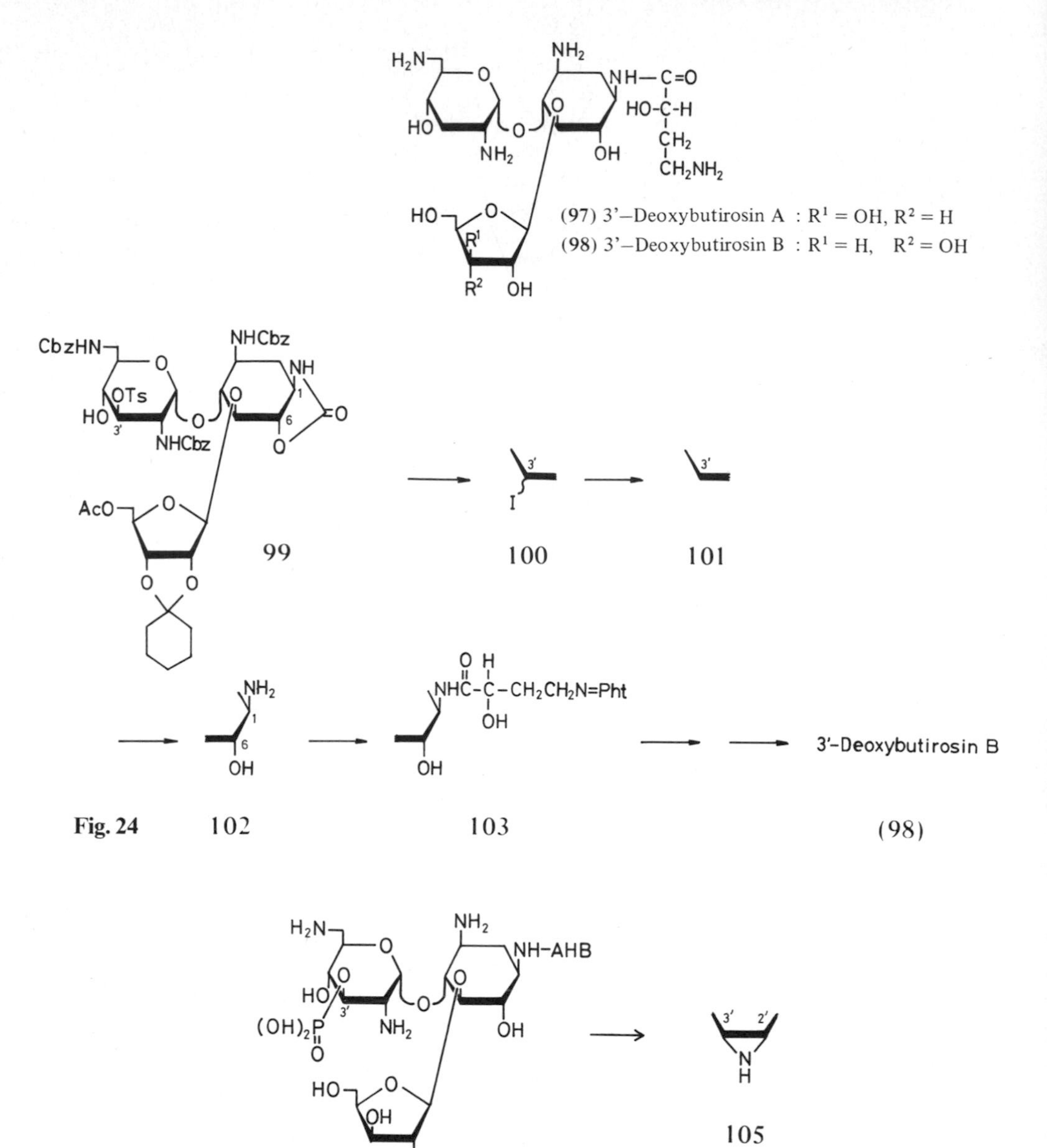

Fig. 24

Fig. 25

tected butirosin A was treated with a mixture of triphenylphosphine, tetrachloromethane, and triethylamine to give the *N*-protected epimine which was then hydrogenolyzed to give the desired compound.

3′-Deoxygenation using Barton's method (BARTON and McCOMBIE 1975) has been reported. A protected butirosin A derivative was treated with *N*,*N*-dimethylbenzamide–phosgene–hydrogen sulfide or with carbon disulfide–methyl iodide to

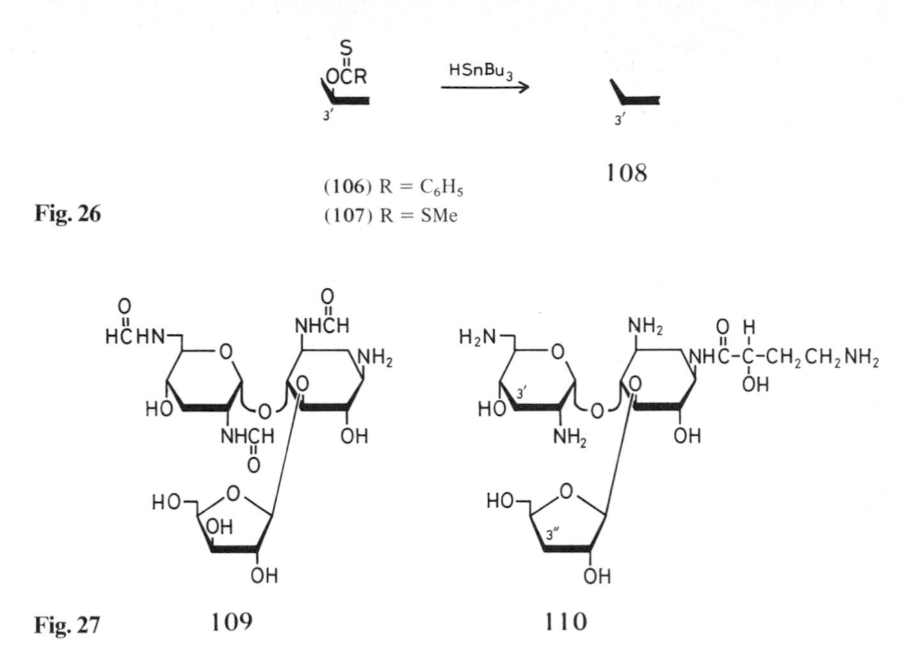

Fig. 26

Fig. 27

give the 3′-thiobenzoate (106) (Fukase et al. 1978) or 3′-(*S*-methyl dithiocarbonate) (107) (Hayashi et al. 1978), respectively. Treatment of either of these with tributylstannane gave the corresponding 3′-deoxy derivative (108) (Fig. 26).

A synthesis of 3′-deoxybutirosin A (97) starting from 3′-deoxyxylostasin by 1-*N*-acylation was reported (Horii et al. 1978). Tetra-*N*-formyl-3′-deoxyxylostasin was treated with 10% aqueous ammonia to give 3′-deoxy-3,2′,6′-tri-*N*-formylxylostasin (109). 1-*N*-Acylation followed by deblocking gave 3′-deoxybutirosin A.

In order to investigate the role of the 3″-hydroxy group in antibacterial activity, 3′, 3″-dideoxybutirosin (110) was prepared (Tsuchiya et al. 1978a) (the difference between butirosin A and B is only the orientation of the hydroxy group at C-3″), and found to have antibacterial activity similar to that of 3′-deoxybutirosin B but slightly lower than that of 3′-deoxybutirosin A. This suggests that the xylose unit in butirosin A is superior to the ribose unit in butirosin B for antibacterial activity.

d) Synthesis of Other Deoxybutirosins

4′-Deoxybutirosins (Kawaguchi et al. 1974; Konishi et al. 1974) were obtained from cultures of *Bacillus circulans* and found to have broader antibacterial activity than butirosins. The synthesis of 4′-deoxybutirosin A was carried out (Fukase et al. 1978) by iodination at C-4′ of a protected butirosin A derivative, followed by reduction with tributylstannane. 6-Deoxybutirosin A was synthesized by Hayashi et al. (1978) and had weaker activity than butirosin A.

e) Synthesis of Epibutirosins

6-Epibutirosin A (Hayashi et al. 1978) and 3′-epibutirosin A (Asako et al. 1978) were synthesized and both showed almost no antibacterial activity.

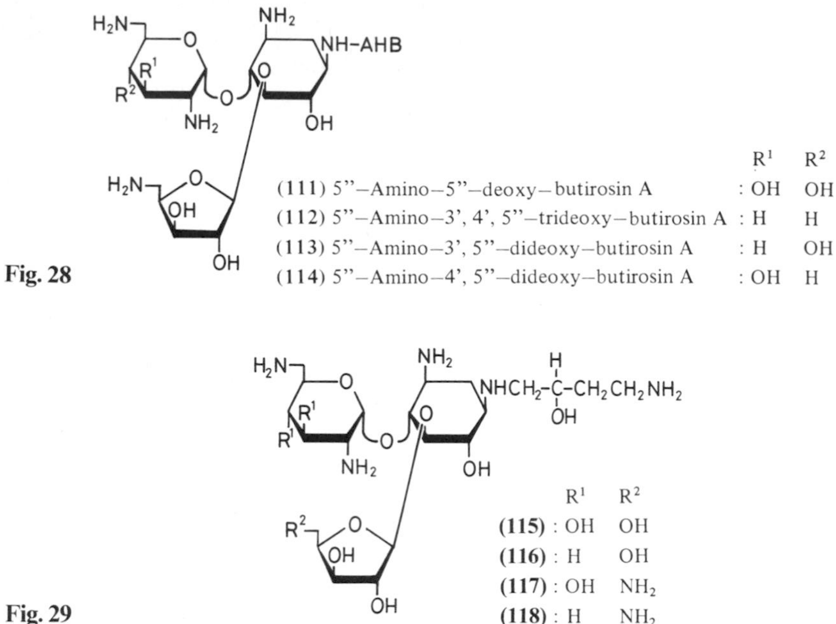

Fig. 28

Fig. 29

f) Synthesis of Amino-deoxy Butirosins

Replacement of the 5″-hydroxy group of butirosin A by an amino group was reported by CULBERTSON et al. (1973); this modification (111) had enhanced antibiotic activity, especially against *Pseudomonas aeruginosa* and *Serratia marcescens*. Two groups of workers prepared 5″-amino-3′,4′,5″-trideoxybutirosin A (112) (WOO 1975; SAEKI et al. 1975) via 3′,4′-unsaturation as a key step. The compound showed activity against some strains resistant to 5″-amino-5″-deoxybutirosin A (111). 5″-Amino-3′,5″-dideoxybutirosin A (113) was prepared through glycosylation (WATANABE et al. 1978) and did not give better activity than 3′-deoxybutirosin A. 5″-Amino-4′,5″-dideoxybutirosin A (114) was prepared by NAITO et al. (1975) (Fig. 28).

g) Synthesis of 1‴-Deoxobutirosins

As described in Sect. C.V.1.1.α, reduction of a 1-*N*-[(*S*)-4-amino-2-hydroxybutyryl] derivative with diborane gave the 1‴-deoxo derivative. The procedure was applied (HAYASHI et al. 1979) to butirosin A, 3′,4′-dideoxybutirosin A, 5″-amino-5″-deoxybutirosin A, and 5″-amino-3′,4′,5″-trideoxybutirosin A to give the corresponding 1‴-deoxo derivatives (115)–(118), which are less active than the parent antibiotics (Fig. 29).

h) Synthesis of Other 1-*N*-Substituted Derivatives

1-*N*-Ethylxylostasin was prepared (HAYASHI et al. 1979) by reduction of the 1-*N*-ethylidene derivative with sodium borohydride and was found to be less active than xylostasin.

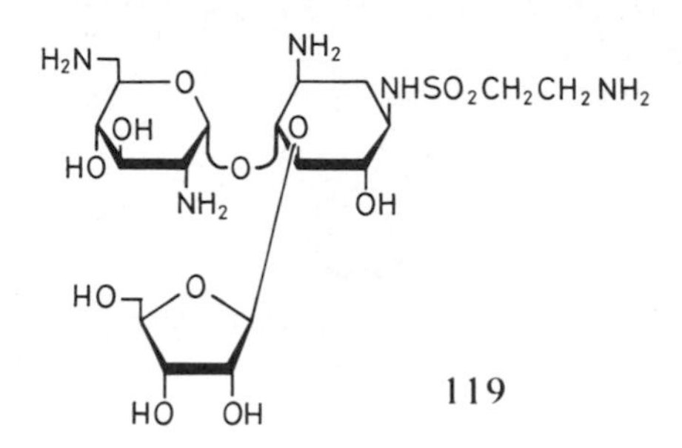

Fig. 30

1-*N*-(2-Aminoethylsulfonyl)ribostamycin (119) (AKITA et al. 1979b), unique analog of butirosin B, was reported to have antibacterial activity similar to that of butirosin B (Fig. 30).

i) Synthesis of *N*-Alkylbutirosins

2′-*N*-Alkyl(methyl, ethyl, and propyl) butirosin A (K. NARA et al. 1979) were prepared from butirosin A by selective 3,6′,4‴-tris(*N*-benzyloxycarbonyl)ation of butirosin A, followed by reductive alkylation of the free 2′-amino group. They showed decreased activity compared to butirosin A; however, 2′-*N*-propylbutirosin A was slightly active for some strains producing 3′-phosphotransferase II. 3′-Deoxy-6′-*N*-methyl- and 3′-deoxy-6-*N*-ethyl-butirosin B (ODA et al. 1978) were also reported.

IV. Pseudotetra- and Pseudopentasaccharides Containing 4,5-Disubstituted 2-Deoxystreptamine – Neomycins, Paromomycins, Lividomycins, and Related Compounds

1. Total Synthesis of Neomycin C

Neomycin (H. UMEZAWA et al. 1948; WAKSMAN and LECHEVALIER 1949) consists of neomycin A (neamine), B, and C. Neomycin C (122) (DUTCHER et al. 1951) was synthesized by S. UMEZAWA and NISHIMURA (1977). The key step of the synthesis was condensation of a protected ribostamycin (120) with a Schiff base derivative of the glycosyl halide (121) as shown in Fig. 31.

2. Synthesis of Analogs of Neomycin, Paromomycin, and Lividomycin B

MORI et al. (1972) prepared lividomycin B from penta-*N*-acetyllividomycin A by treating it with sodium periodate to cleave the D-mannose moiety.

As already described in Sect. C.III.1, periodate oxidation of a suitably protected pseudotetrasaccharide derivative followed by alkaline treatment gave a pseudotrisaccharide. The pseudotrisaccharide (123) was prepared by HANESSIAN et al. (1975, 1978a–c) and found to be slightly antibacterial. A suitably protected derivative of this pseudotrisaccharide could serve as the starting material for the synthesis of analogs of neomycin, paromomycin, or lividomycin.

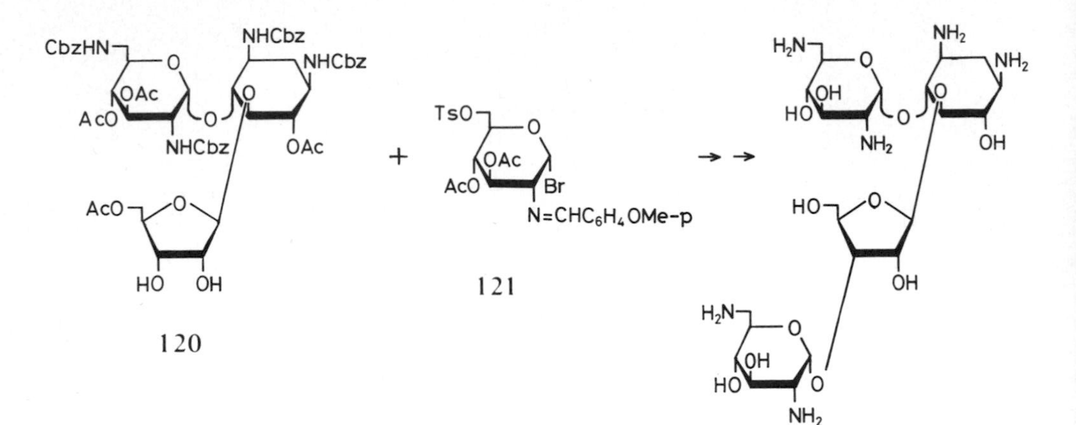

Fig. 31

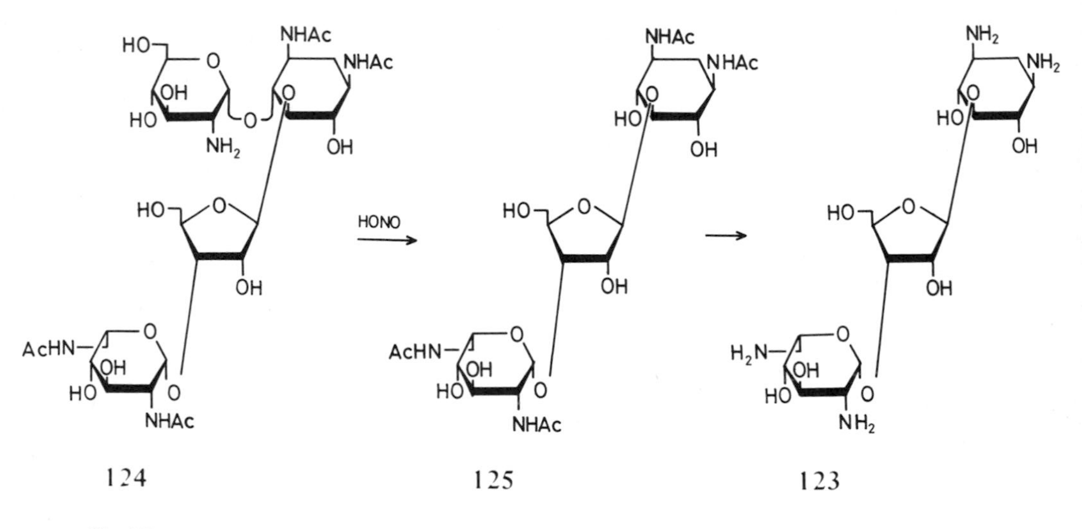

Fig. 32

Another method for the preparation of (123) (CASSINELLI et al. 1978 a, b) utilized 1,3,2‴,6‴-tetra-*N*-acetylparomomycin (124) prepared by selective *N*-acetylation of paromomycin. Nitrous acid deamination of (124) gave (125), which led to (123). By condensation of the suitably protected derivative of (125) with suitably protected glycosyl chlorides, several unnatural pseudotetrasaccharides (126)–(128) have been prepared (CASSINELLI et al. 1978 b). Among the compounds, (126) gave the best antibacterial activity.

The 6‴-deamino-6‴-hydroxy-5‴-epi analog of lividomycin B, that is, 5-*O*-[3-*O*-(2-amino-2-deoxy-α-D-glucopyranosyl)-β-D-ribofuranosyl]-3′-deoxyparomamine

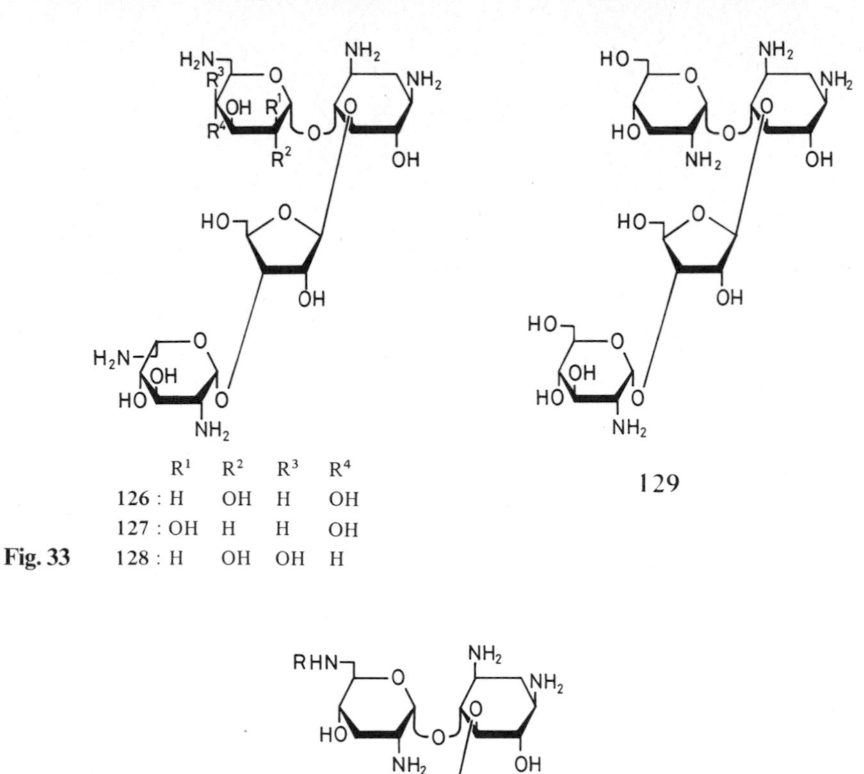

Fig. 33

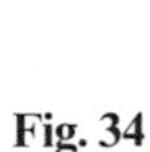

130 : R = H
131 : R = CH_3
132 : R = CH_2CH_2OH

Fig. 34

(129), was synthesized (WATANABE et al. 1977c) by a glycosylation method and had much weaker antibacterial activity than lividomycin B, showing that the presence of the 6‴-amino group in lividomycin B is important for antibacterial activity.

3. Amino-Deoxy Derivatives

6′-Amino-6′-deoxylividomycin B (130), 6′-deoxy-6′-methylaminolividomycin B (131) and 6′-deoxy-6′-(2-hydroxyethylamino)lividomycin B (132) were synthesized by WATANABE et al. (1973b). (130) was the most active among them (more active than neomycin or lividomycin), but was only slightly active against resistant strains producing 3′-phosphotransferase.

5″-Amino-5″-deoxyneomycin B and 5″-amino-5″-deoxyparomomycin B were prepared by HANESSIAN et al. (1977) and shown to have activity similar to the par-

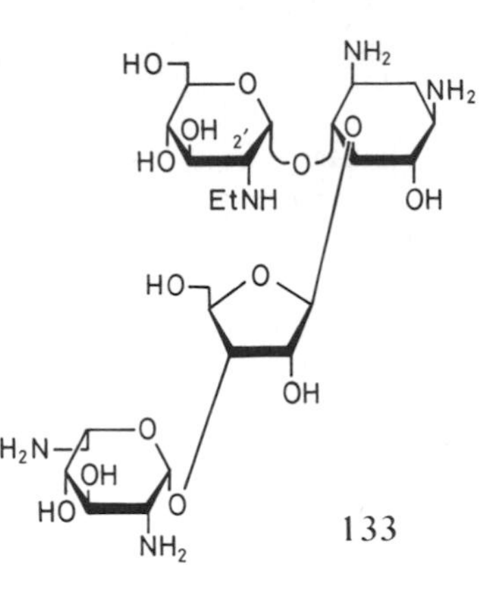

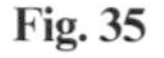
Fig. 35

ent antibiotics. 6′,5″,6‴-Triamino-6′,5″,6‴-trideoxylividomycin A and 6′,5″-diamino-6′,5″-dideoxylividomycin B were prepared (KONDO et al. 1976) and found to be active against lividomycin-resistant strains producing 3′-phosphotransferase I.

4. *N*-Alkyl Derivatives

2′-*N*-Ethylparomomycin (133) was prepared (CASSINELLI et al. 1978a) from (124) (see Sect. C.IV.2) and had activity similar to paromomycin.

5. 1-*N*-Acyl Derivatives

After the discovery of the butirosins, which have a 1-*N*-[(*S*)-4-amino-2-hydroxybutyryl] (AHB) residue, many attempts have been made to introduce this residue into other aminoglycoside antibiotics.

1-*N*-AHB derivatives (NAITO et al. 1974e) of neomycin B and C were more active than the parent antibiotics. The 1-*N*-acyl derivatives (NAITO et al. 1974c) of paromomycins were also reported.

1-*N*-AHB-lividomycin (134) was synthesized by WATANABE et al. (1973a, 1975a) and had a markedly broad antibacterial spectrum against lividomycin-resistant bacteria. 1-*N*-AHB-lividomycin B was also prepared (NAITO et al. 1974d). 6′-Amino-6′-deoxy-1-*N*-AHB-lividomycin A (135) (WATANABE et al. 1975b) also showed broad antibacterial activity but was less active than 1-*N*-AHB-lividomycin A (Fig. 36).

V. Pseudotrisaccharides Containing 4,6-Disubstituted 2-Deoxystreptamine – Kanamycin, Tobramycin, Gentamicin, and Related Compounds

1. Kanamycins and Their Derivatives

a) Total and Partial Synthesis of Kanamycins

The total synthesis of kanamycin A (S. UMEZAWA et al. 1968b; NAKAJIMA et al. 1968a), kanamycin B (S. UMEZAWA et al. 1968c), and kanamycin C (S. UMEZAWA

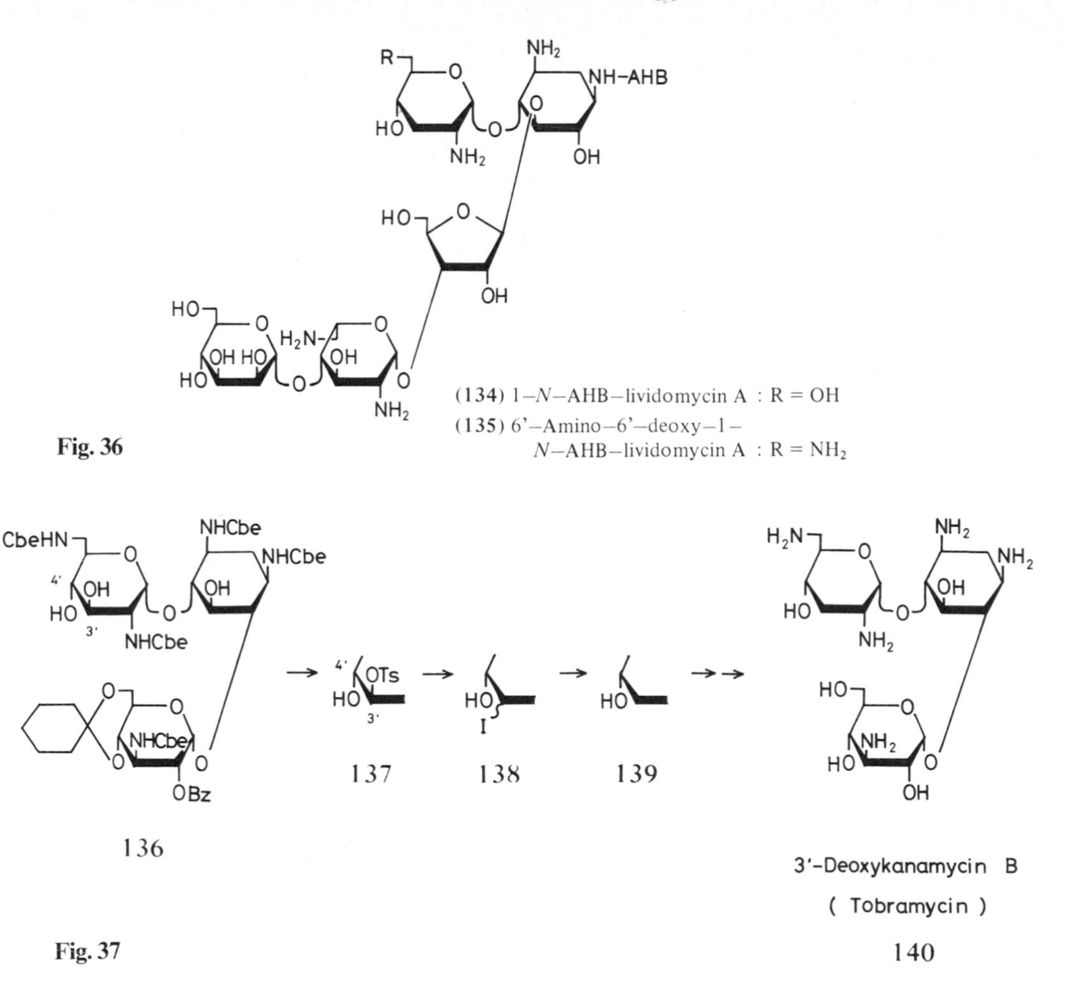

Fig. 36

Fig. 37

et al. 1968 a) was announced in 1968, constituting the first total synthesis of pseudotrisaccharide antibiotics. Kanamycin C was prepared (TODA et al. 1977) by transformation of kanamycin B through nitrous acid deamination of 1,3,3″-tri-*N*-acetylkanamycin B.

b) 3′-Deoxykanamycins

The synthesis of 3′-deoxykanamycin A (S. UMEZAWA et al. 1972 a, c) was accomplished by total synthesis. This synthesis and the synthesis of 3′,4′-dideoxykanamycin B (H. UMEZAWA et al. 1971) led to the finding that they are markedly effective against resistant bacteria including *Pseudomonas aeruginosa* (see Sect. C.V.1.c). Synthesis of 3′-deoxykanamycin A by transformation of kanamycin A was rather difficult and has only recently been accomplished (TSUCHIYA 1979). 3′-Deoxykanamycin B, that is, tobramycin (KOCH and RHOADES 1971), was synthesized (TAKAGI et al. 1973, 1976) from kanamycin B. The key steps of the synthesis include selective deoxygenation of C-3′ of (136), as outlined in Fig. 37. 3′-Deoxykanamycin B

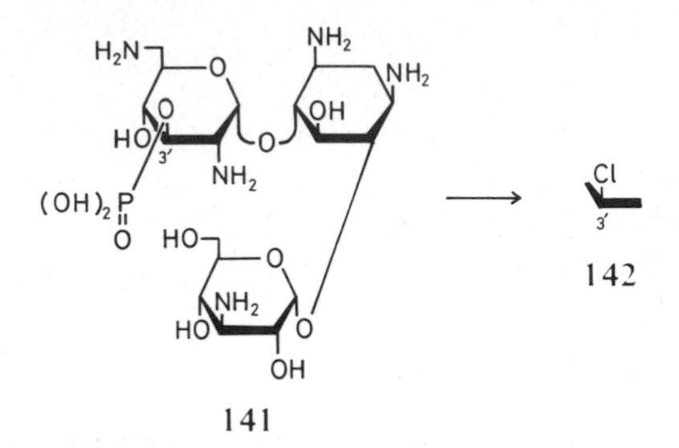

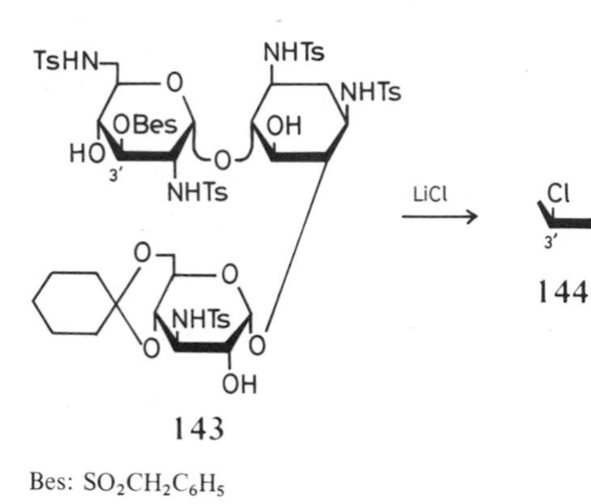

Bes: $SO_2CH_2C_6H_5$

Fig. 38

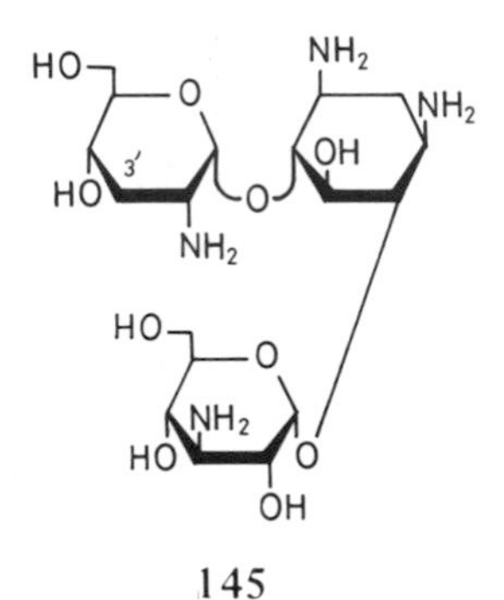

Fig. 39

was also prepared (OKUTANI et al. 1977) from kanamycin B 3′-phosphate (141) obtained by enzymic action. Treatment of (141) with trimethylchlorosilane and hexamethyldisilazane in a mixture of pyridine and hexamethylphosphoric triamide in the presence of triphenylphosphine gave, after hydrolysis, 3′-chloro-3′-deoxykanamycin B (142) which, by hydrogenation, gave 3′-deoxykanamycin B (140). Recently, 3′-deoxykanamycin B was prepared (TSUCHIYA 1979) in high yield via 3′-chlorination of the 3′-*O*-benzylsulfonyl-penta-*N*-tosyl derivative (143) of kanamycin B (Fig. 38). 3′-Deoxykanamycin B was also prepared (KYOTANI et al. 1979) by condensation of suitably protected derivatives of 3-amino-3-deoxy-D-glucopyranose and lividamine (3′-deoxyparomamine) which was easily obtained by hydrolysis of lividomycin. Another synthesis of 3′-deoxykanamycin B involving glycosylation was also reported (TANABE et al. 1977).

3′-Deoxykanamycin C (145) was prepared by KONDO et al. (1977) utilizing 6′-*N*-(*t*-butoxycarbonyl)-3′-deoxykanamycin B (Fig. 39).

c) 3′4′-Dideoxykanamycins

3′,4′-Dideoxykanamycin A (146) has recently been prepared (TSUCHIYA et al. 1979a). 3′,4′-Dideoxykanamycin B (dibekacin) (147) (H. UMEZAWA et al. 1971)

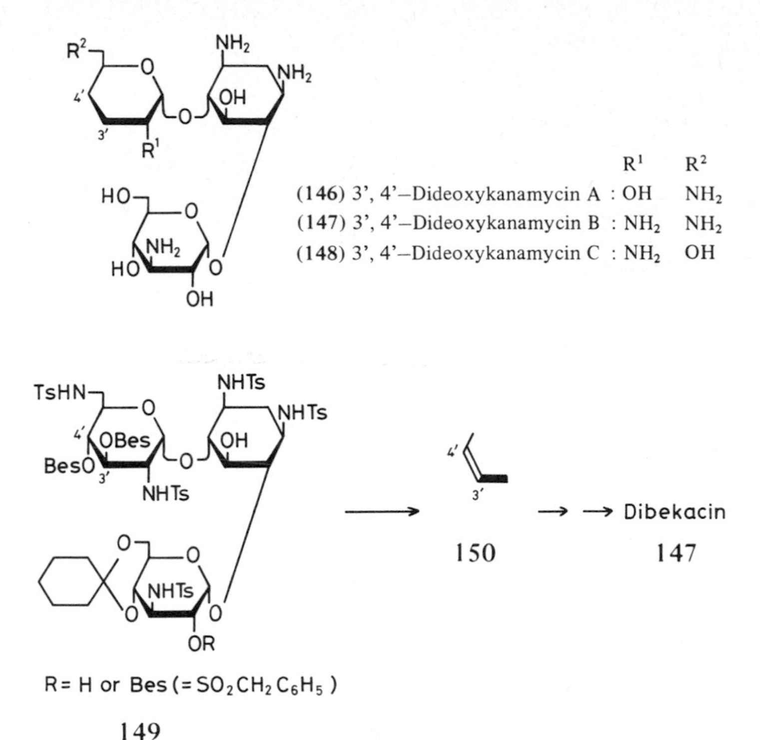

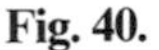
Fig. 40.

was remarkably active against resistant strains, including *Pseudomonas aeruginosa*, and is now in widespread clinical use. Several improved syntheses of dibekacin have been reported. The penta-*N*-tosyl-3′,4′-bis(*O*-benzylsulfonyl) derivative (149) of kanamycin B was treated (Miyake et al. 1976) with sodium iodide in DMF in the absence of zinc dust to give the 3′,4′-unsaturated derivative (150), which was converted to dibekacin by hydrogenation followed by deblocking with sodium in liquid ammonia (Fig. 40). A similar method utilizing the pentakis(*N*-benzyloxycarbonyl) derivative of kanamycin B gave dibekacin in over 50% overall yield from kanamycin B (T. Nishimura et al. 1977). The 3′,4′-unsaturation of kanamycin B was also performed by treatment of the 3′,4′-di-*O*-mesyl derivative with naphthalene-sodium (Hayashi et al. 1977). Another synthesis (Yoneta et al. 1979) of dibekacin (over 40% yield) was performed via the 3′,4′-galacto-epoxide (153) followed by opening of the epoxide with sodium iodide (Fig. 41). 3′,4′-Dideoxykanamycin C (148) was prepared by Kondo et al. (1977).

d) 4′-Deoxykanamycins

In the early stage of the investigation of resistance mechanisms it was thought that 3′-phosphorylation by resistant bacteria might occur by migration from the 4′-phosphate initially formed by resistant bacteria. To check this assumption 4′-deoxykanamycin A (157) was prepared (S. Umezawa et al. 1974b) by total synthesis. However, the compound did not show activity against bacteria producing 3′-phosphotransferase I. Naito et al. (1974a) prepared 4′-deoxykanamycin A start-

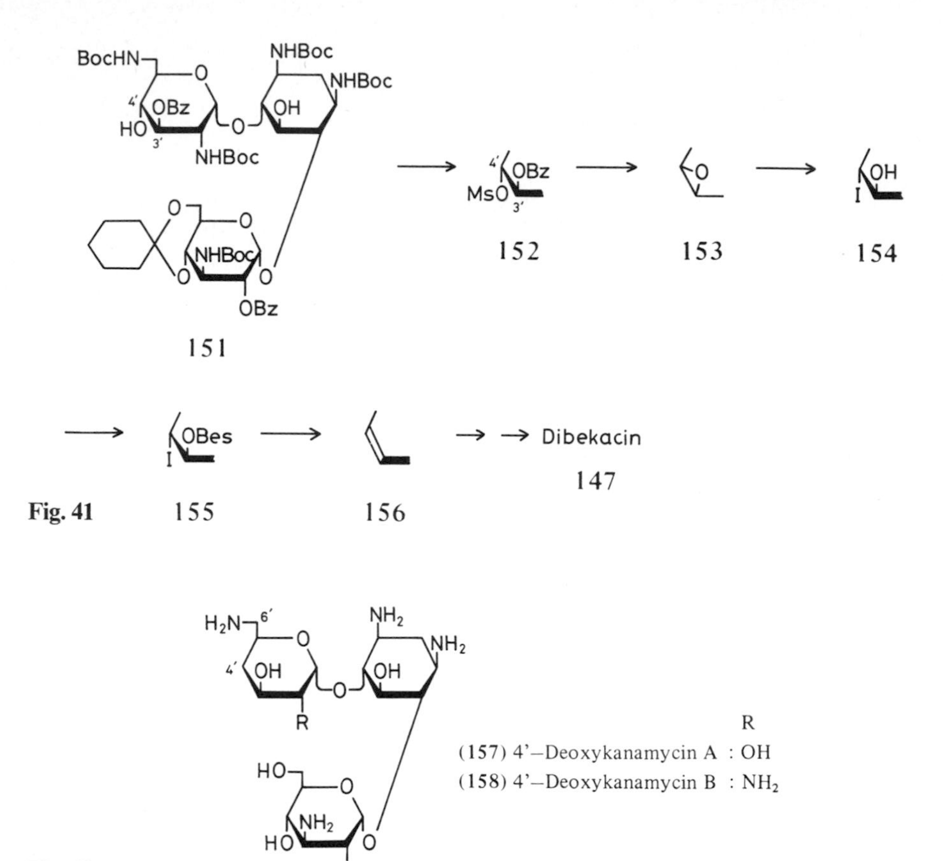

Fig. 41

Fig. 42

ing from kanamycin A. They were led to do so by the fact that 4′-deoxybutirosins (KAWAGUCHI et al. 1974) have a broader antibacterial spectrum than butirosins (Fig. 42).

4′-Deoxykanamycin B (158) was prepared by two groups of workers (MIYAKE et al. 1977; ABE et al. 1977). 6′-*N*-methyl- and 6′-*N*-benzyl-4′-deoxykanamycin A have also been prepared (NAITO et al. 1979).

e) 6′-Deoxykanamycins

6′-Deoxykanamycin C was prepared (TODA et al. 1977) from 1,3,2′,3″-tetra-*N*-acetylkanamycin B by treatment with HBr–$NaNO_2$ followed by hydrogenolysis of the 6′-bromo derivative. The 6′-deoxykanamycin C showed greatly decreased activity compared with kanamycin C, indicating that the 6′-hydroxy group is important for activity.

f) 5-Deoxykanamycins

Total synthesis of 5-deoxykanamycin A (165) (KAVADIAS et al. 1978) was accomplished by the route shown in Fig. 43. The 5-deoxykanamycin A showed an antibacterial spectrum similar to kanamycin, but with about one-half the potency.

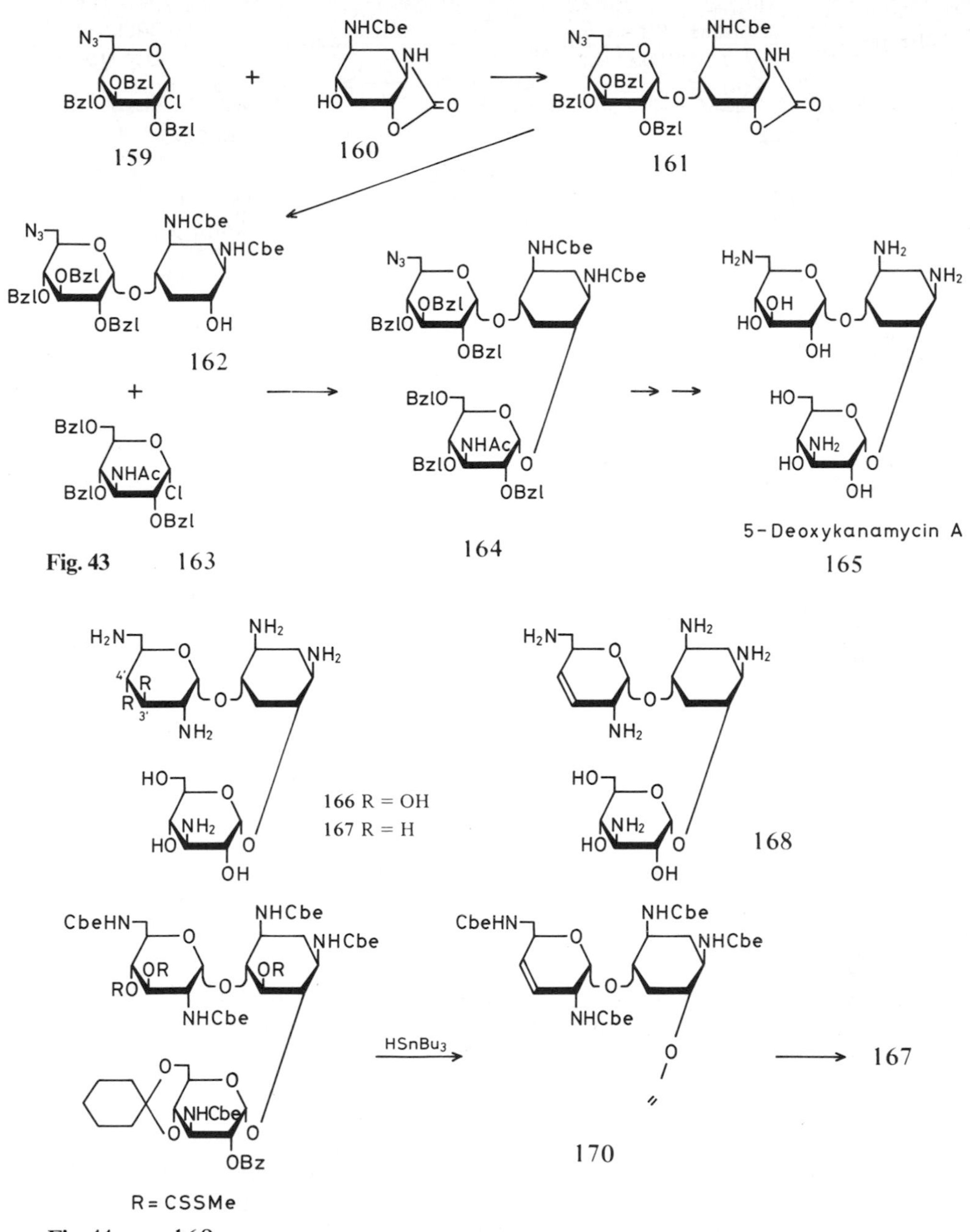

Fig. 43

Fig. 44

5-Deoxykanamycin B (166), 5,3′,4′-trideoxy-3′-enokanamycin B (168), and 5,3′,4′-trideoxykanamycin B (167) have been prepared (HAYASHI et al. 1978) from 5- [in the case of (166)] and 5,3′,4′-tris(*S*-methyldithiocarbonate) [in the case of (167) and (168)] derivatives by treating them with tributylstannane as a key step. The synthesis of (167) is shown in Fig. 44. 5-Deoxykanamycin B (166) showed al-

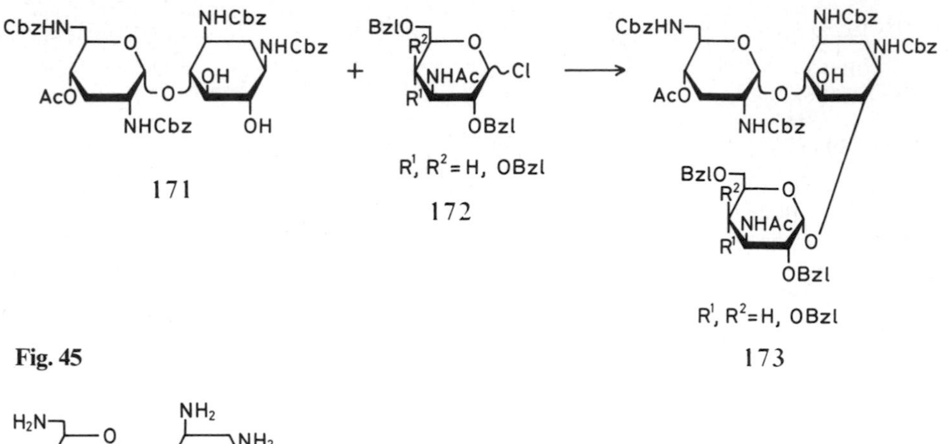

Fig. 45

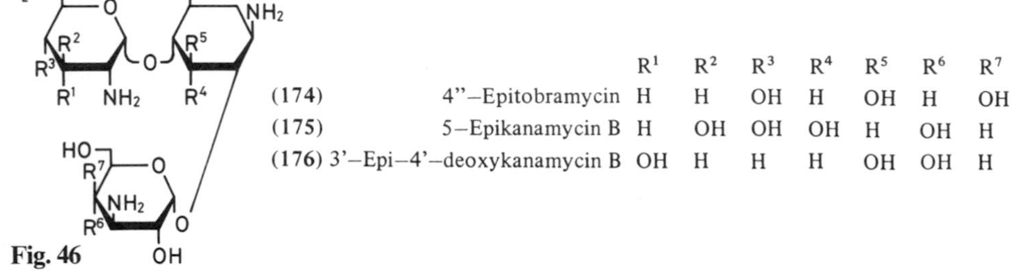

		R^1	R^2	R^3	R^4	R^5	R^6	R^7
(174)	4"–Epitobramycin	H	H	OH	H	OH	H	OH
(175)	5–Epikanamycin B	H	OH	OH	OH	H	OH	H
(176)	3'–Epi–4'–deoxykanamycin B	OH	H	H	H	OH	OH	H

Fig. 46

most the same activity as kanamycin B. 5,3′,4′-Trideoxykanamycin B (167) was slightly less active than dibekacin, and the 3′-eno analog (168) was much less active. 5-Deoxykanamycin B was also prepared (SUAMI et al. 1978b) from a kanamycin B derivative having a free hydroxyl at C-5 by treatment with sulfuryl/chloride, followed by reductive dechlorination of the 5-chloro derivative with tributylstannane.

5,6″-Dideoxykanamycin B was also prepared (SUAMI 1979) and had activity similar to that of kanamycin B.

g) 2″-Deoxykanamycins

2″-Deoxykanamycin B and 2″,3′,4′-trideoxykanamycin B were prepared by REID et al. (1978). The latter was more potent than kanamycin against a group of resistant *Pseudomonas* organisms.

h) Epikanamycins

Tobramycin and 4″-epitobramycin (174) were prepared (TANABE et al. 1977) by condensation of a derivative (171) of nebramine (3′-deoxyneamine) with the glycosyl chlorides (172) of a 3-aminosugar (Fig. 45). The 4″-epitobramycin showed activity similar to that of tobramycin. 5-Epikanamycin B (175) was prepared (SUAMI and NAKAMURA 1979) through inversion at C-5 by treatment of a 5-*O*-mesyl derivative of kanamycin B with sodium acetate. 5-Epikanamycin B was about one-fourth as active as kanamycin B. 3′-Epi-4′-deoxykanamycin B (176) was prepared (AKITA et al. 1979a) through treatment of 2″-*O*-benzoyl-4″,6″-*O*-cyclohexylidene-pentakis(*N*-ethoxycarbonyl)-3′-*O*-tosylkanamycin B (TAKAGI et al. 1973) with sodium borohydride and was less potent than dibekacin (Fig. 46).

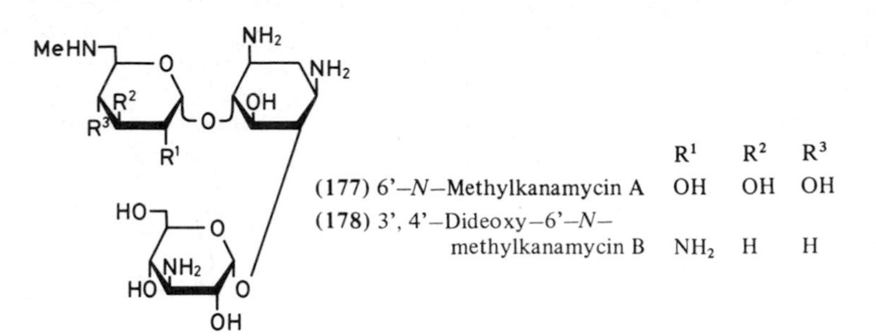

Fig. 47

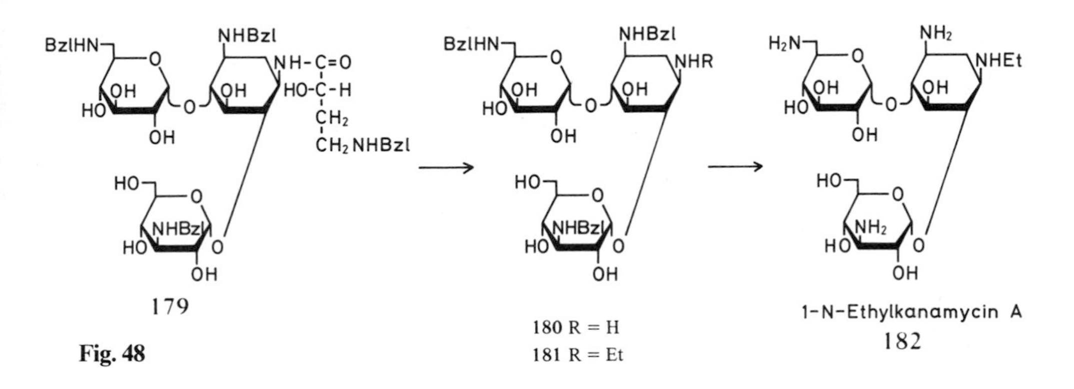

Fig. 48

i) *N*-Alkylkanamycins

In order to obtain variants active against resistant strains producing 6′-*N*-acetyltransferases, 6′-*N*-methylkanamycin A (177) and 3′,4′-dideoxy-6′-*N*-methylkanamycin B (178) were prepared (H. UMEZAWA et al. 1972a) and found to be active against the resistant strains (Fig. 47).

The discovery of 1-*N*-ethylsisomicin (netilmicin) (WRIGHT 1976) a very active aminoglycoside, stimulated the preparation of other *N*-alkylderivatives. 1-*N*-Ethylkanamycin A (182) (NAKAGAWA et al. 1978) was prepared starting from amikacin (KAWAGUCHI et al. 1972) (Fig. 48). Amikacin was treated with benzaldehyde and sodium borohydride to give 3,6′,3″,4‴-tetra-*N*-benzylamikacin (179). Hydrolysis then gave tri-*N*-benzylkanamycin A (180) bearing a free amino group at C-1. Treatment with acetaldehyde and sodium borohydride gave 3,6′,3″-tri-*N*-benzyl-1-*N*-ethylkanamcin A (181). Finally, reductive de-*N*-benzylation gave 1-*N*-ethylkanamycin A (182). 1-,3-,2′-,6′-, and 3″-*N*-Ethylkanamycin B were also prepared. The order of the intrinsic activity of the *N*-ethylkanamycins was: kanamycin A (1), 3″-*N*-ethylkanamycin A (0.66), 1-*N*-ethylkanamycin A (0.29), 6′-*N*-ethylkanamycin A (0.19), 3-*N*-ethylkanamycin A (0.01). 1-*N*-Ethylkanamycin A showed some resistance to the inactivating enzymes, 3′-phosphotransferases, 2″-nucleotidyltransferase, and 3-acetyltransferase II.

6′,3″-Di-*N*-methylkanamycin B (185) was prepared (KUMAR and REMERS 1979) by the route shown in Fig. 49. 6′,3″-Di-*N*-methylkanamycin A, 6′,3″-di-*N*-ethylkanamycin A, and 3″,3″-di-*N*-methylkanamycin A were also prepared and were less active than kanamycin against common strains.

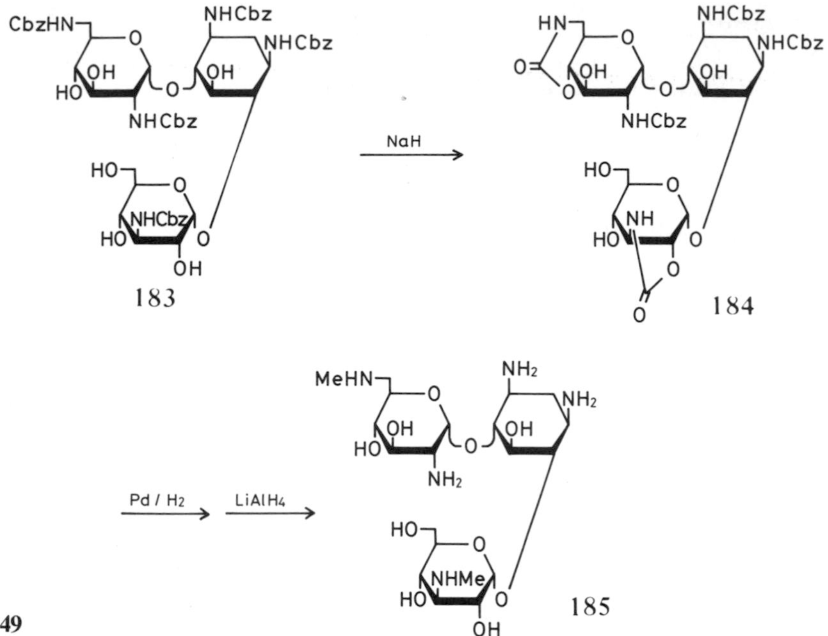

Fig. 49

j) *C*-Alkylkanamycins

6′-*C*-Alkyl derivatives of dibekacin (3′,4′-dideoxykanamycin B) have been prepared (H. UMEZAWA et al. 1979) with the expectation that they would have activity against resistant strains producing 6′-*N*-acetyltransferase. The synthetic route for 6′-(*S*)- and 6′(*R*)-*C*-methyl-3′,4′-dideoxykanamycin B (191) is shown in Fig. 50. Both compounds showed slightly weaker activity than 3′,4′-dideoxykanamycin B; however, both were active against strains producing 6′-*N*-acetyltransferase against which 3′,4′-dideoxykanamycin B is inactive. 6′-*C*-Ethyl derivatives were also prepared. 6′(*R*)- and 6′(*S*)-*C*-Methyltobramycin were also prepared (KONDO 1979) and showed activity similar to that of 3′,4′-dideoxykanamycin B.

k) Deamino-Hydroxykanamycins

Acidic hydrolysis of penta-*N*-formyltobramycin yielded 3,2′6′,3″-tetra-*N*-formyltobramycin (13.2%) (192). Treatment of (192) with 3,5-di-*t*-butyl-1,2-benzoquinone and then with oxalic acid, or with hydrogen peroxide–sodium tungstate followed by hydrolysis, gave the 1-deamino-1-oxo-derivative (193) which, on reduction with sodium borohydride, gave the 1-deamino-1-hydroxytobramycin (194) (IGARASHI 1979) which showed almost no activity, indicating that the 1-amino group is essential for the activity of tobramycin.

l) Amikacin and Related Compounds

The discovery of the 1-*N*-acylated aminoglycosides, butirosins A and B (WOO et al. 1971), and their enhanced activity over ribostamycin suggested an important role for the 1-*N*-[(*S*)-4-amino-2-hydroxybutyryl] residue (AHB). KAWAGUCHI et al.

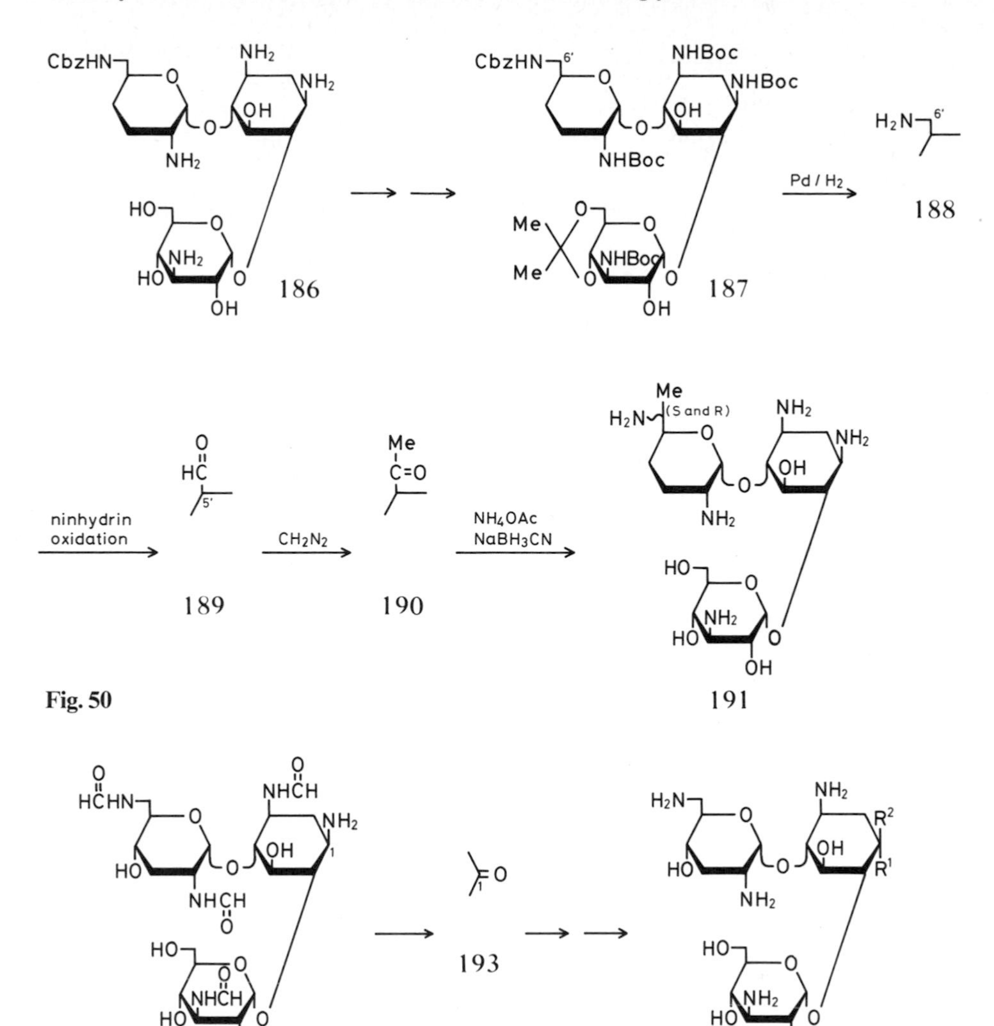

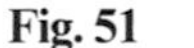

Fig. 51 192 194 $R^1, R^2 = H, OH$

(1972) synthesized 1-*N*-[(*S*)-4-amino-2-hydroxybutyryl]kanamycin A (amikacin), which was found to have remarkable activity against kanamycin-resistant bacteria and, moreover, to show lower acute toxicity than kanamycin A. 1-*N*-AHB-kanamycin B (KONDO et al. 1973) and 1-*N*-AHB-kanamycin C (KONDO et al. 1977) were also prepared.

α) 1-N-Substituted Kanamycins

A number of 1-*N*-acyl analogs of amikacin were prepared (NAITO et al. 1974b). The 1-*N*-acyl residues are: $COCH(OH)(CH_2)_nNH_2$ (n = 1, DL and L; n = 2,3,4, all L), $CO(CH_2)_nNH_2$(n = 1,2,3,4), $COCH(OH)CH(OH)CH_2NH_2$ (DL-erythro), $COCH(OH)CMe_2CH_2NH_2$ (DL), $COCMe(OH)CH_2CH_2NH_2$ (DL),

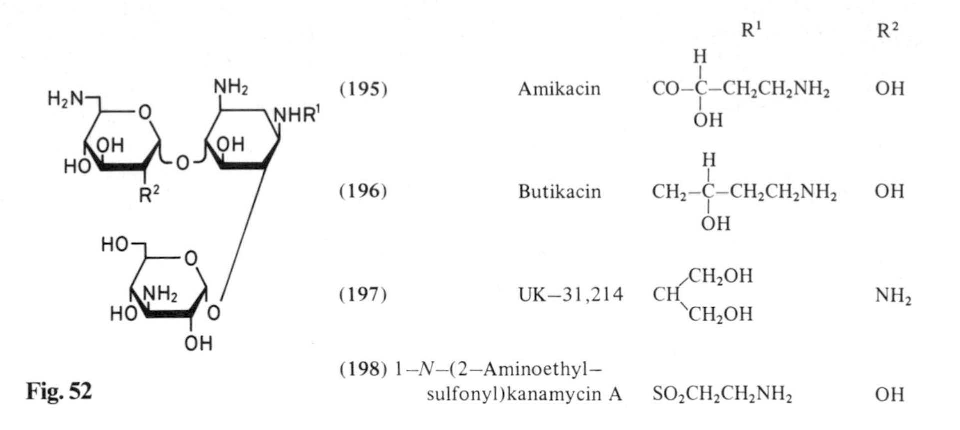

Fig. 52

$COCHR(CH_2)_2NH_2$ [R:H, NH_2(L), OAc(DL)], $COCH_2CH(OH)CH_2NH_2$ (DL), $COCH(OH)(CH_2)_2R$ [R:H(DL), $NHCH_3$(DL), $NHCOCH_2NH_2$ (L), $NHCOCH_3$(L), $CONH_2$(L), COOH(L)], $COCH(NH_2)R$ [R: $CH_2CH_2NH_2$(L), $CH(OH)CH_3$(L), CH_2CH_2OH(DL), CH_2CH_3(L)]. However, all of these are less active than amikacin.

Four 1-*N*-(*S*)-ω-amino-2-hydroxyalkyl derivatives of kanamycin A were prepared (RICHARDSON et al. 1977) by diborane reduction of the corresponding 1-*N*-acyl derivatives. The (*S*)-4-amino-2-hydroxybutyl derivative [UK-18,892, butikacin; (196)] was found to be the most active with almost the same activity as amikacin.

Treatment of 3,2′,6′,3″-tetra-*N*-formylkanamycin B with 1,3-dihydroxyacetone followed by sodium cyanoborohydride gave 1-*N*-(1,3-dihydroxy-2-propyl)kanamycin B [UK-31,214; (197)] (RICHARDSON et al. 1979), which showed activity against *Pseudomonas aeruginosa*.

Another interesting derivative, 1-*N*-(2-aminoethylsulfonyl)kanamycin A (198), was prepared by AKITA et al. (1979 b) and showed activity similar to that of amikacin.

β) On the Selective 1-N-Acylation

The efficient preparation of amikacin from kanamycin A requires selective 1-*N*-acylation. Although the reactivity of the amine groups to normal acylation reactions is similar, except for the reactive primary 6′-amino group, several methods have been found which selectively acylate the secondary amine groups. When kanamycin A was treated with trifluoroacetic anhydride, 6′,3″-bis(*N*-trifluoroacetyl)kanamycin A was obtained (MILLION et al. 1977). Treatment of kanamycin A with copper (II) acetate (0.75–1 mol equiv.) (chelation between the 3″-amino and 4″-hydroxy groups was suggested to occur, thus protecting the 3″-amino group against acylation) and benzyl *p*-nitrophenylcarbonate in aqueous tetrahydrofuran gave 6′-*N*-benzyloxycarbonylkanamycin A (73%). When copper (II) acetate (10 mol equiv.) and *N*-benzyloxycarbonyloxy succinimide (5 mol equiv.) were used, 1,3,6′-tris(*N*-benzyloxycarbonyl)kanamycin A was formed (86%) (HANESSIAN and PATIL 1978), indicating that partial protection of some of the amino groups is possible by metal chelation. When sisomicin, gentamicin -

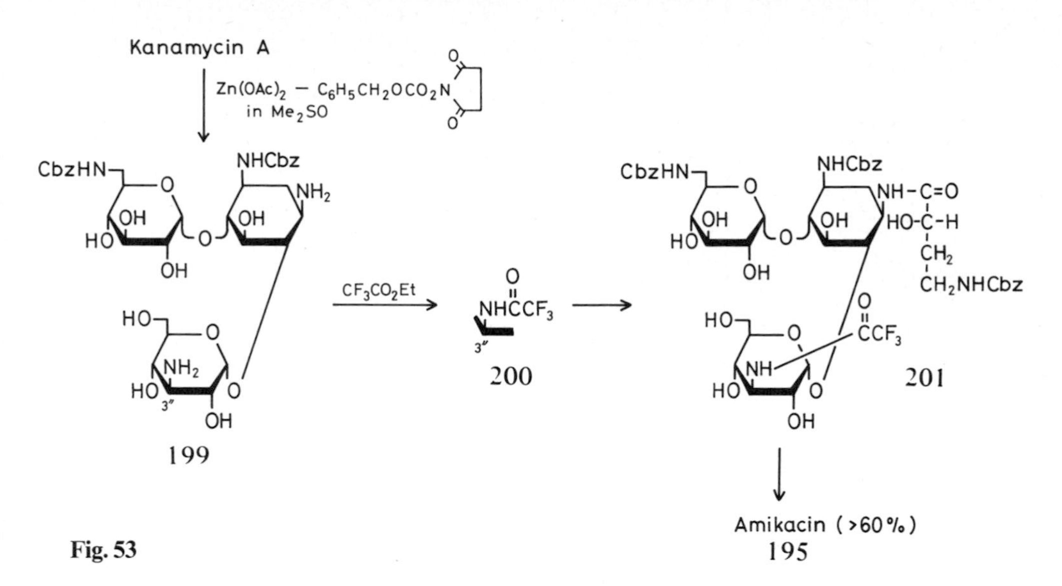

Fig. 53

C_{1a},C_2, or C_1 was treated with an acylating agent in the presence of cobalt (II), nickel (II), or copper (II) acetate (3–4 mol equiv.) in dimethylsulfoxide, the corresponding 3,2′,6′-tri-*N*-acyl derivatives were formed in good yields (NAGABUSHAN et al. 1978c) after removal of the metal ions with hydrogen sulfide. Similarly, from gentamicin B, kanamycin A, and 3′,4′-dideoxykanamycin B, the corresponding 3,6′-di- or 3,2′,6′-tri-*N*-acyl derivatives were obtained. These derivatives were used for preparation of 1-*N*-AHB derivatives (DANIELS et al. 1979) although the 3″-amino groups still remained free. More efficient preparations of amikacin and 1-*N*-AHB-3′,4′-dideoxykanamycin B have recently been carried out (TSUCHIYA et al. 1979b) through 3,6′-bis(*N*-benzyloxycarbonyl)-3″-*N*-trifluoroacetylkanamycin A (200) and 3,2′,6′-tris(*N*-benzyloxycarbonyl)-3′,4′-dideoxy-3″-*N*-trifluoroacetykanamycin B. The two key intermediates were prepared by treatment of kanamycin A or 3′,4′-dideoxykanamycin B with zinc (II) acetate and *N*-(benzyloxycarbonyloxy)succinimide in dimethylsulfoxide, followed by treatment of the resulting di- (199) or tri-*N*-acyl derivatives with ethyl trifluoroacetate. The selective 3″-*N*-trifluoroacetylation was considered to occur by neighboring hydroxy group assistance (Fig. 53).

Another efficient preparation of amikacin was reported (CRON et al. 1979). Treatment of kanamycin A with hexamethyldisilazane in acetonitrile gave polytrimethylsilylkanamycin A which, after treatment with water (10 mol equiv.), was acylated with [(*S*)-4-(benzyloxycarbonylamino)-2-hydroxybutanoyloxy]succinimide to give, after hydrolysis and hydrogenolysis, amikacin (50%).

γ) Deoxyamikacins and Related Compounds

Amikacin is effective against many resistant strains including strains producing 3′-phosphotransferases; however, it is inactivated by some resistant strains by transformation into 3′-*O*-phosphorylamikacin and 4′-*O*-adenylylamikacin (TODA et al. 1978; related references are cited therein). To prevent such inactivation, several deoxy derivatives of amikacin and amikacin analogs have been prepared. 1-*N*-

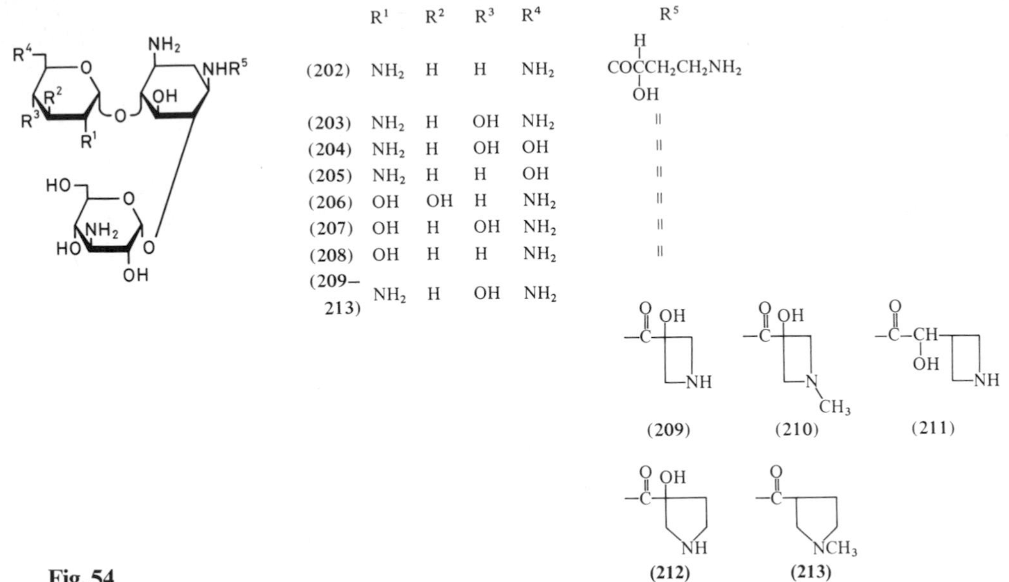

Fig. 54

AHB-3′,4′-dideoxykanamycin B (202) (KONDO et al. 1973), 1-*N*-AHB-tobramycin (203) (BRISTOL-MYERS 1973), 1-*N*-AHB-3′-deoxykanamycin C (204), and 1-*N*-AHB-3′,4′-dideoxykanamycin C (205) (KONDO et al. 1977) were prepared. The kanamycin C derivative (204) was more active than (205). 4′-Deoxyamikacin (206) was prepared by NAITO et al. (1979). 3′-Deoxyamikacin (207) and 3′,4′-dideoxy-amikacin (208) were also prepared by TSUCHIYA et al. (1979 a); the 3′-deoxy derivative (207) was superior to amikacin in both potency and toxicity.

1-*N*-Acyltobramycin derivatives with cyclic amines in the acyl groups (209)–(213) were prepared (IGARASHI 1979), starting from 3,2′,6′,3″-tetra-*N*-formyltobramycin (see Sect. C.V.7.k). Among them (209) was the most active. 1-*N*-Alkyl derivatives of (209) and (212) were prepared by reduction of (209) and (212) with diborane; however, these *N*-alkyl derivatives were much less active than (209) and (212), respectively.

δ) N-Alkylamikacins and Related Compounds

6′-*N*-Methyl- and 6′-*N*-ethyl-amikacins were prepared (H. UMEZAWA et al. 1975 b), and found to be resistant to 6′-*N*-acetyltransferase. 1-*N*-(DL-Isoseryl), 1-*N*-(L-isoseryl), 1-*N*-[(*S*)-4-amino-2-hydroxybutyryl], and 1-*N*-[(*S*)-5-amino-2-hydroxy-*n*-valeryl] derivatives of 3′,4′-dideoxy-6′-*N*-methylkanamycin B were also prepared (H. UMEZAWA et al. 1975 a) and were broadly active against kanamycin-resistant strains producing 3′-phosphotransferases I and II, 2″-nucleotidyltransferase, and 6′-*N*-acetyltransferase. 4′-Deoxy-6′-*N*-methylamikacin was also prepared (NAITO et al. 1979).

ε) Other Analogs of Amikacin

1-*N*-[(*S*)-4-Amino-2-hydroxybutyryl] derivatives of 6′(*S*)- and 6′(*R*)-*C*-methyl-3′,4′-dideoxykanamycin B and 6′(*S*)- and 6′(*R*)-*C*-methyl-3′-deoxykanamycin B

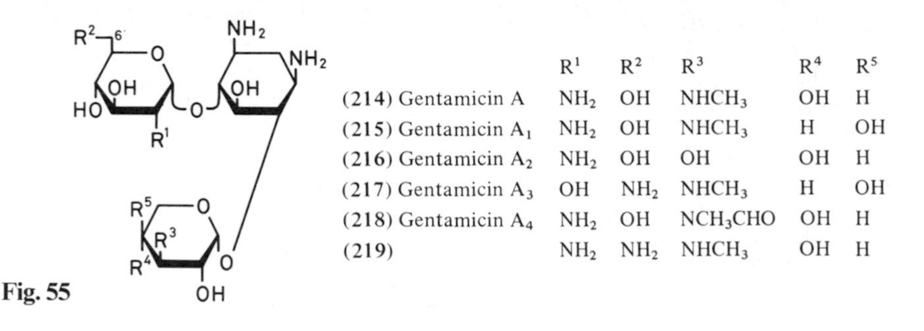

	R^1	R^2	R^3	R^4	R^5
(214) Gentamicin A	NH_2	OH	$NHCH_3$	OH	H
(215) Gentamicin A_1	NH_2	OH	$NHCH_3$	H	OH
(216) Gentamicin A_2	NH_2	OH	OH	OH	H
(217) Gentamicin A_3	OH	NH_2	$NHCH_3$	H	OH
(218) Gentamicin A_4	NH_2	OH	NCH_3CHO	OH	H
(219)	NH_2	NH_2	$NHCH_3$	OH	H

Fig. 55

have been prepared (H. UMEZAWA et al. 1979; KONDO 1979; see Sect. C.V.1.j). 1-*N*-[(*S*)-3-Amino-2-hydroxypropionyl]-5-epikanamycin A was also prepared (DANIELS et al. 1979), but its activity did not exceed that of amikacin.

ζ) Glycosides of Kanamycins

From a phosphate buffer solution (pH 7.6–8.0) of kanamycin A and various sugars incubated at 30 °C–37 °C, kanamycin A glycosides were isolated (PERLMAN et al. 1974). These glycosides were antibacterial although their activity was less than that of kanamycin A. Treatment of a solution of kanamycin A and D-glucose with sodium borohydride gave two *N*-glucosides or *N*-alkyl derivatives (SUZUKI and OHMORI 1979), which showed activity against some kanamycin-resistant strains.

2. Gentamicins and Related Compounds*

The early aspects of the work on this important group of antibiotics have already been reviewed (S. UMEZAWA 1974, 1976; COX et al. 1977). This section is concerned mainly with more recent work carried out between 1975 and 1979.

a) Gentamicin A Derivatives

The structures of gentamicin A (MAEHR and SCHAFFNER 1967, 1970), A_1, A_3, A_4 (NAGABHUSHAN et al. 1975a), and A_2 (NAGABHUSHAN et al. 1975b) have been determined (Fig. 55).

Gentamicin A (214) was transformed into 6′-amino-6′-deoxygentamicin A (219) (NAGABHUSHAN and DANIELS 1974) by a series of reactions including *N*-protection, 6′-*O*-tritylation, *O*-acetylation, detritylation, 6′-*O*-tosylation, and displacement of the tosyloxy group with azide; it had higher activity than gentamicin A.

b) Gentamicin B, X_2, JI-20A, and Their Derivatives

Gentamicin X_2 (221) was synthesized (KUGELMAN et al. 1976b) by condensation of 2′-*O*-acetyl-1,3,3′-tris(*N*-benzyloxycarbonyl)garamine (224) (KUGELMAN et al. 1976a) with the dimer (223) of 3,4,6-tri-*O*-acetyl-2-deoxy-2-nitroso-α-D-glucopyranosyl chloride. By similar condensation, a number of derivatives (225)–(236) were prepared (their activities were not described) (Fig. 56 and 57).

* See also Sect. C.V.4

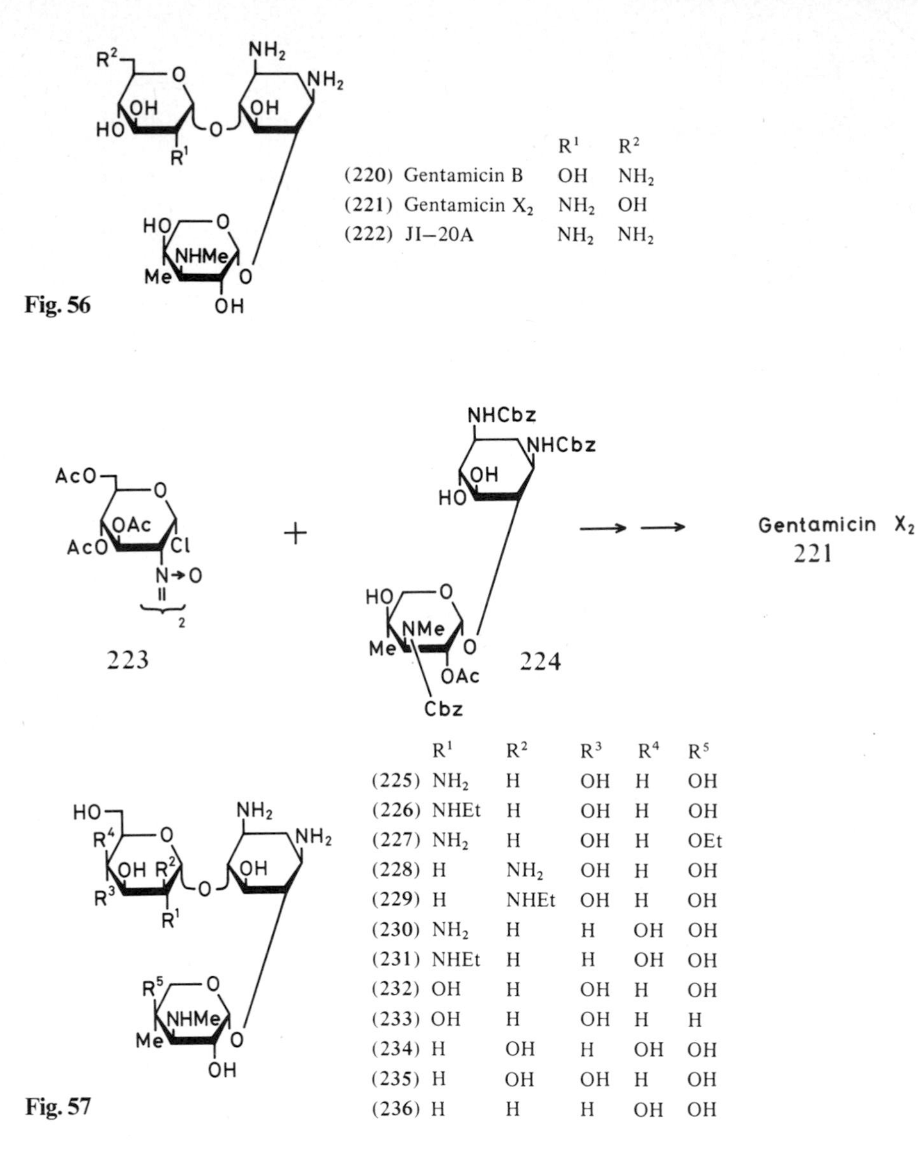

	R¹	R²
(220) Gentamicin B	OH	NH_2
(221) Gentamicin X_2	NH_2	OH
(222) JI–20A	NH_2	NH_2

Fig. 56

	R¹	R²	R³	R⁴	R⁵
(225)	NH_2	H	OH	H	OH
(226)	NHEt	H	OH	H	OH
(227)	NH_2	H	OH	H	OEt
(228)	H	NH_2	OH	H	OH
(229)	H	NHEt	OH	H	OH
(230)	NH_2	H	H	OH	OH
(231)	NHEt	H	H	OH	OH
(232)	OH	H	OH	H	OH
(233)	OH	H	OH	H	H
(234)	H	OH	H	OH	OH
(235)	H	OH	OH	H	OH
(236)	H	H	H	OH	OH

Fig. 57

3′-Deoxygentamicin X_2 was likewise synthesized (KUGELMAN et al. 1976c) by condensation of the protected garamine derivative (238) and dimeric 3-deoxyglycosyl chloride (237) (Fig. 58). Similarly, 3′-epigentamicin X_2 and 3′-*O*-methylgentamicin X_2 were prepared (their antibacterial activities were not described). Gentamicin B (220) and JI-20A (222) were synthesized (KUGELMAN et al. 1976d) by use of (239). Likewise, 3′-deoxygentamicin B, 3′-deoxy-JI-20A, and 6′-*N*-methyl-JI-20A were synthesized (their activities were not described). 3″-De-*N*-methylgentamicin B was reported (NAGABHUSHAN et al. 1978a; see Sect. C.V.2.c).

2′,3′-Dideoxygentamicin B was synthesized (DANIELS et al. 1979) by condensation of (238) and 6-azidoglycal (240) and was more potent than gentamicin against

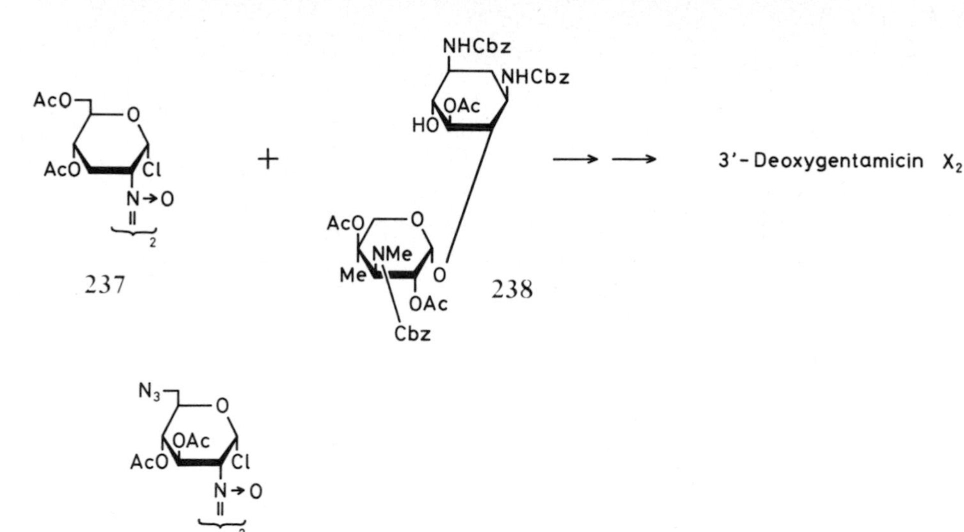

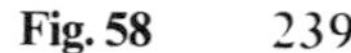

Fig. 58 239

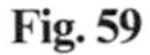

Fig. 59 240

gentamicin-sensitive and gentamicin-resistant strains possessing 3-acetyltransferase I enzymes. It is noteworthy that a compound having no 2′-hydroxy or 2′-amino group showed strong antibacterial activity.

3′,4′-Dideoxygentamicin B (246) was prepared (DANIELS et al. 1979) from gentamicin C_{1a} (248) through 1,3,6′,3″-tretrakis(*N*-benzyloxycarbonyl)gentamicin C_{1a} (243) by oxidative deamination followed by reduction. The intermediate (243) was prepared as follows: Treatment of gentamicin C_{1a} with methanolic nickel (II) acetate followed by 2.1 equiv. of *N*-(2,2,2-trichloroethoxycarbonyloxy)succinimide gave the 2′,6′-di-*N*-protected compound (241). Reaction of the derivative with benzyl chloroformate, followed by removal of the trichloroethoxycarbonyl groups with zinc in acetic acid–methanol, gave (242) which, on treatment with 1 equiv. *N*-(benzyloxycarbonyloxy)phthalimide, gave (243) (Fig. 60).

5-Epigentamicin B was also prepared (DANIELS et al. 1979) and had potency similar to that of gentamicin B.

c) Derivatives of Gentamicin C_1, C_2, C_{1a}, C_{2a}, and C_{2b}

2-Deoxy-4-*O*-(2,6-diamino-2,3,4,6-tetradeoxy-α-D-erythrohexopyranosyl)-6-*O*-(3-deoxy-3-methylamino-α-D-xylopyranosyl)streptamine (254) was prepared (SITRIN et al. 1977) by condensation of (252) and (253) (Fig. 62). Compound (254) resembles gentamicin C_{1a} (248) in structure, the only difference being at position C-4″; however, its potency is only one-fourth to one-eigth that of the gentamicin C complex.

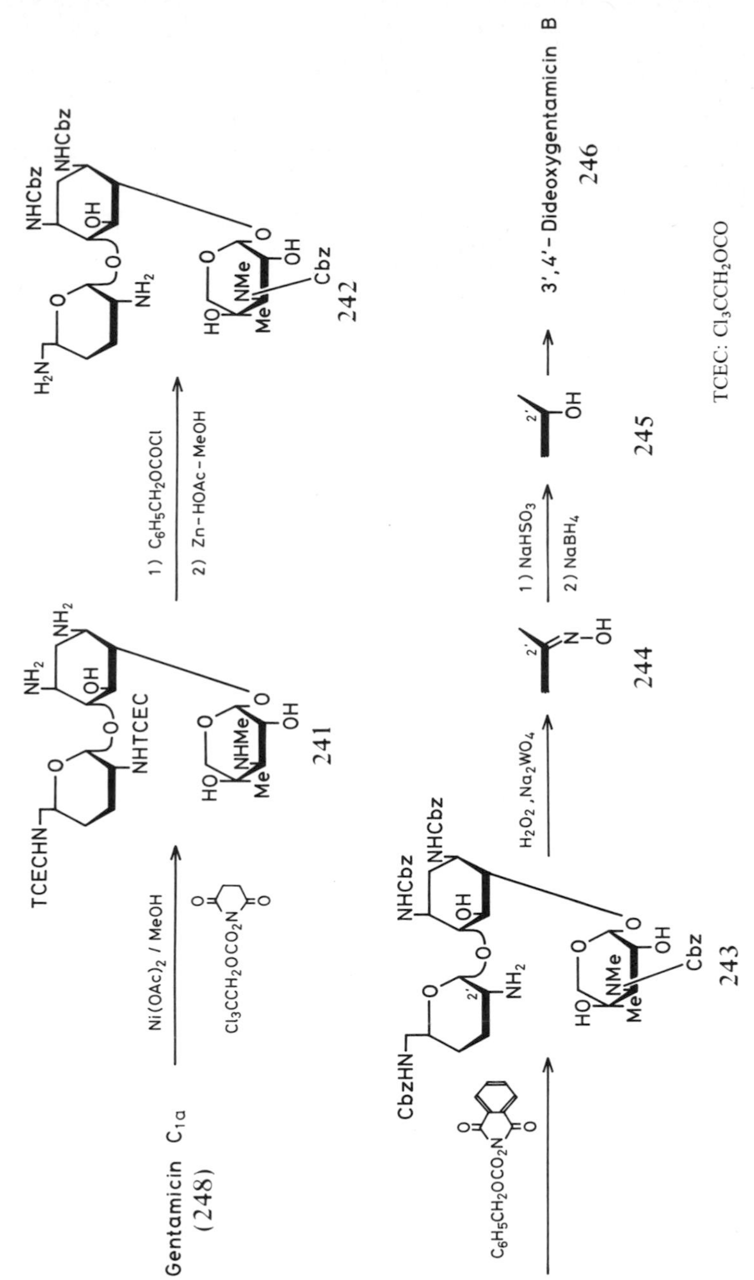

Fig. 60

N-Methylation of gentamicin C_{1a} with methyl *p*-toluenesulfonate gave a mixture of *N*-methyl derivatives, from which 2′-*N*-methylgentamicin C_{1a} and the 6′-*N*-methylisomer (gentamicin C_{2b}) were isolated (DANIELS et al. 1975). 2′-*N*-Methylgentamicin C_{1a} (MATSUSHIMA and MORI 1978e) inhibited the growth of resistant bacteria possessing 2′-acetyltransferase; however, against sensitive strains it was slightly less potent than gentamicin C_{2b}.

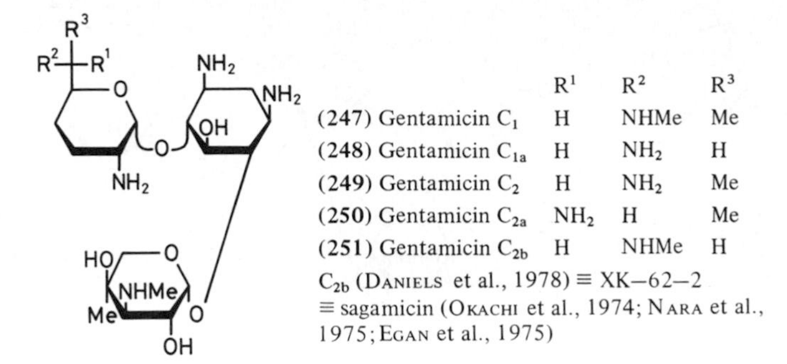

	R^1	R^2	R^3
(**247**) Gentamicin C_1	H	NHMe	Me
(**248**) Gentamicin C_{1a}	H	NH_2	H
(**249**) Gentamicin C_2	H	NH_2	Me
(**250**) Gentamicin C_{2a}	NH_2	H	Me
(**251**) Gentamicin C_{2b}	H	NHMe	H

C_{2b} (DANIELS et al., 1978) ≡ XK–62–2
≡ sagamicin (OKACHI et al., 1974; NARA et al., 1975; EGAN et al., 1975)

Fig. 61

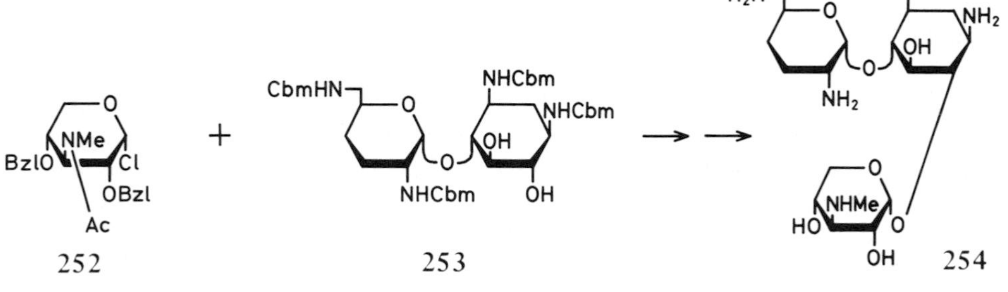

Fig. 62

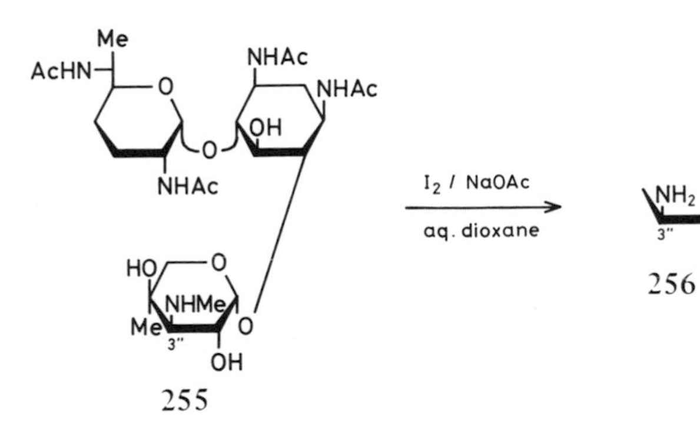

	R
(257) 3"–De–*N*–methylgentamicin C_2	H
(258) 3"–*N*–Ethyl–3"–de–*N*–methylgentamicin C_2	C_2H_5
(259) 3"–De–*N*–methyl–3"–*N*–propylgentamicin C_2	C_3H_7
(260) 3"–*N*–Butyl–3"–de–*N*–methylgentamicin C_2	C_4H_9

Fig. 63

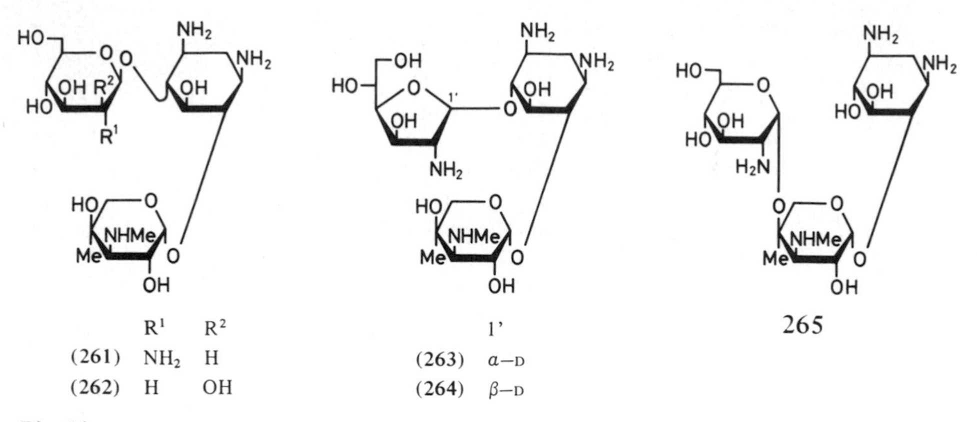

Fig. 64

3″-*N*-Demethyl and 3″-*N*-alkyl (except methyl) derivatives (257)–(260) of gentamicin C_2 were prepared (NAGABUSHAN et al. 1978a) starting from gentamicin C_2. 1,3,2′,6′-Tetra-*N*-acetylgentamicin C_2 (255) was prepared by selective *N*-acetylation by acetic anhydride in methanol containing carbon dioxide and was de-3″-*N*-methylated with I_2–NaOAc. The derivative (256), on 3″-*N*-alkylation, led to 3″-*N*-ethyl-, 3″-*N*-propyl-, and 3″-*N*-butylgentamicin C_2. These four compounds have potency and spectrum similar to those of gentamicin C_2 (249) (Fig. 63).

Similarly de-*N*-methylation afforded 3″-de-*N*-methyl-, 6′-de-*N*-methyl, and 6′,3″-di-de-*N*-methylgentamicin C_{2b} (TOMIOKA and MORI 1976) and 3″-de-*N*-methylgentamicin C_1 (TOMIOKA et al. 1977) from the respective parent antibiotics.

2″-Deoxygentamicin C_{1a} and 2″-deoxygentamicin C_2 were prepared (DANIELS 1975) from the corresponding 2″-ethylthio derivatives by catalytic reduction.

d) Gentamicin Analogs

The following unnatural compounds (261)–(265) were synthesized (KUGELMAN et al. 1976b) (Fig. 64). Their antibacterial activites were not shown.

4-*O*-Pentofuranosylgaramines (266)–(271) and 4-*O*-pentopyranosylgaramines (272)–(276) were prepared (MALLAMS et al. 1976) by condensation of (238) (see Sect. C.V.2.b) and protected pentofuranosyl and pentopyranosyl halogenides (activities were not shown) (Fig. 65).

3. Sisomicin, Its Derivatives, and Related Unsaturated Compounds

Sisomicin(277) is a broad-spectrum antibiotic (WEINSTEIN et al. 1970; REIMANN et al. 1974) isolated from the culture of *Micromonospora inyoensis*. The structure is unique in bearing a double bond between C(4′) and C(5′). As structurally related antibiotics of microbial origin, verdamicin (278) (WEINSTEIN et al. 1975), G-52 (279) (MARQUEZ et al. 1976; DANIELS et al. 1976a), 66-40G (280) (3″-de-*N*-methylsisomicin) (KUGELMAN et al. 1978), 66-40B (281), 66-40D (282) (DAVIES et al. 1975), and 66-40C [a dimeric compound (283)] (DAVIES et al. 1977) have been discovered (Fig. 66). Mutamicins (TESTA et al. 1974) and 5-episisomicin (WAITZ et al. 1978) have been obtained biosynthetically.

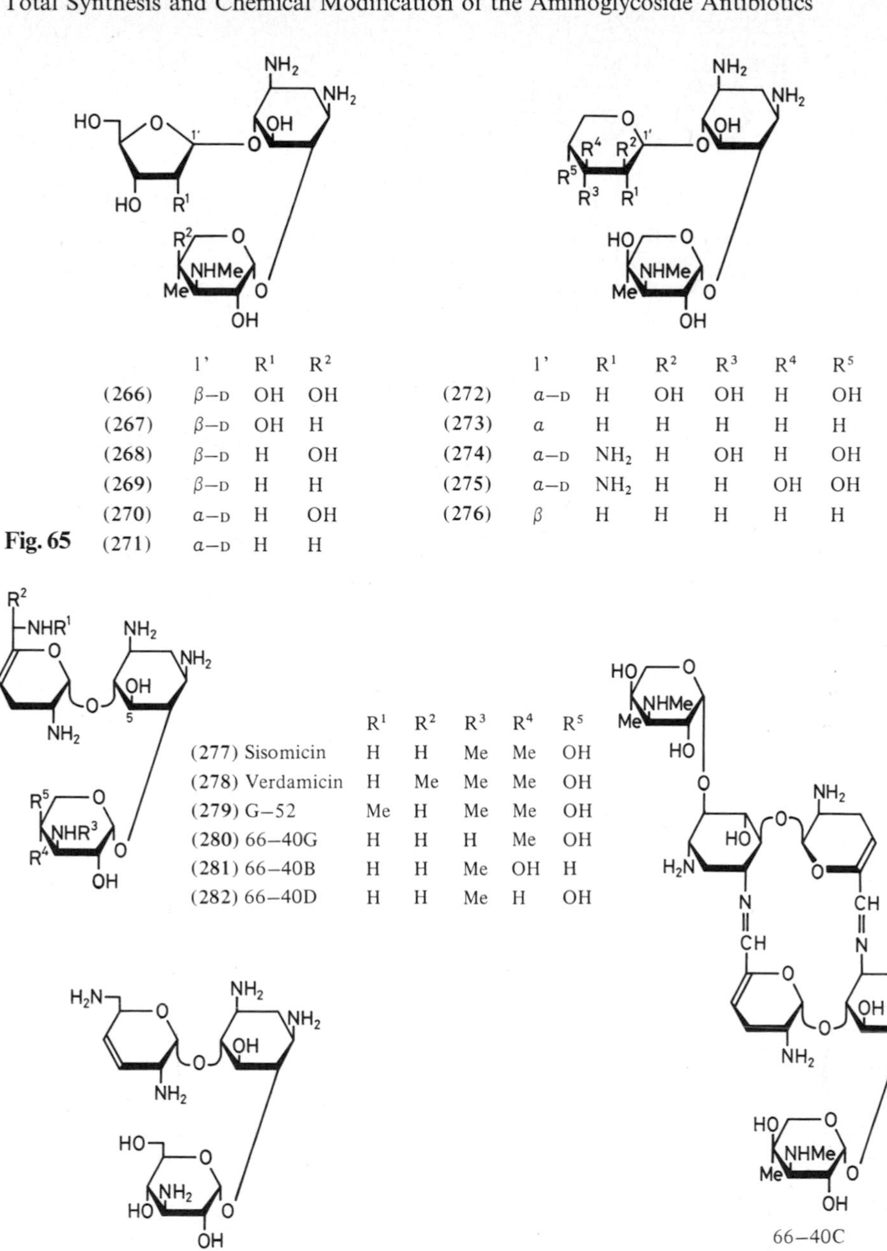

	1'	R^1	R^2
(266)	β–D	OH	OH
(267)	β–D	OH	H
(268)	β–D	H	OH
(269)	β–D	H	H
(270)	α–D	H	OH
(271)	α–D	H	H

	1'	R^1	R^2	R^3	R^4	R^5
(272)	α–D	H	OH	OH	H	OH
(273)	α	H	H	H	H	H
(274)	α–D	NH_2	H	OH	H	OH
(275)	α–D	NH_2	H	H	OH	OH
(276)	β	H	H	H	H	H

Fig. 65

	R^1	R^2	R^3	R^4	R^5
(277) Sisomicin	H	H	Me	Me	OH
(278) Verdamicin	H	Me	Me	Me	OH
(279) G–52	Me	H	Me	Me	OH
(280) 66–40G	H	H	H	Me	OH
(281) 66–40B	H	H	Me	OH	H
(282) 66–40D	H	H	Me	H	OH

Fig. 66

A structurally related compound, 3′,4′-unsaturated kanamycin B (284), was synthesized (S. UMEZAWA 1974) and was less active than kanamycin B.

a) *N*-Alkylsisomicins

1-*N*-Ethylsisomicin (netilmicin) (285) was prepared (WRIGHT 1976) by treating sisomicin sulfate with sodium cyanoborohydride in the presence of acetaldehyde.

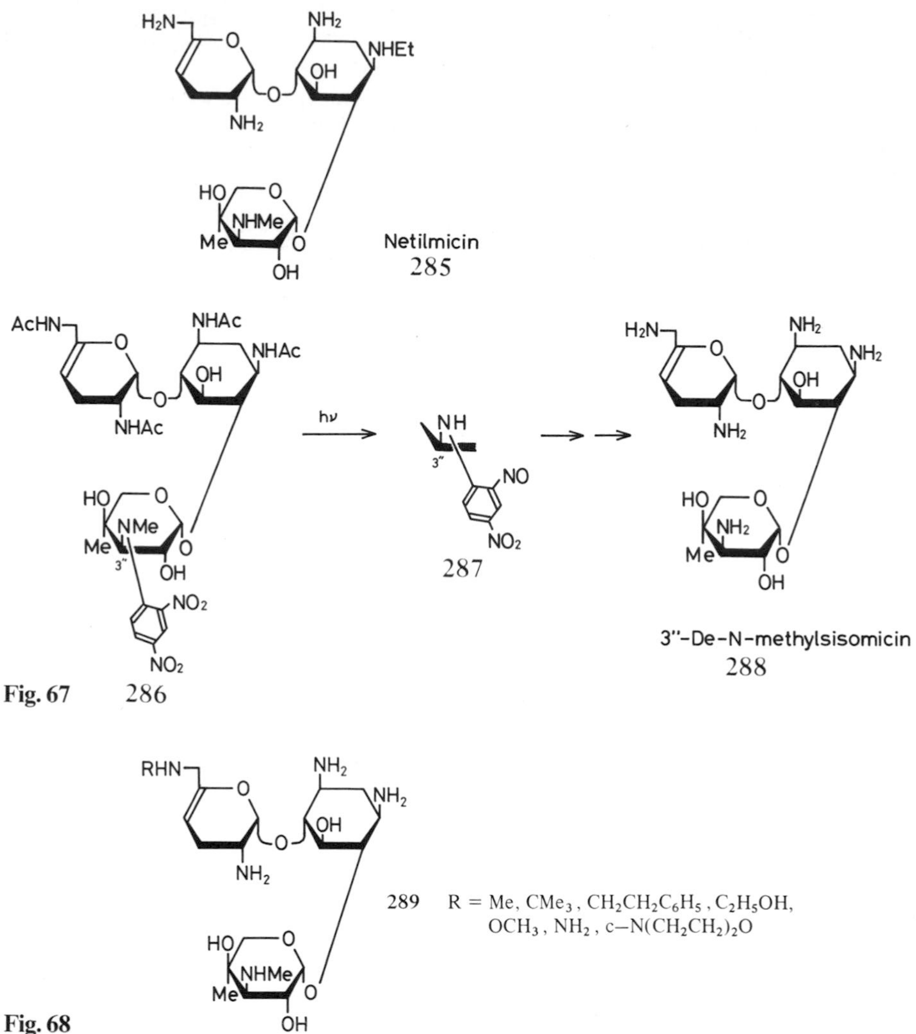

Fig. 67

Fig. 68

Netilmicin is active against many 2″-*O*-adenylylating and 3-*N*-acetylating resistant strains. Netilmicin also shows low chronic toxicity compared to gentamicin and sisomicin. 1-*N*-Methylsisomicin (WEINSTEIN et al. 1978) and 5-deoxysisomicin and 5-deoxy-1-*N*-ethylsisomicin (DANIELS and MCCOMBIE 1977) were also prepared.

3″-De-*N*-methylsisomicin was prepared (NAGABHUSHAN et al. 1978a) from sisomicin by selective 1,3,2′,6′-tetra-*N*-acetylation (as described in Sect. C.III.2.c), dinitrophenylation [to give (286)], and photochemical de-*N*-methylation, and had potency and spectrum similar to those of sisomicin (Fig. 67).

6′-*N*-Substituted analogs (289) of sisomicin were prepared (DAVIES and MALLAMS 1978) from 66-40C (283). Treatment of 66-40C (283) with ammonia, methylamine, hydrazine, and other amines, followed by reduction of the intermediate imines with sodium borohydride, gave sisomicin, 6′-*N*-methylsisomicin, 6′-*N*-aminosisomicin, and other related substances, respectively (Fig. 68).

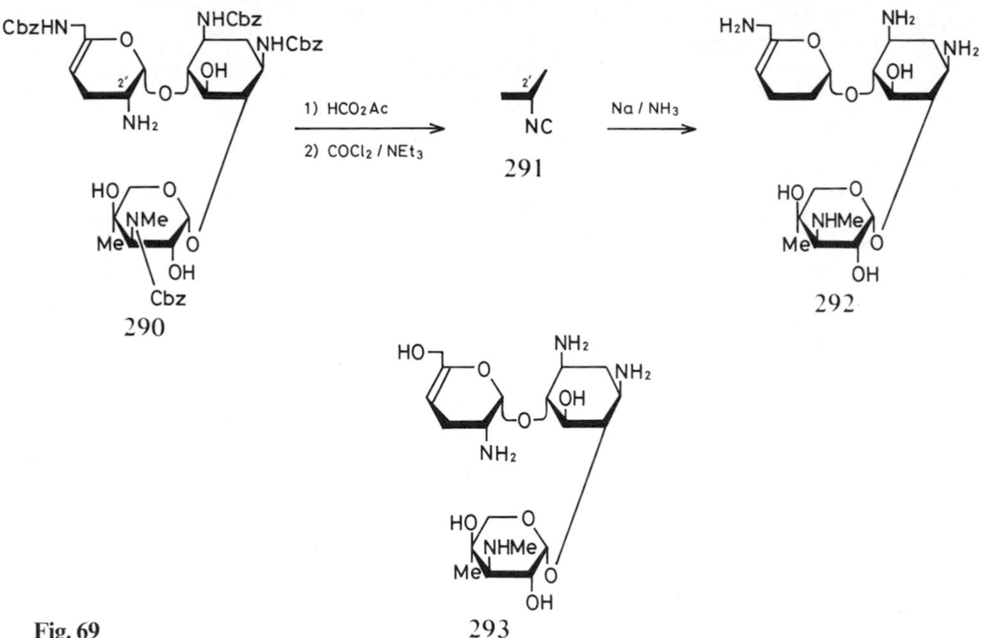

Fig. 69

b) Deamino- and Deamino-Hydroxysisomicins

2′-Deaminosisomicin (292) was prepared (DANIELS et al. 1979) from sisomicin. 1,3,6′,3″-Tetrakis(*N*-benzyloxycarbonyl)sisomicin (290) was prepared by a route similar to that described in the synthesis of 3′,4′-dideoxygentamicin B (see Sect. C.V.2.b) and was 2′-*N*-formylated and dehydrated with phosgene–triethylamine to give the isonitrile (291), which was reduced with sodium in liquid ammonia to give 2′-deaminosisomicin (292).

1-Deamino-1-hydroxy and 1-deamino-1-epi-hydroxysisomicin were prepared (MALLAMS and DAVIES 1978) from sisomicin by a route similar to that described in Sect. C.V.1.k. Protozoacidal 6′-deamino-6′hydroxysisomicin (293) was prepared (MALLAMS and DAVIES 1975) from 66-40C (283) by treatment with aqueous phosphoric acid followed by reduction with sodium cyanoborohydride (Fig. 69).

c) Other Sisomicin-Related Compounds* Including Unsaturated Pseudotrisaccharides

5-Epi-fluoro-5-deoxysisomicin was prepared (DANIELS and RANE 1978) from sisomicin, and was less toxic (LD_{50}, i.v., 160 mg/kg) than sisomicin (30 mg/kg). 1-*N*-Formylsisomicin was reported (VOSS et al. 1978).

Treatment of 1,3,2′,3″-tetrakis(*N*-ethoxycarbonyl)tobramycin (294) with mesitylglyoxal in 90% aqueous DMF gave the 6′-Schiff base (295) which, on treatment with 1,5-diazabicyclo-[3,4,0]-nonene-5, led to the isomeric Schiff base (296). Treatment of (296) with pyruvic acid gave the 6′-aldehyde (297), which on acetylation

* See also Sect. C.V.4

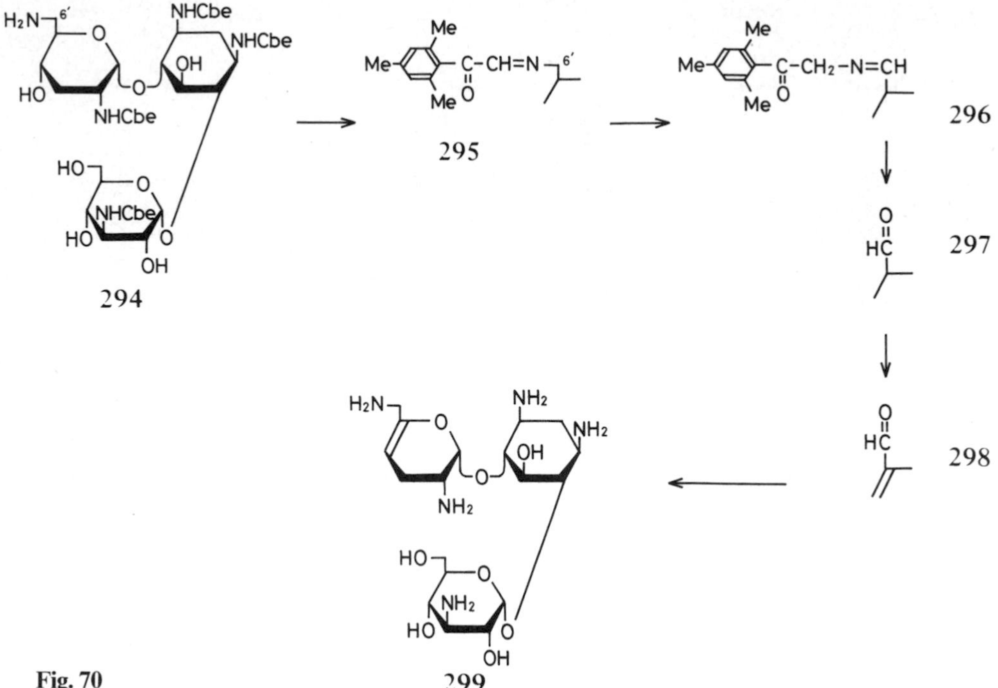

Fig. 70

gave the unsaturated aldehyde (298). Finally, reductive amination gave 4′-deoxy-4′-enotobramycin (299) (IGARASHI 1979). 4′-Deoxy-4′-eno-1-*N*-ethyltobramycin was also prepared. Both 4′-deoxy-4′-eno derivatives were less active than sisomicin (Fig. 70).

4. 1-*N*-Acylgentamicins and 1-*N*-Acylsisomicins

1-*N*-[(*S*)-4-Amino-2-hydroxybutyryl]gentamicin C_1 and 1-*N*-[(*S*)-3-amino-2-hydroxypropionyl]gentamicin C_1 were prepared by DANIELS et al. (1974). Treatment of gentamicin C_1 with ethyl trifluoroacetate (1 mol equiv.) in methanol afforded 2′-*N*-trifluoroacetylgentamicin C_1 which, by repeated treatment with ethyl trifluoroacetate, gave 3,2′-bis(*N*-trifluoroacetyl)gentamicin C_1. Condensation with *N*-[(*S*)-4-benzyloxycarbonylamino-2-hydroxybutyryloxy]succinimide followed by usual workup then gave 1-*N*-AHB-gentamicin C_1. The order of reactivity of the amino groups for trifluoroacetylation was concluded to be $2' > 3 > 1 > 6$ and $3''$.

1-*N*-Acetylsisomicin was prepared directly from half-neutralized sisomicin (sisomicin sulfate and 1 mol equiv. triethylamine) dissolved in aqueous methanol by addition of excess acetic anhydride (WRIGHT et al. 1976). By use of this procedure, a number of 1-*N*-acyl derivatives of sisomicin, gentamicin C_{1a}, and verdamicin having $COCH_2CH_3$, $COCH(OH)CH_2NH_2(S)$ (for sisomicin), $COCH(OH)CH_2NH_2(S)$, $COCH(OH)CH_2CH_2NH_2(S)$ (for gentamicin C_{1a}), and $COCH_3$ (for verdamicin) were prepared. The 1-*N*-acetyl derivatives of sisomicin

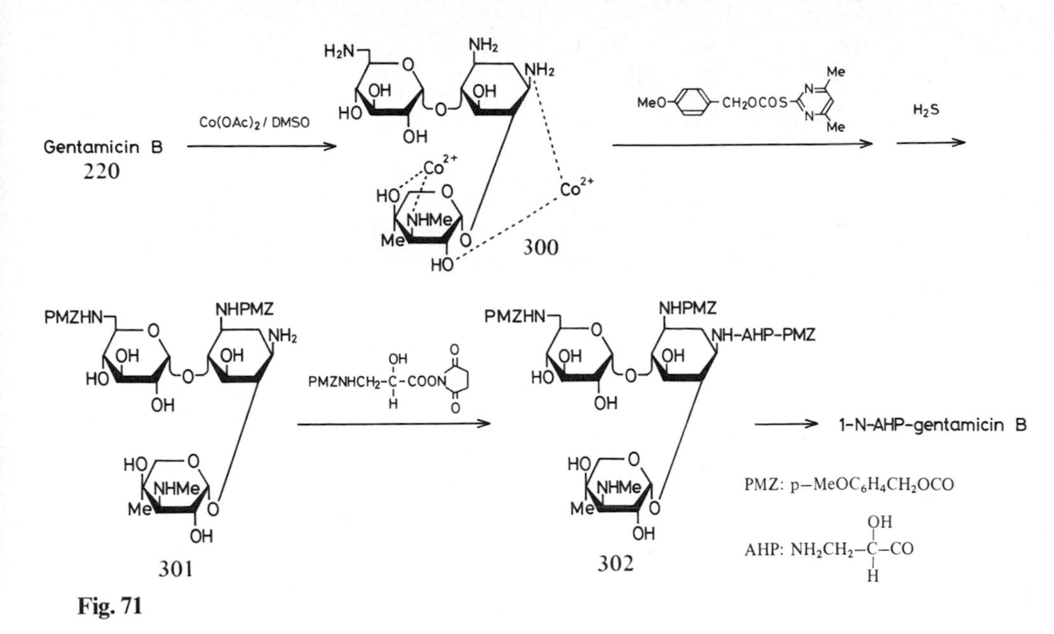

Fig. 71

and verdamicin, which showed similar or slightly reduced potency compared with the parent antibiotics against sensitive organisms, had increased activity against sisomicin-resistant organisms possessing 3-*N*-acetylating and 2″-*O*-nucleotidylating enzymes. 1-*N*-AHB-sisomicin was also prepared by an alternative method (DANIELS 1978). 1-*N*-[(*S*)-3-Amino-2-hydroxypropionyl]gentamicin B (1-*N*-AHP-gentamicin B) (NEU and FU 1978; WATANAKUNAKORN 1978) and 1-*N*-[(*S*)-4-amino-2-hydroxybuytyl]gentamicin B (NAGABHUSHAN et al. 1978 b) have been prepared and were equally active, with amikacin, against both gentamicin-sensitive and gentamicin-resistant strains. Moreover, 1-*N*-AHP-gentamicin B was less toxic (MILLER et al. 1978) than amikacin in a chronic renal function test in rats. A high-yield (60%) synthesis of 1-*N*-AHP-gentamicin B was performed by a process including chelation with cobalt as shown in Fig. 71 (DANIELS et al. 1979).

1-*N*-AHP-2′,3′-dideoxygentamicin B, 1-*N*-AHP-3′,4′-dideoxygentamicin B, and 1-*N*-AHP-2′-deaminosisomicin were also prepared (DANIELS et al. 1979). They had almost the same antibacterial spectra and potency as 1-*N*-AHP-gentamicin B. 1-*N*-AHP-5-epigentamicin B was likewise prepared (DANIELS et al. 1979) from 5-epigentamicin B and was shown to be approximately two to four times more potent than 1-*N*-AHP-gentamicin B, but its nephrotoxicity was increased. 1-*N*-AHP-5-episisomicin ((DANIELS et al. 1979) also showed activity and toxicity similar to 1-*N*-AHP-5-epigentamicin B.

1-*N*-AHB-sagamicin (SHIRAHATA et al. 1975) and 1-*N*-AHB-3″-*N*-demethylsagamicin (TOMIOKA and MORI 1977) were reported.

5. Seldomycin Modifications

Seldomycins have been obtained from the culture of *Streptomyces hofuensis* (NARA et al. 1977). The structures of seldomycin factor 1 [XK-88-1; (303)], factor 2 (XK-

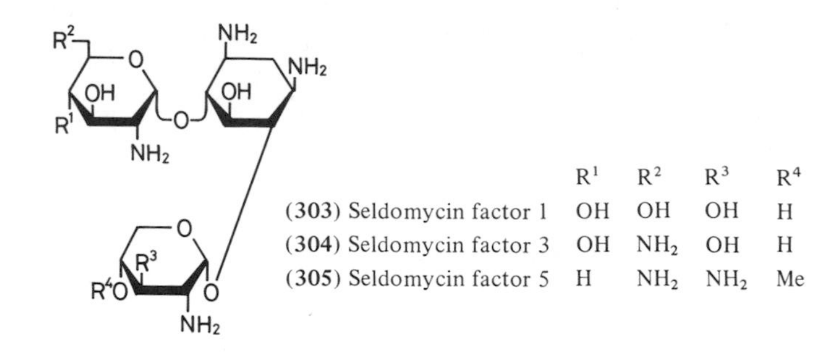

	R^1	R^2	R^3	R^4
(303) Seldomycin factor 1	OH	OH	OH	H
(304) Seldomycin factor 3	OH	NH_2	OH	H
(305) Seldomycin factor 5	H	NH_2	NH_2	Me

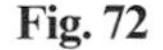
Fig. 72

88-2; 4′-deoxyneamine), factor 3 [XK-88-3; (304)], and factor 5 (305) were determined (EGAN et al. 1977; MCALPINE et al. 1977). Seldomycin factor 5 is the most important therapeutically (Fig. 72).

a) 3′-Modified Seldomycin Factor 5

3′-Deoxyseldomycin factor 5 (306) was prepared by treatment of hexakis(*N*-benzyloxycarbonyl)-3′-*O*-tosylseldomycin factor 5 (310) with sodium borohydride in dimethylsulfoxide followed by deblocking (MATSUSHIMA et al. 1977a), or by treatment (CARNEY et al. 1978) of a 3′-*O*-imidazolylthiocarbonyl derivative (312) with tributylstannane. It was more potent than seldomycin factor 5 against both gram-negative and gram-sensitive bacteria, including *Pseudomonas aeruginosa* and resistant strains which phosphorylate the 3′-hydroxy group of seldomycin factor 5. 2′-Deamino-3′-epiamino-3′-deoxyseldomycin factor 5 (307) and 2′,3′-epimino-2′-deamino-3′-deoxyseldomycin factor 5 (308) were also prepared (MATSUSHIMA et al. 1978) by sodium borohydride reduction; however, both compounds were less active than seldomycin factor 5. 3′-Episeldomycin factor 5 (309) was also prepared (MATSUSHIMA et al. 1977b; CARNEY et al. 1978) from (310) or from the corresponding 3′-*O*-mesyl derivative (311) through the 2′,3′-epicyclic carbamate. It was less active than seldomycin factor 5 against common strains (Fig. 73).

b) *N*-Modified Seldomycin Factor 5

6′-*N*-Methylseldomycin factor 5 (MATSUSHIMA and MORI 1978a), 1-*N*-acyl-derivatives of seldomycin factor 5 (CARNEY and MCALPINE 1978), 1-*N*-[(*S*)-4-amino-2-hydroxybutyryl]seldomycin factor 5 (MATSUSHIMA and MORI 1978b), 2″-*N*-formylseldomycin factor 5 (MATSUSHIMA and MORI 1978c), and 2′-deamino-3′-deoxy-3′-epiaminoseldomycin factor 5 (MATSUSHIMA and MORI 1978d) were synthesized from seldomycin factor 5.

6. Other 4,6-Disubstituted Derivatives

6-*O*-(*β*-D-Ribofuranosyl)paromamine [(314), R=OH] was prepared (ARCAMONE et al. 1974) via condensation of (313) and (67) (see Sect. C.III.1). (314), R=OH was also prepared via a similar condensation by OGAWA et al. (1974) and HANESSIAN et al. (1978c). Unlike 5-*O*-ribosylparomamine (74) (see Sect. C.III.1), (314), R=OH had no activity; however, it was a good substrate (HANESSIAN et al. 1978c) for

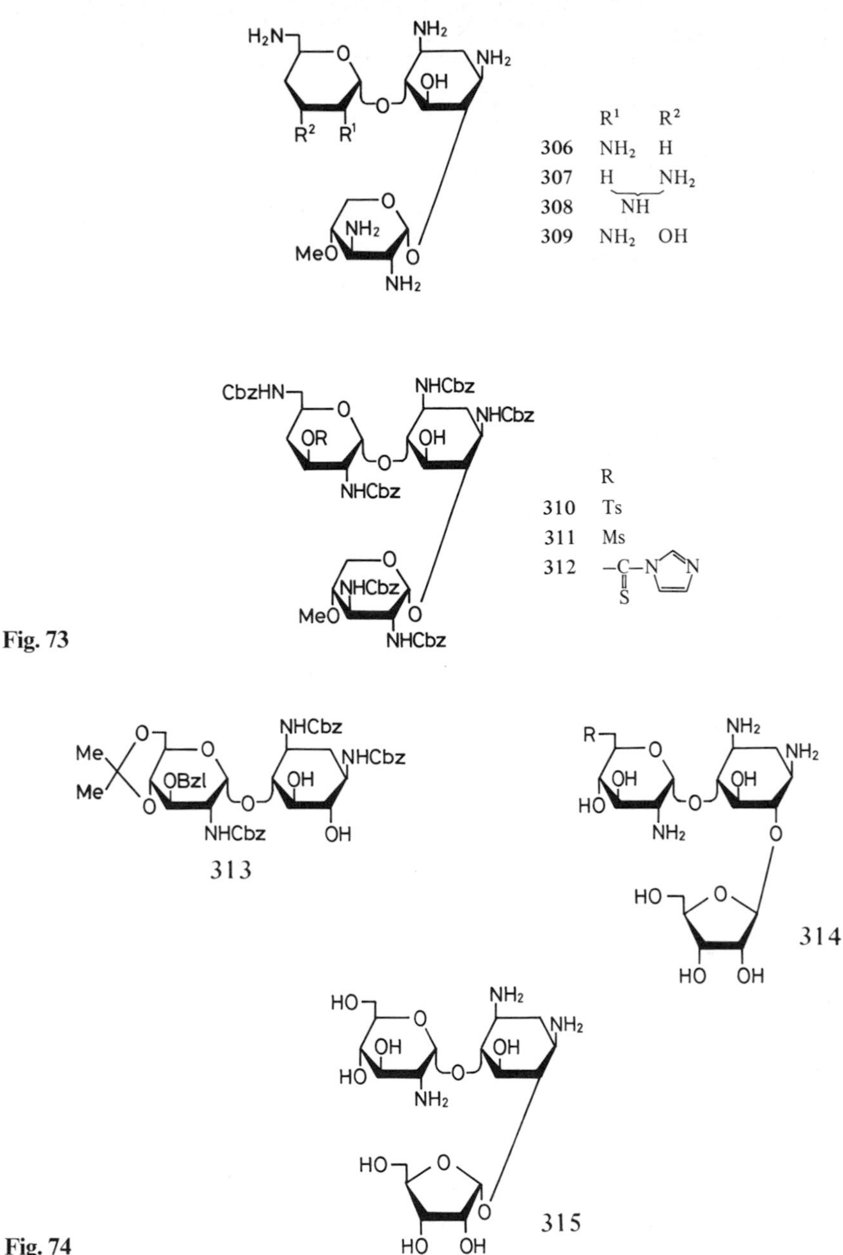

Fig. 73

Fig. 74

3′-phosphotransferases I and II. 6-*O*-(α-D-ribofuranosyl)paromamine (315) was also inactive (HANESSIAN et al. 1978c) (Fig. 74).

6-*O*-(*β*-D-Ribofuranosyl)neamine [(314), $R = NH_2$] was prepared (ARCAMONE et al. 1974; HANESSIAN et al. 1978c) from the above-mentioned condensation products via a series of reactions, including selective 6′-*O*-tosylation or bromination fol-

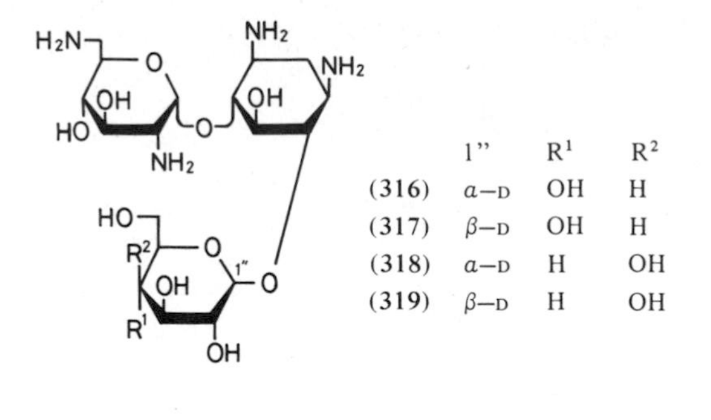

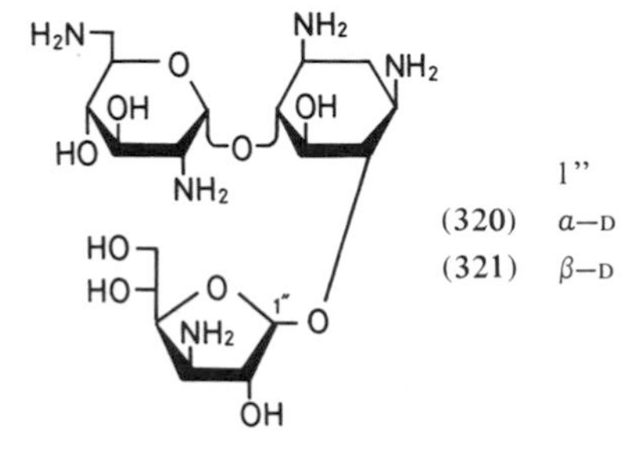

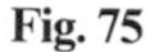
Fig. 75

lowed by amination. Compound [(314), $R = NH_2$] was also prepared (SUAMI et al. 1976) in a similar manner by condensation of 5,3′,4′-tri-*O*-acetyl-tetrakis(*N*-ethoxycarbonyl)neamine and (67). The 6-*O*-(β-D-ribofuranosyl)neamine was much less active than neamine. 6-*O*-(α-D-Glucopyranosyl)neamine (316) (MURASE et al. 1970), 6-*O*-(β-D-glucopyranosyl)- (317), 6-*O*-(α-D-galactopyranosyl)- (318), and 6-*O*-(β-D-galactopyranosyl)neamine (319) were also prepared (SUAMI et al. 1976); (316) and (318) showed activity similar to that of neamine, but (317) and (319) were much less active than neamine.

6-*O*-(3-Amino-3-deoxy-α-D-glucopyranosyl)neamine (320) and 6-*O*-(3-amino-3-deoxy-β-D-glucopyranosyl)neamine (321) were prepared (SITRIN et al. 1978) by similar condensation and were approximately 3% and 1%, respectively, as active as kanamycin B. These results indicate that, for antibacterial activity, substitution at the 6-hydroxyl group of 2-deoxystreptamine with α-D-glycopyranoses gives superior compounds than when other sugars are used (Fig. 75).

Highly active antibacterial compounds (326)–(328) were prepared (CHAZAN and GASC 1976) by condensation of protected neamine or deoxyneamine derivative (323)–(325) with the protected glycosyl halide of the 3-deoxy-3-methylamino sugar (322) derived from ethyl desosaminide via five steps. The 5-deoxy analog of (327) was also prepared (ROUSSEL-UCLAF 1977) (Fig. 76).

Two 4,6-disubstituted pseudotrisaccharides (330) and (331) of 2,5-dideoxystreptamine were prepared (CANAS-RODRIGUEZ and MARTINEZ-TOBED 1979) by condensation of *O*-acetylglucal and (329) which was prepared from di-*N*-benzyl-2-deoxystreptamine via five steps (activity was not described). A position isomer (332) of (331) prepared by CANAS-RODRIGUEZ (1977) was more active than kanamycin A (Fig. 77).

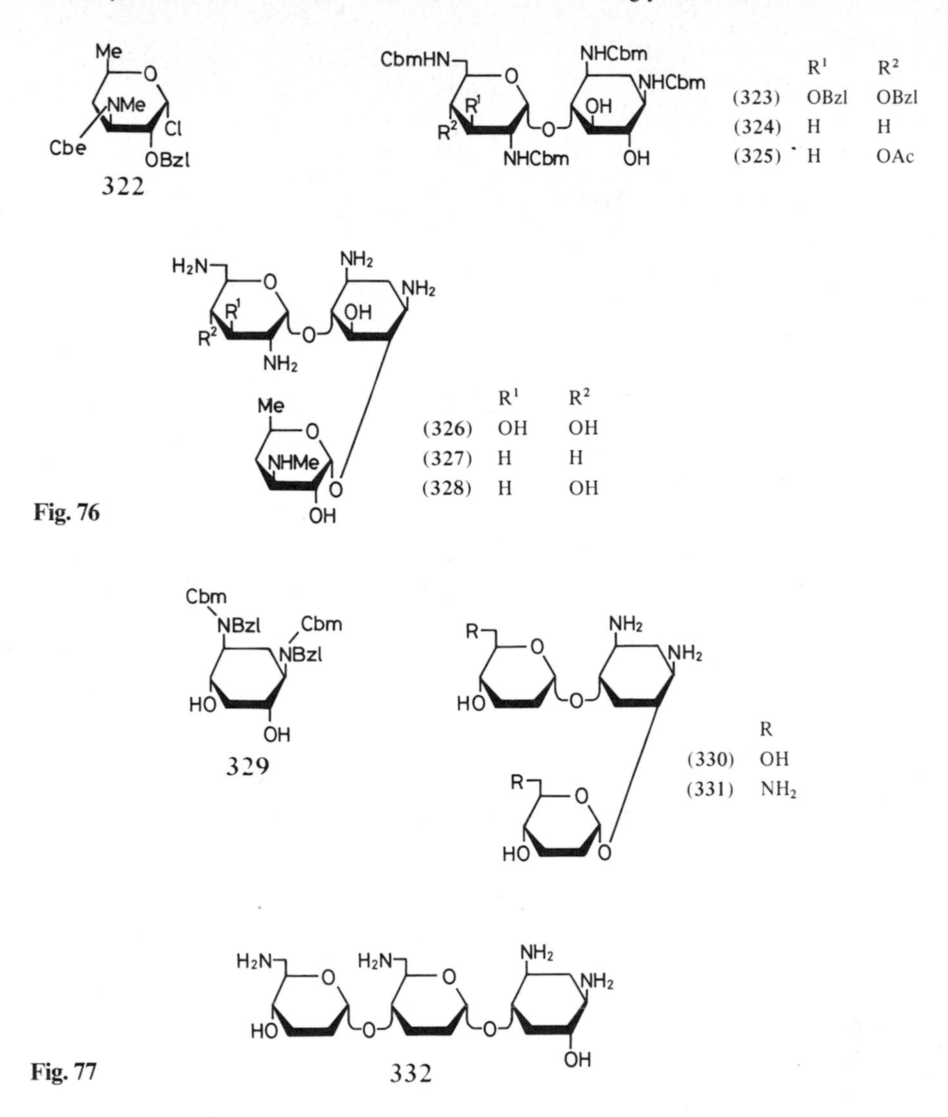

Fig. 76

Fig. 77

VI. Other Groups

1. Kasugamycin and Its Modifications

a) Total Synthesis of Kasugamycin

Kasugamycin has found commercial application as an agrochemical active against *Piricularia oryzae* in rice plants. Partial synthesis of kasugamycin (333) was accomplished by SUHARA et al. (1966) by treatment of kasuganobiosamine (334) with diethyl ester of oxalimidic acid followed by mild hydrolysis. Kasuganobiosamine has been synthesized by two groups of workers. SUHARA et al. (1968, 1972) prepared a nitroso dimer (338) starting from 3,4-dihydro-6-methyl-2*H*-pyran-2-one which, on condensation with a protected (+)-inositol followed by catalytic reduction and deprotection, gave kasuganobiosamine (334). Another synthesis (NAKAJIMA et al.

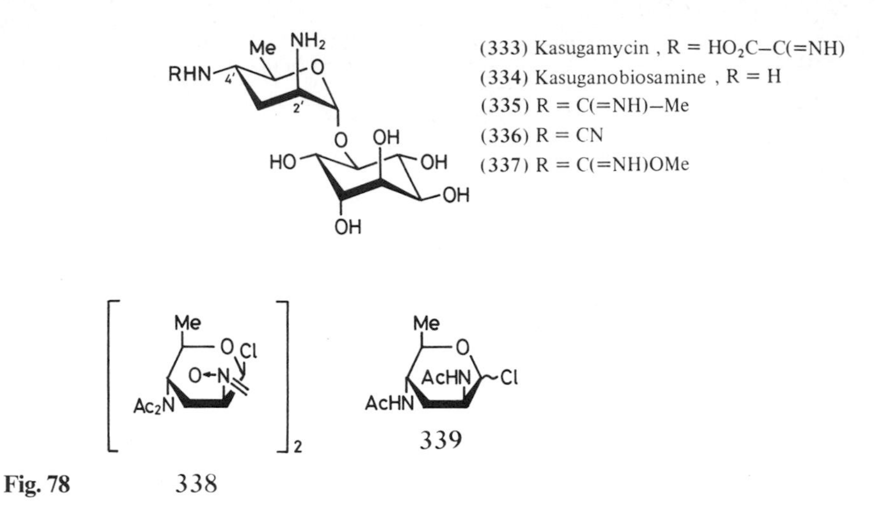

Fig. 78

1968b; KITAHARA et al. 1969) involved condensation of a glycosyl chloride of kasugamine (339) with the protected inositol. Synthesis of an enantiomorph, (–)-kasuganobiosamine was also reported (DAVID and LUBINEAU 1977). Several other syntheses of kasugaminide have been reported (YASUDA et al. 1973; YOSHIMURA et al. 1977) (Fig. 78).

b) Kasugamycin Modifications

The carboxyl group of kasugamycin has been replaced by various alkyl and aryl groups. The 2′-amino group of kasugamycin was protected with dimedone and the oxalamidino group was removed by alkaline hydrolysis. The 4′-amino group thus liberated reacted with a number of imido esters [R-C(=NH)-OEt] to give, after removal of the dimedone group, various guanidino derivatives of kasuganobiosamine (CRON et al. 1969). The methyl derivative (335) was found to be more active than the parent antibiotic. A patent (H. UMEZAWA and SUHARA 1976) for the preparation of similar derivatives involved oxidative decarboxylation of kasugamycin with sodium hypobromite to give a nitrile (336), which was converted into an imido ester (337) by treatment with hydrogen chloride in methanol and finally into various guanidino derivatives by reaction with amines.

2. Spectinomycin Group

a) Total Synthesis of Spectinomycin

Spectinomycin (actinospectacin) (344) has a unique structure including a fused-ring aminocyclitol. Its total synthesis has recently been accomplished by WHITE et al. (1979) (Fig. 79). Condensation of *N,N′*-bis(benzyloxycarbonyl)actinamine with nitroso dimer (340) gave an oxime (341) in which α-glycosylation occurred at the C-5 hydroxyl of actinamine. Deoximation with benzaldehyde then gave the unnatural hemiacetal (342); however, treatment of (342) with anhydrous potassium bicarbonate in acetonitrile successfully generated the desired enoneacetate (343). Finally, hydrolysis followed by catalytic hydrogenation completed the synthesis of spectinomycin (344).

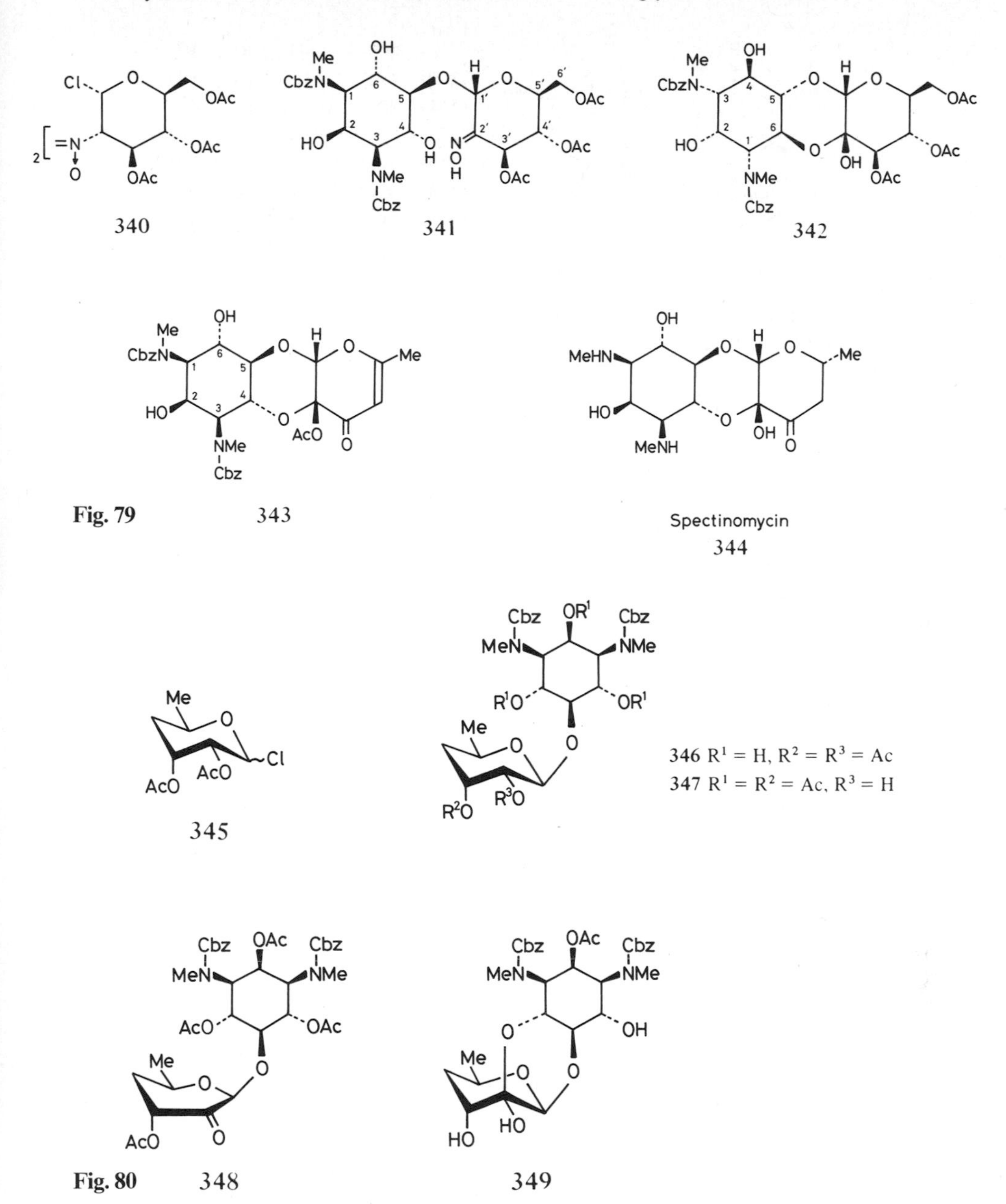

Fig. 79

Fig. 80

HANESSIAN and ROY (1979a, b) have recently described another stereospecific synthesis of spectinomycin. This synthesis involved condensation of *N,N'*-bis(benzyloxycarbonyl)actinamine with 4,6-dideoxy-D-ribohexopyranosyl chloride (345) to give the glycoside (346), which was, after deacetylation, regiospecifically acetylated by the ring opening of the corresponding orthoamide or orthoester derivatives to give (347). Oxidation then gave the keto derivative (348) and this, on con-

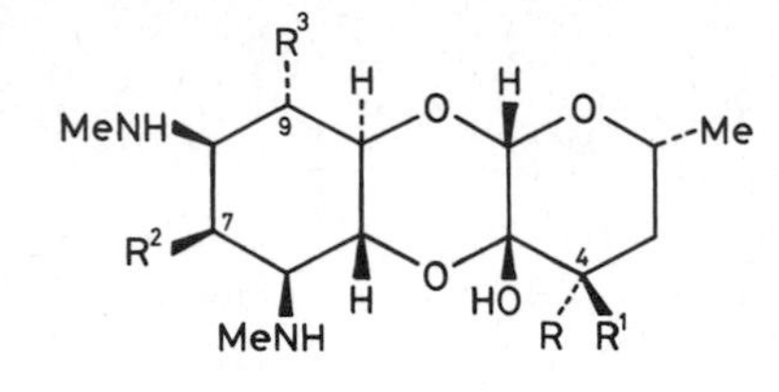

	R	R¹	R²	R³
(350)	OH	H	OH	OH
(351)	H	OH	OH	OH
(352)	H	OH	H	OH
(353)	R and R¹ =O		H	OH
(354)	R and R¹ =O		OH	H
(355)	H	OH	OH	H

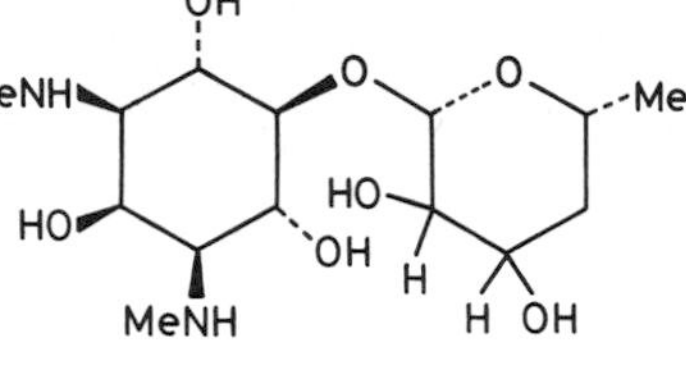
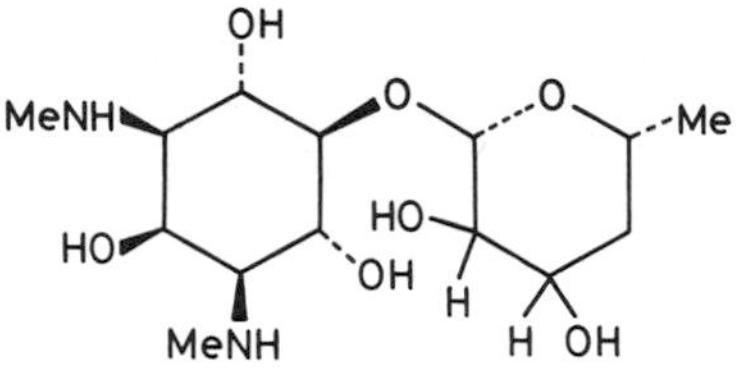

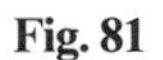

Fig. 81 356

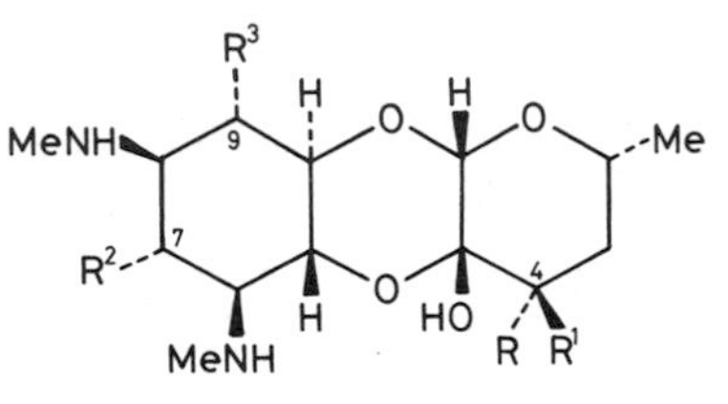

(357) R and R^1 = O, R^2 = OH, R^3 = OH
(358) R = H, R^1 = OH, R^2 = OH, R^3 = H

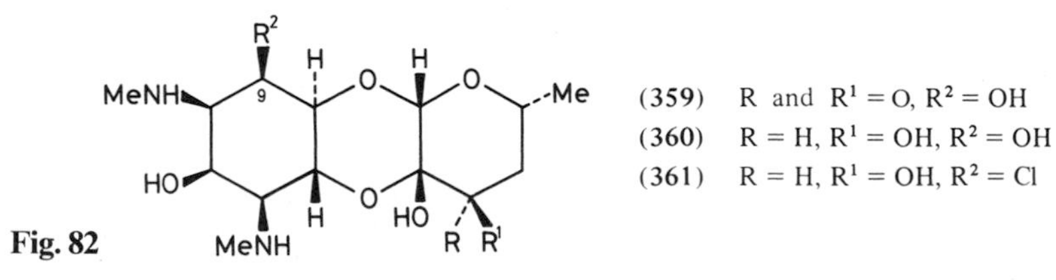

(359) R and R^1 = O, R^2 = OH
(360) R = H, R^1 = OH, R^2 = OH
(361) R = H, R^1 = OH, R^2 = Cl

Fig. 82

trolled deacetylation with sodium methoxide, afforded the desired tricyclic derivative (349), which led to spectinomycin by a sequence of reactions involving the specific oxidation of the axial C-3′ hydroxyl group (Fig. 80).

b) Modification of Spectinomycin

Reduction of spectinomycin with sodium borohydride gave 4(*S*)-dihydrospectinomycin (350) while catalytic hydrogenation gave a mixture of 4(*S*)- and 4(*R*)-dihydrospectinomycin (351) (WILEY et al. 1963), both of which have decreased activity. Further reduction gave four tetrahydrospectinomycins (356) (KNIGHT and HOEKSEMA 1975), one of which was synthesized by a conventional glycoside synthesis (SUAMI et al. 1977c) (Fig. 81).

Several modifications involving the 7- and 9-hydroxyl groups have been reported. 7-Epi-spectinomycin (357) (ROSENBROOK et al. 1975), 7-epi-9-deoxy-4(*R*)-dihy-

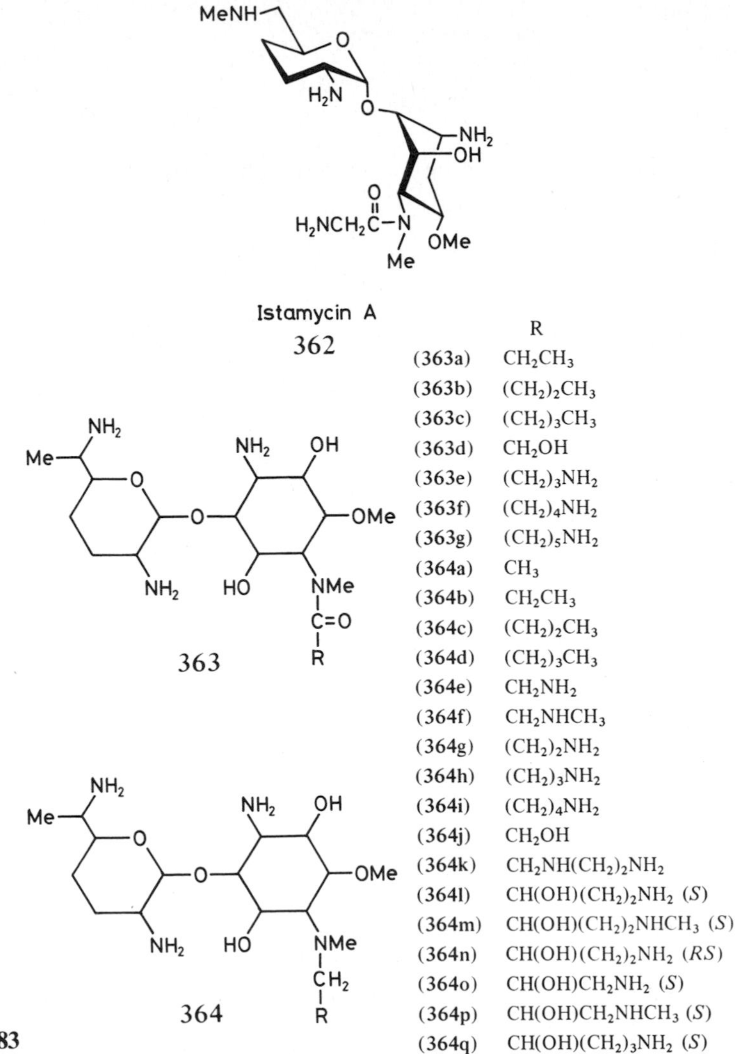

	R
(363a)	CH_2CH_3
(363b)	$(CH_2)_2CH_3$
(363c)	$(CH_2)_3CH_3$
(363d)	CH_2OH
(363e)	$(CH_2)_3NH_2$
(363f)	$(CH_2)_4NH_2$
(363g)	$(CH_2)_5NH_2$
(364a)	CH_3
(364b)	CH_2CH_3
(364c)	$(CH_2)_2CH_3$
(364d)	$(CH_2)_3CH_3$
(364e)	CH_2NH_2
(364f)	CH_2NHCH_3
(364g)	$(CH_2)_2NH_2$
(364h)	$(CH_2)_3NH_2$
(364i)	$(CH_2)_4NH_2$
(364j)	CH_2OH
(364k)	$CH_2NH(CH_2)_2NH_2$
(364l)	$CH(OH)(CH_2)_2NH_2$ (*S*)
(364m)	$CH(OH)(CH_2)_2NHCH_3$ (*S*)
(364n)	$CH(OH)(CH_2)_2NH_2$ (*RS*)
(364o)	$CH(OH)CH_2NH_2$ (*S*)
(364p)	$CH(OH)CH_2NHCH_3$ (*S*)
(364q)	$CH(OH)(CH_2)_3NH_2$ (*S*)

Fig. 83

drospectinomycin (358) (ROSENBROOK and CARNEY 1975), 7-deoxy-4(*R*)-dihydrospectinomycin (352) (ROSENBROOK et al. 1978), 7-deoxyspectinomycin (353), and 7-deoxy-8-epi-4(*R*)-dihydrospectinomycin (FOLEY et al. 1979) were devoid of activity. Attempts to overcome enzymatic adenylylation at the 9 position by preparing 9-deoxyspectinomycin (354), 9-deoxy-4(*R*)-dihydrospectinomycin (355) (FOLEY et al. 1978a), 9-epi-spectinomycin (359), 9-epi-4(*R*)-dihydrospectinomycin (360) (FOLEY et al. 1978b), 9-chloro-9-deoxy-4(*R*)-dihydrospectinomycin (361) (CARNEY and ROSENBROOK 1977), and its 9 epimer resulted in inactive products (Fig. 82).

4(*R*)-Amino-4-deoxydihydrospectinomycin has recently been claimed to have significant activity (MAIER et al. 1979). Recent advances in this field were reviewed by ROSENBROOK (1979).

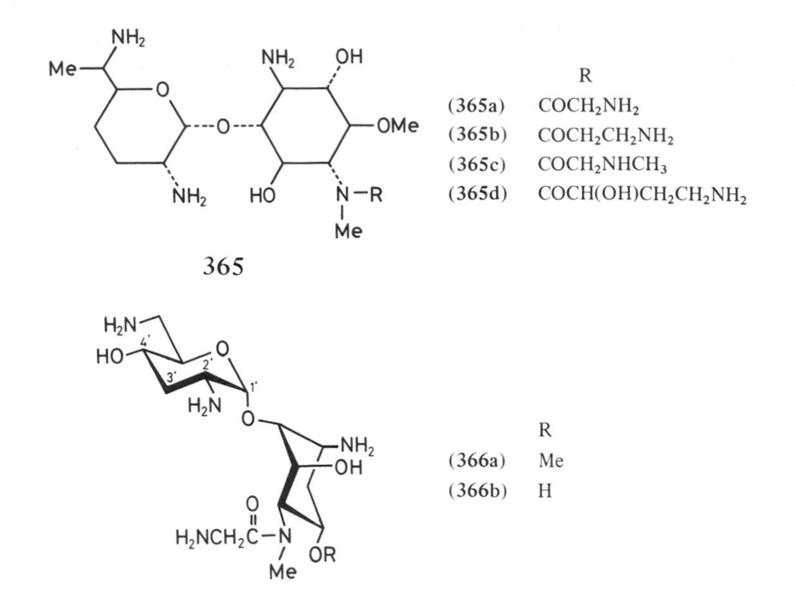

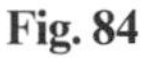
Fig. 84

3. Fortimicins, Istamycins, and Related Compounds

The total synthesis of istamycin A (362) has recently been accomplished by transformation of 3′,4′-dideoxyneamine (D. IKEDA et al. 1979b) (Fig. 83).

SATO and MORI (1979) described the synthesis and antibacterial activities of 4-*N*-acyl and 4-*N*-alkyl derivatives of fortimicin B. The 4-*N*-acyl derivatives, which are relatively unstable to alkaline conditions, were converted into stable 4-*N*-alkyl derivatives by diborane reduction. Derivatives substituted by a simple aliphatic residue (363a)–(363c) and (364a)–(364d) had almost no activity, while introduction of hydroxyl or amino group(s) produced significant activity. 4-*N*-(2-Aminoethyl)- (364e), 4-*N*-[(*S*)-4-amino-2-hydroxybutyl]- (364l), and 4-*N*-[(*S*)-2-hydroxy-4-methylaminobutyl]-fortimicin B (364m) were most potent (Fig. 83).

4-*N*-Glycyl- (365a), 4-*N*-*β*-alanyl- (365b), 4-*N*-sarcosyl- (365c), and 4-*N*-(L-4-amino-2-hydroxybutyryl)-fortimicin E (365d) showed only weak activity against several gram-positive and gram-negative bacteria (KURATH et al. 1979) (Fig. 84).

2-Deoxy-4-*N*-glycyl-6-*O*-(α-nebrosaminyl)fortamine (366a) and 3-de-*O*-methyl-2-deoxy-4-*N*-glycyl-6-*O*-(α-nebrosaminyl)fortamine (366b), which have an additional hydroxyl group at C-4′, have recently been prepared from lividamine by several steps involving transformation of the 2-deoxystreptamine moiety into 4-*N*,3-*O*-didemethyl-2-deoxyfortamine (YAMAGUCHI et al. 1979). These derivatives have a somewhat lower activity than sporaricin A.

4. Sorbistins and Analogs

Sorbistins have unique structures containing a 1,4-diamino-1,4-dideoxyaditol instead of an aminocyclitol moiety. Sorbistin A_1 (367) has been synthesized by OGAWA et al. (1978). The total synthesis involved condensation of a glycosyl chloride (371) having a benzyloxy group at C-2 with a tributyltin alkoxide derivative (372)

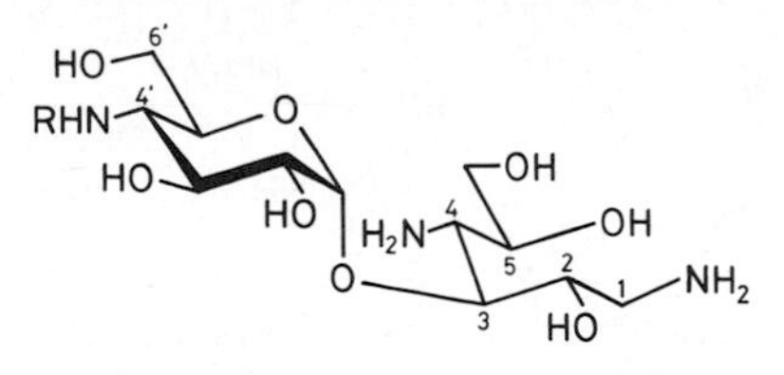

(**367**) Sorbistin A_1 : R = EtCO
(**368**) Sorbistin B : R = MeCO
(**369**) Sorbistin D : R = H
(**370a**~**370p**): see Table 1.

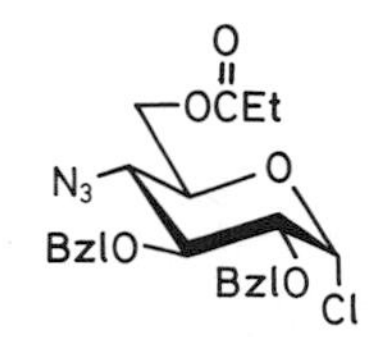

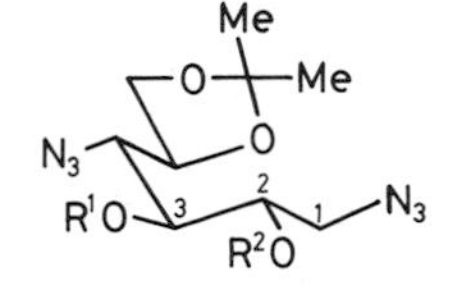

Fig. 85 371 (372) R^1, R^2 = H, $SnBu_3$

Table 1. 4'-*N*-Acyl analogs of sorbistin

Compound	R
(370a)	$—COCH(OH)CH_2CH_2NHCbz$ (L)
(370b)	$—COCH(OH)CH_2CH_2NH_2$ (L)
(370c)	$—COC_6H_5$
(370d)	$—COCH(NHCbz)CH_3$(L)
(370e)	$—COCH(NH_2)CH_3$(L)
(370f)	$—COCH_2CH_2NHCbz$
(370g)	$—COCH_2CH_2NH_2$
(370h)	$—COCH(CH_3)_2$
(370i)	$-COCH(OH)CH_3$(DL)
(370j)	$—COCH(Cl)CH_3$(DL)
(370k)	$—COCH_2NHCbz$
(370l)	$—COCH_2NH_2$
(370m)	$—COCHCl_2$
(370n)	$—COCH_2C_6H_5$
(370o)	—CO—◁
(370p)	$—CO(CH_2)_3CH_3$

in dichloromethane in the presence of tetraethylammonium chloride, followed by column chromatographic separation and subsequent hydrolysis, to give two α-glycosides, namely 3-*O*- and 2-*O*-glycoside. Selective hydrogenation with Lindler catalyst followed by treatment with acetic acid in ethanol (acyl-migration) and catalytic hydrogenolysis (of the benzyl groups) gave sorbistin A_1 and a position isomer.

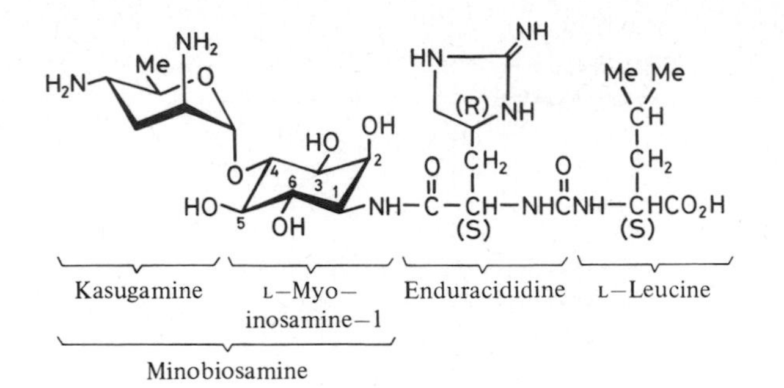

(373) Minosaminomycin

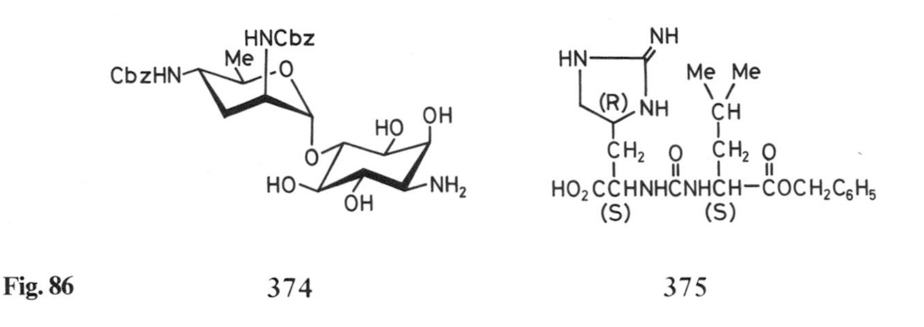

A number of *N*-acyl analogs of sorbistin were prepared via a key intermediate which was derived from sorbistin A_1 and B by blocking the 1- and 4-amino groups of the sorbistins with dimedone followed by deacylation of the 4′-*N*-acyl group. 4′-*N*-Acylation of the intermediate followed by deblocking gave 4′-*N*-acyl analogs (370a)–(370p) (Table 1). 1-*N*-Acyl, 1,4′-*N*,*N*-diacyl, 4-*N*-acyl, and 4,4′-*N*,*N*-diacyl analogs were further prepared. The 4′-*N*-propionyl (sorbistin A_1) and 4′-*N*-cyclopropylcarbonyl (370o) analogs were the most active members of the 4′-*N*-acyl derivatives. 1-*N*- and 4-*N*-Acylation gave inactive products (NAITO et al. 1976).

4′-*N*-Propylsorbistin D and A_1 and 6′-chloro-6′-deoxysorbistin A_1 were prepared and had moderate activities (PONPIPOM et al. 1978). 1-*N*-Alkyl, 4-*N*-ethyl, and 4′-*N*-alkyl analogs of sorbistin A_1 were also prepared by another group of workers (K. NARA et al. 1979).

5. Minosaminomycin

Minosaminomycin (373) is closely related to kasugamycin in that it contains kasugamine and L-*myo*-inosamine-1. The total synthesis of minosaminomycin has been accomplished by IINUMA et al. (1977) (Fig. 86). Minobiosamine, the glycoside portion of minosaminomycin, was synthesized from kasuganobiosamine (334). Catalytic oxidation of 2′,4′-di-*N*-acetylkasuganobiosamine with platinum black followed by treatment with hydroxylamine gave a mixture of ketoximes. Reduction of the mixture with sodium amalgam followed by alkaline hydrolysis gave a mixture containing 4-*O*- and 5-*O*-(α-D-kasugaminyl) glycosides of the inosamine, which were separated by column chromatography. The former was identical to the

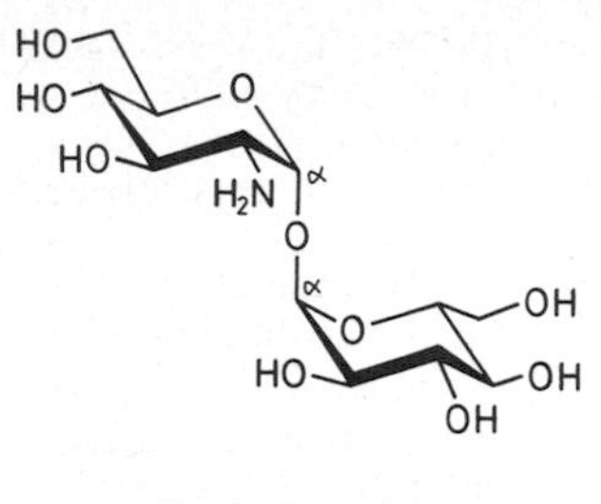

Fig. 87 376

natural minobiosamine. Coupling of 2′,4′-bis(*N*-benzyloxycarbonyl)-minobiosamine (374) with N^{α}[(*S*)-1-(benzyloxycarbonyl)-3-methylbutylcarbamoyl]enduracididine (375) followed by deblocking completed the synthesis of minosaminomycin. Enduracididine found in the antibiotic enduracidin was synthesized by TSUJI et al. (1975).

A diastereomer of minosaminomycin was synthesized from alloenduracididine instead of enduracididine and had about 20% of the bacteriostatic activity of minosaminomycin (IINUMA et al. 1977).

6. Alpha, Alpha-Trehalosamine

Trehalosamine (376) produced by an actinomycete is an unusual antibiotic, being a nonreducing disaccharide and active against acid-fast bacilli (Fig. 87). S. UMEZAWA et al. (1967b) synthesized trehalosamine by condensation of 3,4,6-tri-*O*-acetyl-2-deoxy-2-(*p*-methoxybenzylidene)amino-α-D-gluxopyranosyl chloride with 2,3,4,6-tetra-*O*-benzyl-α-D-glucose followed by hydrolysis and catalytic hydrogenolysis. In another recent synthesis by PAULSEN and SUMFLETH (1979), 6-*O*-acetyl-2-azido-3,4-di-*O*-benzyl-2-deoxy-β-D-glucopyranosyl chloride has been used as a glycosyl halide.

6,6′-Diamino-6,6′-dideoxy-α,α-trehalose (S. UMEZAWA et al. 1967a), 6-amino-6-deoxy-α,α-trehalose (HANESSIAN and LAVALLEE 1972), 3,3′-diamino-3,3′-dideoxy-α,α-trehalose (BAER and BELL 1978) and 3-amino-3-deoxy-α,α-trehalose (BAER and BELL 1979) have also been synthesized.

References

Abe Y, Nakagawa S, Fujisawa K, Naito T, Kawaguchi H (1977) Aminoglycoside antibiotics. XI. synthesis and activity of 4′-deoxykanamycin B. J Antibiot (Tokyo) 30:1004–1007

Akita E, Horiuchi Y, Miyazawa T (1979a) Synthesis of 3′-epi-4′-deoxykanamycin B through 3′-epi-3′,4′-anhydro intermediate. Heterocycles 13:157–162

Akita E, Horiuchi Y, Miyazawa T, Umezawa H (1979b) 1-*N*-(ω-Aminoalkanesulfonyl) derivatives of aminoglycosidic antibiotics. German patent 2,825,289. Chem Abstr 90:204434n

Albano E, Horton D, Tsuchiya T (1966) Synthesis and reactions of unsaturated sugar. IV. Methyl 4,6-*O*-benzylidene-α-D-erythro-hex-2-enopyranoside and its hydrolysis by acid. Carbohydr Res 2:349–362

Arcamone F, Cassinelli G, Cuccia PB, Di Colo G (1974) Synthesis of β-D-ribofuranosyl derivatives of paromamine. Ann Chim 64:485–496
Asako T, Yoshioka K, Mabuchi H, Hiraga K (1978) Chemical transformation of 3′-chloro-3′-deoxyaminoglycosides into new cyclic pseudotrisaccharides. Heterocycles 11:197–202
Baer H, Bell AJ (1978) Synthesis of 3,3′-dinitro and 3,3′-diamino derivatives of α,α-trehalose and its D-gluco, D-manno and D-manno, D-manno isomers. Can J Chem 56:2872–2878
Baer H, Bell AJ (1979) The synthesis of 3-amino-3-deoxy-α-D-glucopyranosyl-α-D-glycopyranoside (3-amino-3-deoxy-α,α-trehalose). Carbohydr Res 75:175–184
Barlow CB, Guthrie RD (1967) Configurational studies on amino-sugars using cuprammonium solutions. J Chem Soc (C) 1194–1197
Barlow CB, Bukhari ST, Guthrie RD, Prior AM (1979) Study of cuprammonium complexing of diols and amino-alcohols using circular dichroism techniques. J Carbohydr Nucleosides Nucleotides 6:81–99
Barrett AGM, Barton DHR, Bielski R (1979) Reactions of relevance to the chemistry of aminoglycoside antibiotics. Part 11. Preparation of olefines from vicinal diols. J Chem Soc [Perkin I] 2378–2381
Barton DHR, McCombie SW (1975) A new method for the deoxygenation of secondary alcohols. J Chem Soc [Perkin I] 1574–1585
Barton DHR, Subramanian R (1977) Reactions of relevance to the chemistry of aminoglycoside antibiotics. Part 7. Conversion of thiocarbonate into deoxy-sugars. J Chem Soc [Perkin I] 1718–1728
Bartz QR, Controulis J, Crooks HM Jr, Rebstock MC (1946) Dihydrostreptomycin. J Am Chem Soc 68:2163–2166
Bell RH, Horton D, Williams DM, Winter-Mihaly E (1977) Photochemical conversion of sugar dimethylthiocarbamates into deoxy sugars. Carbohydr Res 58:109–124
Billingham NC, Jackson RA, Malek F (1977) Radical-initiated reduction of chloroformates to alkanes by tri-*n*-propylsilane: removal of unwanted hydroxyl groups from organic molecules. J Chem Soc Chem Commun 344–345
Bodanszky M (1954) Streptomycin derivatives. Acta Chim Acad Sci Hung 5:97–104; Chem Abstr 50:354
Bristol-Myers Co (1973) γ-Aminoacylation of tobramycin. German patent 2,311,524
Bystricky S, Fric I, Stanek J, Capec K, Jary J, Blaha K (1979) Conformation of 3-acetamido-3,6-dideoxyhexopyranosides: circular dichroism study. Czech Acad Sci 44:174–182
Canas-Rodriguez A (1977) Synthetic aminoglycosides. German patent 2,726,113; Chem Abstr 88:170438 h
Canas-Rodriguez A, Martinez-Tobed A (1979) The synthesis of 2,5-dideoxy-4,6-di-*O*-(2,3-dideoxy-α-D-erythro-hexopyranosyl)streptamine and 4,6-di-*O*-(6-amino-2,3,6-trideoxy-α-D-erythro-hexopyranosyl)-2,5-dideoxystreptamine. Carbohydr Res 68:43–53
Canas-Rodriguez A, Ruiz-Poveda SG (1977) Syntheses of 3′,4′,5,6-tetradeoxyneamine and 5,6-dideoxyneamine. Carbohydr Res 58:379–385
Carney RE, McAlpine JE (1978) Use of copper (II) ion in selective acylation of seldomycin factor 5. Abstracts of the 175th National Meeting of the Am Chem Soc, Anaheim Calif. March 13-17 Paper CARB 46
Carney RE, Rosenbrook W Jr (1977) Spectinomycin modification. III. Chlorodeoxy analogs. J Antibiot (Tokyo) 30:960–964
Carney RE, McAlpine JB, Jackson M, Stanaszek RS, Washburn WH, Cirovic M, Mueller SL (1978) Modification of seldomycin factor 5 at C-3′. J Antibiot (Tokyo) 31:441–450
Cassinelli G, Franceschi G, Dicols G, Arcamone F (1978 a) Semisynthetic aminoglycoside antibiotics. I. New reactions of paromomycin and synthesis of its 2′-*N*-ethyl derivative. J Antibiot (Tokyo) 31:379–381
Cassinelli G, Julita P, Arcamone F (1978 b) Semisynthetic aminoglycoside antibiotics. II. Synthesis of analogues of paromomycin modified in the glucosamine moiety. J Antibiot (Tokyo) 31:382–384
Chazan JB, Gasc JC (1976) Synthese d'antibiotiques aminosidiques á partir de desosamine. Tetrahedron Lett 3145–3148

Claes P, Vanderhaeghe H, Verlody L (1971) Preparation of dideguanylstreptomycylamine and bis-*N*,*N*′-(dideguanylstreptomycyl)-*p*-xylylenediamine. Bull Soc Chim Belg 80:659–667
Cléophax J, Duc DK, Dalaumény JM, Géro SD, Rolland A (1978a) Synthesis of α-linked 3′-deoxy-cyclitol and -aminocyclitol glycosides. J Chem Soc Chem Commun 771–773
Cléophax J, Delaumény JM, Gero SD, Rolland A, Rolland N (1978b) Synthesis of α-linked 3′-deoxy-pseudo-di- and -tri-saccharides related to aminocyclitol-glycoside antibiotics. J Chem Soc Chem Commun 773–773
Collins PM, Munasinghe VRZ (1977) Photochemical preparations of deoxysugars from carbohydrate esters: a simple synthesis of methyl amicetoside. J Chem Soc Chem Commun 927–928
Cox DA, Richardson K, Ross BC (1977) The aminoglycosides. In: Sammes PG (ed) Topics in antibiotic chemistry, vol 1. Wiley & Sons, New York London Sydney Toronto, pp 1–90
Cron MJ, Smith RE, Hooper IR, Keil JG, Ragan EA, Schreiber RH, Schwab G, Godfrey JC (1969) Preparation of semisynthetic kasugamycin derivatives. I. Aliphatic amidino derivatives of kasuganobiosamine. Antimicrob Agents Chemother 219–224
Cron MJ, Keil JG, Lin JS, Ruggeri MV, Walker D (1979) Selective *N*-acylation of kanamycin A. J Chem Soc Chem Commun 266–267
Culbertson TP, Watson DR, Haskell TH (1973) 5″-Amino-5″-deoxybutirosin, a new semisynthetic aminoglycoside antibiotic. J Antibiot (Tokyo) 26:790–793
Daniels PJL (1975) 2″-Deoxyaminoglycosides and 2″-epi-amino-3″-desamino derivatives and intermediates. US patent 3,920,628; Chem Abstr 84:59967h
Daniels PJL (1978) Aminoacyl derivatives of aminoglycoside antibiotics. US patent 4,117,221; Chem Abstr 90:87839k
Daniels PJL, McCombie SW (1977) 5-Deoxy-4,6-di-*O*-(aminoglycosyl)-1,3-diaminocyclitols and their use as antibacterial agents. US patent 4,053,591; Chem Abstr 88:23338x
Daniels PJL, Rane DF (1978) 5-Epifluoro-5-deoxy derivatives. S African patent 7806,385; Chem Abstr 90:104301y
Daniels PJL, Weinstein J, Nagabhushan TL (1974) The syntheses of 1-*N*-[(*S*)-4-amino-2-hydroxybutyryl]gentamicin C_1 and 1-*N*-[(*S*)-3-amino-2-hydroxypropionyl]gentamicin C_1. J Antibiot (Tokyo) 27:889–893
Daniels PJL, Luce C, Nagabhushan TL, Jaret RS, Schumacher D, Reimann H, Ilavsky J (1975) The gentamicin antibiotics. 6. Gentamicin C_{2b}, an aminoglycoside antibiotic produced by *Micromonospora purpurea* mutant JI-33. J Antibiot (Tokyo) 28:35–41
Daniels PJL, Jaret RS, Nagabhushan TL, Turner WN (1976a) The structure of antibiotic G-52, a new aminocyclitol-aminoglycoside antibiotic produced by *Micromonospora zionesis*. J Antibiot (Tokyo) 29:488–491
Daniels PJL, Mallams AK, Weinstein J, Wright JJ (1976b) Mass spectral studies on aminoglycoside antibiotics. J Chem Soc [Perkin I] 1087–1088
Daniels PJL, Cooper AB, McCombie SW, Nagabhushan TL, Rane DF, Wright JJ (1979) Some recent advances in the chemistry of antibiotics of the gentamicin series. Jpn J Antibiot [Suppl] 32:S195–S204
David S, Lubineau A (1977) Cycloaddition as a synthetic method in the field of aminoglycoside antibiotics. Nouv J Chim 1:375–376
Davies DH, Mallams AK (1978) Semisynthetic aminoglycoside antibacterials. 6. Synthesis of sisomicin, antibiotic G-52, and novel 6′-substituted analogues of sisomicin from aminoglycoside 66-40C. J Med Chem 21:189–193
Davies DH, Greeves D, Mallams AK, Morton JB, Tkach RW (1975) Structure of the aminoglycoside antibiotics 66-40B and 66-40D produced by *Micromonospora inyoensis*. J Chem Soc [Perkin I] 814–818
Davies DH, Mallams AK, McGlotten J, Morton JB, Tkach RW (1977) Structure of aminoglycoside 66-40C, a novel unsaturated imine produced by *Micromonospora inyoensis*. J Chem Soc [Perkin I] 1407–1411
Deshayes H, Pete J, Portella C, Scholler D (1975) Photolysis of carboxylic esters: Conversion of alcohols into alkanes. J Chem Soc Chem Commun 439–440

Doi O, Ogura M, Tanaka N, Umezawa H (1968) Inactivation of kanamycin, neomycin, and streptomycin by enzymes obtained in cells of *Pseudomonas aeruginosa*. Appl Environ Microbiol 16:1276–1281
Dorman DE, Paschal JW, Merkel KE (1976) ^{15}N Nuclear magnetic resonance spectroscopy. The nebramycin aminoglycosides. J Am Chem Soc 98:6885–6888
Dutcher JD, Hosansky N, Donin MN, Wintersteiner O (1951) Neomycin B and C, and some of their degradation products. J Am Chem Soc 73:1384–1385
Dyer JR, McGonigal WE, Rice KC (1965) Streptomycin. II. Streptose. J Am Chem Soc 87:654–655
Egan RS, DeVault RL, Mueller SL, Levenberg MI, Sinclair AC, Stanaszek RU (1975) A new antibiotic XK-62-2. III. The structure of XK-62-2, a new gentamicin C complex antibiotic. J Antibiot (Tokyo) 28:29–34
Egan RS, Sinclair AC, De Vault RL, McAlpine JB, Mueller SL, Goodley PC, Stanaszek RS, Cirovic M, Mauritz RJ, Mitscher LA, Shirahara K, Sato S, Iida T (1977) A new aminoglycoside antibiotic complex – the seldomycins. III. The structure of seldomycin factors 1 and 2. J Antibiot (Tokyo) 30:31–38
Endo T, Perlman D (1972) Transglycosylation of neamine. J Antibiot (Tokyo) 25:681–682
Evans ME, Parrish FW, Long L Jr (1967) Acetal exchange reaction. Carbohydr Res 3:453–462
Foley L, Lin JTS, Weigele M (1978a) Spectinomycin chemistry. II. 9-Deoxy-4(*R*)-dihydrospectinomycin and 9-deoxyspectinomycin. J Antibiot (Tokyo) 31:979–984
Foley L, Lin JTS, Weigele M (1978b) Spectinomycin chemistry. III. 9-Epi-4(*R*)-dihydrospectinomycin and 9-epi-spectinomycin. J Antibiot (Tokyo) 31:985–990
Foley L, Lin JTS, Weigele M (1979) Preparation of 7-deoxyspectinomycin and 7-deoxy-8-epi-4(*R*)-dihydrospectinomycin. J Antibiot (Tokyo) 32:418–419
Fukami H, Sano H, Nakajima M (1975) Synthesis of a positional isomer of neamine: 5-*O*-(2,6-diacetamido-2,6-dideoxy-α-D-glucopyranosyl)-*N*,*N'*-diacetyl-2-deoxystreptamine. Agric Biol Chem 39:1097–1101
Fukami H, Kitahara K, Nakajima M (1976) Total synthesis of ribostamycin. Tetrahedron Lett 545–548
Fukami H, Kohno H, Kitahara K, Nakajima M (1977a) Syntheses of ribofuranosyl-2-deoxystreptamines. Agric Biol Chem 41:1685–1688
Fukami H, Ikeda S, Kitahara K, Nakajima M (1977b) Total synthesis of ribostamycin. Agric Biol Chem 41:1689–1694
Fukase H, Mizokami N, Horii S (1978) A new method for the 3'-deoxygenation of butirosin A and B. Carbohydr Res 60:289–302
Golubev VN, Koroleva VG, Vasil'ev VK, Lazareva EN (1970) Long-acting streptomycin. Antibiotiki (in Russian) 15:491–494; Chem Abstr 73:64657j
Hanessian S, Haskell TH (1970) Antibiotics containing sugars. In: Pigmann H, Horton D (eds) The carbohydrates chemistry and biochemistry, vol II A. Academic Press, New York London, pp 139–211
Hanessian S, Lavallée P (1972) Synthesis of 6-amino-6-deoxy-α,α-trehalose: A positional isomer of trehalosamine. J Antibiot (Tokyo) 25:683–688
Hanessian S, Patil G (1978) Aminoglycoside antibiotics – a method for selective *N*-acylation based on the temporary protection of amino alcohol functions as copper chelates. Tetrahedron Lett 1035–1038
Hanessian S, Roy R (1979a) Synthesis of (+)-spectinomycin. J Am Chem Soc 101:5839–5841
Hanessian S, Roy R (1979b) Studies directed toward the total synthesis of antibiotics: (+)-spectinomycin. Jpn J Antibiot (Tokyo) [Suppl] 32:S73–S90
Hanessian S, Butterworth RF, Nakagawa T (1973) Aminoglycoside antibiotics: chemical transformation of paromamine into 3'-epiparomamine. Carbohydr Res 26:261–263
Hanessian S, Takamoto T, Massé R (1975) Aminoglycoside antibiotics: oxidative degradation leading to novel biochemical probes and synthetic intermediates. J Antibiot (Tokyo) 28:835–837
Hanessian S, Massé R, Capmeau ML (1977) Aminoglycoside antibiotics: synthesis of 5''-amino-5''-deoxyneomycin and 5''-amino-5''-deoxyparomomycin. J Antibiot (Tokyo) 30:893–896

Hanessian S, Takamoto T, Massé R, Patil G (1978 a) Aminoglycoside antibiotics: chemical conversion of neomycin B, paromomycin, and lividomycin B into bioactive pseudosaccharides. Can J Chem 56:1482–1491
Hanessian S, Massé R, Ekborg G (1978 b) Aminoglycoside antibiotics: the formation and characterization of dihydroxazine derivatives in the paromomycin series. Can J Chem 56:1492–1499
Hanessian S, Ogawa T, Takamoto T (1978 c) Aminoglycoside antibiotics: synthesis of pseudotrisaccharides derived from neamine and paromamine. Can J Chem 56:1500–1508
Hanessian S, Massé R, Nakagawa T (1978 d) Aminoglycoside antibiotics: studies directed toward the selective modification of hydroxyl groups: synthesis of 3′-epiparomamine and 3′-epineamine. Can J Chem 56:1509–1517
Harayama A, Tsuchiya T, Umezawa S (1979) A synthesis of neamine. Bull Chem Soc Jpn 52:3626–3628
Haskell TH, Woo PWK, Watson DR (1977) Synthesis of deoxy sugars. Deoxygenation of an alcohol utilizing a facile nucleophilic displacement step. J Org Chem 42:1302–1305
Hayashi T, Takeda N, Saeki H, Ohki E (1977) Deoxysugar synthesis. III. Removal of vicinal mesyloxy groups with naphthalene-sodium. Chem Pharm Bull (Tokyo) 25:2134–2137
Hayashi T, Iwaoka T, Takeda N, Ohki E (1978) Deoxysugar synthesis. IV. Deoxygenation of aminoglycoside antibiotics through reduction of their dithiocarbonates. Chem Pharm Bull (Tokyo) 26:1786–1797
Hayashi T, Saeki H, Takeda N, Ohki E (1979) 1-*N*-Alkyl analogs of butirosin. J Antibiot (Tokyo) 32:1280–1287
Heding H (1969) Methylstreptomycin. A new hydrogenation product of streptomycin. Tetrahedron Lett 2831–2832
Heding H, Diedrichsen A (1975) Streptomycylamines. Difference in activity and mode of action between short-chain and long-chain derivatives. J Antibiot (Tokyo) 28:312–316
Heding H, Fredericks GN, Lutzen O (1972) New active streptomycin derivatives. Acta Chem Scand 26:3251–3256
Horii S, Fukase H, Kameda Y, Mizokami N (1978) A new method for selective *N*-acylation of aminoglycoside antibiotics. Carbohydr Res 60:275–288
Igarashi K (1979) Chemical modification of tobramycin. Jpn J Antibiot (Tokyo) [Suppl] 32:S187–S194
Iinuma K, Kondo S, Maeda K, Umezawa H (1977) Total synthesis of minosaminomycin. Bull Chem Soc Jpn 50:1850–1854
Ikeda D, Tsuchiya T, Umezawa S, Umezawa H (1972) Synthesis of butirosin B. J Antibiot (Tokyo) 25:741–742
Ikeda D, Tsuchiya T, Umezawa S, Umezawa H, Hamada M (1973 a) Synthesis of 3′,4′-dideoxybutirosin B. J Antibiot (Tokyo) 26:307–309
Ikeda D, Tsuchiya T, Umezawa S, Umezawa H (1973 b) Synthesis of 3′-deoxyribostamycin. J Antibiot (Tokyo) 26:799–801
Ikeda D, Tsuchiya T, Umezawa S, Umezawa H (1974) Synthesis of butirosin B and its 3′,4′-dideoxy derivative. Bull Chem Soc Jpn 47:3136–3138
Ikeda D, Nagaki F, Umezawa S, Tsuchiya T, Umezawa H (1975) Synthesis of 3′-deoxybutirosin B. J Antibiot (Tokyo) 28:616–618
Ikeda D, Nagaki F, Tsuchiya T, Umezawa S, Umezawa H (1976) Synthesis of 1-*N*-[(*S*)-4-amino-2-hydroxybutyryl]-3′-deoxyribostamycin (3′-deoxybutirosin B). Bull Chem Soc Jpn 49:3666–3668
Ikeda D, Miyasaka T, Yoshida K, Iinuma K, Kondo S, Umezawa H (1979 a) The chemical conversion of gentamine C_{1a} into gentamine C_2 and its 6′-epimer. J Antibiot (Tokyo) 32:1357–1359
Ikeda D, Miyasaka T, Yoshida M, Horiuchi Y, Kondo S, Umezawa H (1979 b) Synthesis of istamycin A. J Antibiot (Tokyo) 32:1365–1366
Ikeda H, Shiroyanagi K, Katayama M, Ikeda H, Fujikami I, Sato T, Sugayama J (1956) Dihydrodeoxystreptomycin, a new reduction product of streptomycin. I. Preparation and characterization. Proc Jpn Acad 32:48–52; Chem Abstr 50:13765
Ireland RE, Muchmore DC, Hengartner U (1972) *N,N,N′N′*-Tetramethylphosphorodiamidate group. A useful function for the protection or reductive deoxygenation of alcohols and ketones. J Am Chem Soc 94:5098–5100

Ito T, Akita E, Tsuruoka T, Niida T (1970) The synthesis of an aminocyclitol antibiotic SF-733. Agric Biol Chem 34:980–981; Antimicrob Agents Chemother 1:33–37
Jikihara T, Tsuchiya T, Umezawa S, Umezawa H (1973) Studies on aminosugars. XXXV. Syntheses of 3′,4′-dideoxyneamine and 3′- and 4′-*O*-methylneamines. Bull Chem Soc Jpn 46:3507–3510
Kavadias G, Dextraze P, Massé R, Belleau B (1978) Aminoglycoside antibiotics. The total synthesis of 5-deoxykanamycin A. Can J Chem 56:2086–2092
Kavadias G, Droghini R, Pépin Y, Ménard M, Lapointe P (1979) Synthesis of a thio-analogue of neamine. The reaction of nitrosochloroadducts of glycals with thiols. Can J Chem 57:1056–1063
Kawaguchi H, Naito T, Nakagawa S, Fujisawa K (1972) BB-K8, a new semisynthetic aminoglycoside antibiotic. J Antibiot (Tokyo) 25:695–708, 709–731 (1972); 26:297–350 (1973); 26:351–357 (1973)
Kawaguchi H, Tomita K, Hoshiya T, Miyaki T, Fujisawa K, Kimeda M, Numata K, Konishi M, Tsukiura H, Hatori M, Koshiyama H (1974) Aminoglycoside antibiotics. V. The 4′-deoxybutirosins (BU-1975 C_1 and C_2), new aminoglycoside antibiotics of bacterial origin. J Antibiot (Tokyo) 27:460–470
Kirby JP, Borders DB, Van Lear GE (1977) Structure of LL-BM 408, an aminocyclitol antibiotic. J Antibiot (Tokyo) 30:175–177
Kishi T, Tsuchiya T, Umezawa S (1979) Photochemical reaction at 3-*O*-functional group of methyl 4,6-*O*-cyclohexylidene-2-deoxy-2-methoxycarbonylamino-α-D-glucopyranoside derivatives. Bull Chem Soc Jpn 52:3015–3018
Kitahara K, Takahashi S, Shibata H, Kurihara N, Nakajima M (1969) Synthesis of methyl kasugaminide. Agric Biol Chem 33:748–754
Knight JC, Hoeksema H (1975) Reduction products of spectinomycin. J Antibiot (Tokyo) 28:136–142
Koch KF, Rhoades JA (1971) Structure of nebramycin factor 6, a new aminoglycosidic antibiotic. Antimicrob Agents Chemother 1970:309–313
Kohno H, Fukami H, Nakajima M (1975) Syntheses of neamine and its diastereomer; the condensation of protected 2,6-diamino-2,6-dideoxy-α-D-glucopyranosyl bromide with a 2-deoxystreptamine derivative. Agric Biol Chem 39:1091–1095
Kondo S (1979) Some chemical modifications of aminoglycoside antibiotics. Jpn J Antibiot [Suppl] 32:S228–S236
Kondo S, Iinuama K, Yamamoto H, Maeda K, Umezawa H (1973) Syntheses of 1-*N*-[(*S*)-4-amino-2-hydroxybutyryl]-kanamycin B and -3′,4′-dideoxykanamycin B active against kanamycin-resistant bacteria. J Anbibiot (Tokyo) 26:412–415
Kondo S, Yamamoto H, Iinima K, Maeda K, Umezawa H (1976) Syntheses of 6′,5″,6‴-triamino-6′,5″,6‴-tri-deoxylividomycin A and 6′,5″-diamino-6′,5″-dideoxylividomycin B. J Antibiot (Tokyo) 29:1134–1136
Kondo S, Miyasaka K, Yoshida K, Iinuma K, Umezawa H (1977) Syntheses and properties of kanamycin C derivatives active against resistant bacteria. J Antibiot (Tokyo) 30:1150–1152
Konishi M, Numata K, Shimoda K, Tsukiura H, Kawaguchi H (1974) Aminoglycoside antibiotics. VI. Structure determination of 4′-deoxybutirosins (BU-1975 C_1 and C_2). J Antibiot (Tokyo) 27:471:483
Kuehl FA, Flynn EH, Holly FW, Mozingo R, Folkers K (1947) Streptomyces antibiotics. XV. *N*-Methyl-L-glucosamine. J Am Chem Soc 69:3032–3035
Kugelman M, Mallams AK, Vernay HF, Crowe DF, Tanabe M (1976a) Semisynthetic aminoglycoside antibacterials. I. Preparation of selectively protected garamine derivatives. J Chem Soc [Perkin I] 1088–1097
Kugelman M, Mallams AK, Vernay HF, Crowe DF, Detre G, Tanabe M, Yasuda DM (1976b) Semisynthetic aminoglycoside antibacterials. II. Synthesis of gentamicin X_2 and related compounds. J Chem Soc [Perkin I] 1097–1113
Kugelman M, Mallams AK, Vernay HF (1976c) Semisynthetic aminoglycoside antibacterials. III. Synthesis of analogues of gentamicin X_2 modified at the 3′-position. J Chem Soc [Perkin I] 1113–1126

Kugelman M, Mallams AK, Vernay HF (1976d) Semisynthetic aminoglycoside antibacterials. IV. Synthesis of Antibiotic JI-20A, gentamicin B and related compounds. J Chem Soc [Perkin I] 1126–1134
Kugelman M, Jaret RS, Mittelman S (1978) The structure of aminoglycoside antibiotic 66-40G produced by *Micromonospora inyoensis*. J Antibiot (Tokyo) 31:643–645
Kumar V, Remers WA (1978) Aminoglycoside antibiotics. I. Regiospecific partial syntheses of ribostamycin and butirosin B. J Org Chem 43:3327–3331
Kumar V, Remers WA (1979) Aminoglycoside antibiotics. 2. *N,N*-Dialkylkanamycins. J Med Chem 22:432–436
Kurath P, Grampovnik D, Tadanier J, Martin JR, Egan RS, Stanaszek RS, Cirvic M, Washburn WH, Hill P, Dunnigan DA, Leonard JE, Johnson P, Goldstein AW (1979) 4-*N*-Aminoacylfortimicins E. J Antibiot (Tokyo) 32:884–890
Kyotani Y, Yamaguchi T, Sato S, Nagakura M, Mori T, Umezawa H, Umezawa S (1979) Tobramycin. Japan Kokai 79 52,060; Chem Abstr 91:193579f
Lazareva EN, Golubev VN, Shneerson AN, Vasienko OS (1968) Biologically active analogs of dihydrostreptomycin containing no guanidino groups, synthesized from dideguanyldihydrostreptomycin. Antibiotiki (in Russian) 13:682–686; Chem Abstr 69:74693
Lemieux RU, Nagabhushan TI, Clemetson KJ, Tucker ICN (1973) Synthesis of kanamycin analogs. I. α-D-Glucopyranosyl derivatives of deoxystreptamine. Can J Chem 51:53–66
Maehr H, Schaffner CP (1967) The chemistry of the gentamicins. I. Characterization and gross structure of gentamicin A. J Am Chem Soc 89:6787–6788
Maehr H, Schaffner CP (1970) Chemistry of the gentamicins. II. Stereochemistry and synthesis of gentosamine. Total structure of gentamicin A. J Am Chem Soc 92:1697–1700
Magerlein BJ (1979) Deoxyneamines. German patent 2,836,913; Chem Abstr 91:5436k
Maier R, Woitun E, Reuter W, Wetzel B, Goeth H, Lechner U (1979) German patent 2756–914
Mallams AK, Davies DH (1975) 4,6-Di-*O*-(aminoglycosyl)-2-deoxystreptamine as an antiprotozoal agent. US patent 3,978,214; Chem Abstr 85:177904d
Mallams AK, Davies DH (1978) 1-Desamino-1-hydroxy and 1-desamino-1-epihydroxy-4,6-di-*O*-(aminoglycosyl)-1,3-diaminocyclitols; 1-desamino-1-oxo-4,6-di-*O*-(aminoglycosyl)-1,3-diaminocyclitols, intermediates and use as antibacterial agents. US patent 4,066,752; Chem Abstr 88:152925k
Mallams AK, Saluja SS, Crowe DF, Detre G, Tanabe M, Yasuda DM (1976)Semisynthetic aminoglycoside antibacterials. V. Synthesis of pentosyl and related derivatives of garamine. J Chem Soc [Perkin I] 1135–1146
Marquez JA, Wagman GH, Testa RT, Waitz JA, Weinstein MJ (1976) A new broad spectrum aminoglycoside antibiotic, G-52, produced by *Micromonospora zionensis*. J Antibiot (Tokyo) 29:483–487
Matsushima H, Mori Y (1978a) 6′-*N*-Methyl derivative of seldomycin factor 5. German patent 2,733,964; Chem Abstr 89:6506d
Matsushima H, Mori Y (1978b) Antibiotic 1-*N*-[L-(-)-α-hydroxy-γ-aminobutyryl]-XK-88-5. Japan Kokai 78 90,244; Chem Abstr 89:215720h
Matsushima H, Mori Y (1978c) 2″-*N*-formyl derivatives of XK-88-5. Japan Kokai 78 79,843; Chem Abstr 90:23603w
Matsushima H, Mori Y (1978d) 2′-Desamino-3′-epiamino-3′-deoxy derivative of antibiotic XK-88-5, Japan Kokai 78 79,842; Chem Abstr 90:23604x
Matsushima H, Mori Y (1978e) Chemical transformation of gentamicin C_{1a} into 2′-*N*-methylgentamicin C_{1a}, active against *Providencia* 164. J Antibiot (Tokyo) 31:621–622
Matsushima H, Mori Y, Kitaura K (1977a) Synthesis of 3′-deoxyseldomycin factor 5. J Antibiot (Tokyo) 30:890–892
Matsushima H, Kitaura K, Mori Y (1977b) Chemical transformation of seldomycin 5 into 3′-episeldomycin 5 and its antibacterial activity. Bull Chem Soc Jpn 50:3039–3042
Matsushima H, Mori Y, Kitaura K (1978) Chemical transformation of seldomycin factor 5 into 3′-deoxyseldomycin factor 5 and related compounds. Bull Chem Soc Jpn 51:3553–3558

McAlpine JB, Sinclair AC, Egan RS, De Vault RL, Stanaszek RS, Cirovic M, Mueller SL, Goodley PC, Mauritz RJ, Wideburg NE, Mitscher LA, Shirahata K, Matsushima H, Sato S, Iida T (1977) A new aminoglycoside antibiotic complex – the seldomycins. IV. The structure of seldomycin factor 5. J Antibiot (Tokyo) 30:39–49

Miller GH, Chiu PJS, Waitz JA (1978) Biological activity of Sch 21420, the 1-*N*-*S*-α-hydroxy-β-aminopropionyl derivative of gentamicin B. J Antibiot (Tokyo) 31:688–695

Million WA, Plews RM, Richardson K (1977) Compounds for use in manufacturing aminoglycoside antibiotic. German patent 2,716,533; Chem Abstr 88:51128x

Miyake T, Tsuchiya T, Umezawa S, Umezawa H (1976) A synthesis of 3′,4′-dideoxykanamycin B. Carbohydr Res 49:141–151

Miyake T, Tsuchiya T, Umezawa S, Umezawa H (1977) Syntheses of 4′-deoxykanamycin and 4′-deoxykanamycin B. Bull Chem Soc Jpn 50:2362–2368

Mori T, Kyotani Y, Watanabe I, Oda T (1972) Chemical conversion of lividomycin A into lividomycin B. J Antibiot (Tokyo) 25:149–150

Murase M, Ito T, Fukatsu S, Umezawa H (1970) Studies on kanamycin related compounds produced during fermentation by mutants of *Streptomyces kanamyceticus*. Isolation and properties. Prog Antimicrob Anticancer Chemother 2:1098–1110

Nagabhushan TL, Daniels PJL (1974) Synthesis and biological properties of 6′-amino-6′-deoxygentamicin A. J Med Chem 17:1030–1031

Nagabhushan TL, Turner WN, Daniels PJL, Morton JB (1975a) The gentamicin antibiotics. 7. Structures of the gentamicin antibiotics A_1, A_3, and A_4. J Org Chem 40:2830–2834

Nagabhushan TL, Daniels PJL, Jaret RS, Morton JB (1975b) The gentamicin antibiotics. 8. Structure of gentamicin A_2. J Org Chem 40:2835–2836

Nagabhushan TL, Wright JJ, Cooper AB, Turner WN, Miller GH (1978a) Chemical modification of some gentamicins and sisomicin at the 3″-position. J Antibiot (Tokyo) 31:43–54

Nagabhushan TL, Cooper AB, Tsai H, Daniels PJL, Miller GH (1978b) The syntheses and biological properties of 1-*N*-(*S*-4-amino-2-hydroxybutyryl)-gentamicin B and 1-*N*-(*S*-3-amino-2-hydroxypropionyl)-gentamicin B. J Antibiot (Tokyo) 31:681–687

Nagabhushan TL, Cooper AB, Turner WN, Tsai H, McCombie S, Mallams AK, Rane D, Wright JJ, Reichert P, Boxler DL, Weinstain J (1978c) Interaction of vicinal and non-vicinal amino-hydroxy group pairs in aminoglycoside-aminocyclitol antibiotics with transition metal cations. Selective N protection. J Am Chem Soc 100:5253–5254

Naito T, Nakagawa S, Abe Y, Fujisawa K, Kawaguchi H (1974a) Aminoglycoside antibiotics. VIII. Synthesis and activity of 4′-deoxykanamycin A. J Antibiot (Tokyo) 27:838–850

Naito T, Nakagawa S, Narita Y, Toda S, Abe Y, Oka M, Yamashita H, Yamasaki T, Fujisawa K, Kawaguchi H (1974b) Aminoglycoside antibiotics. IX. Structure-activity relationship in 1-*N*-acyl-derivatives of kanamycin A (amikacin analogs). J Antibiot (Tokyo) 27:851–858

Naito T, Nakagawa S, Toda S (1974c) Antibiotic derivatives. Japan Kokai 74 85,048; Chem Abstr 82:73423t

Naito T, Nakagawa S, Toda S (1974d) Antibiotic lividomycin B derivatives. Japan Kokai 74 92,043; Chem Abstr 82:125570k

Naito T, Nakagawa S, Toda S (1974e) Antibiotic neomycin B and C derivatives. Japan Kokai 74 92,044; Chem Abstr 82:125569s

Naito T, Nakagawa S, Toda S (1975) 5″-Amino-4′-5″-dideoxybutirosin A. Japan Kokai 75 35,132; Chem Abstr 83:97868p

Naito T, Nakagawa S, Harita Y, Kawaguchi H (1976) Chemical modification of sorbistin. I. *N*-Acyl analogs of sorbistin. J Antibiot (Tokyo) 29:1286–1296

Naito T, Nakagawa S, Toda S, Fujisawa K, Kawaguchi H (1979) Aminoglycoside antibiotics. XIII. Synthesis and activity of 4′-deoxy-6′-*N*-methylamikacin and related compounds. J Antibiot (Tokyo) 32:659–664

Nakagawa S, Toda S, Abe Y, Yamashita H, Fujisawa K, Naito T, Kawaguchi H (1978) Aminoglycoside antibiotics. XII. Effect of *N*-alkylation in kanamycin antibiotics. J Antibiot (Tokyo) 31:675–680

Nakajima M, Hasegawa H, Kurihara N, Shibata H, Ueno T, Nishimura D (1968a) Total synthesis of kanamycin A. Tetrahedron Lett 623–627

Nakajima M, Shibata H, Kitahara K, Takahashi S, Hasegawa A (1968b) Synthesis of kasuganobiosamine. Tetrahedron Lett 2271–2274

Nara K, Yoshioka K, Kida M (1979) Chemical modification of aminoglycoside antibiotics. Some *N*-alkyl derivatives of sorbistin A_1 (P-2563P) and butirosin A. Chem Pharm Bull (Tokyo) 27:65–75

Nara T, Kawamoto I, Okachi K, Takasawa S, Yamamoto M, Sato S, Sato T, Morikawa A (1975) New antibiotic XK-62-2(sagamicin). II. Taxonomy of the producing organism, fermentative production and characterization of sagamicin. J Antibiot (Tokyo) 28:21–28

Nara T, Yamamoto M, Takasawa S, Sato S, Sato T, Kawamoto I, Okachi R, Takahashi I, Morikawa A (1977) A new aminoglycoside antibiotic complex – the seldomycins. I. Taxonomy, fermentation and antibacterial properties. J Antibiot (Tokyo) 30:17–24; see also J Antibiot (Tokyo) 30:25–30

Neu HC, Fu KP (1978) 1-N-HAPA Gentamicin B, a new aminoglycoside active against gentamicin resistant isolates – activity compared to other aminoglycosides. J Antibiot (Tokyo) 31:385–393

Nishimura T, Tsuchiya T, Umezawa S, Umezawa H (1977) A synthesis of 3′,4′-dideoxykanamycin B. Bull Chem Soc Jpn 50:1580–1583

Nishiyama S, Ishikawa Y, Yamazaki M, Suami T (1978) Chemical modification of neamine. 5. Preparation of aminodeoxyneamines. Bull Chem Soc Jpn 51:555–558

Oda T, Mori T, Kyotani Y (1971) Studies on new antibiotic lividomycins. III. Partial structure of lividomycin A. J Antibiot (Tokyo) 24:503–510

Oda T, Mori T, Yamaguchi T, Umezawa H, Umezawa S, Tsuchiya T (1978) 3′-Deoxybutirosin B and its 6′-*N*-alkyl derivatives. Japan Kokai 78 90,245; Chem Abstr 90:23606z

Ogawa T, Takamoto T, Hanessian S (1974) Aminoglycoside antibiotics: Synthesis of 6-*O*-(β-D-ribofuranosyl)paromamine. Tetrahedron Lett 4013–4016

Ogawa T, Katano K, Matsui M (1978) A synthesis of sorbistin A_1 and a position isomer thereof. Carbohydr Res 60:C13–C17

Oida S, Saeki H, Ohhashi Y, Ohki E (1975) Deoxysugar synthesis. I. Lithium-ethylamine reduction of carbohydrate phosphorodiamidates. Chem Pharm Bull (Tokyo) 23:1547–1551

Okachi R, Kawamoto I, Takasawa S, Yamamoto M, Sato S, Sato T, Nara T (1974) A new antibiotic XK-62-2. I. Isolation, physicochemical and antibacterial properties. J Antibiot (Tokyo) 27:793–800

Okutani T, Asako T, Yoshioka K, Hiraga K, Kida M (1977) Conversion of aminoglycoside antibiotics: novel and efficient approaches to 3′-deoxyaminoglycosides via 3′-phosphoryl esters. J Am Chem Soc 99:1278–1279

Paulsen H, Sumfleth B (1979) Synthese von Trehalosamin Mannotrehalosamin und verwendeten $\alpha,\alpha(1\rightarrow1)$-verknüpften Disacchariden. Chem Ber 112:3203–3213

Paulsen H, Tödter F, Banaszek A, Stadler P (1977) Synthese des Dihydrostreptosyl-desoxystreptamins. Chem Ber 110:1916–1924

Paulsen H, Lockhoff O, Schröder B, Stenzel W (1979) Stereoselektive Synthese von α-verknüpften Polyaminodeoxy-Zucker-Disacchariden mit der Azid-Methode. Carbohydr Res 68:239–255

Peck RL, Hoffhine CE Jr, Gale P, Folkers K (1949) Streptomyces antibiotics. XXIII. Isolation of neomycin A. J Am Chem Soc 71:2590–2591

Pennington FC, Guercio PA, Solomons IA (1953) Streptohydrazid. J Am Chem Soc 75:2261

Perlman D, Endo T, Hinz RS, Cowan SK, Endo S (1974) Properties of glycosides of neamine, kanamycin A and gentamicin C_1. J Antibiot (Tokyo) 27:525–528

Pete J, Portella C, Monneret C, Florent J, Khuong-Huu Q (1977) A general and convenient photochemical method for the preparation of deoxysugars. Synthesis 774–776

Pfeiffer F, Schmidt SJ, Kinzig CM, Hoover JRE, Weisbach JA (1979) 3′- and 4′-axial and equatorial amino and hydroxy derivatives of neamine. Carbohydr Res 72:119–137

Polglase WJ (1962) Alkaline degradation of dihydrostreptomycin. J Org Chem 27:1923
Ponpipom MM, Bugianesi RL, Shen T (1978) Chemical modification of 1,4-diamino-1,4-dideoxy-3-*O*-(4-deoxy-4-propionamido-α-D-glucopyranosyl)-D-glucitol. J Med Chem 2:221–225
Reeves RE (1951) Cuprammonium-glycoside complexes. Advan Carbohydr Chem Biochem 61:107–134
Reid RJ, Mizsak SA, Reineke LM, Zurenko GE, Magerlein BJ (1978) Chemical modifications of aminoglycosides. I. Synthesis of 2″-deoxykanamycin B and 2″,3′,4′-trideoxykanamycin B. 176th ACS National Meeting (Miami), Medicinal Chemistry Division No. 18
Reimann H, Cooper DJ, Mallams AK, Jaret RS, Yehaskel A, Kugelman M, Vernay HF, Schumacher D (1974) The structure of sisomicin, a novel unsaturated aminocyclitol antibiotic from *Micromonospora inyoensis*. J Org Chem 39:1451–1457
Richardson K, Jevons S, Moore JW, Ross BC, Wright JR (1977) Synthesis and antibacterial activities of 1-*N*-[(*S*)-ω-amino-2-hydroxyalkyl]kanamycin A derivatives. J Antibiot (Tokyo) 30:843–846
Richardson K, Brammer KW, Jevons S, Plews RM, Wright JR (1979) Synthesis and antibacterial activity of 1-*N*-(1,3-dihydroxy-2-propyl)kanamycin B (UK-31,214). J Antibiot (Tokyo) 32:973–977
Rosenbrook W Jr (1979) Chemistry of spectinomycin. Jpn J Antibiot [Suppl] 32:S211–S227
Rosenbrook W Jr, Carney RE (1975) Spectinomycin modification. I. 7-Epi-9-deoxy-4 (*R*)-dihydrospectinomycin. J Antibiot (Tokyo) 28:953–959
Rosenbrook W Jr, Carney RE, Egan RS, Stanaszek RS, Cirovic M, Nishinaga T, Mochida K, Mori Y (1975) Spectinomycin modification. II. 7-Epispectinomycin. J Antibiot (Tokyo) 28:960–964
Rosenbrook W Jr, Carney RE, Egan RS, Stanaszek RS, Cirovic M, Nishinaga T, Mochida K, Mori Y (1978) Spectinomycin modification. IV. 7-Deoxy-4-(*R*)-dihydrospectinomycin. J Antibiot (Tokyo) 31:451–455
Roussel-UCLAF (1977) Streptamine derivative and its salts. French patent 2,351,660; Chem Abstr 89:180302u
Saeki H, Shimada Y, Ohashi Y, Tajima M, Sugawara S, Ohki E (1974) Synthesis of 3′,4′-dideoxybutirosin A, active against resistant bacteria. Chem Pharm Bull (Tokyo) 22:1145–1150
Saeki H, Shimada Y, Ohki E, Sugawara S (1975) Synthesis of aminotrideoxybutirosin A, a chemically modified antibiotic active against butirosin-resistant bacteria. J Antibiot (Tokyo) 28:530–536
Saeki H, Hayashi T, Shimada Y, Takeda N, Ohki E (1977) Selective *O*-benzoylation in aminoglycoside antibiotics. Chem Pharm Bull (Tokyo) 25:2089–2097
Sano H, Tsuchiya T, Kobayashi S, Hamada M, Umezawa S, Umezawa H (1976) Synthesis of 3″-deoxydihydrostreptomycin active against resistant bacteria. J Antibiot (Tokyo) 29:978–980
Sano H, Tsuchiya T, Kobayashi S, Umezawa H, Umezawa S (1977) Synthesis of a masked derivative of 3′-deoxydihydrostreptobiosamine, a precursor for the synthesis of 3″-deoxydihydrostreptomycin. Bull Chem Soc Jpn 50:975–978
Sato M, Mori Y (1979) Chemical modification of fortimicins: preparation of 4-*N*-substituted fortimicin B. J Antibiot (Tokyo) 32:371–378
Shirahata K, Tomioka S, Nara T, Matsushima H, Matsubara I (1975) Gentamicin derivatives. German patent 2,458,921; Chem Abstr 83:147704e
Sinay P (1978) Recent advances in glycosylation reactions. Pure Appl Chem 50:1437–1452
Sitrin RD, Cooper DJ, Weisback JA (1977) The aminoglycoside antibiotics. I. Synthesis and biological evaluation of an analog of gentamicin. J Antibiot (Tokyo) 30:836–842
Sitrin RD, Cooper DJ, Weisbach JA (1978) Aminoglycoside antibiotics. 3. Synthesis of a furanosyl isomer of kanamycin B from a protected 3-amino-3-deoxyglucofuranosyl chloride. J Org Chem 43:3048–3052
Suami T (1979) Modifications of aminocyclitol antibiotics. Jpn J Antibiot [Suppl] 32:S91–S102

Suami T, Nakamura K (1979) Modification of aminocyclitol antibiotics. 7. Preparation of 5-epikanamycin B. Bull Chem Soc Jpn 52:955–956

Suami T, Nishiyama S, Ishikawa Y, Katsura S (1976) Chemical modification of aminocyclitol antibiotics. Carbohydr Res 52:187–196

Suami T, Nishiyama S, Ishikawa Y, Katsura S (1977a) Chemical modification of neamine. Carbohydr Res 53:239–246

Suami T, Nishiyama S, Ishikawa Y, Katsura S, (1977b) Chemical modification of neamine Part III. Carbohydr Res 56:415–418

Suami T, Nishiyama S, Ishikawa H, Okada H, Kinoshita T (1977c) Synthesis of tetrahydrospectinomycin. Bull Chem Soc Jpn 50:2754–2757

Suami T, Nishiyama S, Ishikawa Y, Katsura S (1978a) Chemical modification of neamine. Carbohydr Res 65:57–64

Suami T, Nishiyama S, Ishikawa Y, Umemura E (1978b) Modification of aminocyclitol antibiotics. 6. Preparation of 5-deoxykanamycin B. Bull Chem Soc Jpn 51:2354–2357

Suhara Y, Maeda K, Umezawa H, Ohno M (1966) Chemical studies of kasugamycin. V. The structure of kasugamycin. Tetrahedron Lett 1239–1244

Suhara Y, Sasaki F, Maeda K, Umezawa H, Ohno M (1968) The total synthesis of kasugamycin. J Am Chem Soc 90:6559–6560

Suhara Y, Sasaki F, Koyama G, Maeda K, Umezawa H, Ohno M (1972) The total synthesis of kasugamycin. J Am Chem Soc 94:6501–6507

Suzuki Y, Ohmori H (1979) Preparation and some microbiological properties of novel kanamycin-glucoside derivatives. J Antibiot (Tokyo) 32:753–755

Takagi Y, Miyake T, Tsuchiya T, Umezawa S, Umezawa H (1973) Synthesis of 3′-deoxykanamycin B. J Antibiot (Tokyo) 26:403–406

Takagi Y, Miyake T, Tsuchiya T, Umezawa S, Umezawa H (1976) Synthesis of 3′-deoxykanamycin B (tobramycin). Bull Chem Soc Jpn 49:3649–3651

Takamoto T, Hanessian S (1974) Aminoglycoside antibiotics: chemical transformation of paromomycin into a bioactive pseudotrisaccharide. Tetrahedron Lett 4009–4012

Tanabe M, Yasuda DM, Detre G (1977) Aminoglycoside antibiotics: synthesis of nebramine, tobramycin and 4″-epi-tobramycin. Tetrahedron Lett 3607–3610

Testa RT, Wagman GH, Daniels PJL, Weinstain MJ (1974) Mutamicins; biosynthetically created new sisomicin analogues. J Antiobiot (Tokyo) 27:917–921

Tipson RS, Cohen A (1965) Action of zinc dust and sodium iodide in *N*,*N*-dimethylformamide on contiguous, secondary sulfonyloxy groups: a simple method for introducing nonterminal unsaturation. Carbohydr Res 1:338–340

Toda S, Nakagawa S, Naito T (1977) Aminoglycoside antibiotics. X. Chemical conversion of kanamycin B to kanamycin C and 6′-deoxykanamycin C. J Antibiot (Tokyo) 30:1002–1003

Toda S, Nakagawa S, Naito T, Kawaguchi H (1978) Stucture determination of amikacin derivatives modified by enzymes from resistant *S. aureus* strains. Tetrahedron Lett 3917–3920

Tomioka S, Mori Y (1976) Demethylation of aminoglycoside antibiotic. German patent 2,550,168; Chem Abstr 85:47016e

Tomioka S, Mori Y (1977) 3″-*N*-Demethyl analogs of 1-*N*-(L-(-)-α-hydroxy-δ-aminobutyryl)sagamicin. Japan Kokai 77 83,515; Chem Abstr 88:7307f

Tomioka S, Fukuhara T, Mori Y (1977) 3″-Demethyl analogs of gentamicin C_1. Japan Kokai 77 83,516; Chem Abstr 88:7306e

Tsuchiya T (1979) Deoxygenation of aminoglycosides. Jpn J Antibiot [Suppl] 32:S129–S135

Tsuchiya T, Watanabe I, Nakamura F, Hamada M, Umezawa S (1978a) Synthesis of 3′,3″-dideoxybutirosin. J Antibiot (Tokyo) 31:933–935

Tsuchiya T, Watanabe I, Yoshida M, Nakamura F, Usui T, Kitamura M, Umezawa S (1978b) 3-Deoxygenation of methyl α-D-glucopyranosides by treatment of their 3-*O*-(*N*,*N*-dimethylsulfamoyl) derivatives with sodium metal in liquid ammonia. Tetrahedron Lett 3365–3368

Tsuchiya T, Jikihara T, Miyake T, Umezawa S, Hamada M, Umezawa H (1979a) 3′-Deoxyamikacin and 3′,4′-dideoxyamikacin and their antibacterial activities. J Antibiot (Tokyo) 32:1351–1353

Tsuchiya T, Takagi Y, Umezawa S (1979 b) 1-*N*-Acylation of aminocyclitol antibiotics *via* zinc chelation and regiospecific *N*-trifluoroacetylation. Tetrahedron Lett 4951–4954
Tsuji S, Kusumoto S, Shiba T (1975) Synthesis of enduracididine, a component amino acid of antibiotic enduracidin. Chem Lett 1281–1284
Tsukiura H, Saito K, Kobaru S, Konishi M, Kawaguchi H (1973) Aminoglycoside antibiotics. IV. BU-1709 E_1 and E_2, new aminoglycoside antibiotics related to the butirosins. J Antibiot (Tokyo) 26:386–388
Umezawa H (1970) Mechanism of inactivation of aminoglycoside antibiotics by enzymes of resistant organisms of clinical origin. Progr Antimicrob Anticancer Chemother 2:567–571
Umezawa H (1974) Biochemical mechanism of resistance to aminoglycosidic antibiotics. Adv Carbohyd Chem Biochem 30:183–225
Umezawa H (1979) Studies on aminoglycoside antibiotics: enzymatic mechanism of resistance and genetics. Jpn J Antibiot [Suppl] 32:S1–S14
Umezawa H, Suhara Y (1976) Guanidino derivatives of kasugamycin. US patent 3,968,100
Umezawa H, Hayano S, Ogata Y (1948) Classification of antibiotic strains of streptomyces and their antibiotic substances on the basis of their antibacterial spectra. Jpn Med J 1:504–511
Umezawa H, Umezawa S, Tsuchiya T, Okazaki Y (1971) 3′,4′-Dideoxykanamycin B active against kanamycin-resistant *Escherichia coli* and *Pseudomonas aeruginosa*. J Antibiot (Tokyo) 24:485–487
Umezawa H, Nishimura Y, Tsuchiya T, Umezawa S (1972 a) Syntheses of 6′-*N*-methylkanamycin and 3′,4′-dideoxy-6′-*N*-methylkanamycin B active against resistant strains having 6′-*N*-acetylating enzymes. J Antibiot (Tokyo) 25:743–745
Umezawa H, Tsuchiya T, Muto R, Umezawa S (1972 b) The synthesis of 3′-*O*-methylkanamycin. Bull Chem Soc Jpn 45:2842–2847
Umezawa H, Iinuma K, Kondo S, Hamada M, Maeda K (1975 a) Synthesis of 1-*N*-acyl derivatives of 3′,4′-dideoxy-6′-*N*-methylkanamycin B and their antibacterial activities. J Antibiot (Tokyo) 28:340–343
Umezawa H, Iinuma K, Kondo S, Maeda K (1975 b) Synthesis and antibacterial activity of 6′-*N*-alkyl derivatives of 1-*N*-[(*S*)-4-amino-2-hydroxybutyryl]-kanamycin. J Antibiot (Tokyo) 28:483–485
Umezawa H, Ikeda D, Miyasaka T, Kondo S (1979) Syntheses and properties of the 6′-*C*-alkyl derivatives of 3′,4′-dideoxykanamycin B. J Antibiot (Tokyo) 32:1360–1364
Umezawa S (1974) Structures and syntheses of aminoglycoside antibiotics. Adv Carbohydr Chem Biochem 30:111–182
Umezawa S (1976) Sugar-containing antibiotics. MTP (Med Tech Publ Co) Int Rev Sci Ser Two Org Chem 7:149–200
Umezawa S (1979) Total synthesis of aminoglycoside antibiotics. Jpn J Antibiot [Suppl] Symp. 32:S60–S72
Umezawa S Synthesis of aminocyclitol antibiotics. ACS (Am Chem Soc) Symp Ser 125:15–41
Umezawa S, Koto S (1966) The synthesis of paromamine. Bull Chem Soc Jpn 39:2014–2017
Umezawa S, Nishimura Y (1977) Total synthesis of neomycin C. J Antibiot (Tokyo) 30:189–191
Umezawa S, Tsuchiya T, Fujita H (1966 a) Structure of (2-amino-2-deoxy-α-D-glucosyl)-deoxystreptamine produced by acid reversion. J Antibiot (Tokyo) A19:222–228
Umezawa S, Tsuchiya T, Tatsuta K (1966 b) Configurational studies of aminosugar glycosides and aminocyclitols by a copper complex method. Bull Chem Soc Jpn 39:1235–1243
Umezawa S, Tsuchiya T, Nakada S, Tatsuta K (1967 a) Studies of aminosugars. XIV. Synthesis of 6,6′-diamino-6,6′-dideoxy-trehalose. Bull Chem Soc Jpn 40:395–401
Umezawa S, Tatsuta K, Muto R (1967 b) Synthesis of trehalosamine. J Antibiot (Tokyo) A20:388–389
Umezawa S, Tatsuta K, Tsuchiya T, Kitazawa E (1967 c) Synthesis of neamine. J Antibiot (Tokyo) A20:53–54
Umezawa S, Koto S, Tatsuta K, Tsumura T (1968 a) The total synthesis of kanamycin C. J Antibiot (Tokyo) 21:162–163

Umezawa S, Tatsuta K, Koto S (1968b) The total synthesis of kanamycin A. J Antibiot (Tokyo) 21:367–368
Umezawa S, Koto S, Tatsuta K, Hineno H, Nishimura Y, Tsumura T (1968c) The total synthesis of kanamycin B. J Antibiot (Tokyo) 21:424–425
Umezawa S, Tsuchiya T, Muto R, Nishimura Y, Umezawa H (1971a) Synthesis of 3′-deoxykanamycin effective against kanamycin-resistant *Escherichia coli* and *Pseudomonas aeruginosa*. J Antibiot (Tokyo) 24:274–275
Umezawa S, Tsuchiya T, Jikihara T, Umezawa H (1971b) Synthesis of 3′,4′-dideoxyneamine active against kanamycin-resistant *E. coli* and *P. aeruginosa*. J Antibiot (Tokyo) 24:711–712
Umezawa S, Takagi Y, Tsuchiya T (1971c) A new method for the simultaneous protection of amino and hydroxyl groups in aminosugars and aminocyclitols. Bull Chem Soc Jpn 44:1411–1415
Umezawa S, Miyazawa T, Tsuchiya T (1972a) Synthesis of paromamine. J Antibiot (Tokyo) 25:530–534
Umezawa S, Tsuchiya T, Ikeda D, Umezawa H (1972b) Synthesis of 3′,4′-dideoxy and 3′,4′,5″-trideoxyribostamycin active against kanamycin-resistant *E. coli* and *P. aeruginosa*. J Antibiot (Tokyo) 25:613–616
Umezawa S, Nishimura Y, Hineno H, Watanabe K, Koike S, Tsuchiya T, Umezawa H (1972c) The synthesis of 3′-deoxykanamycin. Bull Chem Soc Jpn 45:2847–2851
Umezawa S, Okazaki Y, Tsuchiya T (1972d) Synthesis of 3,4-dideoxy-3-enosides and the corresponding 3,4-dideoxy sugars. Bull Chem Soc Jpn 45:3619–3624
Umezawa S, Umezawa H, Okazaki Y, Tsuchiya T (1972e) Synthesis of 3′,4′-dideoxykanamycin B. Bull Chem Soc Jpn 45:3624–3628
Umezawa S, Ikeda D, Tsuchiya T, Umezawa H (1973) Synthesis of 1-*N*-[(*S*)-4-amino-2-hydroxybutyryl]-3′,4′-dideoxyneamine. J Antibiot (Tokyo) 26:304–306
Umezawa S, Tsuchiya T, Yamasaki T, Sano H, Takahashi Y (1974a) Total synthesis of dihydrostreptomycin. J Am Chem Soc 96:920–921
Umezawa S, Nishimura Y, Hata Y, Tsuchiya T, Yagisawa M, Umezawa H (1974b) Synthesis of 4′-deoxykanamycin and its resistance to kanamycin phosphotransferase II. J Antibiot (Tokyo) 27:722–725
Umezawa S, Takahashi Y, Usui T, Tsuchiya T (1974c) Total synthesis of streptomycin. J Antibiot (Tokyo) 27:997–999
Umezawa S, Yamasaki T, Kubota Y, Tsuchiya T (1975) Total synthesis of dihydrostreptomycin. Bull Chem Soc Jpn 48:563–569
Usui T, Tsuchiya T, Umezawa S (1978) 1- and 3-Deamidino derivatives of dihydrostreptomycin and some 1-*N*-acyl derivatives. J Antibiot (Tokyo) 31:991–996
Vass G, Rolland A, Cleophax J, Mercier D, Quiclet B, Gero SD (1979) Synthesis of α-linked 2′,3′-dideoxy-2′-fluoro-pseudo-disaccharides related to aminocyclitol-glycoside antibiotics. J Antibiot (Tokyo) 32:670–672
Voss E, Metzger K, Petersen U, Stadler P (1978) 1-*N*-Formylsisomicin. German patent 2,726,208; Chem Abstr 90:187285y
Waitz JA, Miller GH, Moss E Jr, Chiu PJS (1978) Chemotherapeutic evaluation of 5-episisomicin (Sch 22591), a new semisynthetic aminoglycoside. Antimicrob Agents Chemother 13:41–48
Waskman SA, Lechevalier HA (1949) Neomycin a new antibiotic active against streptomycin-resistant bacteria, including tuberculosis organisms. Science 109:305–307
Watanabe I, Tsuchiya T, Umezawa S, Umezawa H (1973a) Synthesis of 1-*N*-[(*S*)-4-amino-2-hydroxybutyryl]lividomycin A. J Antibiot (Tokyo) 26:310–312
Watanabe I, Tsuchiya T, Umezawa S, Umezawa H (1973b) Synthesis of 6′-amino-6′-deoxylividomycin B and 6′-deoxy-6′-methylamino- and 6′-deoxy-6′-(2-hydroxymethylamino)-lividomycin B. J Antibiot (Tokyo) 26:802–804
Watanabe I, Tsuchiya T, Umezawa S, Umezawa H (1975a) Synthesis of 1-*N*-[(*S*)-4-amino-2-hydroxybutyryl]lividomycin A. Bull Chem Soc Jpn 48:2124–2126
Watanabe I, Ejima A, Tsuchiya T, Umezawa S, Umezawa H (1975b) Synthesis of 6′-amino-1-*N*-[(*S*)-4-amino-2-hydroxybutyryl]-6′-deoxylividomycin A. Bull Chem Soc Jpn 48:2303–2305

Watanabe I, Ejima A, Tsuchya T, Ikeda D, Umezawa S (1977a) A synthesis of 3′-deoxybutirosin B. Bull Chem Soc Jpn 50:487–490

Watanabe I, Tsuchiya T, Umezawa S (1977b) Improved syntheses of 3′-deoxybutirosin A and B. Bull Chem Soc Jpn 50:972–974

Watanabe I, Tsuchiya T, Takase T, Umezawa S, Umezawa H (1977c) Synthesis of a lividomycin B analogue, 5-*O*-[3-*O*-(2-amino-2-deoxy-α-D-glucopyranosyl)-β-D-ribofuranosyl]-3′-deoxyparomamine. Bull Chem Soc Jpn 50:2369–2374

Watanabe I, Tsuchiya T, Nakamura F, Hamada M, Umezawa S (1978) Synthesis of 5″-amino-3′,5″-dideoxybutirosin A. J Antibiot (Tokyo) 31:863–867

Watanakunakorn C (1978) Comparative *in vitro* activity of a semisynthetic derivative of gentamicin B (Sch 21420) and five other aminoglycosides. J Antibiot (Tokyo) 31:1063–1064

Weinstein MJ, Marquex JA, Testa RT, Wagman GH, Oden EM, Waitz JA (1970) Antibiotic 6640, a new Micromonospora-produced aminoglycoside antibiotic. J Antibiot (Tokyo) 23:551–554; see also 23:555–558 and 559–569

Weinstein MJ, Wagman GH, Marquez JA, Testa RT, Waitz JA (1975) Verdamicin, a new broad spectrum aminoglycoside antibiotic. Antimicrob Agents Chemother 7, 246–249

Weinstein MJ, Daniels PJL, Wagman GH, Testa RT, Mallams AK, Wright JJ, Nagabhushan TL (1978) Pseudotrisaccharides. Swiss patent 601,340; Chem Abstr 89:215718p

White DR, Birkenmeyer RD, Thomas RC, Mizsak SA, Wiley VH (1979) The stereospecific synthesis of spectinomycin. Tetrahedron Lett 2723–2740

Wiley PF, Argoudelis AD, Hoeksema H (1963) The chemistry of actinospectacin. IV. The determination of the structure of actinospectacin. J Am Chem Soc 85:2652

Wolfrom ML, Polglase WJ (1948) A synthesis of streptidine. J Am Chem Soc 70:1672–1673

Wolfrom ML, Olin SM, Polglase WJ (1950) Synthesis of streptidine. J Am Chem Soc 72:1724–1729

Woo PWK (1975) 5″-Amino-3′,4′-5″-trideoxybutirosin A, a new semisynthetic aminoglycoside antibiotic. J Antibiot (Tokyo) 28:522–529

Woo PWK, Dion HW, Bartz QR (1971) Butirosin A and B, aminoglycoside antibiotics. I. Structural units. Tetrahedron Lett 2617–2620; see also 2624, 2625–2628

Wright JJ (1976) Synthesis of 1-*N*-ethylsisomicin: a broad-spectrum semisynthetic aminoglycoside antibiotic. J Chem Soc Chem Commun 206–208

Wright JJ, Cooper A, Daniels PJL, Nagabhushan TL, Rane D, Turner WN, Weinstein J (1976) Selective *N*-acylation of gentamicin antibiotics – synthesis of 1-*N*-acyl derivatives. J Antibiot (Tokyo) 29:714–719

Yagisawa M, Yamamoto H, Naganawa H, Kondo S, Takeuchi T, Umezawa H (1972) A new enzyme in *Escherichia coli* carrying R-factor phosphorylating 3′-hydroxyl of butirosin A, kanamycin, neamine and ribostamycin. J Antibiot (Tokyo) 25:748–750

Yamaguchi T, Tsuchiya T, Umezawa S (1977a) Syntheses of 6′-*C*-aminomethyl-3′-deoxyparomamines. J Antibiot (Tokyo) 30:71–75

Yamaguchi T, Kamiya K, Mori T, Oda T (1977b) Deneosaminyllividomycin B. J Antibiot (Tokyo) 30:332–333

Yamaguchi T, Kyotani Y, Watanabe I, Sato S, Takahashi Y, Nagakura M, Mori T (1979) Synthesis of sporaricin analogues, 3-deoxy-4-*N*-glycyl-6-*O*-(α-nebrosaminyl)fortamine and its 3-de-*O*-methyl compound. J Antibiot (Tokyo) 32:1137–1146

Yamasaki T, Tsuchiya T, Umezawa S (1978) A synthesis of dihydrostreptomycin. J Antibiot (Tokyo) 31:1233–1237

Yasuda S, Ogasawara T, Kawabata S, Iwataki I, Matsumoto T (1969) A synthesis of α-diacetylmethylkasugaminide. Tetrahedron Lett 3969–3972

Yasuda S, Ogasawara T, Kawabata S, Iwataki I, Matsumoto T (1973) Synthesis of methyl *N*,*N*-diacetyl-α-D-kasugaminide. Tetrahedron 29:3141–3147

Yoneta T, Shibahara S, Matsuno T, Tohma S, Fukatsu S, Seki S, Umezawa H (1979) An improved synthesis of 3′,4′-dideoxy-kanamycin B. Bull Chem Soc Jpn 52:1131–1134

Yoshimura J, Sato K, Hashimoto H, Shimizu K (1977) A facile synthesis of benzyl α- and β-kasugaminides *via* the corresponding abequosides. Bull Chem Soc Jpn 50:3305–3309

CHAPTER 3

Biosynthesis and Mutasynthesis of Aminoglycoside Antibiotics

T. OKUDA and Y. ITO

A. Introduction

I. Historical Background

The discovery of streptomycin by WAKSMAN in 1944 contributed significantly to the therapy of tuberculosis and initiated the era of aminoglycoside antibiotic research. Following the discovery of streptomycin, neomycin (1949) and kanamycin (1957) were discovered and applied to the control of infections caused by gram-negative bacteria. In addition to these aminoglycoside antibiotics (aminoglycosides), paromomycin (1959), spectinomycin (1961), gentamicin (1963), ribostamycin (1970), sisomicin (1970), and tobramycin (1971) are now in widespread clinical use. Butirosin (1971), lividomycin (1971), apramycin (1973), sagamicin (1974), fortimicin (1976), and seldomycin (1977) are under clinical investigation. The aminoglycosides kasugamycin (1965), destomycin (1965), and validamycin (1971) are now widely used for agricultural and veterinary purposes.

Aminoglycosides are mainly produced by actinomycetes including *Streptomyces*, *Streptoverticillium*, *Nocardia*, *Micromonospora*, *Streptoalloteichus*, etc. Some *Bacillus* species also produce aminoglycosides. These organisms often produce simultaneously several structurally related antibiotics which are mutually convertible by chemical, enzymatic, or microbiologic procedures and give valuable information on the biosynthesis of these aminoglycosides.

Once a clinically promising aminoglycoside is found and the structure is determined by chemical, spectroscopic, or X-ray crystallographic procedures, biosynthetic studies on the antibiotic and its subunits soon commence. Such studies are of academic interest, and of great practical use in increasing the productivity of the new antibiotic fermentation. Recent progress in biosynthetic research includes the development of "mutational biosynthesis (mutasynthesis)" which is used to create improved antibiotics.

Research on aminoglycoside biosynthesis started before 1950, soon after streptomycin had been found to contain three unique subunits i.e., streptidine, streptose, and *N*-methyl-L-glucosamine. Since then, numerous papers have been published in the field including reviews by RINEHART and STROSHANE (1976), NARA (1977, 1978), GRISEBACH (1978), NOMI (1978), and RINEHART (1979). This chapter deals with biosynthetic and mutasynthetic studies on the major aminoglycosides up to the beginning of 1980, including work on plasmid involvement in biosynthesis, a recent active field of research.

II. Methodology

Microorganisms undergoing fermentation produce various metabolites which, following BU'LOCK (1965), are generally classified as primary or secondary metabolites. Primary metabolism is involved with providing cells with energy and macromolecules such as proteins and nucleic acids, substances essential for the life, growth, and multiplication of living cells. In most cases, the study of biosynthetic mechanisms has elucidated the role of the primary metabolites. Contrary to this, secondary metabolism is concerned with products, although their function in the growth and multiplication of microorganisms has not yet been defined. The term "secondary metabolites" was first used in plant physiology for plant products which had no obvious function in the growth of plants. The term "microbial secondary metabolites" was used by H. UMEZAWA (1977) for microbial products which have no obvious function in, or are not essential for, the growth of microbial cells.

Primary metabolism in living cells is fundamentally the same in all microorganisms and metabolic regulation is so finely balanced that the accumulation of a primary intermediate is rare. Secondary metabolites are generally peculiar to species or strains of microorganisms and frequently accumulate in large amounts in the fermentation broth or in the mycelia of a specific microorganism. As cited by TURNER (1971), BU'LOCK (1967) suggested that microorganisms rarely produce secondary metabolites while primary metabolism is fully operational (trophophase). However, when cell growth and replication decline (idiophase), a variety of metabolic changes occur and enzymes are produced which convert primary metabolites into secondary metabolites such as antibiotics. The enzymes involved in antibiotic production were termed antibiotic-committed enzymes (QUEENER et al. 1978).

The procedures used to elucidate metabolic pathways are common to both primary and secondary metabolism, except for the application of mutant strains.

1. Application of Labeled Compounds

Studies of secondary metabolism have been dominated by the use of isotopically labeled compounds. Though constituent sugars or aminosugars are unique, they are usually assumed to originate from glucose. Therefore, at the beginning of a study, randomly labeled D-glucose (D-[U-^{14}C]-glucose) is added to a growing culture of the producing strain and the resulting antibiotic is examined for the incorporation of radioactivity. When incorporation is observed, D-glucose labeled at a specific atom is used and the resulting labeled antibiotic is degraded into its subunits which are further selectively degraded to determine the location of the labeled atom. Application of a doubly labeled precursor with ^{14}C, ^{2}H, ^{3}H, or ^{15}N is useful to avoid errors due to the change or decomposition of a labeled precursor before incorporation and also to determine the biosynthetic mechanism more positively. If the ratio of the radioactivity of the two isotopes shown by a precursor is equal to that shown by the resulting metabolite, the precursor was probably incorporated into the product without fragmentation. But, if the ratio is different, fragmentation or some biochemical change involving a labeled atom may be occurring. Application of a ^{13}C-labeled precursor is of great advantage in avoiding the above problems. The distribution position of ^{13}C in the product is readily assigned by comparing the ^{13}C-NMR spectrum of an enriched product (antibiotic or subunit) with the natural abundance spectrum. The application of ^{13}C-isotopes to antibiotic biosynthesis has been reviewed by NEUSS (1975). RINEHART et al. (1974) first applied this technique in elucidation of the biosynthesis of the aminoglycoside antibiotic neomycin, as described later.

Although tracer experiments with ^{15}N-amino acid had been reported as early as 1937 for biosynthetic studies, this procedure was not applied to aminoglycosides until RINEHART (ROLLS et al. 1975) utilized it for the study of neomycin biosynthesis. Recent developments in mass, NMR, and other spectroscopy make it possible to more easily measure incorporation of ^{15}N, thus increasing the usefulness of this isotope.

Incorporation studies with labeled glucose or glucosamine may suggest potential intermediates but in order to establish the sequence between glucose and antibiotic, it may be necessary to examine the incorporation of many potential intermediates. Since it is often difficult to prepare numbers of such compounds in large quantities, the following indirect methods are often used.

1. The first method is to compare the incorporation rate of a labeled substrate with or without exogenous supplementation of an unlabeled potential intermediate. If biosynthesis proceeds according to the following pathway, an exogenously added intermediate (B_{ex}) is incorporated more readily than an intermediate (B_{en}) endogenously produced from labeled substrate (A^*_{ex}), so exogenous intermediate will interfere with incorporation of labeled substrate. With this method it is not necessary to have labeled intermediate B.

$$\begin{array}{c} A^*_{ex} \rightarrow B_{en} \rightarrow C_{en} \rightarrow \text{Antibiotic}^* \\ \uparrow \\ B_{ex} \end{array}$$

This method is called the "isotope competition method." For example, incorporation of D-[^{14}C]glucose into streptidine, a subunit of streptomycin, decreases when *myo*-inositol is simultaneously present, suggesting that streptidine is synthesized from glucose via *myo*-inositol.

2. Another method involves determining the labeling order among intermediates in the biosynthetic sequence. When a biosynthesis starts from labeled A^*_{ex}, as shown in the above scheme. B_{en} is labeled earlier that C_{en}. Therefore, it is possible to determine the sequence of biosynthetic steps by comparing the radioactivity of the intermediates isolated from the culture broth at various times.

As described above, the application of isotopes is useful in studying the biosynthetic pathway of a subunit but it is not effective in determining the mechanism for the assembly of subunits.

2. Application of Cell-Free Extracts of Mycelia or Enzymes

It is impossible to introduce a precursor or an intermediate directly into cells and also it is uncertain whether or not an exogenous precursor passes through the cell wall and membrane. Even if they penetrate the cell, exogenous substrates are said to be generally less accessible to the active sites of antibiotic-committed enzymes than in the case of primary metabolism (QUEENER et al. 1978). Moreover, labeled precursor may be diluted by degradation by other enzymes in the cells. Thus, it may be better to use cell-free extracts of the mycelia which contain the enzymes or enzyme systems, together with cofactors essential for biosynthesis. If possible, it is better to use a possible precursor together with purified enzymes and well-defined cofactor(s). Although this approach has frequently been applied to primary metabolism, it has not been useful for the study of secondary metabolites for several reasons. Often enzymes involved in secondary metabolism are vulnerable to extraction procedures, since such enzymes are often aggregates which readily undergo inactivation by dissociation. An antibiotic-producing strain may produce a protease which may decompose the antibiotic-producing enzymes. Difficulties in finding suitable assay methods for intermediates often restrict the application of this approach.

This technique has been used in studies of the biosynthetic pathway of streptidine from glucose-6-phosphate, and also in following the linkage of dTDP-dihydrostreptose to streptidine-6-phosphate to form a pseudodisaccharide.

3. Application of Mutants

As reviewed by QUEENER et al. (1978), a sequence of biosynthetic steps may be elucidated by using mutants blocked in one or more biosynthetic steps.

a) Auxotroph and Idiotroph

Regulator genes concerned with the biosynthesis of essential enzymes for primary or secondary metabolism are susceptible to mutation. The resulting blocked mutants, auxotrophs or idiotrophs, may be isolated under appropriate conditions. According to QUEENER et al. (1978), "a mutant with an inheritable lesion blocking the synthesis of an essential metabolite that it must obtain exogenously to grow" is called an auxotroph. In contrast to this, a strain in which the biosynthetic pathway of a secondary metabolite is genetically blocked is called an idiotroph. According to NAGAOKA and DEMAIN (1975), "an idiotroph (*idio*, peculiar; *troph*, nutrition; a mutant requiring a special nutrient to produce a product peculiar to that organism) is a mutant which grows in minimal medium but fails to produce an idiolite (secondary metabolite) unless supplemented with a precursor of that secondary metabolite."

b) Selection of an Idiotroph

Auxotrophs have been widely used in the study of primary metabolism (UMBARGER and DAVIS 1962). However, idiotrophs have been less widely used in the study of secondary metabolism, probably for the following reasons. In primary metabolism, a block on the pathway to an essential metabolite is easily detectable, because growth is not possible unless the essential metabolite or a blocked intermediate is supplied in the medium. In contrast, the loss of the ability to produce a secondary metabolite is rather difficult to detect, but idiotrophs can be selected from mutagenized colonies by modifying the procedure adapted for the isolation of an auxotroph. Selection of an idiotroph blocked in the aminoglycoside pathway was first reported by SHIER et al. (1969). They succeeded in isolating from mutagenized colonies of neomycin-producing *Streptomyces fradiae* an idiotroph which could produce neomycin only when 2-deoxystreptamine was added to the culture medium. Such an idiotroph may be designated by the precursor necessary for antibiotic production, for example, 2-deoxystreptamine-requiring idiotroph, 2-deoxystreptamine-negative mutant (simply DOS^- mutant), or 2-deoxystreptamine-dependent mutant.

Genes controlling the biosynthesis of primary metabolites are coded on chromosomal DNA, but those concerning secondary metabolism are not only coded on chromosomal DNA, but also on extrachromosomal DNA in a plasmid. Plasmids are readily eliminated from the cells by treating the cells with a plasmid-curing agent such as acriflavine, ethidium bromide, etc.

The possibilities of isolating a blocked mutant due to depression or inactivation of an enzyme involved in one step of the biosynthetic sequence are greater in strains with point mutations or short deletions than in strains with large deletions. Thus, a mutant useful for the study of biosynthesis of an antibiotic may be isolated from strains mutagenized by DNA-alkylating agents or by UV irradiation. Mutants obtained by treatment with a plasmid-curing agent are not always suitable, as these mutants are often deficient in the entire plasmid involving several steps of biosynthesis

c) Cosynthesis

When two antibiotic-nonproducing mutants are cultivated together, the original antibiotic is often produced. This phenomenon is called "cooperative biosynthesis" or "cosynthesis" and is attributed to the conversion by one strain of an intermediate secreted by the other strain into the antibiotic (DELIC et al. 1969). Cosynthesis can be examined in a liquid medium or on an agar plate.

α) Cosynthesis in a Liquid Medium (Mixed Fermentation). Cosynthesis may be observed in a liquid medium by inoculating and cultivating two blocked mutants together in the usual medium, and looking for antibiotic production. Cosynthesis of streptomycin in a liquid medium was reported with a pair of blocked mutants of *Actinomyces streptomycini* (*Streptomyces griseus*) (BOROSOWA and IVKINA 1968; SHEVCHENKO et al. 1977). KRASILNIKOVA et al. (1978b) also reported that a pair of streptidine-requiring idiotrophs could produce streptomycin by cosynthesis. LEE et al. (1978) found that two aminocyclitol-requiring idiotrophs representing two different species of *Micromonospora* produced gentamicin A, X_2, C_{1a}, and C_{2b}, when they were paired and cofermented in a liquid medium. These results indicate that one of the two blocked mutants accumulates an intermediate from which the other strain can produce an antibiotic. However, it is impossible to determine which is producing the intermediate and which is converting it to the antibiotic.

β) Cosynthesis on Agar. The method for detecting cosynthesis on an agar plate was first devised by DELIC et al. (1969) in a study of tetracycline biosynthesis. Later, the Tanabe Seiyaku group applied this technique to the study of biosynthesis of butirosin (FURUMAI et al. 1979). In this experiment, cosynthesis abilities by 9 butirosin-nonproducing mutants of *Bacillus circulans* were tested with 36 possible pairs as shown in the following example.

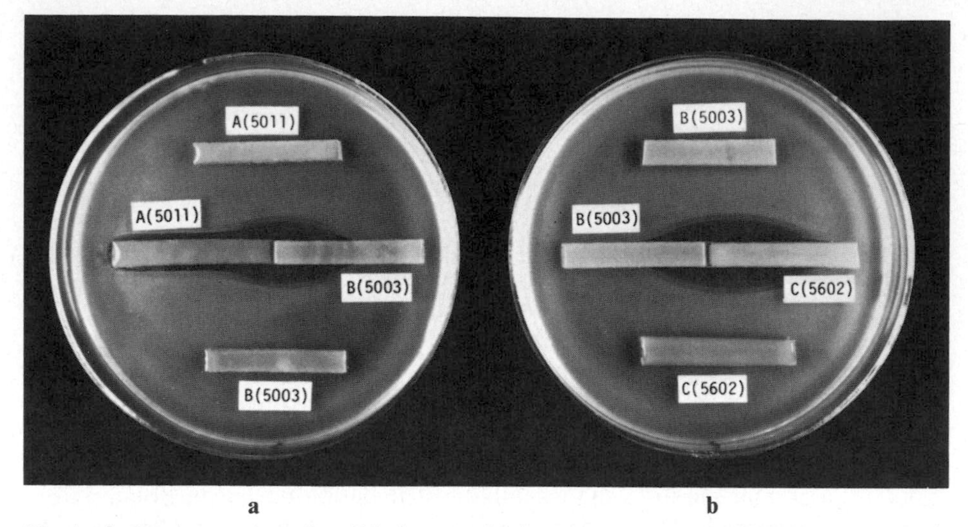

Fig. 1 a, b. Demonstration of antibiotic cosynthesis among mutants MCRL 5011 (group A), 5003 (group B), and 5602 (group C). **a** Plate 1 (left); **b** Plate 2 (right)

Cosynthesis between two mutants, for example between mutants MCRL 5003 and 5011, was examined as follows: Three agar plates were prepared. On the surface of the first and second plates, mutants MCRL 5003 and 5011 were streaked with a glass spreader. On the third plate, each mutant was streaked over one-half of the agar surface, separated 2 mm from each other. After incubation an agar strip (5–6 mm × 50–60 mm) was cut from the third plate, perpendicular to the center line of separation, and placed on an assay plate seeded with *Pseudomonas aeruginosa* No. 12. Agar strips from the first and second plates were also placed on the assay plate for comparison. After incubation of the assay plate it was examined for inhibition and when observed, it was noted on which side of the agar strip the inhibition was found. Plate 1 in Fig. 1 shows the results. Both mutants alone produced no inhibitory zone, while the agar strip cut from the third plate showed an inhibition zone on the side corresponding to mutant MCRL 5003. This result showed that MCRL 5011 produced (or accumulated) a metabolite which was converted to the antibiotic (butirosin) by the paired mutant MCRL 5003. In other words, MCRL 5011 was blocked in a biosynthetic step nearer to the final product, butirosin, than MCRL 5003. Plate 2 in Fig. 1 shows the results obtained by pairing the two mutants MCRL 5003 and 5602. In this case, the inhibition zone is observed on the side corresponding to 5602. With this combination, MCRL 5003 behaved as a secretor and MCRL 5602 acted as a converter, indicating that MCRL 5003 was blocked nearer to butirosin than MCRL 5602. The blocked sites of these three mutants in the biosynthetic pathway to butirosin are as follows:

Precursor →| | ——→ | | ——→ | | ——→ Butirosin
MCRL 5602   MCRL 5003   MCRL 5011

As a result of the cosynthesis experiments carried out with the above-mentioned nine blocked mutants of *B. circulans*, these mutants were classified into seven groups (A to F and exceptional groups). The complementation patterns of these mutants are shown in Fig. 2.

Recently, FUJIWARA et al. (1980a) modified the method for cosynthesis on an agar plate and characterized 2-deoxystreptamine-requiring mutants of *B. circulans* B15M.

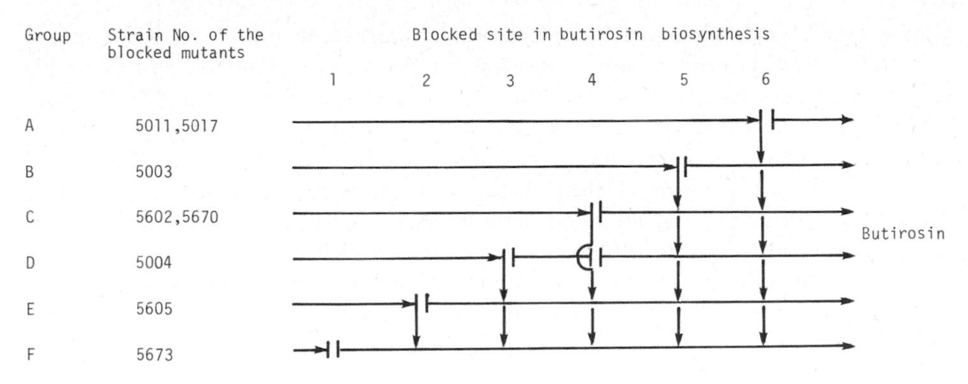

Fig. 2. Complementation pattern of the blocked mutants for the biosynthesis of butirosins. →| |→ shows the blocked site and *vertical arrows* show the processes along which butirosins are cosynthesized by a pair of blocked mutants

d) Utilization of Mutants for Biosynthesis

As described later, an idiotroph of an aminoglycoside-producing strain was originally developed by SHIER et al. (1969) for the purpose of mutasynthesis. Idiotrophs have also been useful in the study of the biosynthesis of this group of antibiotics.

Assuming a sequence of the steps A→B→C→D (2-deoxystreptamine)→ →E→F→G→H (antibiotic) in the biosynthesis of 2-deoxystreptamine-containing aminoglycosides, one may suppose that even if one of the enzymes participating in 2-deoxystreptamine formation is inactivated, the enzymes involved in the steps from 2-deoxystreptamine to antibiotic may remain intact. Consequently, such a mutant is of use to determine whether a compound E, F, or G is a real intermediate or not. If a 2-deoxystreptamine-requiring idiotroph produces antibiotic when fed with the compound F, compound F may be an intermediate located between 2-deoxystreptamine and the antibiotic.

With aminoglycosides, the above method (sometimes referred to as a feeding experiment with an idiotroph) was first applied by TESTA and TILLEY (1975) to the biosynthetic study of sisomicin and then broadly to studies of gentamicin, neomycin, butirosin, and sagamicin.

On the other hand, if the step from 2-deoxystreptamine to compound E is interrupted in a mutant, accumulation of 2-deoxystreptamine may occur, and isolation of 2-deoxystreptamine from the broth indicates that 2-deoxystreptamine is an intermediate.

III. Plasmid Involvement

1. General Aspects

The plasmid is an autonomously replicating extrachromosomal genetic element in the cells of microorganisms. UMEZAWA and OKANISHI first assumed that at least part of the biosynthesis of antibiotics may be controlled by a plasmid specific for each antibiotic (OKANISHI et al. 1970; OKANISHI and UMEZAWA 1978). This assumption was derived from the following evidence. First, antibiotic-nonproducing mutants were readily obtained by cultivating a slant culture at high temperature (37 °C). Secondly, antibiotics with the same or chemically related structures are often produced by microorganisms belonging to taxonomically quite different species. Thirdly, species which, genetically speaking, belong to the same genospecies often include various nomenspecies which produce chemically different antibiotics. Based on these observations, they initiated the study of plasmid involvement in antibiotic production and obtained the following experimental results which support the above assumption (OKANISHI and UMEZAWA 1978).

1. Treatment of the producers of chloramphenicol, aureothricin, kasugamycin, streptomycin, and chlortetracycline with either acriflavine or the highest temperature permitting growth always caused an increased incidence of antibiotic-nonproducing mutants.

2. A gene or genes involved in chloramphenicol production, which were lost by acriflavine treatment, were not linked with the normal chromosomal markers.

3. Three types of plasmid DNAs presumably involved in chloramphenicol, kasugamycin, and aureothricin production were isolated and detected in *Streptomyces venezuela* and *Streptomyces kasugaensis*.

The HOPWOOD group (KIRBY et al. 1975; WRIGHT and HOPWOOD 1976) confirmed the involvement of a plasmid in the production of methylenomycin. NOACK et al. (see reference 14 in OKANISHI and UMEZAWA 1978) also suggested that production of tunicamycin might be caused by a plasmid. Plasmid involvement in antibiotic production was reviewed by HOPWOOD (1978), OKANISHI and UMEZAWA (1978), and OKANISHI (1978, 1979).

Recently, based on studies of the pharmacologically active metabolites (leupeptin, pepstatin, etc.) produced by *Streptomyces*, UMEZAWA demonstrated that plasmid involvement is possible not only in the biosynthesis of antibiotics but also in the biosynthesis of other microbial secondary metabolites. UMEZAWA proposed that secondary metabolites are plasmid products, defined as a product that is biosynthesized at least in part, under the control of a plasmid (H. UMEZAWA 1976).

The plasmid is considered to have no function in the growth of microorganisms, but as shown in Table 1, it is concerned with numerous morphological and biologic properties (phenotypes and functions) of organisms.

2. Plasmid Involvement in Aminoglycoside Synthesis

Since OKANISHI et al. (1970) demonstrated the involvement of a plasmid in the biosynthesis of kasugamycin by *S. kasugaensis*, plasmids have been implicated in the synthesis of other aminoglycosides.

Plasmids may affect antibiotic production in the following respects (OKANISHI 1971): (1) As structural genes for enzymes involved in antibiotic synthesis; (2) as regulatory genes for induction or activation of biosynthetic enzymes; (3) as governing the function of antibiotic excretion or membrane permeability; (4) as repressor or inhibitor of enzymes involved with the decomposition of antibiotics. In aminoglycosides plasmids have been reported to be involved in the synthesis of kasugamycin, istamycin, and 2-deoxystreptamine, as well as showing resistance to neomycin in the fermentation of these compounds. In neomycin synthesis, plasmids may govern membrane permeability.

Table 1. Events controlled by plasmids. (OKANISHI and UMEZAWA 1978)

A. Low molecular weight products
- H_2S (*Escherichia coli*)
- Nisin (*Streptococcus lactis*)
- Melanin (*Streptomyces scabies*)
- Antibiotics (*Streptomyces*)

B. High molecular weight products
- Antibiotic-inactivating enzymes (Enterobacteriaceae, *Pseudomonas*, and Staphylococci)
- Lipase (*Staphylococcus aureus*)
- Proteinase (*Streptococcus lactis*)
- Urease (*Streptococcus faecium*)
- α and β Hemolysin (*E. coli*)
- Enterotoxin (*E. coli*)
- Toxin (*Staphylococcus aureus*)
- Exfoliative toxin (*Staphylococus aureus*)
- Hemolysin (*Streptococcus faecalis* var. *zymogenes*)
- Erythrogenic toxin (Group A Streptococci)
- Botulinus toxin C and D (*Clostridium botulinum*)
- Diphteria toxin (*Corynebacterium diphteriae*)
- Pyocin (*Pseudomonas aeruginosa*)
- Colicins (*E. coli*)
- Staphylococcin (*Staphylococcus aureus*)
- Vibrilcin (*Vibrio*)
- Megacin = Phospholipase (*Bacillus megaterium*)

C. Cell constituents
- Antigen (*Pseudomonas aeruginosa*)
- K 88 antigen (*E. coli*)
- Antigen I (*Shigella flexneri*)
- Antigen IV (*Shigella flexneri*)
- Antigen 3 and 15 (*Salmonella anatum*)
- M protein (Group A Streptococci)

D. Biologic functions
- Sexuality (Enterobacteriaceae, *Pseudomonas*, *Vibrio*, and *Streptomyces coelicolor*)
- Plant virulence (*Erwinia amylovora*)
- Heavy metal resistance (*Staphylococcus aureus*)
- Antibiotic resistance (Enterobacteriaceae, *Pseudomonas*, *Staphylococcus*, *Streptococcus*, *Haemophilus*, and *Bordetella*)
- Glutamic acid excretion (*Citrobacter intermedium*)
- Inhibition of sporulation (*Bacillus pumilus*)
- Competence of transformation (*Neisseria menigitidis*)

E. Utilization of special substrates
- Camphor oxidation (*Pseudomonas putida*)
- Degradation of octane (*Pseudomonas*)
- Benzoic acid and m-toluate degradation (*Pseudomonas arvilla*)
- N_2 fixation (*Klebsiella*, *E. coli*)
- Sucrose utilization (*Salmonella*)
- Lactose utilization (*Salmonella*, Streptococci, and *Serratia liquefaciens*)

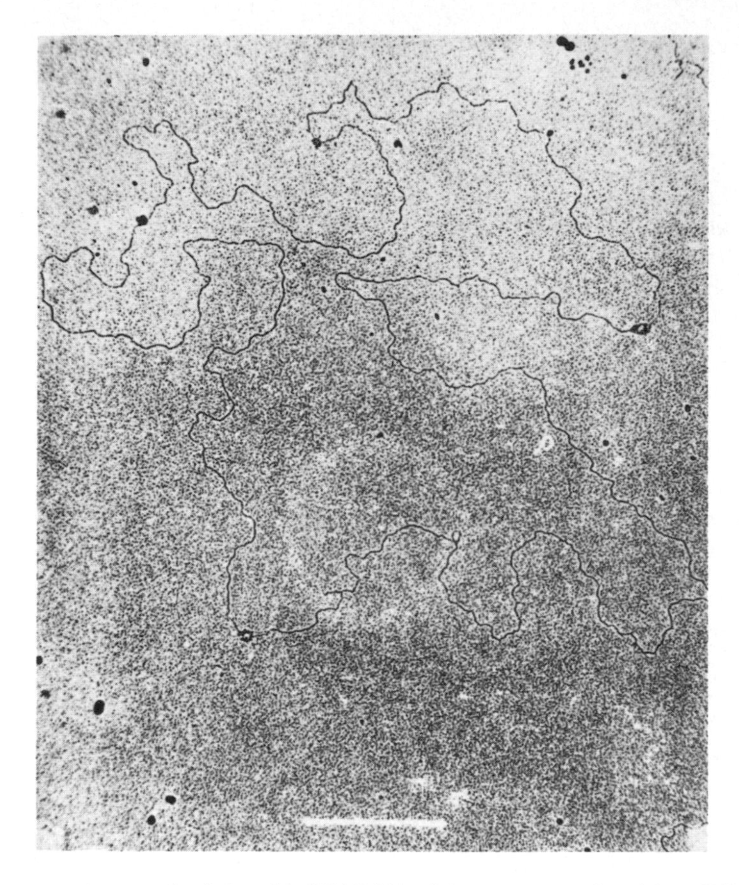

Fig. 3. Electron micrograph of plasmid pSR1 DNA of *Streptomyces ribosidificus* KCC S-0923. *Bar* corresponds to 1 μm. (Courtesy of Dr. M. OKANISHI)

3. Experimental Methods

In addition to high-temperature treatment, elimination of plasmid is carried out by treating the strain with a so-called plasmid-curing agent, such as acridine dyes (acriflavine, acridine orange, etc.), and ethidium bromide.

A general procedure reported by OKANISHI et al. (1980) will be useful for the isolation and detection of plasmid from the cells of aminoglycoside-producing *Streptomyces*.

Figure 3 exhibits the supercoiled plasmid DNA (mol. wt: 49–56 megadaltons) isolated from ribostamycin-producing *S. ribosidificus*.

Generally, an antibiotic-nonproducing strain, if antibiotic production is controlled by plasmids, lacks one or more of the plasmid DNAs in a parental strain.

Final proof of plasmid involvement is ideally given by confirming the physiologic function of such DNA by transformation into plasmid-deficient mutants, though this approach has not been successful in aminoglycoside-producing strains.

B. Biosynthesis of Major Aminoglycosides

In this section, the biosynthesis of subunits and their assembly are considered, followed by discussion of plasmid involvement and other special subjects.

I. Streptomycin and Bluensomycin

Streptomycin produced by *S. griseus* and many other *Streptomyces* species is a pseudotrisaccharide composed of three unique subunits, streptidine, streptose, and *N*-methyl-L-glucosamine, linked with α-L-glycosidic bonds. The structure of streptomycin and related antibiotics is shown in Fig. 4.

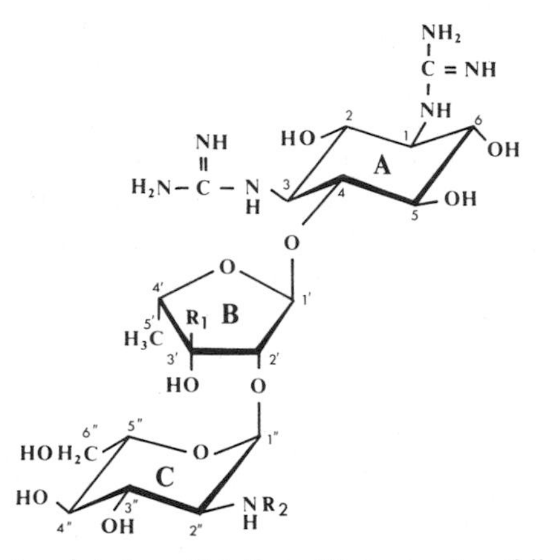

Fig. 4. Streptomycin and related antibiotics. *Ring A*, streptidine; *Ring B*, streptose [R_1=CHO], dihydrostreptose [R_1=CH_2OH]; *Ring C*, *N*-methyl-L-glucosamine [R_2=CH_3], L-glucosamine [R_2=H]; *Ring B+C*, streptobiosamine [R_1=CHO, R_2=CH_3], dihydrostreptobiosamine [R_1=CH_2OH, R_2=CH_3]; *Ring A+B+C*, streptomycin [R_1=CHO, R_2=CH_3], dihydrostreptomycin [R_1=CH_2OH, R_2=CH_3], *N*-demethylstreptomycin [R_1=CHO, R_2=H]

As reviewed by LEMIEUX and WOLFROM (1948), the structural determination of streptomycin was almost completely accomplished by 1948, soon after its discovery; however, in spite of much research, the biosynthetic pathway has not yet been elucidated thoroughly.

The investigation of the biosynthesis of streptomycin started with isotope incorporation studies. KAROW et al. (1952) first reported the preparation of ^{14}C-labeled streptomycin by feeding labeled glucose or starch to the growing culture of *S. griseus*, then HUNTER and HOCKENHULL (1955) found that about 5% of D-[^{14}C]glucose supplied to a 60-h culture of *S. griseus* was incorporated into streptomycin with the radioactivity equally distributed into the three subunits (streptidine, 34.1%; streptose, 31.7%; and *N*-methyl-L-glucosamine, 34.8%). Thereafter, ^{14}C-labeled compounds were used extensively as discussed in review articles by HOCKENHULL (1960), MENDICINO and PICKEN (1966), HORNER (1967), AKAMATSU (1968), and DEMAIN and INAMINE (1970).

In addition to ^{14}C-labeled compounds, MUNRO et al. (1975) used D-[6-^{13}C]glucose. This technique confirmed the location of labeled carbons which had been determined by chemical degradation of [^{14}C]streptomycin. After *S. griseus* MA-4583 was grown in a medium containing D-[6-^{13}C]glucose, ^{13}C-enriched streptomycin was isolated and studied by NMR spectroscopy. Assignment of the signals in enriched streptomycin and comparison of these signals with those of the natural abundance spectrum showed that ^{13}C-enrichment was observed at C-6 in streptidine, C-5 in streptose, and C-6 in *N*-methyl-L-glucosamine moieties. These tracer experiments with [^{14}C]- and [^{13}C]glucose demonstrated that all the subunits of streptomycin are synthesized from D-glucose, as is true for other aminoglycosides.

1. Biosynthesis of Subunits

a) Streptidine

Streptidine is a diguanidine derivative of *scyllo*-inositol, derived from glucose as discussed above. The correlation of the carbon atoms of glucose with those of streptidine was accomplished as follows (BRUCE et al. 1968; HORNER and RUSS 1971; RUSS 1975): Samples of streptidine were prepared from *S. griseus* grown on D-glucose labeled with ^{14}C in positions 1, 2, 3–4, or 6. Alkaline hydrolysis of streptidine to streptamine followed by benzoylation and de-*O*-benzoylation gave *N,N*-dibenzoyl streptamine, which upon periodate oxidation gave a hemiacetal and formic acid. When [1-^{14}C]glucose was administered, a majority of the label was lost as formic acid from C-5 of streptidine, and when [2-^{14}C]-, [3, 4-^{14}C]-, or [6-^{14}C]glucose was fed, a majority of the label was retained in the hemiacetal. Subsequently, from the above results and from studies on the incorporation of tritium from D-[1-^{3}H]- and D-[3-^{3}H]glucoses, HORNER and RUSS (1971) showed that C-5 and C-3 of streptidine are derived from C-1 and C-3 of glucose, respectively. A correlation of C-6 of glucose with C-6 of streptidine was provided by feeding experiments with D-[6-^{13}C]glucose (MUNRO et al. 1975).

S. MAJUMDAR and KUTZNER (1962) suggested that *myo*-inositol is a precursor of the streptidine moiety, because *myo*-inositol, especially in combination with arginine, enhanced the production of streptomycin by two mutants (L118 and 230) of *S. griseus*, and decreased the incorporation of [^{14}C]glucose into streptomycin, particularly into the streptidine moiety. The favorable effects shown by a combination of *myo*-inositol and arginine were also demonstrated with washed mycelium.

Later, HORNER (1964b) and HEDING (1964) confirmed the above suggestion using *myo*-[U-^{14}C]inositol feeding. All of the incorporated isotope was found in the streptidine moiety. Feeding with *myo*-[^{14}C]inositol and D-[^{14}C]glucose gave different radioactivity distribution patterns in the streptidine moiety, indicating that *myo*-inositol is incorporated directly and not via glucose. The utility of *myo*-inositol as a precursor of streptidine was also demonstrated by BRUTON et al. (1967), who observed that 8.1% of *myo*-[U-^{14}C]inositol fed to the growing culture of *S. griseus* on the 5th day was incorporated into streptomycin. They further isolated *myo*-inositol from the acid hydrolyzate of mycelium grown in medium containing D-[1-^{14}C]glucose. The specific activity of *myo*-inositol was much greater than that of the streptidine moiety, suggesting that *myo*-inositol is biosynthesized from D-glucose by *S. griseus*. RUSS (1975) also isolated *myo*-inositol from the acid hydrolyzate of mycelium of *S. griseus* grown in the presence of D-[^{14}C]glucose.

Myo-Inositol may be bioconverted from D-glucose via D-glucose-6-phosphate by ring closure between C-1 and C-6, as was found for cell-free extracts of yeast (CHEN and CHARALAMPOUS 1965a, b, 1966a, b, 1967; KINDL et al. 1965), but not yet confirmed in *Streptomyces*.

BRUTON et al. (1967) also found that addition of *scyllo*-[2-^{3}H]inositol with 0.02% of arginine to *S. griseus* resulted in 7.1%–7.8% incorporation of tritium into streptomycin with all the incorporated tritium located in the streptidine. This finding suggested the possibility that *scyllo*-inositol is a precursor to streptidine. Interconversion between *myo*-inositol and *scyllo*-inositol, with equilibrium in favor of *myo*-inositol, was also demonstrated. Later, this interconversion by *S. griseus* was proposed by HORNER and THAKER (1968) to take place via *scyllo*-inosose, which is now considered to be a precursor to *scyllo*-inosamine in streptidine biosynthesis:

myo-Inositol⇌*scyllo*-Inosose⇌*scyllo*-Inositol.

However, HORNER and RUSS (1969) considered *scyllo*-inositol an unlikely intermediate in streptidine biosynthesis, since BRUCE et al. (1968) found that isotope incorporation into streptidine from D-glucose specifically labeled with ^{14}C was not random. If it were an intermediate, formation of symmetrical *scyllo*-inositol from D-glucose would cause randomization of the isotope.

The role of *scyllo*-inosose as a direct intermediate to *scyllo*-inosamine involved in streptidine biosynthesis was established by HORNER and RUSS (1969). If *scyllo*-inosamine was bioconverted from *myo*-inositol via *scyllo*-inosose, loss of tritium would occur during the oxidation of *myo*-[2-^{3}H]inositol to *scyllo*-inosose and thus streptidine should be unlabeled. To confirm this, a mixture of *myo*-[2-^{3}H]inositol and *myo*-[2-^{14}C]inositol was fed to *S. griseus*. Streptomycin isolated after 24-h incubation was degraded to streptidine which was analyzed for ^{3}H:^{14}C ratio. In duplicate experiments, the ratios in the starting *myo*-inositol mixture were 25.4 and 2.22, while those in the streptidine moiety were 1.3 and 0. Thus, tritium incorporation into streptidine was very slight, indicating that *scyllo*-inosose is an intermediate in streptomycin formation.

As the result of experiments with cell-free extracts of the mycelium of *S. griseus*, *S. bikiniensis*, and *S. glebosus*, WALKER and collaborators proposed the biosynthetic pathway of streptidine-6-phosphate from glucose-6-phosphate shown in Fig. 5 (J. WALKER 1958, 1978; M. WALKER and J. WALKER 1964, 1965, 1971; J. WALKER and M. WALKER 1967b, c, 1968, 1969; WALKER and SKORVAGA 1973b). Details of the individual enzyme reactions were described in his contribution to *Methods in Enzymology* (J. WALKER 1975) and summarized in his review (J. WALKER 1971).

The biosynthetic sequence shown in Fig. 5 is: D-glucose-6-phosphate (1) is first cyclized to *myo*-inositol-phosphate (2) and dephosphorylated to give *myo*-inositol (3). Then, (3) is oxidized at C-2 (corresponding to C-5 of the original glucose) to *scyllo*-inosose (4), which goes to *scyllo*-inosamine (5) by transamination from L-glutamine. Subsequently, *scyllo*-inosamine (5) is phosphorylated at the hydroxyl group *para* to the amino group, which is then transamidinated from arigine to yield *N*-amidino-*scyllo*-inosamine-phosphate (7). *N*-Amidino-keto-*scyllo*-inosamine (9), resulting from (7) by dephosphorylation followed by oxidation of the hydroxyl group β to the amidino group, is converted into *N*-amidino-streptamine (10) by

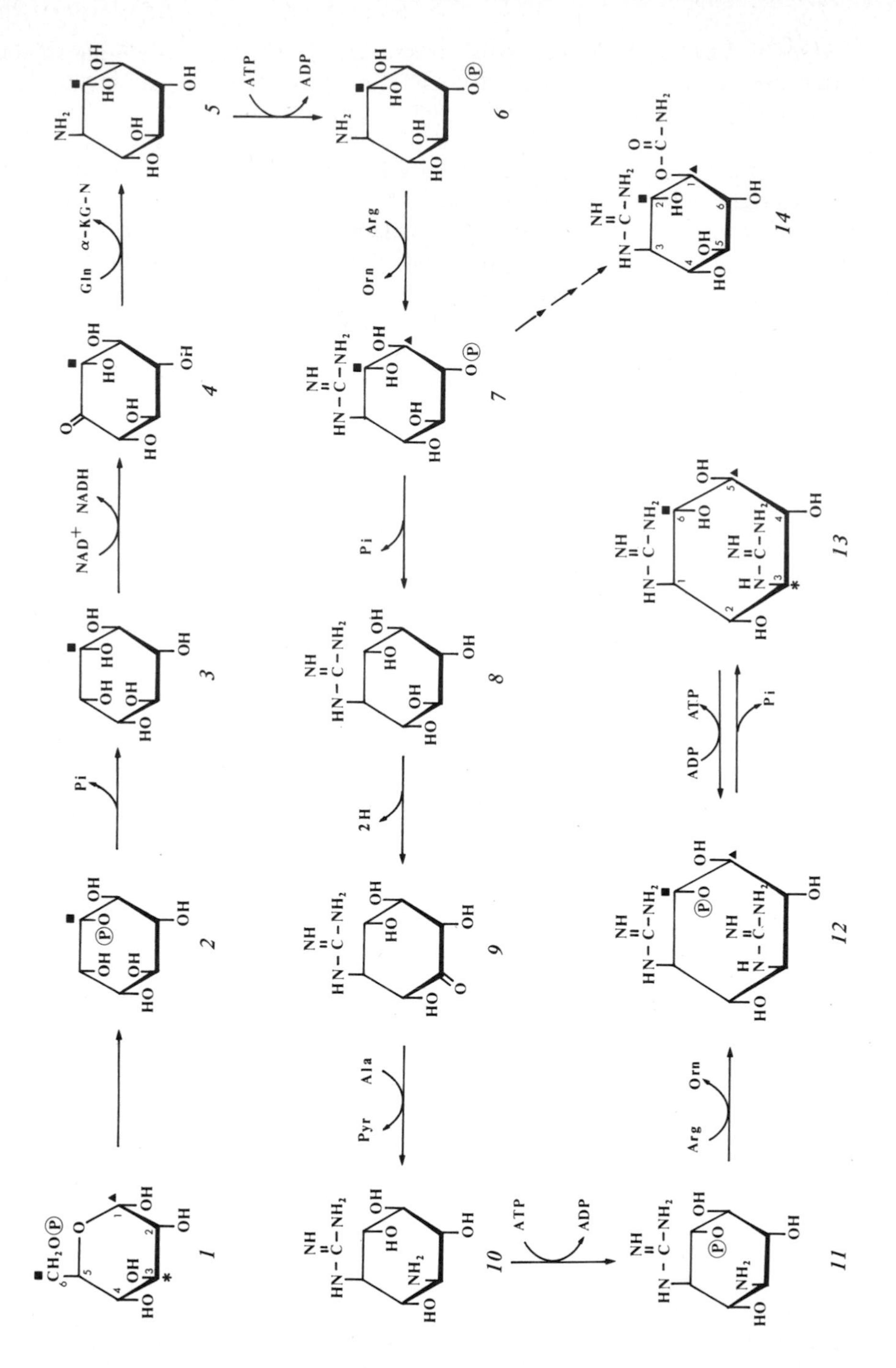

Fig. 5. Biosynthetic pathway of streptidine or bluensidine. Gln, glutamine; α-KG-N, α-ketoglutaramate; Orn, ornithine; Arg, arginine; Ala, alanine; ⓟ, phosphate; Pyr, pyruvate; Pi, orthophosphoric acid

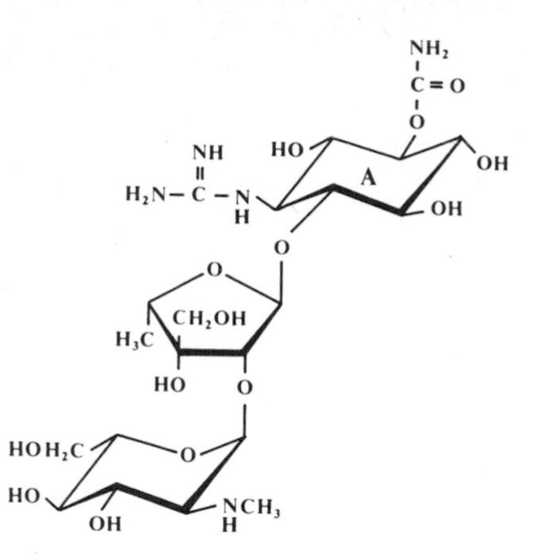

Fig. 6. Bluensomycin (glebomycin). *Ring A*, bluensidine

transamination from alanine. (10) is again phosphorylated to (11) which undergoes a second transamidination from arginine to give streptidine-6-phosphate (12). Finally, (12) is converted to streptomycin or hydrolyzed to streptidine (13) by streptomycin-(streptidino)-phosphate phosphatase found in streptomycin-producing strains of *Streptomyces*.

The above sequence was in accordance with the observation that, when labeled *myo*-inositol was fed to *S. griseus*, labeled (5)–(8), (11), and (12) were isolated from hot-water extracts of mycelium (J. WALKER and M. WALKER 1967a; M. WALKER and J. WALKER 1967; RUSS 1975). When L-[guanidino-^{14}C]arginine was supplied instead of *myo*-[^{14}C]inositol, amidino-streptamine-phosphate (11) and streptidine-6-phosphate (12) labeled in the guanidine function were obtained (HORNER 1964a; M. WALKER and J. WALKER 1966).

Bluensomycin (glebomycin) (Fig. 6) produced by *S. hygroscopicus* forma *glebosus* is a monoguanidinated analog of dihydrostreptomycin. In bluensomycin, the streptidine moiety of dihydrostreptomycin is replaced by bluensidine (ring A in Fig. 6). Bluensidine and streptidine differ only in the substituent at C-1, a carbamoyl group in bluensidine and a guanidine group in streptidine.

According to J. WALKER (1974), bluensidine (14) is synthesized from *myo*-inositol via *scyllo*-inosamine, which may undergo oxidation, transamination, phosphorylation, dephosphorylation, and transamidination by the enzyme system of streptomycin biosynthesis. Bluensidine biosynthesis, however, involves a carbamoylation step. It has not yet been established where, between *scyllo*-inositol and bluensidine-6-phosphate, carbamoylation takes place.

b) Streptose

Streptose is a C-3 formyl derivative of 5-deoxy-L-lyxose, a unique branched deoxypentose.

A biosynthetic pathway for streptose from D-glucose first proposed by BADDILEY and his collaborators is shown in Fig. 7 (BLUMSON and BADDILEY 1961; BADDILEY et al. 1961). They isolated thymidine diphospho-rhamnose (dTDP-rham-

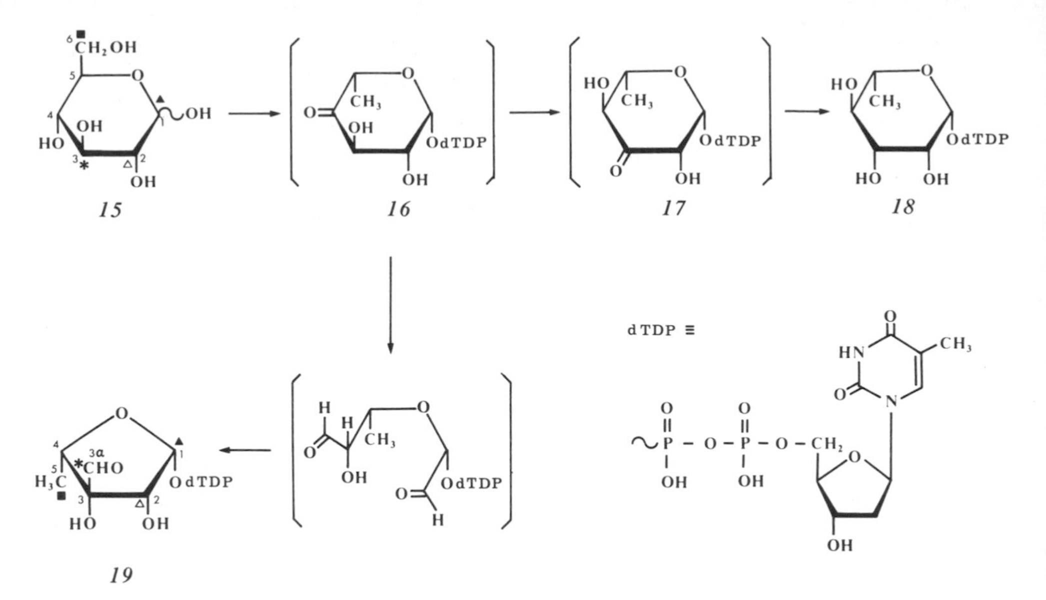

Fig. 7. Postulated biosynthetic pathway of dTDP-streptose and dTDP-L-rhamnose. (BLUMSON and BADDILEY 1961)

nose) (18) from the mycelium of *S. griseus* and proved the formation of dTDP-rhamnose from dTDP-glucose by using cell-free preparations. They suggested that this reaction proceeded via two carbonyl intermediates, dTDP-6-deoxy-L-arabino-4-hexulose (16) and dTDP-6-deoxy-L-arabino-3-hexulose (17), and further assumed that dTDP-streptose (19) might be formed by a single rearrangement of either one of these two carbonyl intermediates. Subsequently, they (CANDY et al. 1964; CANDY and BADDILEY 1965) demonstrated that C-1, C-3, and C-6 of glucose corresponded to C-1, C-3α (the formyl carbon), and C-6 (the methyl carbon), respectively, and assumed that the 4-hexulose (16) might be an intermediate from D-glucose. The above assumption was supported by BRUTON and HORNER (1966, 1969) who showed that C-2 of streptose arose from C-2 of glucose. Thus, it was concluded that the whole carbon chain of glucose is incorporated intact into the streptose molecule via the route shown in Fig. 7. The origin of C-5 of streptose was later confirmed by MUNRO et al. (1975) who carried out feeding experiments with D-[6-^{13}C]glucose.

A biosynthetic pathway for dihydrostreptose and its dTDP-derivative from D-glucose was later proposed by GRISEBACH and his group, based on enzymatic studies, indicating that streptomycin may be biosynthesized from dihydrostreptomycin (ORTMAN et al. 1974; WAHL et al. 1975; WAHL and GRISEBACH 1979). When dTDP-D-[U-^{14}C]glucose was incubated with a cell-free extract of streptomycin-producing *S. griseus* in the presence of nicotinamide adenine dinucleotide phosphate (NADPH), nucleotide sugars were produced which, on hydrolysis, gave radioactive dihydrostreptose together with rhamnose and 4-keto-6-deoxy-D-glucose (6-deoxy-D-*xylo*-4-hexosulose). Labeled dTDP-4-keto-6-deoxy-glucose was formed from dTDP-D-[U-^{14}C]glucose by incubation with an enzyme extract of *S. griseus*

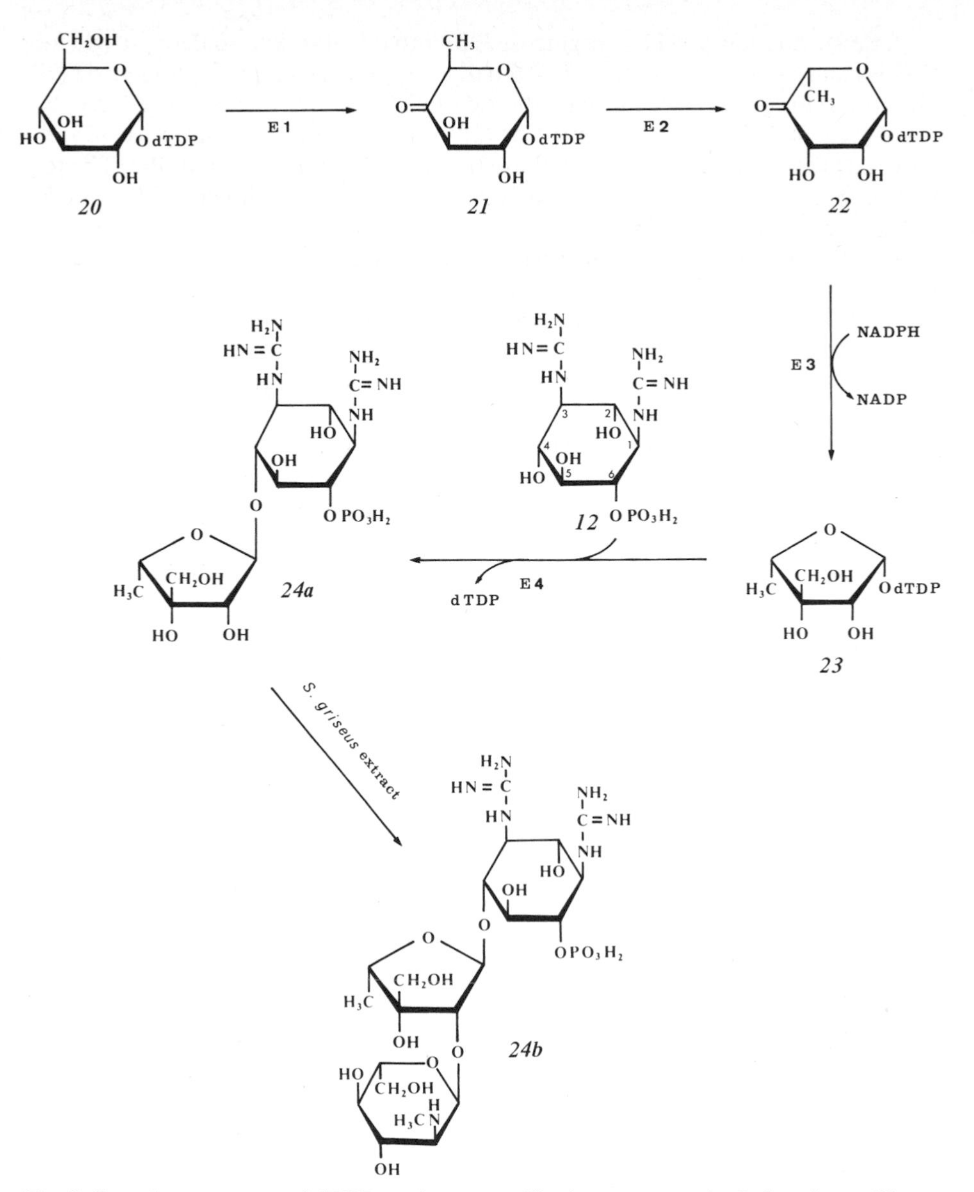

Fig. 8. Reaction sequence of dTDP-D-glucose to dihydrostreptomycin 6-phosphate. (GRISEBACH 1980). Enzyme; *E1*, dTDP-glucose 4,6-dehydratase; *E2*, dTDP-4-keto-L-rhamnose 3,5-epimerase; *E3*, dTDP-dihydrostreptose synthase; *E4*, dTDP-L-dihydrostreptose: streptidine 6-phosphate dihydrostreptosyltransferase

even in the absence of exogenous NADPH. dTDP-4-keto-6-deoxy-glucose (21) thus obtained gave labeled dTDP-L-rhamnose (18) and dTDP-dihydrostreptose (23) by incubation with a cell-free extract in the presence of NADPH. Consequently, the reaction would proceed from dTDP-D-glucose (20) to dTDP-dihydrostreptose (23) according to the sequence shown in Fig. 8.

Transformation of dTDP-D-glucose (20) into dTDP-4-keto-6-deoxy-D-glucose (21) is catalyzed by dTDP-glucose-4,6-dehydratase (E_1), epimerization to dTDP-4-keto-L-rhamnose (22) occurs with the aid of dTDP-4-keto-L-rhamnose-3,5-epimerase (E_2), and final rearrangement of (22) into dTDP-dihydrostreptose (23) involves dTDP-dihydrostreptose-synthase (E_3) in the presence of NADPH. The formation of dTDP-4-keto-L-rhamnose (22) from glucose was shown by *Escherichia coli* Y10 which possessed the former two enzymes, E_1 and E_2, but lacked enzyme E_3. dTDP-4-keto-L-[U-^{14}C]rhamnose bioconverted from dTDP-D-[U-^{14}C]glucose by strain Y10 was identified by reduction with NaB^3H_4 into 6-deoxy-[U-^{14}C, ^{3}H]-talose. L-Rhamnose, another expected reduction product from dTDP-4-keto-L-rhamnose (22), was difficult to identify on paper chromatograms, because the R_F-value was so close to that of 6-deoxyglucose, a reduction product from dTDP-4-keto-6-deoxy-glucose (21).

Enzymic transformation of dTDP-D-glucose to dTDP-4-keto-6-deoxy-D-glucose by *E. coli* was considered in detail by GABRIEL and LINDQUIST 1968), MELO et al. (1968), and recently by SNIPES et al. (1977), and it was shown that the reaction is catalyzed by dTDP-D-glucose oxidoreductase containing an essential NAD$^{\oplus}$ moiety. In particular, SNIPES et al. studied the stereochemistry involved in the reaction, using partially purified oxidoreductase isolated from late log phase cells of *E. coli* (ATCC 11303) and nucleotide glucose doubly labeled with deuterium and tritium, namely dTDP-(6R)- and (6S)-[4-^{2}H, 6-^{3}H]glucose, as substrate. They proposed a stereochemical course for the dTDP-glucose oxidoreductase reaction as shown in Fig. 9. Exogenous NADPH was not necessary for the reaction and elimination of water from C-5 and C-6 was formally *syn*, whereas the reduction of the resulting double bond formally involves an *anti* addition of H$^{\oplus}$ and H$^{\ominus}$, thus bringing on the change of chirality around C-6. A similar reaction has been report-

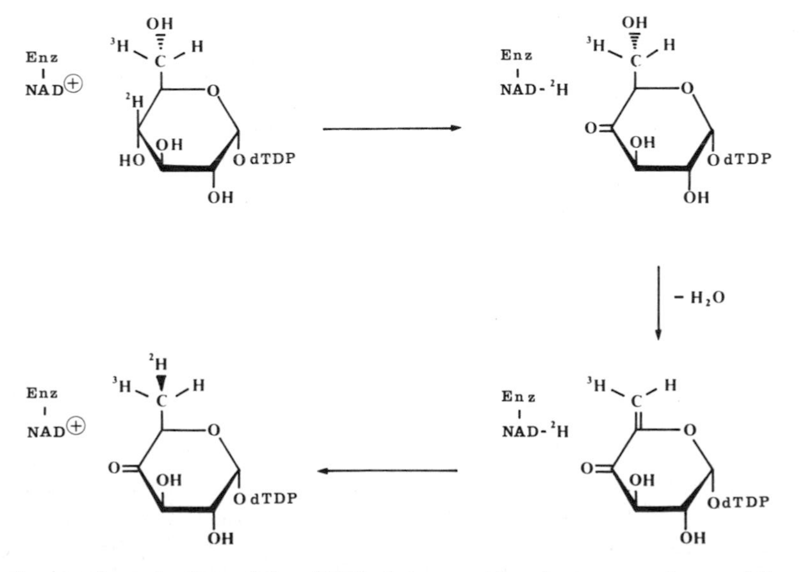

Fig. 9. Proposed mechanism of the dTDP-glucose oxidoreductase reaction and its stereochemical course. (GABRIEL and LINDQUIST 1968; SNIPES et al. 1977)

ed for the inversion of UDP-D-glucuronic acid to UDP-D-apiose catalyzed by UDP-apiose/UDP-xylose synthase (GRISEBACH 1978). The significance of dihydrostreptose in the biosynthesis of streptomycin will be discussed later.

c) *N*-Methyl-L-Glucosamine

As already mentioned, it was shown that *N*-methyl-L-glucosamine originated from D-glucose involving the interesting transformation of a D-sugar into an L-sugar. The mechanism remained obscure until recently.

HUNTER and HOCKENHULL (1955) observed that 15.5% of *N*-methyl-L-[U-^{14}C]glucosamine added to a 60-hr culture of *S. griseus* was incorporated into streptomycin, and about 75% of the incorporated radioactivity was found in the *N*-methyl-L-glucosamine moiety. Incorporation of D-[U-^{14}C]glucose was very low (5%). According to BRUTON et al. (1967), L-[1-^{14}C]glucose added in place of D-[1-^{14}C]glucose was not incorporated into streptomycin, while D-[1-^{14}C]glucosamine was efficiently incorporated into streptomycin with 59%–64% of the incorporated radioactivity detected in *N*-methyl-L-glucosamine. Moreover, 76% of the radioactivity in this aminosugar was concentrated in C-1 of the molecule. In addition, the higher distribution ratio (59%–64%) of D-glucosamine into *N*-methyl-L-glucosamine excluded the possibility of bioconversion of D-glucosamine to D-glucose prior to incorporation into streptomycin. From these data, the pathway D-glucose→D-glucosamine→L-glucosamine (or *N*-methyl-L-glucosamine) was assumed.

Labeled positions in *N*-methyl-L-glucosamine (25) after the administration of specifically labeled glucoses were determined by the degradation procedure shown in Fig. 10. By this procedure, SILVERMAN and RIEDER (1960) determined which carbon atoms of *N*-methyl-L-glucosamine were labeled after feeding [1-^{14}C]- or [6-^{14}C]glucose. Later, BRUTON et al. (1967) also studied feeding of D-[1-^{14}C]-, [2-^{14}C]-, [3, 4-$^{14}C_2$]-, or [6-^{14}C]glucose to *S. griseus* cultures. The results of both groups may be summarized as follows. The carbons at C-1, C-2, and C-6 of D-glucose are concentrated in C-1, C-2 and C-6 of *N*-methyl-L-glucosamine, respectively, and [3, 4-$^{14}C_2$]glucose is mainly incorporated into C-3 and C-4 (or C-5) of the aminosugar. The finding by MUNRO et al. (1975) that D-[6-^{13}C]glucose enriched the C-6 of the aminosugar agreed with the above observations. These results indicate that six-carbon chain of D-glucose is incorporated as a unit into *N*-methyl-L-glucosamine and the individual carbon atoms of this hexosamine originate from the corresponding carbons of D-glucose, though the configuration of the asymmetric centers is extensively altered.

Several hypothetical mechanisms for the biotransformation of D-glucose to this hexosamine have been summarized by RINEHART and STROSHANE (1976), but the above results eliminated all the suspected mechanisms except one involving multiple inversions of the asymmetric carbon atoms of D-glucose or D-glucosamine leading to *N*-methyl-L-glucosamine. A similar sequence was suggested by VOLK (1959) for the conversion of L-arabinose to D-arabinose-5-phosphate.

GRISEBACH (1978) suggested a possible sequence based on analogy with similar reactions. Epimerization of UDP-2-acetamido-2-deoxy-D-glucose by the enzyme which was found in *E. coli* (KAWAMURA et al. 1975) may afford first UDP-2-acetamido-2-deoxy-D-mannose, which is oxidized to the corresponding 4-ketosugar.

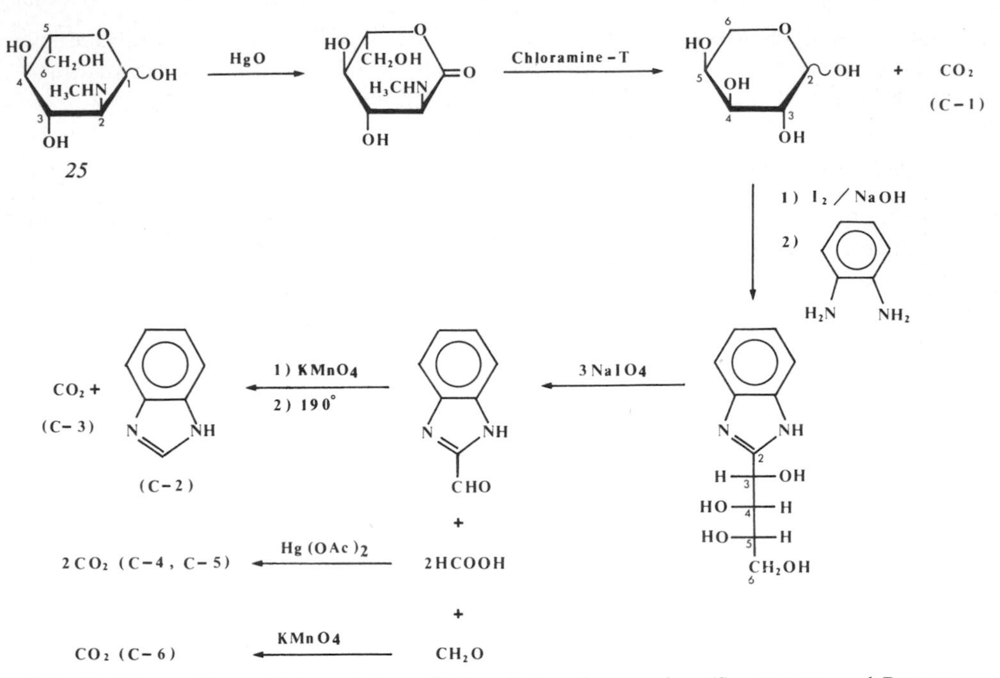

Fig. 10. Scheme for total degradation of *N*-methyl-L-glucosamine. (SILVERMAN and RIEDER 1960; BRUTON et al. 1967)

Then, a second epimerization of 4-ketosugar by a 3,5-epimerase and stereospecific reduction of the C-4 carbonyl could led to inversion at all chiral centers of D-glucosamine.

KUMAGAI and AKAMATSU (1977) suggested the possibility of epimerization via keto-enol interconversion. They simultaneously fed D-[1-^{14}C]glucose and D-[6-^{3}H]glucose at various ratios to cultures of *S. griseus* ME936-B3 and isolated labeled streptomycin. The *N*-methyl-L-glucosamine obtained was analyzed for the ^{3}H:^{14}C ratio. The ^{3}H:^{14}C ratio for *N*-methyl-L-glucosamine was the same as that of the administered D-glucose. This suggested that D-glucose was not cleaved during the conversion to an L-aminosugar. They further studied mixtures with varying amounts of D-[1-^{14}C]glucose and D-[3-^{3}H]glucose and found that the ^{3}H:^{14}C ratios in *N*-methyl-L-glucosamine recovered were lower than those in the starting mixtures. From these results, they concluded that the hydrogen atom at C-3 of D-glucose must be involved in the steps from D-glucose to L-aminosugar, presumably in an epimerization step by keto-enol interconversion.

Finally, CANDY et al. (1964) demonstrated that the *N*-methyl group of *N*-methyl-L-glucosamine arises from the *S*-methyl group of methionine and not from formate by experiments with L-[CH_3-^{14}C]methionine and other labeled compounds. These results explain the previous observations by GALANINA and AGATOV (1959) and S. MAJUNDAS and KUTZNER (1962) that under certain conditions L-methionine stimulated streptomycin production. The following observation by HEDING (1968) is also in agreement with the above conclusion. He isolated demethylstreptomycin from a culture of *S. griseus* grown in synthetic medium supplemented with ethionine, a competitive inhibitor of methionine. Later, HEDING and BAJPAI (1973) found that both *N*-demethylstreptomycin and dihydro-*N*-demethylstreptomycin were methylated by *S. griseus* to give streptomycin and dihydrostreptomycin. They concluded that the last step in the biosynthesis of streptomycin is *N*-methylation. On the contrary, RUSS (1975) reported that *N*-methyl-L-glucosamine may be preformed and then incorporated into streptomycin, because a strain of *S. griseus* produced *N*-methyl-L-glucosamine whose molar concentration was nearly twice as high as that of streptomycin in the broth.

Besides the timing of *N*-methylation, many problems remain to be solved before the biosynthesis of L-glucosamine or *N*-methyl-L-glucosamine is completely understood.

2. Subunit Assembly

The incorporation of *N*-methyl-L-[U-^{14}C]glucosamine into streptomycin has already been described. No report has appeared on the incorporation of labeled streptose, probably because of the instability of streptose which makes it difficult to isolate this moiety from the degradation of labeled streptomycin. The successful isolation of a streptidine-requiring idiotroph (mutant MIT-AS) of *S. griseus* by NAGAOKA and DEMAIN (1975) indicated that streptidine is capable of incorporation into streptomycin. ANISOVA et al. (1976) also isolated a streptidine-requiring idiotroph of *S. griseus* by chemical mutagenesis and demonstrated that this mutant utilized exogenously supplemented [^{14}C]-streptidine to produce streptomycin with labeled streptidine.

Idiotrophs of aminoglycoside-producing strains have provided much information concerning subunit assembly. However, no data are available for streptomycin biosynthesis because incorporation experiments by idiotrophs with pseudodi- or trisaccharides have not been conducted.

M. WALKER and J. WALKER (1971) speculated that L-streptose and *N*-methyl-L-glucosamine are first converted into nucleosides: nucleoside-streptose is transferred to streptidine-6-phosphate to give *O*-α-L-streptose-(1→4)-streptidine-6-phosphate to which nucleoside-*N*-methyl-L-glucosamine is transferred forming streptomycin-6-phosphate.

NOMI and his group (NOMI et al. 1968, 1969; NOMI and NIMI 1969; NIMI et al. 1971 b, c) also assumed streptomycin-6-phosphate to be a natural precursor in streptomycin biosynthesis, since streptomycin-6-phosphate is produced in the culture broth by keeping the pH below neutrality so as to prevent the action of alkaline phosphatase. Also [^{32}P]streptidine-6-phosphate is converted intact into [^{32}P]streptomycin-6-phosphate by resting cells. However, mycelium, especially at a late stage when the cells extensively excreted streptomycin, contained a large amount of a phosphorylating enzyme inside the cell (NIMI et al. 1971 a, b), so that the possibility remains that streptomycin phosphate is formed by phosphorylation of streptomycin which has been excreted outside the cell.

PIWOWARSKI and SHAW (1976) also found that a cell-free extract of *S. bikiniensis*, especially in the stationary phase, contained an adenosine 5′-triphosphate-dependent kinase which inactivates streptomycin and dihydrostreptomycin by phosphorylation at the hydroxyl group at C-6 of the streptidine moiety. In addition, streptomycin-3″-kinase was detected in the extract of another strain of *S. griseus* (J. WALKER and SKORVAGA 1973a). It is unknown whether or not such a streptomycin-inactivating enzyme is participating in the biosynthesis of streptomycin. Streptomycin-6-kinase will be dealt with further in connection with plasmids.

On the other hand, GRISEBACH and his group proposed the following steps for streptomycin biosynthesis: (a) transfer of dihydrostreptose to streptidine-6-phosphate (12) to form *O*-α-L-dihydrostreptose (1→4)-streptidine-6-phosphate (24a); (b) transfer of *N*-methyl-L-glucosamine to (24a) to give dihydrostreptomycin-6-phosphate (24b); (c) oxidation of dihydrostreptomycin-6-phosphate to streptomycin-6-phosphate; (d) hydrolysis of streptomycin-6-phosphate to streptomycin (Fig. 8).

In this respect, KNIEP and GRISEBACH (1976) first observed that a cell-free extract of *S. griseus* transferred dTDP-L-[U-^{14}C]dihydrostreptose to (12) and they recently (1980a) obtained a highly purified enzyme involved in this step, dTDP-L-dihydrostreptose : streptidine-6-phosphate dihydrostreptosyltransferase from frozen cells of *S. griseus*. The transferase activity in the course of fermentation runs parallel to those of dTDP-dihydrostreptose synthase and arginine:x-amidinotransferase, and reaches a maximum just before the appearance of streptomycin.

Incubation of (24a) with a protein-free extract from *S. griseus* as endogenous donor and a cell-free extract from this organism led to the formation of dihydrostreptomycin-6-phosphate (24b), demonstrating the pathway (b) (KNIEP and GRISEBACH 1980b). *N*-Methyl-L-glucosamine was detected in the acid hydrolyzate of the above protein extract. The presence of *N*-methyl-L-glucosamine was also demonstrated in the sugar nucleotide fraction of *S. griseus*.

On step (c), MAIER et al. (1975) had already suggested that dihydrostreptomycin was oxidized to streptomycin at the outer cell membrane or by an exoenzyme in the fermentation broth, because both streptomycin and dihydrostreptomycin were detected in the broth, whereas inside the mycelium only dihydrostreptomycin was detected throughout all stages of the fermentation.

More recently, MAIER and GRISEBACH (1979) gave additional proof for the enzymic oxidation of dihydrostreptomycin or its 6-phosphate to streptomycin or streptomycin-6-phosphate. Dihydrostreptomycin was oxidized to streptomycin by resting cells, permeabilized cells (obtained by dimethylsulfoxide treatment), and also protoplasts of *S. griseus* and the dihydrostreptomycin oxidoreductase activity was concentrated in the $10^6 \times g$ particulate fraction consisting mainly of membrane vesicles. Thus, they considered that the enzyme was localized in the cell membrane. It was shown that both dihydrostreptomycin and dihydrostreptomycin-6-phosphate underwent oxidation by the oxidoreductase, the phosphate being a better substrate in the cell-free system. As shown later, dephosphorylation of streptomycin-6-phosphate in the cells of the producing strain seemed to be the last step in streptomycin biosynthesis (MILLER and WALKER 1969, 1970; NIMI et al. 1970). Therefore, MAIER and GRISEBACH (1979) concluded that the pathway from dihydrostreptomycin-6-phosphate to streptomycin via streptomycin-6-phosphate is consistent with all of the above results.

However, there are some experimental findings which do not fit with the above conclusion. According to the suggestion of HEDING and BAJPAI (1973), *N*-methylation is the final step of the biosynthesis of streptomycin. GRISEBACH's (1978) data do not support this, since he could not show *N*-methylation of dihydro-*N*-demethylstreptomycin or *N*-demethylstreptomycin by *S*-adenosyl-L-[CH_3-^{14}C] methionine with a cell-free extract of *S. griseus*.

KRASILNIKOVA et al. (1978a) isolated low-producing mutants of *Actinomyces streptomycini* by mutation with nitrosomethylbiuret and found that most of these mutants produced about 1,000 μg/ml of streptomycin in the presence of streptobiosamine (ring A+B in Fig. 1), but in a medium containing *N*-methyl-L-glucosamine showed no increase in streptomycin production.

3. Correlation with Cell Wall Biosynthesis

As mentioned previously, *N*-methyl-L-glucosamine is biosynthesized from D-glucose via D-glucosamine. D-Glucosamine is also utilized as a precursor of other aminoglycosides. On the other hand, D-glucosamine as a primary metabolite is a precursor of cell wall mucopeptides. Therefore, a regulation mechanism must be present to control the utilization of D-glucosamine for cell wall formation and antibiotic production.

A close correlation between streptomycin production and cell wall mucopeptide formation was pointed out by NIMI et al. (1976). They found that streptomycin was produced by suspending the mycelium of *S. griseus* in glucose solution containing 0.5% NaCl and shaking at 28 °C for at least 24 h. Addition of certain amino acids to the above system enhanced the production of streptomycin and depressed the incorporation of L-[U-^{14}C]alanine into cell mucopeptide. L-Phenylalanine was the most active in this regard and also inhibited the incorporation of D-[U-^{14}C]glucosamine into mucopeptide but increased the incorporation of glucosamine into streptomycin. Even greater effects were observed when a cell wall synthesis inhibitor, such as bacitracin or enduracidin, was added along with L-phenylalanine. IKEDA et al. (1977) carried out similar studies with resting cells. The biosynthesis of cell walls rapidly decreased after the addition of an inhibitor to the medium and glucosamine-6-phosphate and *N*-acetyl-glucosamine-1-phosphate accumulated. The cells exhibited the strongest streptomycin biosynthetic ability 4 h later. D-[1-^{14}C]Glucosamine fed simultaneously with the addition of the cell wall inhibitor was incorporated mostly into *N*-methyl-L-glucosamine, but labeled glucosamine fed 6 h later was distributed equally between *N*-methyl-L-glucosamine and streptose moieties and that fed 12 h later was mostly incorporated into streptose.

The above findings suggested that D-glucosamine was preferentially utilized for cell wall synthesis in the normally growing mycelium, but if cell wall synthesis is depressed, utilization of D-glucosamine is shunted toward streptomycin production. This is one of the reasons for the vigorous production of streptomycin in the stationary phase of growth.

Penicillin, a well-known inhibitor of cell wall synthesis, at a subinhibitory concentration (1–5 μg/ml) increased streptomycin production about twofold when added to older cultures (BARABÁS and SZABÓ 1977). However, when added to younger cultures it decreased production, so that penicillin seems not to control the utilization of D-glucosamine in young cells, but influences the permeability of the mature cell wall.

VITÁLIS et al. (1963) observed a morphological difference between streptomycin-producing and -nonproducing strains, caused by the depression of cell wall biosynthesis. This phenomenon was also observed in glucosamine-requiring auxotrophs of butirosin-producing *Bacillus circulans* as described in Sect. B.III.

4. Plasmid Involvement

Plasmids are thought to be involved in the biosynthesis of streptomycin by *S. griseus* and *S. bikiniensis*.

SHAW and PIWOWARSKI (1977; PIWOWARSKI and SHAW 1979) incubated the spores of streptomycin-producing *S. bikiniensis* which is resistant to streptomycin in a medium containing ethidium bromide (5 μg/ml) or acriflavine (2μg/ml). Colonies isolated from the medium were examined for (1) sensitivity to streptomycin, (2) streptomycin production, (3) pigment production, and (4) aerial mycelium formation. It was found that 2%–16% of the isolated colonies were deficient in streptomycin production, lacked streptomycin-6-kinase activity at all stages of growth, and had lost their resistance to streptomycin. Some were temporarily unable to form aerial mycelium. The production of brown–black pigment was not affected by ethidium bromide or acriflavine. These results indicated that plasmids are involved in streptomycin production and also in resistance to streptomycin. However, isolation of plasmids from the cells was not reported.

XUE et al. (1978) reported on work with a valine auxotroph (strain 45-706) derived from streptomycin-producing and penicillin-sensitive *S. griseus* 45. High-temperature treatment of strain 45–706 at 36 °C for 8 days induced mutants which were unable to form aerial mycelium or produce streptomycin, and which were resistant to penicillin in some cases.

The compound termed A-factor may be significant in streptomycin biosynthesis. A-factor (Fig. 11) was first isolated by KHOKHLOV et al. (1967) from the fermentation broth of a streptomycin-nonproducing mutant of *A. streptomycini* 1439, and later identified as 2(*S*)-isocapryloyl-3(*R*)-hydroxymethyl-γ-butyrolactone (KLEINER et al. 1976). It was synthesized as a racemate by KLEINER et al. (1977). A-factor was produced only by *A. streptomycini* and *S. bikiniensis*, irrespective of their ability to produce streptomycin, but not by other streptomycin-producers such as *S. galbus* and *S. mashuensis* and other aminoglycoside-producing strains (KORNITSKAYA et al. 1976b).

Mutants of the streptomycin-producing strains from which A-factor had been eliminated were examined by KHOKHLOV et al. (1973) and KORNITSKAYA et al. (1975, 1976a). These mutants were asporogenous and unable to produce streptomycin, but A-factor added to fermentation medium during inoculation of seed cultures resulted in the biosynthesis of streptomycin. When A-factor was added to a

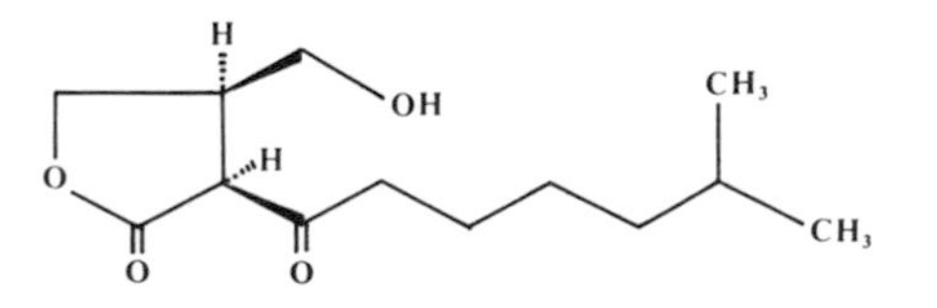

Fig. 11. A-factor

1- or 2-day-old culture, 10 times more A-factor was required, because of high non-specific absorption by the mycelium. Parallel to the restoration of streptomycin productivity, transamidinase activity participating in streptidine biosynthesis in the cells became measurable. A-factor normalized the properties of A-factor-deficient mutants with respect to spore formation, coloration of colonies, and enzymes involved in primary metabolism. Consequently, A-factor was considered to primarily affect enzymes involved in primary metabolism and thus influence the production of secondary metabolites such as streptomycin. It would be interesting from a genetic standpoint to reinvestigate this factor.

II. Neomycin and Paromomycin

As shown in Fig. 12, neomycin and paromomycin are 4,5-disubstituted-2-deoxystreptamine antibiotics with four cyclic subunits: 2-deoxystreptamine (ring A), D-ribose (ring C), and two aminosugars (rings B and D). One of the aminosugars (ring B) of neomycin is neosamine C (paromose II) (2,6-diamino-2,6-dideoxy-D-glucose) which is replaced in the paromomycin by D-glucosamine. The other aminosugar (ring D) of both neomycin B and paromomycin I is neosamine B (paromose I) (2,6-diamino-2,6-dideoxy-D-idose), while that of neomycin C and paromomycin II is a second neosamine C.

RINEHART and his collaborators have summarized their work on neomycin biosynthesis in their review articles (RINEHART and SCHIMBOR 1967; RINEHART and STROSHANE 1976). On the other hand, biosynthetic studies on paromomycin are limited, so the paromomycins are considered here with the neomycins. The biosynthesis of ribostamycin, which comprises a part of the neomycin molecule, will be dealt with in Sect. B.III.

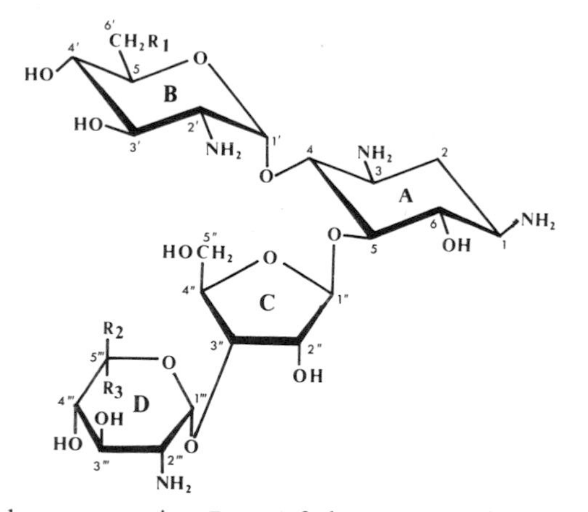

Fig. 12. Neomycins and paromomycins. *Ring A*, 2-deoxystreptamine; *Ring B*, D-glucosamine [R_1=OH], neosamine C (paromose II) [$R_1=NH_2$]; *Ring C*, D-ribose; *Ring D*, neosamine B (paromose I) [R_2=H, $R_3=CH_2NH_2$], neosamine C (paromose II) [$R_2=CH_2NH_2$, R_3=H]; *Ring A+B*, neamine [$R_1=NH_2$], paromamine [R_1=OH]; *Ring C+D*, neobiosamine B [R_2=H, $R_3=CH_2NH_2$], neobiosamine C [$R_2=CH_2NH_2$, R_3=H]; *Ring A+B+C+D*, neomycin B [$R_1=NH_2$, R_2=H, $R_3=CH_2NH_2$], neomycin C [$R_1=NH_2$, $R_2=CH_2NH_2$, R_3=H], paromomycin I [R_1=OH, R_2=H, $R_3=CH_2NH_2$], paromomycin II [R_1=OH, $R_2=CH_2NH_2$, R_3=H]

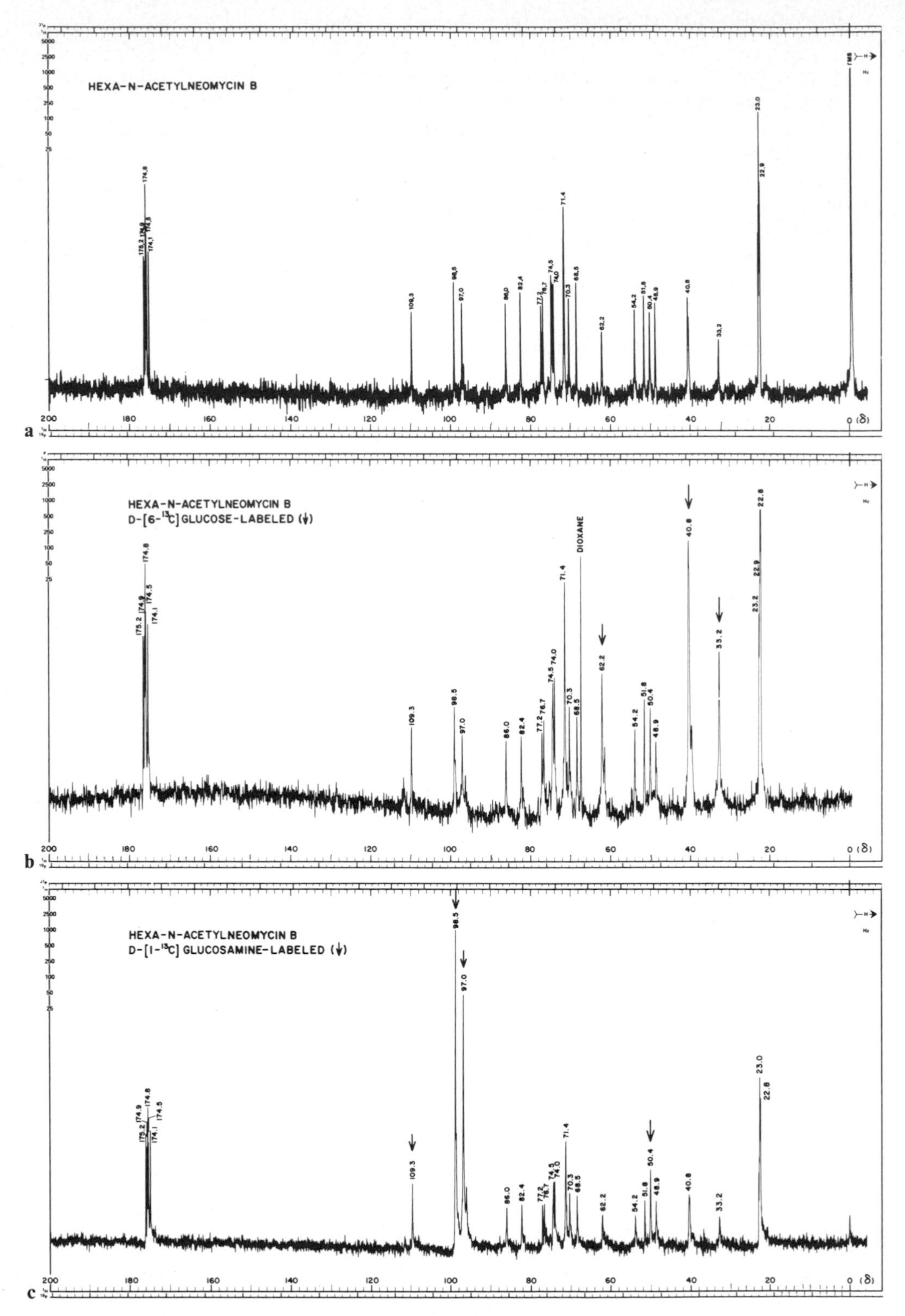

HEXA-N-ACETYLNEOMYCIN B
a
HEXA-N-ACETYLNEOMYCIN B
D-[6-¹³C] GLUCOSE-LABELED (↓)
DIOXANE
b
HEXA-N-ACETYLNEOMYCIN B
D-[1-¹³C] GLUCOSAMINE-LABELED (↓)
c

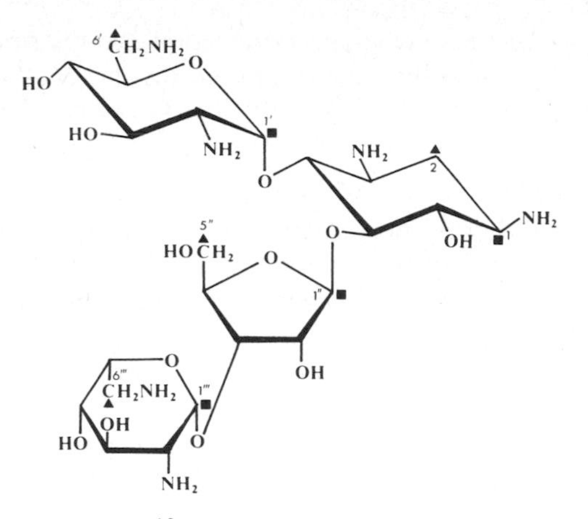

Fig. 14. Distribution of enriched ^{13}C-isotopes in neomycin B. ▲, enrichment due to [6-^{13}C] glucose; ■, enrichment due to [1-^{13}C] glucosamine

1. Biosynthesis of Subunits

The first studies on the biosynthesis of neomycin involved the incorporation and distribution of a labeled glucose, such as D-[U-^{14}C]-, [1-^{14}C]-, and [6-^{14}C]glucose and D-[1-^{14}C]glucosamine, into neomycin and the subunits (RINEHART and STROSHANE 1976). Glucose was incorporated into neomycin (1.4%–3.6%) and all subunits (ribose, 8.6%–19.3% of total incorporated, and each of the remaining three subunits, 23%–32.9%). Glucosamine was incorporated better than glucose (14.4%). However, the distribution of radioactivity in the subunits varied (ribose, 1.6%; neosamine B, 44.8%; neosamine C, 24.0%; 2-deoxystreptamine, 29.6%). Recently ^{13}C-NMR spectroscopy and ^{13}C-enriched compounds have made it possible to analyze specific carbon atoms in the subunits and in the parent antibiotics. [6-^{13}C]Glucose (63% ^{13}C) and [1-^{13}C]glucosamine (63% ^{13}C) were incorporated in neomycin B fermentation. The ^{13}C-NMR spectra of the *N*-hexaacetyl neomycin derivatives are shown in Fig. 13. Signals due to the individual carbons in the neomycin B derivative were assigned by off-resonance decoupling experiments, standard chemical shift data, and by comparison with the *N*-acetyl derivatives of structurally related compounds. As seen in Fig. 13, when the spectrum of neomycin B *N*-acetate derived from D-[6-^{13}C]glucose was compared with that of unprecursored neomycin B *N*-acetate, ^{13}C enrichment was observed for signals assigned to C-2 of 2-deoxystreptamine, C-6′ of neosamine C, C-6‴ of neosamine B, and C-5″ of ribose. In the same manner, it was found that [1-^{13}C]glucosamine enriched the C-1 of each subunit. The ^{13}C-enriched carbons in neomycin were as depicted in Fig. 14 (RINEHART et al. 1974).

With regard to the paromomycins, D-[U-^{14}C]glucose und D-[U-^{14}C]glucosamine fed to *Streptomyces albus* var. *metamycinus* were incorporated into parom-

◄ **Fig. 13a–c.** Proton-decoupled ^{13}C-NMR spectrum of hexa-*N*-acetylneomycin B. **a** unlabeled; **b** labeled by D-[6-^{13}C] glucose; **c** labeled by D-[1-^{13}C] glucosamine. (Courtesy of Prof. K. L. RINEHART, Jr.)

omycin I and II. As with neomycin, the label was evenly distributed in the four subunits. Glucosamine was either incorporated intact (56.1%) or converted to paromose (43.3%) (KÖSTER et al. 1975, 1977; REUTER et al. 1977).

a) Neosamine (Paromose)

It has been suggested that the neosamine C moiety (ring B) in neomycin is derived from the glucosamine moiety of paromamine. The biosynthetic pathway for neosamine B or the second neosamine C (ring D) in the neobiosamine moiety has not yet been clarified.

Periodate degradation of neosamine B and C and the neosaminols indicated that the labeled atoms of D-[1-^{14}C]glucose and [6-^{14}C]glucose were incorporated into C-1 and C-6 of the neosamines, respectively, and that of D-[1-^{14}C]glucosamine (a more efficient precursor than glucose) was introduced into C-1. These findings were confirmed with the ^{13}C-labeled precursor as shown in Fig. 14. In addition, [^{15}N]glucosamine was found to be incorporated into neosamine without any fragmentation of the carbon skeleton and enriched the 2-amino nitrogen of neosamine (ROLLS et al. 1975).

KÖSTER et al. (1977) speculated that the D-glucosamine-6-phosphate derived from D-glucose was converted into paromose I and II (neosamine B and C), which were phosphorylated and linked to the other subunits.

The well-known pathway from D-glucose to D-glucosamine is not dealt with here (cf. LOWTHER and ROGERS 1956).

b) Ribose

D-[1-^{14}C]- and [6-^{14}C]glucose were fed to *S. fradiae* and the isotope distribution pattern in the ribose of the neomycin was analyzed by chemical degradation. It was found that D-[1-^{14}C]- and [6-^{14}C]glucose labeled C-1 and C-5 of ribose, respectively.

It is well known that in microorganisms D-ribose may be derived from D-glucose by two alternative pathways, one via glucuronate and the other through the hexosemonophosphate shunt (RINEHART and STROSHANE 1976). If the ribose is synthesized via the glucuronate route, C-6 of glucose will be split off as carbon dioxide and C-1 will become C-1 of ribose. If ribose is synthesized by the second pathway, C-1 is lost and C-6 of glucose is retained as C-5 of ribose. Since retention of radioactivity was observed at both C-1 and C-5 of ribose, it is suggested that both pathways are involved in the biosynthesis of ribose in *S. fradiae*. As described earlier, this incorporation pattern was confirmed with ^{13}C-feeding experiments.

Incorporation of glucosamine in ribose was inferior to that of the other subunits. Therefore, glucosamine might be first converted to D-glucose and then into ribose. The conversion of D-glucosamine to D-glucose in microorganisms is also well established (cf. AXELROD 1960).

c) 2-Deoxystreptamine

Chemical degradation of labeled 2-deoxystreptamine indicated that D-[1-^{14}C]- and [6-^{14}C]glucose labeled C-1, C-2, or C-3 of 2-deoxystreptamine but could not indicate the exact location of the label. However, feeding experiments with

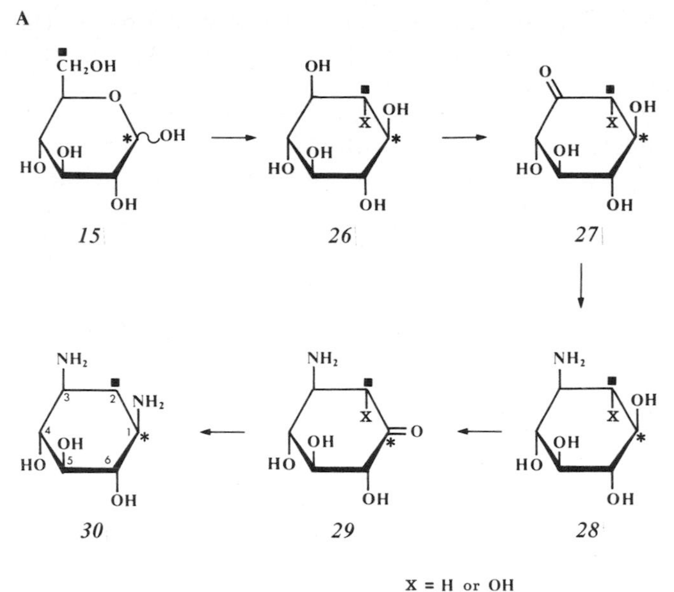

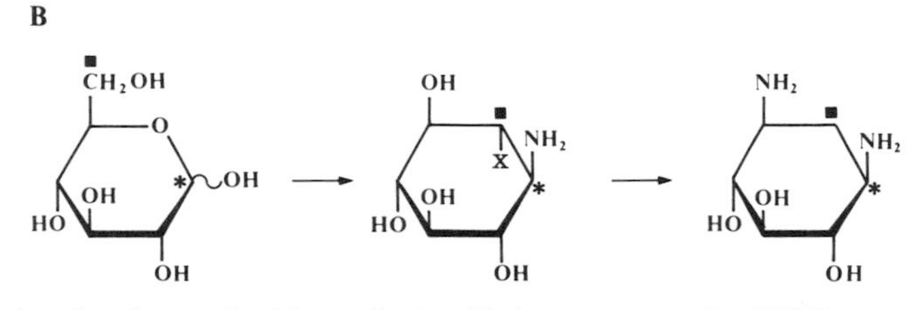

Fig. 15. Postulated pathways for biosynthesis of 2-deoxystreptamine (30) from D-glucose (15). (RINEHART and STROSHANE 1976) X=H or OH. 2-deoxy-*scyllo*-inosose (27 a) [X=H in 27]; 2-deoxy-*scyllo* inosamine (28 a) [X=H in 28]; monoamino-deoxy-*scyllo*-inosose (29 a) [X=H in 29]

D-[6-^{13}C]glucose and [1-^{13}C]glucosamine demonstrated that these isotopes enriched C-2 and C-1 of 2-deoxystreptamine, respectively, as depicted in Fig. 14.

D-Glucose labeled 2-deoxystreptamine more efficiently than did D-glucosamine, suggesting that D-glucosamine is first converted to D-glucose and then to 2-deoxystreptamine. [^{15}N]Glucosamine fed to *S. fradiae* enriched the neosamine subunits, but not 2-deoxystreptamine (RINEHART and STROSHANE 1976; ROLLS et al. 1975). RINEHART and STROSHANE (1976) proposed the pathway from D-glucose to 2-deoxystreptamine shown as route A in Fig. 15. X in this scheme is a hydroxyl group or a hydrogen atom. In this sequence, D-glucose (15) is first converted to a cyclitol (26), which is oxidized at the carbon corresponding to C-5 of glucose and then reductively aminated to give a monoaminocyclitol (28). The carbon atom corresponding to C-1 of glucose in (28) undergoes a second oxidation and amination to form 2-deoxystreptamine (30) through monoamino-inosose (29). The second amination takes place in a clockwise direction. However, they did not exclude an alternative pathway (route B), in which the hydroxyl group at the carbon atom derived from C-1 of glucose undergoes oxidation and amination, then the second oxidation–amination takes place in an anticlockwise direction at the carbon atom corresponding to C-5 of glucose.

J. WALKER (1971) proposed that an inositol-type intermediate similar to that reported for streptomycin might be involved in the route from glucose to 2-deoxystreptamine, but *myo*-inositol has been found not to be an intermediate in neomycin synthesis.

Recently, 2-deoxy-*scyllo*-inosose (27a) and 2-deoxy-*scyllo*-inosamine (28a) were demonstrated to be intermediates in the biosynthesis of gentamicin (DAUM et al. 1977b) and butirosin (FURUMAI et al. 1979). Consequently, the hydroxyl group corresponding to that on C-6 of glucose may be eliminated in an earlier step of biosynthesis. This will be discussed in Sect. B.X.

Glutamine was suggested to be the donor of the amino group in this pathway (CHEN and WALKER 1977).

2. Subunit Assembly

a) Neomycin

To examine the possibility of the direct involvement of the subunits themselves in neomycin biosynthesis, RINEHART and SCHIMBOR (1976) administered labeled subunits to *S. fradiae*, and found that [1-^{14}C]ribose was incorporated into ribose (32%), neosamine C (23%), 2-deoxystreptamine (30%), and neosamine B (15%) moieties of neomycin B. Since the ribose moiety was the most heavily labeled and C-1 of the precursor was retained, it was felt that ribose is directly incorporated. Moieties other than ribose might be derived from glucose formed from the [^{14}C]ribose. [1-^{14}C]Deoxystreptamine was incorporated exclusively into the 2-deoxystreptamine moiety of neomycin B (85%). [1-^{14}C]Neosamine C was not incorporated into neomycin B.

Experiments with a 2-deoxystreptamine-requiring idiotroph of the producing strain indicated the order of assembly of the subunits. PEARCE et al. (1976, 1978) first prepared ^{3}H- and ^{14}C-labeled neamines as follows: ^{3}H-labeled neamine composed of labeled 2-deoxystreptamine and labeled neosamine C was obtained by hydrolysis of neomycin produced in medium containing [6-^{3}H]glucose, and neamine labeled only in the neosamine C moiety was obtained from ^{14}C-labeled neomycin produced by a 2-deoxystreptamine-requiring idiotroph of *S. fradiae* in medium supplemented with 2-deoxystreptamine and [U-^{14}C]glucose. A mixture of the two labeled neamines was converted into neomycin (not paromomycin) by a 2-deoxystreptamine-requiring idiotroph of *Streptomyces rimosus* forma *paromomyceticus* with a 30% yield. The ^{3}H:^{14}C ratio in this neomycin preparation was the same as that in neamine obtained by hydrolysis of neomycin, and in unused neamine reisolated from the incubation medium. The ^{3}H:^{14}C ratio in neomycin was not affected by the presence of unlabeled 2-deoxystreptamine during cultivation, and the radioactivity in neomycin was ascribed only to the neosamine C and 2-deoxystreptamine moieties. Thus, it was concluded that the supplemented neamine was incorporated into neomycin intact. From these findings, the first step in the subunit assembly of neomycin is assumed to be the formation of neamine (PEARCE et al. 1976).

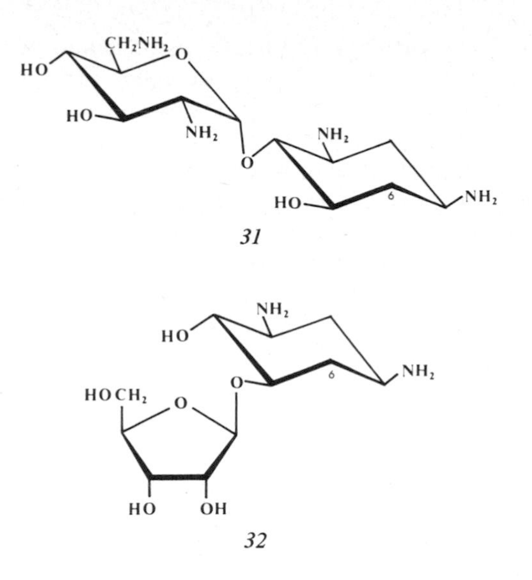

31

32

Furthermore, this 2-deoxystreptamine-requiring idiotroph incorporated 6-deoxyneamine (31) to produce an antibiotically active compound, but did not convert 5-*O*-*β*-D-ribofuranosyl-2,6-dideoxystreptamine (32) to any antibiotic substance. Thus, PEARCE et al. (1978) suggested that the binding of neosamine C with 2-deoxystreptamine takes place first to give neamine which then binds with D-ribose. Since the antibiotic consisting of neosamine C, 2-deoxystreptamine, and D-ribose, namely ribostamycin, was known to be produced by *Streptomyces* sp., they considered that the fourth aminosugar subunit (neosamine C or B) was attached to the ribose moiety of ribostamycin. The biosynthesis of ribostamycin will be discussed in Sect. B.III.2.

BAUD et al. (1977) found a mutant of neomycin-producing *S. fradiae* (strain N_4C_2), which produced ribostamycin instead of neomycin. By mutagenic treatment of strain N_4C_2, they succeeded in isolating the neomycin-producing revertant which no longer accumulated ribostamycin. Thus, they suggested that strain N_4C_2 was blocked in one of the last steps from ribostamycin to neomycin and that neomycin is formed by linking a second neosamine to ribostamycin. Thus, neomycins were thought to be synthesized as follows:

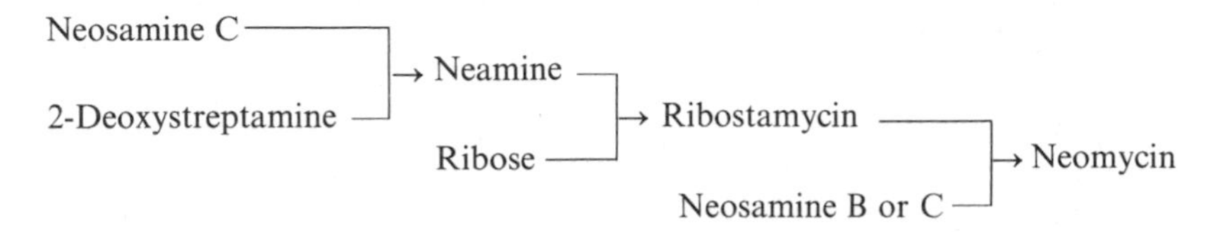

However, neosamine C is not directly incorporated into neomycin. Therefore, taking into account the information available on the biosynthesis of paromomycin and butirosin, the following sequence may be most likely for the biosynthetic pathway of neomycin:

2-Deoxystreptamine→Paromamine→Neamine→Ribostamycin→Neomycin

In Sect. B.X, the above pathway will be discussed again, but there are some experimental findings which do not fit with the above conclusion.

The first contradictory phenomenon was observed with a 2-deoxystreptamine-requiring idiotroph of neomycin-producing *S. fradiae*. This strain incorporated streptamine and 2-*epi*streptamine to produce four new antibiotics, hybrimycin A_1 and A_2 from the former and Hybrimycin B_1 and B_2 from the latter (SHIER et al. 1969, 1972), but could not incorporate 2-deoxystreptamine-containing pseudo-disaccharides such as neamine and paromamine assumed to be derived from 2-deoxystreptamine in neomycin biosynthesis (SHIER et al. 1974). PEARCE et al. (1978) explained this as follows: "One attractive possibility is that in the experimental conditions used these potential precursors are unable to enter the region of the cell where subunit assembly occurs. It seems probable, however, that neamine has access to at least some intracellular processes because at high concentration neamine is toxic to *S. fradiae*."

The second contradiction was the detection of irrational metabolites in the neomycin fermentation products. In addition to neomycin, an industrial strain of *S. fradiae* produced as minor metabolites the following antibiotics or related compounds: paromamine, neamine, 3-mono-*N*-acetylneamine(LP-A), diamino-dideoxyhexosyl-*myo*-inositol, 5-*O*-(neobiosaminyl)-2-deoxystreptamine, paromomycin I, paromomycin II, 3-mono-*N*-acetylneomycin B (LP-B), and 3-mono-*N*-acetylneomycin C (LP-C) (HESSLER et al. 1970; CLAES et al. 1974). The presence of diamino-dideoxyhexosyl-*myo*-inositol and 5-*O*-(neobiosaminyl)-2-deoxystreptamine cannot be explained by the biosynthetic pathway proposed above.

Also, STROSHANE (1976) demonstrated the concurrent synthesis of neamine and neobiosamine during fermentation. This indicates the possibility of an alternate route for neomycin biosynthesis. Therefore, more studies are needed to fully elucidate the pathway.

Neomycin-inactivating and -reactivating enzymes may also participate in neomycin biosynthesis. M. MAJUMDAR and S. MAJUMDAR (1969, 1970) obtained neomycin C and a phosphoamide derivative of an aminosugar antibiotic by cultivating *S. fradiae* in medium containing certain amino acids, particularly glycine and serine. They identified the phosphoamide as a complex of neomycin B pyrophosphate, neomycin C pyrophosphate, and neomycin C dipyrophosphate. Examining the relationship between alkaline phosphatase and neomycin formation in *S. fradiae* 3535, M. MAJUMDAR and S. MAJUMDAR (1971) concluded that neomycin is finally derived from phosphoamides or phosphates by hydrolysis (dephosphorylation) with alkaline phosphatase produced in the culture broth.

Biosynthesis of an antibiotic is often accomplished by formation of antibiotic-inactivating and -reactivating enzymes. Among the numerous neomycin-inactivating enzymes, aminoglycoside-3′-phosphotransferase[APH(3′)] was found to be produced by neomycin-producing *S. fradiae* and also *Micromonospora chalcea* (BENVENISTE and DAVIES 1973; YAGISAWA et al. 1978; DAVIES et al. 1979; GANELIN et al. 1979; PETYUSHENKO et al. 1979). Acetyltransferase was also produced by *S. fradiae* (DAVIES et al. 1979) and may be connected with the production of 3-*N*-acetylneomycin B and C reported by RINEHART (1961) from the broth of neomycin-producing *S. fradiae*. As will be considered in Sect. B.II.3, YAGISAWA et al. (1978) postulated the participation of 3′-phosphotransferase in the biosynthesis of neomycin, though the participation of acetyltransferase was thought to be unlikely.

b) Paromomycin

After feeding [^{14}C]deoxystreptamine and D-[^{14}C]ribose, paromomycin was isolated from cultures of *S. albus* var. *metamycinus* and analyzed for the distribution of these isotopes. It was found that 2-deoxystreptamine was incorporated intact and approximately 50% of the ribose was incorporated per se. Ribose also labeled 2-deoxystreptamine, glucosamine, and paromose. These results were all consistent with those obtained in neomycin biosynthesis (REUTER et al. 1977).

SHIER et al. (1973) examined 29 2-deoxystreptamine analogs and three 2-deoxystreptamine-containing pseudodisaccharides [neamine, paromamine, and 6-(kanosaminyl)-2-deoxystreptamine] for incorporation into paromomycin or other antibiotics by a 2-deoxystreptamine-requiring idiotroph of *S. rimosus* forma *paromomycinus*. Their results were of little use in clarifying the biosynthetic sequence from 2-deoxystreptamine to paromomycin, because no compounds except 2-deoxystreptamine and streptamine yielded any antibiotically active substances.

On the other hand, in addition to paromomycin I and II, ribosylparomamine (identical with 6′-deamino-6′-hydroxyribostamycin, see Sect. B.III) was detected as a direct fermentation product of a paromomycin-producing *Streptomyces* (KIRBY et al. 1977). In analogy to the role of ribostamycin in neomycin biosynthesis, the coexistence of ribosylparomamine and paromomycin suggests that ribosylparomamine is an intermediate in paromomycin biosynthesis. Subunit assembly in paromomycin biosynthesis may proceed as follows:

2-Deoxystreptamine→Paromamine→Ribosylparomamine→Paromomycin

The fact that paromomycin I and II are produced as minor components by neomycin-producing strains, including *S. fradiae* 3535 (HESSLER et al. 1970), may support this pathway.

3. Plasmid Involvement

YAGISAWA et al. (1978) and DAVIES et al. (1979) reported on a plasmid which may carry a gene for the neomycin-inactivating enzyme, 3′-phosphotransferase[APH(3′)], and a gene for 2-deoxystreptamine formation. By treating the neomycin-producing *S. fradiae* ATCC 10745 with acridine dye, they obtained three stable nonproducing variants. These variants (AO 80, AO 83, and AO 144) and one additional neomycin-nonproducing mutant (CMP 487), together with the parent strain, were examined for sensitivity to neomycin, production of two neomycin-inactivating enzymes, neomycin 3′-phosphotransferase[APH(3′)] and acetyltransferase (AAC), and utilization of exogenous 2-deoxystreptamine for neomycin formation. The results are summarized in Table 2.

Based on sensitivity to neomycin, these variants can be divided into two groups, a neomycin-sensitive group (AO 80 and AO 83) and a resistant group (AO 144 and CMP 487). Strains of the sensitive group did not produce APH(3′), but those of the resistant group did. AAC production was not related to sensitivity to neomycin. This suggested that resistance of *S. fradiae* to neomycin requires the produc-

Table 2. Characteristics of neomycin-producing and -nonproducing *Streptomyces fradiae*

	Minimum inhibitory concentration of neomycin	Production of		Neomycin production	
		APH(3′)[a]	AAC[b]	Without supplement of 2-deoxy-streptamine	With supplement of 2-deoxy-streptamine
Neomycin-producing parent strain					
ATCC 10745	>100	+	+	+	+
Neomycin-nonproducing variants					
AO 80	1.56	−	+	−	−
AO 83	1.56	−	+	−	−
AO 144	100	+	+	−	+
CMP 487	>100	+	+	−	±

[a] Neomycin 3′-phosphotransferase
[b] Aminoglycoside acetyltransferase

tion of APH(3′) and the gene for this enzyme may be coded on a plasmid in the neomycin-producing strain.

Furthermore, it was revealed that variants AO 144 and CMP 487 (to a much lesser extent) produced neomycin, when 2-deoxystreptamine was fed to 2-day-old cultures of these strains, while AO 80 and AO 83, which are both sensitive to neomycin, did not convert 2-deoxystreptamine into neomycin. This result also suggested the involvement of plasmids with the genes for 2-deoxystreptamine production.

Plasmids pSF 1 and pSF 2 were isolated from the logarithmically growing cells of strain ATCC 10745. These plasmids had molecular weights from contour length measurement of 14.9 and 21.9 megadaltons, respectively, and were assumed to be concerned with APH(3′) production, since they were not isolated from the neomycin-nonproducing variants, AO 80 and AO 83.

Isolation of plasmid DNA from neomycin-producing strains was also reported by CHUNG and MORRIS (1978), STEPNOV et al. (1978), and HAYAKAWA et al. (1979). CHUNG and MORRIS isolated two plasmid DNA peaks (76 S and 49 S) from lysates of *S. fradiae* and showed, by electron microscopic analysis, that the 76 S peak was covalently closed circular DNA and the 49 S fraction was open circular DNA. According to OKANISHI (1978), the molecular weight of these two plasmid DNAs was 55 and 34 megadaltons, respectively.

STEPNOV et al. (1978) prepared plasmid DNA from neomycin-producing *Actinomyces fradiae* 676, and showed that it contained circular plasmid DNA with a molecular weight of 5.9 megadaltons. Recently, HAYAKAWA et al. (1979) found that neomycin-producing *Streptomyces* sp. 7068-CC_1 harbored at least two kinds of plasmids which are covalently closed circular DNA molecules with S-values of 51.7 and 75.1 and molecular weight of 22.2 and 47.0 megadaltons. Physiologic functions were not determined for the above plasmids.

Recently, OKANISHI (1979, 1980) postulated a plasmid which regulates the function of the cell membrane in neomycin biosynthesis. This speculation was based on the following experimental findings reported by ARIMA et al. (1973) and OKAZAKI et al. (1973, 1974) on neomycin-producing *S. fradiae* IFO 3123 and its neomycin-nonproducing mutant ST-5 B.

The parent strain, whose cellular fatty acid spectra are of the 14-methyl-pentadecanoate-type (iso 16:0-type) or normal hexadecanoate-type (normal 16:0-type), had amino acid and hexosamine pools which were two to six times larger than those of mutant ST-5 B, which has the 12-methyl-tetradecanoate-type (anteiso 15:0-type) cellular fatty acid spectrum. The major amino acid was L-glutamic acid in either type of cells. When cultivated in medium containing more than 0.5% L-glutamic acid, the mutant could produce neomycin, although the fatty acid spectrum of the cells was unchanged; so the difference in neomycin production ability was ascribed to the pool size of L-glutamic acid in the cell. The difference in pool size probably resulted from the difference in fatty acid composition of the cell membranes. The ability for L-glutamine uptake was markedly reduced in anteiso 15:0-type cells and accumulated glutamate was easily washed out by buffer. Mutant ST-5 B could also produce neomycin under supplementation with oleic acid, palmitic acid, or a high concentration of sodium chloride. Cells grown under these conditions showed the same fatty acid spectrum and glutamic acid levels as the parent strain. These results may be rationalized as follows: Addition of oleate, palmitate, or sodium chloride caused some change of fatty acids in the membrane of the mutant. This change altered the glutamate permeability and resulted in higher glutamate levels. This situation induced the initiation of neomycin biosynthesis, which is dependent on a certain level of glutamate in the cells. Similar results were found by OKANISHI (1980) for aureothricin biosynthesis by *S. kasugaensis* MB 273.

WHITE and DAVIES (1978) reported that treatment of paromomycin-producing *S. rimosus* forma *paromomycinus* with acridine orange gave stable antibiotic-nonproducing mutants. Some of these mutants were deficient in the ability to form aerial mycelium and changed in morphology. Some were 2-deoxystreptamine-requiring idiotrophs. After examining resistance to paromomycin, the presence of aminoglycoside phosphotransferase and acetyltransferase activities, and 2-deoxystreptamine utilization, they suggested that plasmids are involved in the biosynthesis of paromomycin.

III. Ribostamycin, Xylostasin, and Butirosin

Ribostamycin is an antibiotic produced by *S. ribosidificus*, while butirosin and xylostasin are produced by *Bacillus* species. In spite of the distinct taxonomic differences of the producing strains, the biosynthetic pathways appear to be closely related, because mutants of butirosin-producing *B. circulans* also produced ribostamycin and/or xylostasin (FUJIWARA et al. 1978; FURUMAI et al. 1979). Therefore, biosynthesis of these antibiotics and related compounds are considered together in this section.

These antibiotics are 4,5-disubstituted-2-deoxystreptamine antibiotics with three subunits. As shown in Fig. 16, ribostamycin is identical to ribosylneamine,

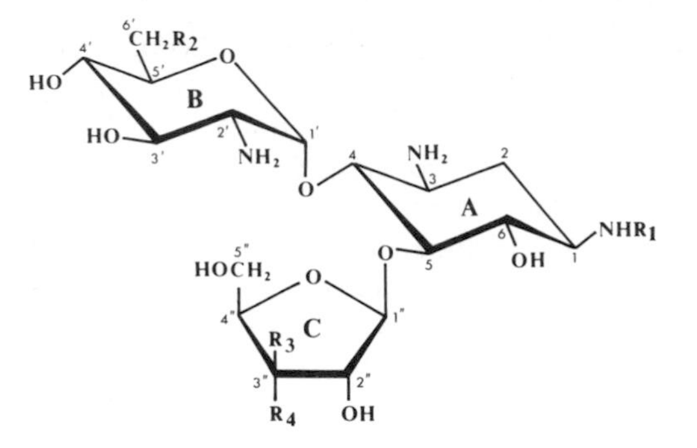

Fig. 16. Ribostamycin, xylostasin, butirosin, and related compounds. *Ring A*, 2-deoxystreptamine (DOS) [$R_1=H$], (*S*)-(−)-4-amino-2-hydroxybutyryl (AHB)-DOS [$R_1=COCH(OH)CH_2CH_2NH_2$]; *Ring B*, D-glucosamine [$R_2=OH$], neosamine C[$R_2=NH_2$]; *Ring C*, D-xylose [$R_3=OH$, $R_4=H$], D-ribose [$R_3=H$, $R_4=OH$]; *Ring A+B*, paromamine [$R_1=H$, $R_2=OH$], neamine [$R_1=H$, $R_2=NH_2$], (AHB)-paromamine [$R_1=AHB$, $R_2=OH$], (AHB)-neamine [$R_1=AHB$, $R_2=NH_2$].
Ring A+B+C,

	R_1	R_2	R_3	R_4
Ribostamycin	H	NH_2	H	OH
Xylostasin	H	NH_2	OH	H
Butirosin A	$COCH(OH)CH_2CH_2NH_2$	NH_2	OH	H
Butirosin B	$COCH(OH)CH_2CH_2NH_2$	NH_2	H	OH
DAH-butirosin A* (Bu-1709 E_1)	$COCH(OH)CH_2CH_2NH_2$	OH	OH	H
DAH-butirosin B* (Bu-1709 E_2)	$COCH(OH)CH_2CH_2NH_2$	OH	H	OH
DAH-ribostamycin* (LL-BM408)	H	OH	H	OH
DAH-xylostasin*	H	OH	OH	H
2‴-Deoxybutirosin A (Z-1159-5)	$COCH_2(CH_2)_2NH_2$	NH_2	OH	H

* DAH = 6′-Deamino-6′-hydroxy

the pseudotrisaccharide portion of neomycin. Xylostasin is xylosylneamine in which the ribosyl moiety in ribostamycin is replaced by a xylosyl moiety. Butirosin, a mixture of butirosin A and B, is characterized by the presence of an (*S*)-(−)-4-amino-2-hydroxybutyryl side chain attached to the amino group at C-1 of the 2-deoxystreptamine moiety.

6′-Deamino-6′-hydroxybutirosin (DAH-butirosin) (TSUKIURA et al. 1973; TAKEDA et al. 1978b, c), 6′-deamino-6′-hydroxyxylostasin, and antibiotic Z-1159-5 (2‴-deoxybutirosin A) (NOGAMI et al. 1974) are produced by some strains of *Bacillus* species. 6′-Deamino-6′-hydroxyribostamycin was found in the broth of an unidentified *Streptomyces* which produced paromomycin I and II.

1. Biosynthesis of Subunits

No papers on the application of labeled precursors for biosynthetic studies have been published, except for KOJIMA's (1974) brief report on ribostamycin, in which he reported that D-[U-^{14}C]glucose, D-[1-^{14}C]glucosamine, *N*-acetyl-D-[1-^{14}C]glucosamine, and D-[U-^{14}C]ribose were incorporated into ribostamycin. Thus, as with other aminoglycosides, D-glucose, D-glucosamine, and D-ribose are the primary starting metabolites for ribostamycin. The radioactivity from supplemented ribose was distributed not only in the ribose moiety, but also in the neamine moiety.

The biosynthesis of (*S*)-(−)-4-amino-2-hydroxybutyric acid, a unique constitutional amino acid of butirosin, will be discussed in Sect. B.III.2.

The biosynthetic pathway of 2-deoxystreptamine in butirosin biosynthesis was studied by the Tanabe Seiyaku group which demonstrated that the pathway is the same as in neomycin, which has already been described, and in gentamicin, which will be discussed in detail later.

By treatment with *N*-methyl-*N'*-nitro-*N*-nitrosoguanidine, TAKEDA et al. (1978c) isolated a number of butirosin-nonproducing mutants from a strain of *B. circulans* which normally produced butirosin and a trace amount of 6'-deamino-6'-hydroxybutirosin. Later, FURUMAI et al. (1979) examined nine stable mutants selected from the above butirosin-nonproducing mutants for their interaction in antibiotic cosynthesis. These mutants were classified into seven groups (A to F and exceptional group), based on their complementation patterns (Fig. 2). Two mutants (MCRL 5001 and 5017) of group A produced des-(4-amino-2-hydroxybutyryl)butirosin (a mixture of xylostasin and ribostamycin), whereas mutant MCRL 5003 of group B was a neamine-requiring idiotroph and accumulated 2-deoxystreptamine in the fermentation broth. Five mutants belonging to groups C to F could produce butirosin from 2-deoxystreptamine as well as from neamine, so they were all 2-deoxystreptamine-requiring idiotrophs. Information from the above mutants suggested that the biosynthetic pathway of 2-deoxystreptamine in *B. circulans* comprises more than four steps. Five mutants of groups C to F were then examined for their ability to produce butirosin from 2-deoxystreptamine-related cyclitols assumed to be intermediates leading to 2-deoxystreptamine.

Studies were done with *myo*-inositol, conduritol B [DL-5-cyclohexene-1,3/2,4-tetrol], 1-deoxy-*scyllo*-inositol [1,3,5/2,4-cyclohexanepentol] and its pentaacetate, 2-deoxy-*scyllo*-inosose [DL-2,4/3,5-tetrahydroxy-cyclohexanone], 2-deoxy-*scyllo*-inosamine [DL-(1,3,5/2,4)-5-amino-1,2,3,4-cyclohexanetetrol] and its pentaacetate. All mutants could convert 2-deoxy-*scyllo*-inosamine, and mutants MCRL 5605 (group E) and MCRL 5673 (group F) produced butirosin from 2-deoxy-*scyllo*-inosose. The latter two mutants could also produce 2-hydroxybutirosin from *scyllo*-inosose [2,4,6/3,5-pentahydroxy-cyclohexanone], *scyllo*-inosamine [1-amino-1-deoxy-*scyllo*-inositol], and streptamine. The other compounds were not utilized at all.

These results and the complementation patterns shown by the above mutants indicated that in *B. circulans*, 2-deoxystreptamine is synthesized from glucose according to the following sequence: glucose→2-deoxy-*scyllo*-inosose→2-deoxy-*scyllo*-inosamine↠2-deoxystreptamine. This sequence was the same as that proposed for the biosynthesis of neomycins (Fig. 15 in Sect. B.II). Consequently, a part of the postulated sequence in Fig. 15 is experimentally supported by the above results. Though not isolated, at least one of the intermediates accumulated by the mutants of group C and D may be 2-deoxy-*scyllo*-inosamine or its derivative (phosphate).

Recently, FUJIWARA et al. (1980a) isolated a 2-deoxystreptamine precursor, S-11-P, from the fermentation broth of the 2-deoxystreptamine-requiring idiotroph (strain S-11) derived from a xylostasin-producing *B. circulans*. The structure of S-

11-P was determined to be (1L)-1,3,5/2,4-5-aminocyclohexanetetrol (IGARASHI et al. 1980), indicating that route A in Fig. 15 is the real pathway in 2-deoxystreptamine biosynthesis by *B. circulans*.

2. Subunit Assembly

According to KOJIMA (1974), tritium-labeled 2-deoxystreptamine and neamine are so readily incorporated into ribostamycin that these compounds may be direct precursors of ribostamycin. KOJIMA and SATOH (1973) also found that the 2-deoxystreptamine-requiring idiotroph (AF-1) of *S. ribosidificus*, in contrast to that from neomycin-producing *S. fradiae*, could convert neamine into ribostamycin. Consequently, binding of ribose with preformed neamine was assumed to be the last step in ribostamycin biosynthesis.

CLARIDGE et al. (1974) and TAYLOR and SCHMITZ (1976) used 2-deoxystreptamine-requiring idiotrophs (strains 61a and 76b) derived from *B. circulans* 301 to study butirosin synthesis. However, these idiotrophs were of no use in studying assembly, because they could convert 2-deoxystreptamine or its analogs such as streptidine, streptamine, and 2,5-dideoxystreptamine into butirosin and its analogs but could not convert the following key pseudodi- or trisaccharides: neamine, 1-*N*-[(*S*)-(−)-4-amino-2-hydroxybutyryl]-2-deoxystreptamine, 1-*N*-[(*S*)-(−)-4-amino-2-hydroxybutyryl]-neamine, ribostamycin, and xylostasin (cf. Fig. 16).

a) (*S*)-(−)-4-Amino-2-hydroxybutyryl Moiety

VIRTANEN and HIETALA (1955) reported that a mutant of *E. coli* could decarboxylate γ-hydroxyglutamic acid to 4-amino-2-hydroxybutyric acid. As described later, acylation was suggested by TAKEDA et al. (1978b, 1979) to take place on xylostasin or ribostamycin, so that this amino acid, or a related derivative, are apparently preformed before the acylation reaction.

According to MATSUMURA et al. (1978) who examined the incorporation of amino acids and peptides into butirosin by nonproliferating cells of a mutant (strain BA 44) derived from *Bacillus vitellinus* Z-1159, not only (*S*)-(−)-4-amino-2-hydroxybutyric acid but also DL-2,4-diaminobutyric acid and 4-aminobutyric acid hardly affected butirosin production. Therefore, it is not certain what kind of amino acid derivative participates in this acylation reaction. Simultaneous production of antibiotic Z-1159-5 (2‴-deoxybutirosin A) and xylostasin by *B. vitellinus* Y-1456 reported by NOGAMI et al. (1974) indicates that this strain may be blocked at the hydroxylation of the α position, but does not indicate whether butirosin A is derived by hydroxylation at C-2‴ of 2‴-deoxybutirosin A or not.

b) Ribostamycin, Xylostasin, and Butirosin

Subunit assembly to form the antibiotics of this series was elucidated by the Tanabe Seiyaku group. Using the neamine-requiring idiotroph MCRL 5003 and 2-deoxystreptamine-requiring idiotroph MCRL 5004, TAKEDA et al. (1978b, 1979) examined the conversion of plausible biosynthetic intermediates and characterized the products.

Table 3. Production of butirosin and related antibiotics from 2-deoxystreptamine and 2-deoxystreptamine-containing compounds. (TAKEDA et al. 1979)

Precursors [a]	Strain MRCL 5003		Strain MCRL 5004	
	Antibiotics produced	Conversion yield to butirosin (mol %)	Antibiotics produced	Conversion yield to butirosin (mol %)
2-Deoxystreptamine	None	0	Butirosin (A: 80%–90%)	78
Paromamine	Butirosin (A: 80%–90%)	75	Butirosin (A: 80%–90%)	76
Neamine	Butirosin (A: 80%–90%)	74	Butirosin (A: 80%–90%)	30
Ribostamycin	Butirosin (A: 40%–60%)	70	Butorison (A: 40%–60%)	24
Xylostasin	Butirosin A	67	Butirosin A	24
AHB-2-Deoxystreptamine	None	0	None	0
AHB-Paromamine	AHB-Neamine	0	AHB-Neamine	0
AHB-Neamine	Butirosin A (trace) and neamine (trace)	3	None (unchanged)	0
DAH-Xylostasin	DAH-Butirosin A	0	DAH-Butirosin A	0
DAH-Butirosin B	DAH-Butirosin A	0	DAH-Butirosin A	0
DAH-Butirosin A	None (unchanged)	0	None (unchanged)	0
Butirosin B	Butirosin A	(~50)	Butirosin A	(~50)
Butirosin A	None (unchanged)	–	None (unchanged)	–

[a] AHB = 4-amino-2-hydroxybutyryl; DAH = 6′-deamino-6′-hydroxy

Table 4. Products from 2-deoxystreptamine, paromamine, neamine, ribostamycin, and xylostasin. (TAKEDA et al. 1979)

Strain	MCRL 5004	MCRL 5003			
Precursor (100 μg/ml)	2-Deoxystreptamine	Paromamine	Neamine	Robostamycin	Xylostasin
Products isolated [a] (yield, μg/ml broth)	Butirosin (114), DAH-butirosin (7) [b], ribostamycin (5), and xylostasin (2)	Butirosin (49), DAH-butirosin (22) [b], ribostamycin (3), xylostasin (2), and neamine (1)	Butirosin (64), ribostamycin (0.4), and xylostasin (trace)	Butirosin (48) and xylostasin (0.3)	Butirosin A (42)

[a] The products were isolated from broths by adsorption on Amberlite IRC-50 resin and separated by chromatography on Amberlite CG-50 and CM-Sephadex C-25

[b] A mixture of DAH-butirosin A (80%–90%) and DAH-butirosin B (10%–20%)

Mutants MCRL 5003 and 5004 were fed with the 2-deoxystreptamine-containing compounds shown in Table 3 (for structures see Fig. 16) and the yield of butirosin as well as the ratio of butirosin A to butirosin B were determined.

The experimental results are summarized in Table 3 and 4. From these data, the following conclusions about the biosynthesis of butirosin and 6′-deamino-6′-hydroxybutirosin can be drawn.

1. 2-Deoxystreptamine, paromamine, neamine, ribostamycin, xylostasin, and butirosin B are possible intermediates of butirosin A, because these compounds were efficiently bioconverted to butirosin A by idiotrophs MCRL 5003 (except for 2-deoxystreptamine) and MCRL 5004. However, 6′-deamino-6′-hydroxybutirosin (DAH-butirosin) may be a shunt metabolite in the biosynthesis of butirosin.

2. Insertion of the 6′-amino group of butirosins must take place before pseudotrisaccharide formation, since DAH-xylostasin and DAH-butirosin were not converted into butirosin.

3. The 4-amino-2-hydroxybutyryl (AHB) group is probably introduced after the formation of a pseudotrisaccharide, because AHB-2-deoxystreptamine, AHB-paromamine, and AHB-neamine were not significantly converted to butirosin by either idiotroph.

4. Isomerization probably takes place only from *ribo*-isomer to *xylo*-isomer, because ribostamycin and butirosin B were converted to butirosin A, but xylostasin and butirosin A were not converted to butirosin B.

5. Butirosin and DAH-butirosin are derived from paromamine, because DAH-butirosin was produced only from 2-deoxystreptamine and paromamine, and not from neamine, ribostamycin, and xylostasin.

6. The route from paromamine to neamine, involving amino substitution of the hydroxyl group of paromamine at the C-6′ position, is postulated, because neamine was isolated as one of the minor products converted from paromamine.

7. The following three routes are probably involved in the formation of butirosin A from neamine: (i) neamine → xylostasin → butirosin A, (ii) neamine → ribostamycin → butirosin B → butirosin A, and (iii) neamine → ribostamycin → xylostasin → butirosin A. These pathways are inferred from identification of the products from neamine, ribostamycin, xylostasin, and butirosin B.

8. Among the two routes involving xylosylation and ribosylation of neamine at C-5, the route from neamine to xylostasin seems to be predominant from comparison of the A:B ratios in butirosin converted from ribostamycin (A = 40%–60%), xylostasin (A = 100%), and butirosin B (A = ~50%) with those of butirosin bioconverted from 2-deoxystreptamine, paromamine, and neamine (A = 80%–90% in all precursors). If the route from neamine to ribostamycin were predominant, butirosin converted from neamine would have an A:B ratio similar to that from ribostamycin (Table 3).

9. The routes from paromamine to DAH-butirosin A are suggested by analogy with the routes from neamine to butirosin A.

Additional evidence for the participation of xylostasin and ribostamycin as intermediates was the fact that other blocked mutants (strains MCRL 5011 and 5017) accumulated both xylostasin and ribostamycin in the fermentation broth.

The biosynthetic pathways for butirosin and 6′-deamino-6′-hydroxybutirosin which involve ribostamycin, xylostasin, and their 6′-deamino-6′-hydroxy derivatives are summarized in Fig. 17. The mutants are blocked at the sites shown.

The above findings eliminate the possibility that a pseudodi- or trisaccharide exogenously supplied is hydrolyzed into subunits which are then reused for synthesis of butirosin. If hydrolysis occurred, the A:B ratio in the butirosin would be similar, irrespective of the pre-

Fig. 17. Possible biosynthetic pathway for butirosin and DAH-butirosin in *Bacillus circulans* MCRL 5001. *DAH*, 6′-deamino-6′-hydroxy; →| |→, the step where a mutant was blocked; (a), amino substitution at C-6′; (b), *N*-acylation at C-1; (c), epimerization at C-3″ ▶

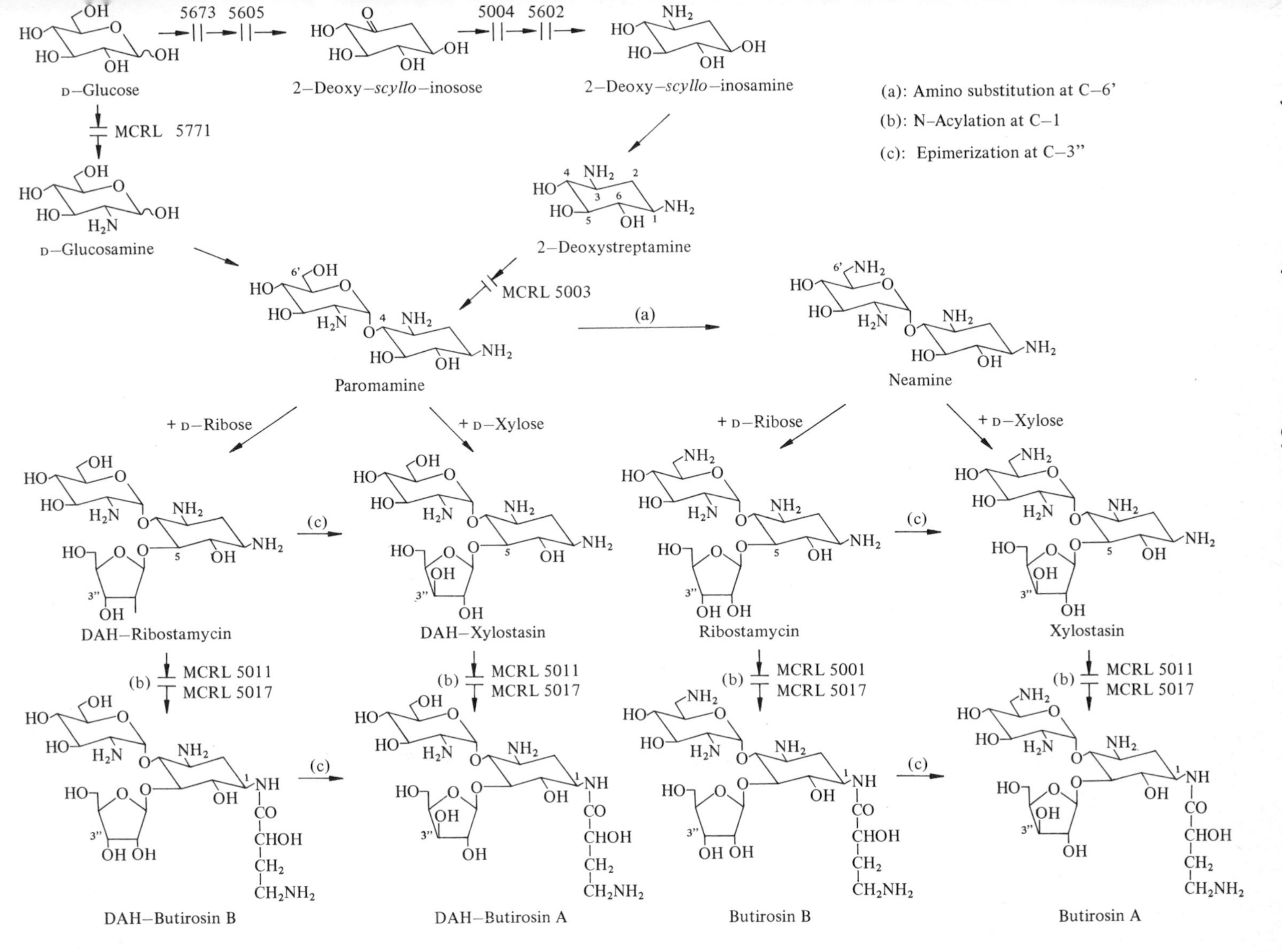
D-Glucose
5673 5605
2-Deoxy-scyllo-inosose
5004 5602
2-Deoxy-scyllo-inosamine
(a): Amino substitution at C-6'
(b): N-Acylation at C-1
(c): Epimerization at C-3''
MCRL 5771
D-Glucosamine
2-Deoxystreptamine
MCRL 5003
(a)
Paromamine
Neamine
+ D-Ribose
+ D-Xylose
+ D-Ribose
+ D-Xylose
(c)
(c)
DAH-Ribostamycin
DAH-Xylostasin
Ribostamycin
Xylostasin
(b) MCRL 5011 MCRL 5017
(b) MCRL 5011 MCRL 5017
(b) MCRL 5001 MCRL 5017
(b) MCRL 5011 MCRL 5017
(c)
(c)
DAH-Butirosin B
DAH-Butirosin A
Butirosin B
Butirosin A

cursors added (Table 3). Also, 6′-deamino-6′-hydroxybutirosin was derived only from 2-deoxystreptamine and paromamine, and not from neamine, ribostamycin, and xylostasin (Table 4). Furthermore, as will be shown in Sect. C, these mutants directly converted neamine analogs to butirosin analogs without any fragmentation.

Antibiotic-inactivating enzymes or inactive derivatives of an antibiotic often have some connection with the biosynthesis of the antibiotic. KOJIMA et al. (1973, 1975a, b) isolated two inactive derivatives of ribostamycin from the broth of *S. ribosidificus* cultivated in the presence of D-xylose as a carbon source and identified them as *N*-carboxymethyl- and *N*-acetyl-ribostamycins. SHIRAFUJI et al. (1977) isolated two inactive compounds, 6′-*N*-pyrophosphamido butirosin A and 6′-*O*-pyrophospho-6′-deamino-6′-hydroxybutirosin A, from the mutant strains P-15 and AP-165 which were derived from *B. vitellinus* Z-1159, and were blocked in phosphatase synthesis. However, it is not certain if these inactive metabolites participate in ribostamycin or butirosin synthesis.

DAVIES et al. (BENVENISTE and DAVIES 1973; see also DAVIES et al. 1979) found that ribostamycin- und butirosin-inactivating phosphorylating enzymes are produced by antibiotic-producing *S. ribosidificus* and *B. circulans*. NAKAHAMA et al. (1977) found two intracellular enzymes in the cells of *B. vitellinus*, a butirosin producer. One catalyzed the phosphorylation of butirosin and the other the decomposition of butirosin phosphate into the original antibiotic. The former was purified and characterized as butirosin A 3′-phosphotransferase. As this enzyme showed a higher affinity for butirosin A than for substrates which are thought to be precursors of butirosin, for example, neamine, ribostamycin, and xylostasin, they assumed that this enzyme is responsible for resistance to butirosin. Independently, MATSUHASHI et al. (1977) also found butirosin 3′-phosphotransferase and an alkaline phosphatase in the cells of butirosin-producing *B. circulans* (NRRL B-3313). The phosphorylating enzyme was identified as an aminoglycoside 3′-phosphotransferase and was differentiated from those found in aminoglycoside-resistant strains by immunologic behavior. This enzyme showed similar activity for phosphorylation of butirosin A and ribostamycin. During fermentation of *B. circulans*, butirosin began to appear in the broth on the sixth day. Phosphotransferase activity was highest on the first day of cultivation and decreased gradually, while phosphatase activity showed a peak on the second day and decreased but then showed a second peak on the fifth day and then gradually decreased. The role of these enzymes in butirosin synthesis needs further study.

3. Glucosamine Auxotroph and Butirosin Biosynthesis

TAKEDA et al. (1979) succeeded in isolating a D-glucosamine auxotroph MCRL 5771 of *B. circulans* MCRL 5001. MCRL 5771 could utilize either D-glucosamine or *N*-acetyl-D-glucosamine as the sole carbon source for growth, but could not convert D-glucose to D-glucosamine. It could produce butirosin even if the concentration of D-glucosamine (less than 100 μg/ml) was insufficient for normal growth of the strain. Under these conditions, the cells showed an abnormal round (protoplast-like), protuberant, or filamentous form. As shown in Table 5, mutant MCRL 5771 utilized D-glucosamine more effectively than *N*-acetyl-D-glucosamine for butirosin production. Glucosamine could be replaced by *N*-acetyl-D-

Table 5. Production of butirosin from D-glucosamine and its derivatives by glucosamine auxotroph MCRL 5771. (TAKEDA et al. 1979)

Precursor (μg/ml)		Butirosin activity in 7-day broth (μg/ml)	Morphological characteristic of cells [a]	Conversion yield to butirosins (mol %)
D-Glucosamine	(50)	15	Abnormal	11
	(200)	168	Normal	30
	(500)	260	Normal	19
N-Acetyl-D-glucosamine	(50)	13	Abnormal	10
	(200)	28	Normal	5
	(500)	105	Normal	8
Methyl *N*-acetyl-α-D-glucosaminide	(200)	115	–	23
Methyl *N*-acetyl-β-D-glucosaminide	(200)	132	–	26
Benzyl *N*-acetyl-α-D-glucosaminide	(200)	265	–	69
None		0	Abnormal	0

[a] The shape of the cells in 3-day broth was inspected in the phase contrast microscope; normal cells were observed as short rod form and abnormal cells were observed as round (protoplasting), protuberant, or filamentous form. – = not observed

glucosaminides such as methyl-*N*-acetyl-α (or β)-D-glucosaminide(s) and benzyl *N*-acetyl-α-D-glucosaminide.

However, this mutant was unable to use glucosamine analogs such as 3-deoxy-D-glucosamine, 3,4-dideoxy-D-glucosamine, purpurosamine C, 6-*N*-methylpurpurosamine C, 6-*N*-methylneosamine C, or their 2-*N*-acetyl derivatives, or their methyl or benzyl glucosaminides for antibiotic production, when they were added to medium containing a limited amount of D-glucosamine (50–200 μg/ml). Therefore, either one or both of the hydroxy groups of D-glucosamine at C-3 and C-6 positions are essential for the incorporation of D-glucosamine into butirosin.

4. Plasmid Involvement

Plasmids in the ribostamycin-producing *S. ribosidificus* were isolated and characterized by two groups, though the functions of these plasmids were not determined.

OKANISHI et al. (1980) isolated plasmid pSR 1 from ribostamycin-producing *S. ribosidificus* KCC S-0923 and characterized it as a supercoiled DNA (see Fig. 3) with molecular weight of 49–56 megadaltons. This plasmid was cut into 8, 4, and 8 fragments by hydrolysis with *Eco* RI, *Hind* III, and *Bam* HI, respectively.

Independently, NOJIRI et al. (1980) isolated and characterized three plasmids, one from ribostamycin-producing *S. ribosidificus* ATCC 211294 and two from ribostamycin-nonproducing variants AF-1 and AFM-1. Variant AF-1 was resistant to ribostamycin and a 2-deoxystreptamine-requiring idiotroph, while strain AFM-1 was sensitive to ribostamycin (minimum inhibition concentration = 5 μg/ml), deficient in sporulation ability, and did not produce ribostamycin. The molecular weights of these three plasmids were approximately the same (52 ± 2 megadaltons). Moreover, these plasmids were found to be similar by electron microscopy and DNA restriction endonuclease digestion. These plasmids gave eight fragments by digestion with *Eco* RI, but fragments by *Bam* I, *Hind* III, *Sal* I, and *Sma* I were too small to be detected on agarose gels.

IV. Kanamycin

Kanamycin, produced by *Streptomyces kanamyceticus*, is a 4,6-disubstituted-2-deoxystreptamine-containing antibiotic built up from three subunits, 2-deoxystreptamine and two aminosugars. As shown in Fig. 18, kanamycin A, B, and C all contain the 3-amino-3-deoxy-D-glucose (kanosamine) moiety, which is glycosidically bound to the hydroxyl group at C-6 of 2-deoxystreptamine. They are, however, differentiated by the second aminosugar on the hydroxyl group at C-4 of 2-deoxystreptamine; 6-amino-6-deoxy-D-glucose in kanamycin A, 2,6-diamino-2,6-dideoxy-D-glucose (neosamine C) in kanamycin B, and D-glucosamine in kanamycin C.

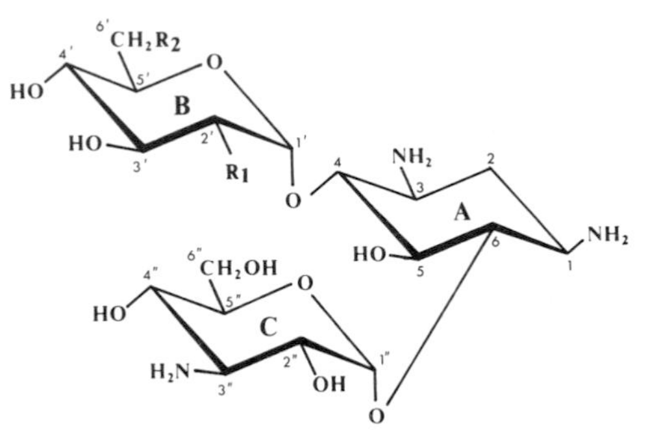

Fig. 18. Kanamycins. *Ring A*, 2-deoxystreptamine; *Ring B*, 6-amino-6-deoxy-D-glucose [$R_1 = OH$, $R_2 = NH_2$], 2,6-diamino-2,6-dideoxy-D-glucose [$R_1 = R_2 = NH_2$], D-glucosamine [$R_1 = NH_2$, $R_2 = OH$]; *Ring C*, kanosamine; *Ring A+B*, kanamine [$R_1 = OH$, $R_2 = NH_2$], neamine [$R_1 = R_2 = NH_2$], paromamine [$R_1 = NH_2$, $R_2 = OH$]; *Ring A+B+C*, kanamycin A [$R_1 = OH$, $R_2 = NH_2$], kanamycin B [$R_1 = R_2 = NH_2$], kanamycin C [$R_1 = NH_2$, $R_2 = OH$]

When H. UMEZAWA (1967) reviewed the biosynthesis of kanamycins, the subunits of kanamycin were assumed to be independently synthesized and directly combined with 2-deoxystreptamine to form kanamycin. For example, UDP-3-amino-3-deoxy-D-glucose and NucDP-6-amino-6-deoxy-D-glucose independently synthesized were linked with 2-deoxystreptamine to form kanamycin A.

In recent years studies on the other aminoglycosides such as gentamicin, sisomicin, and butirosin have raised the possibility that the D-glucosamine is first attached to 2-deoxystreptamine to give paromamine, which is then directly, or after modification on the glucosamine moiety, converted into a kanamycin-related precursor or kanamycin. This new concept will be the basis for the present discussion.

1. Biosynthesis of Subunits

KOJIMA et al. (1968) fed D-[1-^{14}C]glucose to a growing culture of *S. kanamyceticus* at various times. Incorporation was highest (3.8%) when the labeled glucose was added at an early stage (25 h) of growth and the subunits were almost equally labeled. They also found that D-[1-^{14}C]glucosamine was incorporated well into kanamycin A. Maximal incorporation was observed when the glucosamine was added at a later time (96 h) and incorporation (38%) was much higher than that of labeled glucose. The label was limited to the 6-amino-6-deoxy-D-glucose moiety of kanamycin A. This finding suggested that 6-amino-6-deoxy-D-glucose was derived from glucose via glucosamine, though the mechanism remains unknown.

To date, the pathways from glucose to both 2-deoxystreptamine and kanosamine have not been demonstrated with kanamycin-producing strains. However, the biosynthetic pathway of 2-deoxystreptamine proposed by RINEHART et al. (1974) for neomycin-producing strains may be present in kanamycin producers as well (cf. Sect. B.II.1).

Concerning the biosynthesis of kanosamine, the following pathway found in *Bacillus aminoglucosidicus* may be relevant. S. UMEZAWA et al. (1968) added sodium [U-^{14}C]pyruvate, [1-^{14}C]glycerol, sodium [1-^{14}C]acetate, or D-[^{14}C]glucose to a 16-h culture of this kanosamine-producing organism (S. UMEZAWA et al. 1967) and 4 h later isolated kanosamine. D-Glucose was incorporated into kanosamine to a much greater extent (about ten times greater) than glycerol, pyruvate, or acetate. Similar incorporation was obtained with D-[1-^{14}C]-, [2-^{14}C]-, and [6-^{14}C]glucoses, indicating that the carbon skeleton of D-glucose was incorporated without fragmentation. They also studied a cell-free system from *B. aminoglucosidicus*. When D-[U-^{14}C]glucose was incubated at 28 °C for 30 min in a reaction mixture containing the cell-free extract together with ATP, UTP, glutamine, magnesium sulfate, NAD (nicotinamide adenine dinucleotide), and pH 6.0 phosphate buffer, radioactive kanosamine was obtained. Since kanosamine could be formed from UDP-D-glucose in the same reaction mixture in the absence of D-glucose, ATP, UTP, and magnesium ion, D-glucose was shown to be first converted to UDP-glucose and then to kanosamine. Moreover, the requirement for NAD in this reaction suggested that UDP-D-glucose was oxidized to UDP-3-keto-D-glucose (not yet isolated). Based on the above findings, the following pathway was proposed: D-glucose → D-glucose-1-phosphate → UDP-D-glucose → [UDP-3-keto-D-glucose] → [UDP-3-amino-3-deoxy-D-glucose] → 3-amino-3-deoxy-D-glucose. A pathway involving 3-keto-D-glucose was unlikely because 3-keto-D-[^{14}C]glucose was not converted to kanosamine in the same cell-free system.

Recently kanosamine was found to be produced by a *Streptomyces* species (DOLAK et al. 1980).

2. Subunit Assembly

Few papers deal with the subunit assembly of kanamycin. KOJIMA et al. (1968) examined the incorporation of some labeled subunits of kanamycin by feeding them to a 3- to 4-day culture of *S. kanamyceticus* and found that tritium-labeled 2-deoxystreptamine was specifically incorporated into kanamycin A, B, and C with earlier addition giving higher incorporation. However, [U-^{14}C]kanosamine, 6-amino-6-deoxy-D-[U-^{14}C]glucose, and [U-^{14}C]paromamine were not incorporated into kanamycin. SHIER et al. (1973) and RINEHART (1977) studied the incorporation of 2-deoxystreptamine-related compounds with a 2-deoxystreptamine-requiring idiotroph of *S. kanamyceticus*. Among the compounds tested, 2-deoxystreptamine was well incorporated, but pseudodisaccharides such as neamine, paromamine, kanamine, and 6-*O*-(3-amino-3-deoxy-D-glucopyranosyl)-2-deoxystreptamine were not incorporated.

In addition to labeled kanamycin components, labeled paromamine was detected in a 5-day culture broth which had been fed D-[1-^{14}C]glucosamine at the third day of incubation (KOJIMA et al. 1969). The label was found only in glucosamine, suggesting that 2-deoxystreptamine is first glycosidated with glucosamine to yield paromamine.

The results of SATOH et al. (1975b) suggest that kanamine is a precursor of kanamycin A. The washed cells (1 g) of *S. kanamyceticus* (36 h growing cells) in 10 ml of Tris-HCl buffer (0.1 *M*, pH 8.0) containing glucose (0.5%), glutamine (0.1%), and magnesium sulfate (0.01 *M*) were incubated for 48 h. In this system, 8–10 μg/ml of kanamycin production was observed. Addition of kanamine (0.25 m*M*) to this system significantly stimulated the production of kanamycin (48 μg/ml), while addition of kanamycin itself (0.02 m*M*) inhibited the production of kanamycin. Addition of kanosamine alone showed almost no effect on kanamycin production (5.5 μg/ml potency). Interestingly, the inhibition of kanamycin production by kanamycin was partly counteracted by the addition of kanamine (0.25 m*M*) and 30 μg/ml of kanamycin was produced. Further addition of kanosamine (0.25 m*M*) gave a yield (50 μg/ml) similar to that obtained by the addition of kanamine only. These data suggested that kanamine might be glycosidated with kanosamine to form kanamycin A. As described later, studies on the participation of kanamycin acetylating and deacetylating enzymes in kanamycin biosynthesis supported the above conclusion.

An alternative possibility for linking the third residue is that glucose first links to pseudodisaccharide and then amino substitution takes place at C-3″. In addition to kanamycin A, B, and C accumulated, 2-deoxystreptamine, paromamine, neamine, kanamine, 6-*O*-glucosylneamine, and 4,6-(diglucosyl)-2-deoxystreptamine were detected in the fermentation broth of a mutant strain of *S. kanamyceticus* (MURASE et al. 1970). To account for the occurrence of these compounds, the present authors postulate a so-called metabolic grid for kanamycin biosynthesis which is shown in Fig. 19. In this pathway, paromamine is assumed to be a key precursor of kanamycin biosynthesis. Substitution of the hydroxyl group at C-6′ in paromamine with an amino group (amino substitution) gives neamine. This reaction was shown to be present in butirosin biosynthesis. Glucosidation of the hydroxyl group at C-6 of neamine gives rise to 6-*O*-glucosylneamine, which undergoes subsequent amino substitution at C-3″ to yield kanamycin B. Substitution of the amino group at C-2′ of neamine with a hydroxyl group (deamino hydroxylation) will afford kanamine, which may also be produced by deamino hydroxylation at C-2′ and amino substitution at C-6′ of paromamine, though the intermediate, 4-*O*-glycosyl-2-deoxystreptamine, was not reported by MURASE et al. (1970). If the deamino hydroxylation reaction at C-2′ takes place at the pseudotrisaccharide stage, kanamycin A is assumed to be derived from kanamycin B or 6-*O*-glucosylneamine via 6-*O*-glucosylkanamine. Kanamycin C may be produced by glucosidation at C-6 of paromamine and subsequent amino substitution at C-3″.

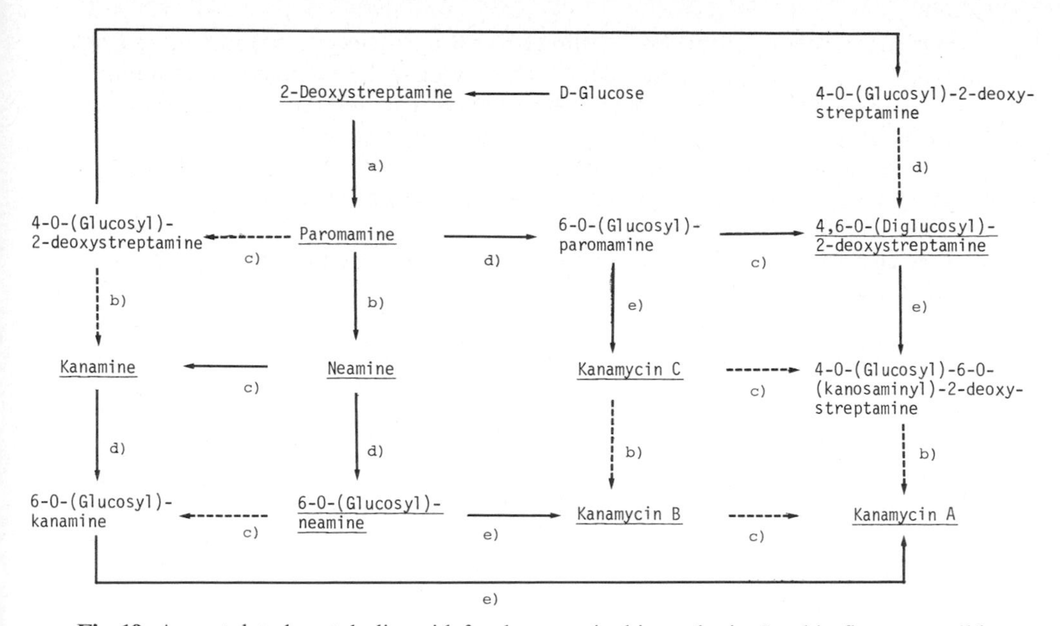

Fig. 19. A postulated metabolic grid for kanamycin biosynthesis. In this figure, possible correlations between the compounds actually detected or assumed are shown. The *compound underlined* is the product detected by MURASE et al. (1970). The steps shown by *solid lines* are most probable and those shown with *dotted lines* more speculative. *DOS*, 2-deoxystreptamine. Reactions: a) *O*-glycosidation with D-glucosamine at C-4; b) amino substitution at C-6′; c) deaminohydroxylation at C-2′; d) *O*-glucosidation at C-6; e) amino substitution at C-3″

In studies of the biosynthesis of gentamicin and sisomicin, it was shown that a pseudotrisaccharide containing paromamine underwent amino substitution at C-6′, yielding a neamine-containing pseudotrisaccharide. These findings indicate the presence of an additional route for production of kanamycin B from kanamycin C. A direct glucosidation mechanism was also proposed in the biosynthetic pathway for gentamicin and sisomicin, in which paromamine was first glycosidated by a neutral sugar (xylose).

4,6-*O*-(Diglucosyl)-2-deoxystreptamine found in the broth of the mutant is presumably derived from 6-*O*-glucosylparomamine by deamino hydroxylation at C-2′ or by the direct glucosidation at C-6 of 4-*O*-(glucosyl)-2-deoxystreptamine. Finally, there is the possibility that kanamycin A is produced by amino substitution at C-6′ of 4-*O*-(glucosyl)-6-*O*-(kanosaminyl)-2-deoxystreptamine.

By mutational biosynthesis with a 2-deoxystreptamine-requiring idiotroph of *S. kanamyceticus*, KOJIMA and SATOH (1973) obtained 4-*O*-(α-D-glucopyranosyl)-6-*O*-(kanosaminyl)-1-*N*-methyl-2-deoxystreptamine and 4-*O*-(α-D-glucopyranosyl)-6-*O*-(kanosaminyl)-2-*epi*-streptamine from 1-*N*-methyl-2-deoxystreptamine and 2-*epi*-streptamine, respectively. Modifications at C-1 and C-2 in 2-deoxystreptamine may cause repression of the amino substitution reaction at C-6′ (step b in Fig. 19) and result in accumulation of derivatives of 4-*O*-(glucosyl)-6-*O*-(kanosaminyl)-2-deoxystreptamine.

Similarly, YASUDA et al. (1978) showed that a 2-deoxystreptamine-requiring idiotroph of *S. kanamyceticus* could bioconvert 3.5 g of 2,5-dideoxystreptamine into 5-deoxykanamycin A (128 mg), 5-deoxykanamine (406 mg), and 6-*O*-(glucosyl)-5-deoxykanamine (462 mg). These results suggest that 6-*O*-glucosylkanamine is an intermediate from kanamine to kanamycin A and that deoxygenation at C-5 of 2-deoxystreptamine suppressed 6-*O*-glucosidation and amino substitution at C-3″ (steps d and e in Fig. 19).

It is difficult to formulate a precise pathway for kanamycin biosynthesis at present. However, the following scheme seems most probable:

$$\begin{array}{ccccc} \text{Glucose} \rightarrow \text{Paromamine} & \rightarrow & \text{Neamine} & \rightarrow & \text{Kanamine} \\ \downarrow & & \downarrow & & \downarrow \\ \text{Kanamycin C} & \rightarrow & \text{Kanamycin B} & \rightarrow & \text{Kanamycin A} \end{array}$$

Paromamine or neamine, key precursors in this scheme, have not been incorporated into kanamycin in experiments with *S. kanamyceticus* or 2-deoxystreptamine-requiring idiotrophs (KOJIMA et al. 1969; SHIER et al. 1973). Therefore, final conclusions must await the discovery of a mutant or cell-free system which incorporates the pseudodisaccharides. The type of sugar derivative involved in the glycosidation of the pseudodisaccharide is also unknown.

Kanamycin biosynthesis may also involve kanamycin-inactivating enzymes. SATOH et al. (1975a) found kanamycin-6′-*N*-acetyl transferase (KAT) and *N*-acetyl-kanamycin-amidohydrolase (NAKA) in cell-free extracts of *S. kanamyceticus*. They also observed that 6′-*N*-acetylkanamycin A was accumulated inside or outside cells of the producing strain. SATOH et al. (1975b, 1976) discussed the possible participation of these enzymes in the biosynthesis of kanamycin. Acetylation of kanamycin by KAT (produced only at an early phase of the fermentation) might be a prerequisite for kanosamine to bind with kanamine, giving 6′-*N*-acetylkanamycin A, and kanamycin A might be liberated by the action of NAKA produced at the idiophase of the kanamycin fermentation and excreted outside the cells. Recently, BASAK and MAJUMDAR (1978) found that alkaline phosphatase is produced late in the fermentation of *S. kanamyceticus* and that kanamycin formation is directly related to the activity of this enzyme.

3. Plasmid Involvement

Plasmids are probably involved in 2-deoxystreptamine formation. HOTTA et al. (1977) isolated kanamycin-nonproducing mutants of *S. kanamyceticus* by cultivating the strain in the presence of acriflavine (0–30 μg/ml). These mutants showed loss of kanamycin productivity and weakened ability to form aerial mycelium, but showed no decrease in kanamycin acetyltransferase and *N*-acetylkanamycin-amidohydrolase activity. These mutants produced kanamycin in medium supplemented with 2-deoxystreptamine, thus it was suggested that plasmids control the formation of enzymes involved in 2-deoxystreptamine synthesis. The detection of plasmid DNA, however, has not yet been reported.

CHANG et al. (1978) also examined the effects of plasmid-curing agents (acriflavine, 5–10 μg/ml; acridine orange, 5–10 μg/ml; and ethidium bromide, 2.5–

5 μg/ml) and incubation at high temperature (35 °C) on the occurrence of kanamycin-nonproducing colonies derived from fragmented (by sonication) mycelia or conidia of an industrial strain of *S. kanamyceticus*, and observed a high incidence of nonproducing colonies (five to tenfold increase), compared to no treatment. These mutants were found to be 2-deoxystreptamine-requiring idiotrophs, suggesting that active kanamycin production, 2-deoxystreptamine, and other cultural characteristics are controlled by plasmid genes in this organism. Plasmid DNA was not detected.

V. Gentamicin and Sisomicin

Gentamicin, sisomicin, and their relatives are pseudotrisaccharides containing 4,6-disubstituted-2-deoxystreptamine and are produced mostly by various species of *Micromonospora*.

Gentamicin C, a complex consisting mainly of gentamicin C_1, C_2, and C_{1a}, and sisomicin are now commercially available.

As shown in Figs. 20 and 22, gentamicin C and sisomicin contain 2-deoxystreptamine and two aminosugar moieties. Garosamine (ring C), common to both gentamicin C and sisomicin, is glycosidically linked to the hydroxyl group at C-6 of 2-deoxystreptamine to form a pseudodisaccharide, garamine (ring A+C). The second aminosugar linked at C-4 of garamine is purpurosamine (ring B) in gentamicin C and in sisomicin is a 4,5-unsaturated aminosugar. Gentamicin C_1, C_2, and C_{1a}, contain purpurosamine A, B, and C, respectively. The structures of gentamicin- and sisomicin-related antibiotics are shown in Figs. 21 and 22.

1. Biosynthesis of Subunits

a) 2-Deoxystreptamine

The biosynthetic sequence of 2-deoxystreptamine formation in gentamicin-producing microorganisms was examined by feeding 2-deoxystreptamine analogs or possible intermediates to a 2-deoxystreptamine-requiring idiotroph of the gentamicin-producing strain.

Daum et al. (1977a) found that a 2-deoxystreptamine-requiring idiotroph of *M. purpurea* produced the gentamicin complex (C_1, C_2, and C_{1a}) when 2-deoxy-*scyllo*-inosose was fed. This mutant also produced 2-hydroxygentamicin C_1 and C_2, when *scyllo*-inosose, *scyllo*-inosamine, or streptamine was added to the fermentation medium. At the same time, it was found that *scyllo*-inosose was converted to streptamine, whereas *myo*-inositol, a precursor of streptidine, was not converted to the antibiotic by this organism.

These findings suggested the presence in *M. purpurea* of the following pathway postulated in *Streptomyces* by Rinehart and Stroshane (1976): 2-Deoxy-*scyllo*-inosose → 2-Deoxy-*scyllo*-inosamine →→ 2-Deoxystreptamine [(27a) → (28a) →→ (30) in Fig. 15].

The isolation of 2-deoxy-*scyllo*-inosamine from the fermentation broth of a mutant of *M. sagamiensis*, a producer of gentamicin C_1 and C_{2b} (sagamicin), supports the above sequence (Kase et al. 1980).

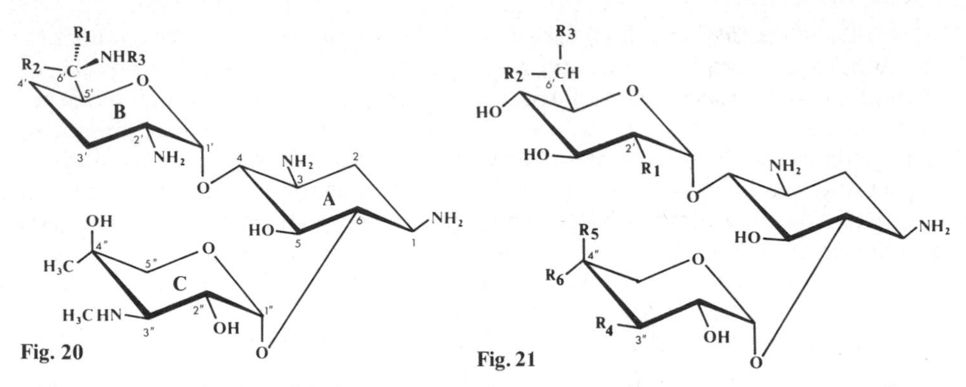

Fig. 20. Gentamicin C antibiotics. *Ring A*, 2-deoxystreptamine; *Ring B*, purpurosamine A [$R_1=H, R_2=CH_3, R_3=CH_3$], purpurosamine B [$R_1=H, R_2=CH_3, R_3=H$]; purpurosamine C [$R_1=H, R_2=H, R_3=H$], 6-*epi*-purpurosamine B [$R_1=CH_3, R_2=H, R_3=H$], *N*-methyl-purpurosamine C [$R_1=H, R_2=H, R_3=CH_3$]; *Ring C*, garosamine; *Ring A+B*, gentamine C_1 [$R_1=H, R_2=CH_3, R_3=CH_3$], gentamine C_2 [$R_1=H, R_2=CH_3, R_3=H$], gentamine C_{1a} [$R_1=H, R_2=H, R_3=H$]; *Ring A+C*, garamine; *Ring A+B+C*, gentamicin C_1 [$R_1=H, R_2=CH_3, R_3=CH_3$], gentamicin C_2 [$R_1=H, R_2=CH_3, R_3=H$], gentamicin C_{1a} [$R_1=H, R_2=H, R_3=H$], gentamicin C_{2a} [$R_1=CH_3, R_2=H, R_3=H$], gentamicin C_{2b} [$R_1=H, R_2=H, R_3=CH_3$] (sagamicin)

Fig. 21. Gentamicin-related antibiotics

	R_1	R_2	R_3	R_4	R_5	R_6
Gentamicin A	NH_2	H	OH	$NHCH_2$	H	OH
Gentamicin A_1	NH_2	H	OH	$NHCH_3$	OH	H
Gentamicin A_2	NH_2	H	OH	OH	H	OH
Gentamicin A_3	OH	H	NH_2	$NHCH_3$	OH	H
Gentamicin B	OH	H	NH_2	$NHCH_3$	OH	CH_3
Gentamicin B_1	OH	CH_3	NH_2	$NHCH_3$	OH	CH_3
Gentamicin X_2	NH_2	H	OH	$NHCH_3$	OH	CH_3
Antibiotic G-418	NH_2	CH_3	OH	$NHCH_3$	OH	CH_3
Antibiotic JI-20A	NH_2	H	NH_2	$NHCH_3$	OH	CH_3
Antibiotic JI-20B	NH_2	CH_3	NH_2	$NHCH_3$	OH	CH_3

CHEN and WALKER (1977) suggested the possibility that at least one of the amino groups of 2-deoxystreptamine is donated from L-glutamine by an amino-transferase in the mycelium of *M. purpurea*.

b) Garosamine and Purpurosamine

GRISEBACH (1978) speculated on the biosynthetic pathway from D-glucose to L-garosamine. However, it has not been demonstrated whether garosamine and purpurosamine are synthesized before or after binding with 2-deoxystreptamine.

2. Subunit Assembly

The biosynthetic pathways from 2-deoxystreptamine to gentamicin–sisomicin group antibiotics are summarized in Fig. 23.

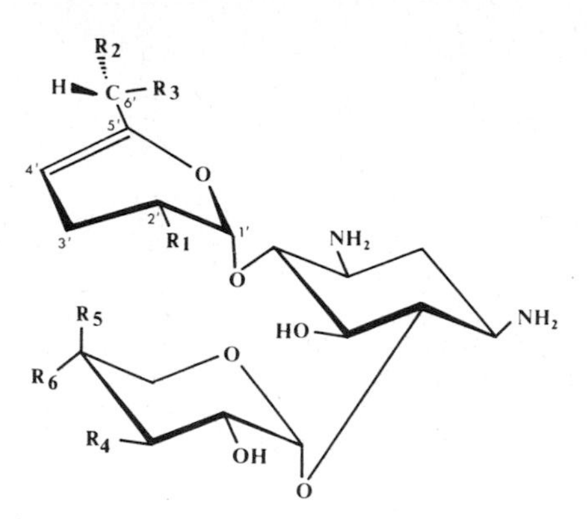

Fig. 22. Sisomicin and related antibiotics

	R_1	R_2	R_3	R_4	R_5	R_6
Sisomicin	NH_2	H	NH_2	$NHCH_3$	OH	CH_3
Verdamicin	NH_2	CH_3	NH_2	$NHCH_3$	OH	CH_3
Antibiotic G-52	NH_2	H	$NHCH_3$	$NHCH_3$	OH	CH_3
Antibiotic 66-40B	NH_2	H	NH_2	$NHCH_3$	H	OH
Antibiotic 66-40D	NH_2	H	NH_2	$NHCH_3$	OH	H
Antibiotic 66-40G	NH_2	H	NH_2	NH_2	OH	CH_3

a) Studies on Gentamicin-Producing Strains

A biosynthetic pathway for gentamicin C was first proposed by TESTA and TILLEY (1976) who examined the bioconversion of various gentamicin-related antibiotics into gentamicin by mutant Paro 346 of *M. purpurea*. This mutant did not produce gentamicin, but accumulated paromamine. In this experiment, gentamicin A, B, C_1, C_2, C_{1a}, and X_2, and related antibiotics, JI-20A, JI-20B, and G-418, were tested and the products were analyzed by paper chromatography. The results were as follows:

1. Gentamicin A afforded bioactive spots corresponding to gentamicin C_1, C_2, and C_{1a}.
2. Gentamicin X_2 gave gentamicin C_{1a}, C_2, and C_1.
3. Antibiotic JI-20A (6′-aminogentamicin X_2) gave gentamicin C_{1a} and C_{2b}.
4. Antibiotic G-418 (6′-*C*-methylgentamicin X_2) or antibiotic JI-20B (6′-*C*-methyl JI-20A) yielded gentamicin C_2 and C_1.
5. Gentamicin C_{1a} gave gentamicin C_{2b}.
6. Gentamicin C_2 gave gentamicin C_1.
7. Gentamicin B, B_1, and C_1 were not converted to any other antibiotics.

Based on the above findings, TESTA and TILLEY (1976) proposed the following pathway for gentamicins: Paromamine is first converted to gentamicin X_2 via gentamicin A. From gentamicin X_2, the pathway branches into two routes. One leads to JI-20A (by amino substitution at C-6′), gentamicin C_{1a} (by 3′,4′-dideoxygenation), and finally to gentamicin C_{2b} (by *N*-methylation at C-6′). The second pathway leads to G-418 (by *C*-methylation at C-6′), JI-20B (by amino substitution at C-6′), gentamicin C_2 (by 3′,4′-dideoxygenation followed by epimerization at C-

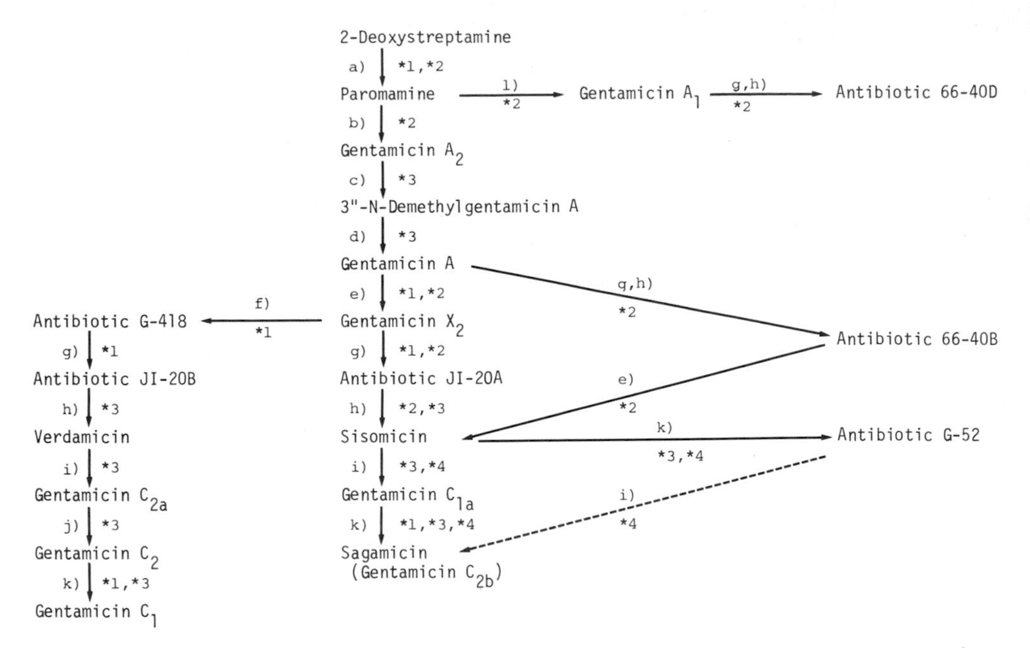

Fig. 23. Biosynthetic pathways proposed for gentamicin–sagamicin–sisomicin group antibiotics. (TESTA and TILLEY 1975, 1976; KASE et al. 1980; LEE et al. 1977). Reactions: a) *O*-glycosidation with D-glucosamine at C-4; b) *O*-glycosidation with D-xylose at C-6; c) amino substitution at C-3″; d) *N*-methylation at C-3″; e) *C*-methylation with epimerization at C-4″; f) *C*-methylation at C-6′; g) amino substitution at C-6′; h) 3′,4′-dideoxygenation and 4′,5′-unsaturation; i) (4′,5′)-hydrogenation; j) epimerization at C-6′; k) *N*-methylation at C-6; l) glycosidation with 4-*N*-demethylgarosamine at C-6.
A step *asterisked* shows a pathway demonstrated by feeding experiments with *M. purpurea* or its mutant (*1), M. inyoensis or its mutant (*2), *M. sagamiensis* or its mutant (*3), and *M. rhodorangea* (*4)

6′), and then to gentamicin C_1 (by *N*-methylation at C-6′). In these sequences, the steps from gentamicin X_2 to G-418 and from gentamicin C_{1a} to gentamicin C_{2b} required cobalt ions, indicating that *C*-methylation and *N*-methylation at C-6′ are cobalt dependent. Furthermore, the step from gentamicin A to X_2, involving *C*-methylation with epimerization at C-4″, is also cobalt dependent (GRISEBACH 1978; TESTA and TILLEY 1979).

Labeling experiments with L-[CH_3-^{14}C]methionine indicated that the methyl groups in gentamicin were all derived from the methionine methyl (LEE et al. 1973, 1975, 1976, 1979). Labeling experiments with L-[CH_3-^{14}C]- and L-[CH_3-^{2}H] methionine simultaneously applied also supported the above conclusion (DANIELS et al. 1976).

Recently, OKA et al. (1979) found that when kanamycin B was fed to a 24-h growing culture of gentamicin-non- or low-producing mutants of *M. echinospora* or other *Micromonospora*, the antibiotic was converted to 3″-*N*-methyl-4″-*C*-methyl-3′,4′-dideoxy-6′-*N*-methylkanamycin B (designated compound I-B_1; Fig. 24), or 3″-*N*-methyl-4″-*C*-methyl-3′,4′-dideoxykanamycin B, depending on the strain used. Likewise, kanamycin A was transformed into 3″-*N*-methyl-4″-*C*-

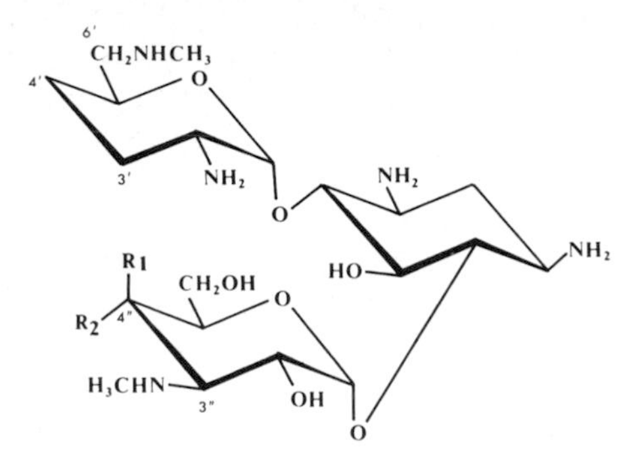

Fig. 24. Compound I–B_1 bioconverted from kanamycin B by the mutant strain of *Micromonospora* sp. R_1=OH, R_2=CH_3 or R_1=CH_3, R_2=OH. (OKA et al. 1979)

methyl-3',4'-dideoxykanamycin A. Though the configuration at C-4" of the resulting antibiotics was not determined, they may be epimeric at C-4". This finding indicates that the enzymes involved in the above reaction have broad substrate specificity.

b) Studies on Sisomicin-Producing Strain

Using the same technique as for gentamicin biosynthesis, TESTA and TILLEY (1975) examined the bioconversion of 6 2-deoxystreptamine-containing pseudodisaccharides and 12 pseudotrisaccharides by a 2-deoxystreptamine-requiring idiotroph of sisomicin-producing *M. inyoensis*. The pseudodisaccharides paromamine and neamine were converted to sisomicin, but 6'-*C*-methylneamine, 3',4'-dideoxyneamine (gentamine C_{1a}), 6'-*C*-methyl-6'-*N*-methylgentamine C_{1a} (gentamine C_1), and garamine were not converted into any antibiotic. On the other hand, pseudotrisaccharides such as gentamicin A, X_2, and JI-20A, which were convertible to gentamicin, could be transformed to sisomicin as well.

These results suggested that a route, gentamicin A→X_2→JI-20A, is present in *M. inyoensis* as in *M. purpurea*. Gentamicin A_2 (6-*O*-xylosylparomamine) and antibiotic 66-40B (4"-demethyl-*xylo*-isomer of sisomicin) were also converted to sisomicin, whereas gentamicin A_1 (4" epimer of gentamicin A) was converted not to sisomicin, but to antibiotic 66-40D (4"-demethylsisomicin). Conversion was not observed with G-418, JI-20B, 66-40D, gentamicin B, B_1, and sisomicin. Based on these results, they proposed the following biosynthetic pathway from 2-deoxystreptamine to sisomicin: 2-Deoxystreptamine is converted to gentamicin A via paromamine and gentamicin A_2. From gentamicin A, the pathway has two branches. The first leads to sisomicin via gentamicin X_2 and JI-20A. The second leads to sisomicin via 66-40B.

c) Studies on Sagamicin-Producing Strains

The transformation of gentamicin C_{1a} to C_{2b} (sagamicin) was studied by DEGUCHI et al. (1977). They found that resting cells of *M. sagamiensis* could convert gentamicin C_{1a} to sagamicin in the presence of L-[CH_3-^{14}C]methionine or *S*-adenosyl-L-[CH_3-^{14}C]methionine. This finding indicates that the step from gentamicin C_{1a} to C_{2b} is the same in *M. sagamiensis* and in *M. purpurea*.

More recently, KASE et al. (1980) developed a 2-deoxystreptamine-requiring idiotroph (KY 11525) from a parent strain of *M. sagamiensis*. The parent strain normally produces sagamicin (gentamicin C_{2b}) as a major product and gentamicin C_1, C_2, and C_{1a} as minor products. Applying the feeding method of TESTA and TILLEY (1975, 1976), they confirmed the biosynthetic pathway for gentamicin which had been proposed by TESTA and TILLEY. In other experiments, a conversion system using washed cells of 2-deoxystreptamine-requiring idiotroph (strain KY 11525) was devised and used.

2-Deoxystreptamine, paromamine, gentamicin A, and X_2 were all converted to sagamicin and trace amounts of gentamicin C_1, C_2, and C_{1a}. Antibiotic JI-20A was converted to sagamicin and gentamicin C_{1a}, while antibiotic G-418 and JI-20B were transformed to gentamicin C_1 and C_2. Also this mutant could convert gentamicin C_{1a} and C_2 to sagamicin and gentamicin C_1, respectively, but could not transform sagamicin and gentamicin C_1 to any other antibiotic. These results are in accordance with the biosynthetic pathways proposed by TESTA and TILLEY, therefore similar pathways are present in *M. sagamiensis* and *M. purpurea*. At the same time, these researchers also isolated two sagamicin-nonproducing mutants of *M. sagamiensis*. One of them (KY 11565) could produce gentamicin X_2 and antibiotic G-418, indicating that the mutant was blocked at the stage of amino substitution at C-6′. The other mutant (KY 11533) produced gentamicin A_2 and 3″-*N*-demethylgentamicin A, both of which are expected to be intermediates for gentamicin A. These products were then converted to sagamicin and gentamicin C_{1a} by the 2-deoxystreptamine-requiring idiotroph (strain KY 11525), suggesting a possible route from A_2 to A via 3″-demethylgentamicin A. It was also shown that mutant KY 11533 could coproduce a series of 3″-demethyl derivatives of gentamicin–sisomicin group antibiotics, i.e., 3″-demethyl derivatives of gentamicin A and C_{1a}, JI-20A, G-52, sagamicin, sisomicin, and 3″-*N*-acetylsisomicin. These results suggested that the strain was blocked at the step of *N*-methylation at C-3″.

d) Biosynthetic Correlation in Gentamicin–Sisomicin Group Antibiotics

LEE et al. (1977) reported that sisomicin was converted to gentamicin C_{2b} by *M. rhodorangea*, an organism producing antibiotic G-418. Since this conversion requires *N*-methylation at C-6′ and (4′-5′)-hydrogenation, gentamicin C_{1a} or antibiotic G-52 may be an intermediate in this sequence.

Recently, KASE et al. (1980) followed the time course of the conversion of sisomicin and verdamicin by resting cells of the 2-deoxystreptamine-requiring idiotroph (KY 11525) of sagamicin-producing *M. sagamiensis*. They confirmed the following two pathways: Sisomicin→Gentamicin C_{1a}→Gentamicin C_{2b}, and Verdamicin→Gentamicin C_{2a}→Gentamicin C_2→Gentamicin C_1 (see also NAKAYAMA et al. 1979d).

They further suggested that sisomicin and verdamicin participate in the biosynthesis of gentamicin and sagamicin as intermediates. Among mutants deficient in (4′-5′)-hydrogenation activity, a mutant (KY 11535) of *M. sagamiensis* was isolated, which accumulated antibiotic G-52 as a major component and sisomicin as a minor component. This mutant, by further mutation, gave another 2-deoxystreptamine-requiring idiotroph (KY 11536) which converts sisomicin to antibiotic G-

52. In addition, mutant KY 11536 could convert both 2-deoxystreptamine and antibiotic JI-20A to antibiotic G-52 and sisomicin, and also antibiotic JI-20B to verdamicin. Furthermore, KY 11536 could convert gentamicin C_{1a} and C_2 to sagamicin and gentamicin C_1, respectively. These results strongly indicated that sisomicin and verdamicin are intermediates on the biosynthetic pathway of the gentamicin–sagamicin group antibiotics and that sisomicin and gentamicin antibiotics are biosynthetically related to each other. The presence of sisomicin as a minor product of gentamicin-producing strain was previously pointed out by BERDY et al. (1977).

KASE et al. (1980) proposed the biosynthetic pathways for sagamicin, gentamicin, and sisomicin antibiotics shown in Fig. 23, in which the pathways involving antibiotics 66-40B and 66-40D are those of TESTA and TILLEY (1975).

They presented additional proof which supported the above pathways. They isolated two additional mutants of *M. sagamiensis*. One of the mutants (KY 11564) produced sagamicin and gentamicin C_{2a}, but not gentamicin C_1. The other (KY 11566) produced gentamicin C_{1a} and C_{2a} together with trace amounts of gentamicin C_2, but not sagamicin and gentamicin C_1. These results indicated that mutant KY 11564 was blocked at the epimerization step at C-6′, while mutant KY 11566 was blocked at the *N*-methylation step at C-6′.

Gentamicin production was significantly enhanced by the addition of cobalt to the production medium. In the sagamicin fermentation, the addition of $CoCl_2$ enhanced gentamicin production and depressed sagamicin production. As described previously, the *C*-methylation and *N*-methylation steps at C-6′ involved in gentamicin biosynthesis are cobalt dependent so that, if a mutant is obtained which cannot produce gentamicin C_2 even in medium with added $CoCl_2$, the sole production of sagamicin with higher yields might be expected. KASE et al. (1980) succeeded in isolating such a mutant (KY 11538), which was capable of producing only sagamicin in the presence of $CoCl_2$. This mutant could convert antibiotic G-418, JI-20B, and gentamicin C_2 into gentamicin C_1, but could not convert gentamicin A_2 and X_2 into gentamicin C_1. From these results, the blocked step in this mutant is assumed to be *C*-methylation at C-6′.

The biosynthetic correlation of gentamicins with other related antibiotics, such as 3″-*N*-demethyl and 4″-*C*-demethyl derivatives, and 1-amino-1-hydroxy derivatives of gentamicin will be discussed again in Sect. B.X.

Gentamicin A_3, B, and B_1 differ from other gentamicins in the hydroxyl substituent at C-2′. No reports have been published on the biosynthesis of these gentamicins, but it will be interesting to know whether they are synthesized from 4-*O*-glucosyl-2-deoxystreptamine or produced by the substitution of the amino function at C-2′ in gentamicin with a hydroxyl function.

For example, are antibiotics JI-20A and JI-20B converted to gentamicin B and B_1? In kanamycin biosynthesis described in Sect. B.IV, the possibility of the formation of kanamycin A from kanamycin B by a similar substitution is suggested.

e) Additional Findings on Biosynthesis

LEE et al. (1979) reported data contradictory to the above biosynthetic pathway for gentamicin. They found that the incubation of *M. purpurea* SC 1210, a producer of antibiotic JI-20A, with L-[CH_3-^{14}C]methionine yielded [CH_3-^{14}C]gentamicin A and [CH_3-^{14}C]JI-20A in a molar radioactivity ratio of 9:2. However, [CH_3-^{14}C]gentamicin X_2, which was expected to be an intermediate in gentamicin biosynthesis, could not be isolated. On the other hand, when the [CH_3-^{14}C]JI-20A was fed to a 2-deoxystreptamine-requiring idiotroph (SC 1124) of gentamicin-producing *M. purpurea*, the substrate was converted into gentamicin C_{1a} and C_{2b} in variable molar radioactivity ratios (JI-20A added: gentamicin C_{1a} produced: gentamicin C_{2b} produced = 10:3–8:7–9). They concluded that the pathway, gentamicin A→gentamicin X_2→JI-20A→gentamicin C_{1a}→gentamicin C_{2b}, proposed by TESTA and TILLEY was not supported by these data, because the radioactivity ratios in the converted products were so varied. Consequently, they suggested that (1) JI-20A is not derived from gentamicin A or X_2, and (2) JI-20A is converted to gentamicin C_{1a} and C_{2b} independently, and questioned whether gentamicin C_{1a} and C_{2b} are biosynthesized independently or via the same pathway.

KASE et al. (1980) found that 3″-*N*-demethylgaramine is produced by a sagamicin-nonproducing mutant (KY 11533) or *M. sagamiensis*. It is not reported whether this metabolite is converted into any antibiotic, but formation of this metabolite cannot be explained by the above biosynthetic sequence. Perhaps it is an artifact from hydrolysis of 3″-*N*-demethyl pseudotrisaccharide.

From the culture broth of a gentamicin C-producing *Micromonospora*, BERDY et al. (1971) isolated the following minor components: 4′-demethylgentamicin C_1, C_2, and C_{1a}, and the unique compound (33). KUGELMAN et al. (1978) also reported the production of minor components of sisomicin, including 3″-demethylsisomicin

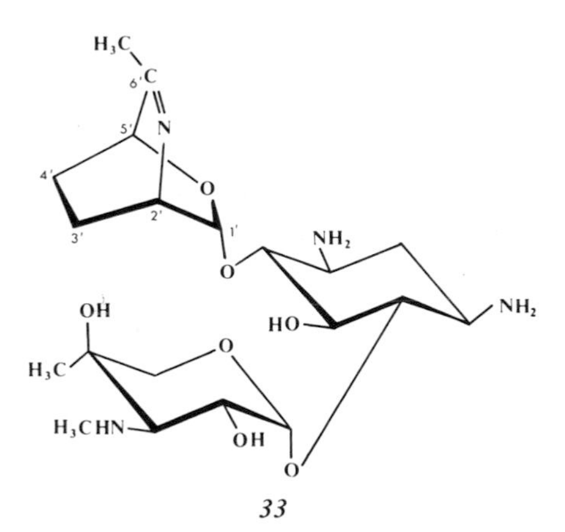

33

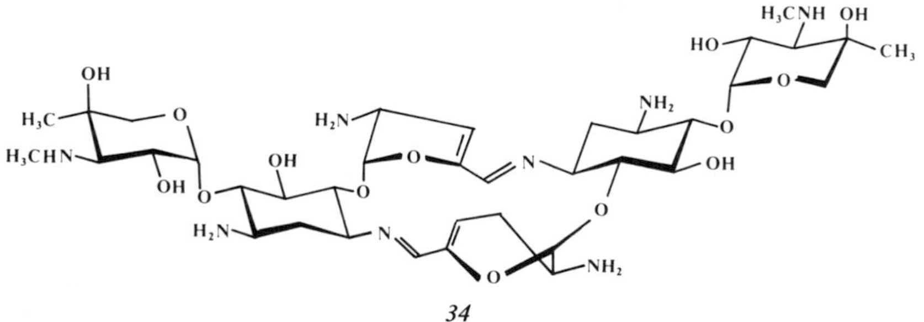

34

and 66-40C (34) by *M. inyoensis*. It is not clear how these minor components participate in the biosynthetic mechanism. Therefore, further investigations are necessary to establish the biosynthetic pathway of the gentamicin–sagamicin–sisomicin antibiotics, including these metabolites.

VI. Spectinomycin (Actinospectacin)

Spectinomycin (35 a) produced by a variety of *Streptomyces*, such as *S. spectabilis*, *S. flavopersicus*, and others, possesses an unique structure (Fig. 25) in which a single sugar component (actinospectose; ring C) is fused to a diaminocyclitol (actinamine, ring A) by both a β-glycosidic bond and a hemiketal bond to form a 1,4-dioxin ring (ring B). In aqueous solution, the carbonyl group is present in the hydrated form (35 b).

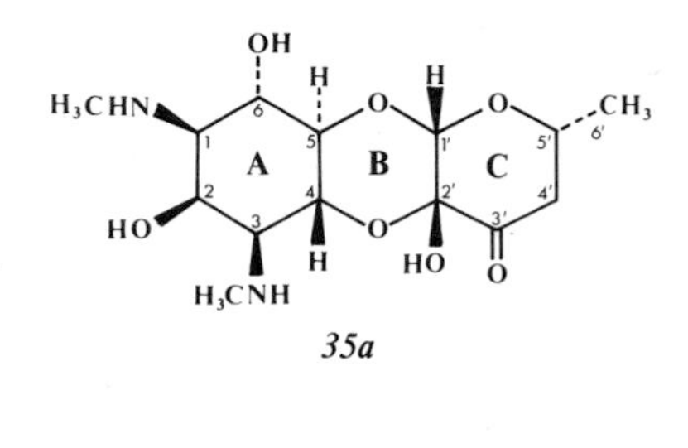

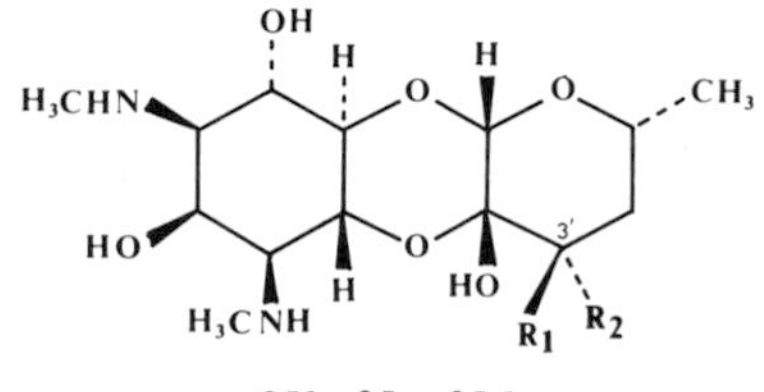

Fig. 25. Spectinomycin and dihydrospectinomycin. *Ring A*, actinamine; *Ring C*, actinospectose. Spectinomycin (35a); spectinomycin hydrated (35b) [$R_1=R_2=OH$]; dihydrospectinomycin isomer (35c) [$R_1=H$, $R_2=OH$]; dihydrospectinomycin isomer (35d) [$R_1=OH$, $R_2=H$]

1. Biosynthesis of Subunits

MITSCHER et al. (1971) examined the incorporation of several labeled compounds by *S. flavopersicus* and the distribution of the label in the subunits with the results shown in Table 6. Later, STROSHANE et al. (1976) studied the incorporation of D-[6-^{13}C]glucose by *S. spectabilis*. As with other aminoglycosides, glucose is introduced equally into both subunits.

a) Actinamine

Of the radioactivity incorporated from [6-^{13}C]glucose into spectinomycin, 2.4% was found in C-6 of actinamine (ring A) and the two *N*-methyl carbons. As shown

Table 6. Incorporation and distribution of label in spectinomycin and its subunits. (MITSCHER et al. 1971)

	Incorporation into spectinomycin (%)	Distribution of incorporated radioactivity (%)	
		Actinamine (N-Me)	Actinospectose (C-Me)
L-[CH_3-^{14}C]Methionine	38.8	91.1–94.2 (92.1)	0
D-[6-^{3}H]Glucose	3.5	46.1–49.5 (ND [a])	36.9–37.5 (36.9–37.5)
myo-[2-^{14}C]Inositol	46.8–47.0	88.0–91.1 (ND)	0
[2-^{14}C]Actinamine	6.6	ND [a]	ND
[2-^{14}C]Acetic acid	0.3	ND	ND

[a] ND = not determined

in Table 6 and also as demonstrated by SLECHTA and COATS (1974), methionine is a direct donor of these *N*-methyl groups. Therefore, enrichment of the *N*-methyl groups by [6-^{13}C]glucose probably results from the conversion of glucose to methionine via [3-^{13}C]serine and [methylene-^{13}C]tetrahydrofolic acid.

myo-Inositol was well incorporated into spectinomycin and selectively distributed into the actinamine moiety. Since the incorporation of actinamine itself was very low, it was not clear whether *myo*-inositol (3) was converted to actinamine (38) before or after binding with actinospectose.

Successful isolation of an actinamine-requiring idiotroph of *S. spectabilis* and feeding experiments with this mutant carried out by SLECHTA and COATS (1974) not only demonstrated that exogenous actinamine is directly incorporated into spectinomycin, but also suggested a conversion sequence from glucose to actinamine. The idiotroph could incorporate *N,N*-didemethylactinamine (36) into spectinomycin. When cultured in the presence of non-radioactive actinamine with [CH_3-^{13}C]methionine, it produced non-labeled spectinomycin. However, when fed [CH_3-^{13}C]methionine and either *N,N*-didemethylactinamine (*myo*-inosadiamine-1,3) (36) or *N*-monodemethylactinamine (*N*-methyl-*myo*-inosadiamine-1,3) (37), the mutant produced antibiotic labeled in the *N*-methyl group. These facts confirmed the role of methionine as a donor of two *N*-methyl groups and suggested that *myo*-inosadiamine-1,3 is methylated just before actinamine is linked to actinospectose or a precursor. The biosynthetic pathway from glucose (15) to actinamine (38) via *myo*-inositol (3) is summarized in Fig. 26. This pathway is similar to that from *myo*-inositol to streptidine in streptomycin, but in streptidine the first *N*-guanidinylation occurs before the second amino group is introduced, while *N*-methylation in actinamine biosynthesis occurs after both amino groups are introduced into the cyclitol.

When *myo*-inosadiamine-1,3 was replaced by *scyllo*-inosadiamine-1,3, the mutant produced 2-*epi*-spectinomycin which showed no antibacterial activity.

During the synthesis from D-glucose to actinamine via *myo*-inositol, an inversion of configuration at C-4 of glucose is involved. Tritium attached at C-4 was completely lost during the incorporation of glucose into the actinamine moiety (FLOSS et al. 1978; see Table 7 and Fig. 27).

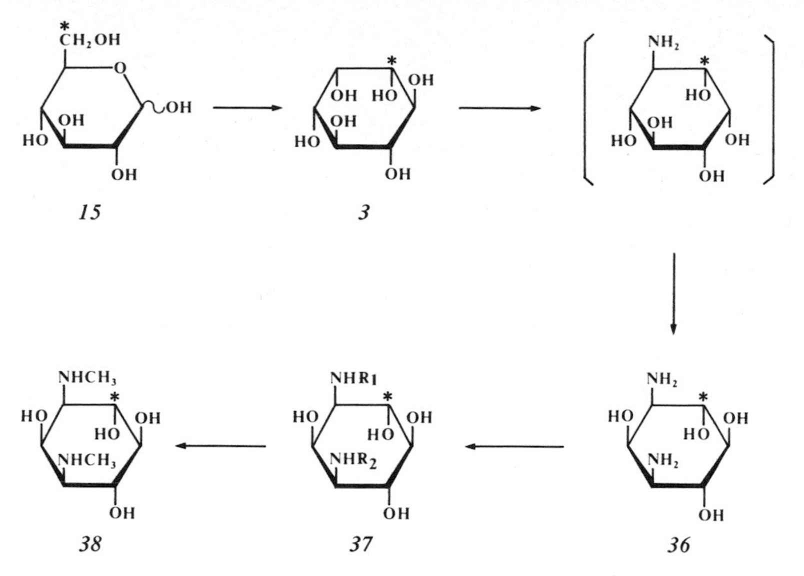

Fig. 26. Biosynthetic pathway from D-glucose (15) to actinamine (38) via *myo*-inositol (3)

b) Actinospectose

Radioactivity incorporated from D-[6-^{3}H]- and D-[6-^{13}C]glucose to actinospectose was found only in the hydrogen atoms or carbon atom of the C-6′ methyl group (MITSCHER et al. 1971; STROSHANE et al. 1976).

Recently, FLOSS et al. (1978) carried out feeding experiments with [6-^{14}C, 6-^{3}H]- and [6-^{14}C, 4-^{3}H]glucose with the results shown in Table 7. In contrast to the actinamine moiety, where one-half of the tritium at C-6 and all the tritium at C-4 of glucose are lost during incorporation, almost all the tritium at C-6 and about two-thirds of that at C-4 are retained during incorporation into the actinospectose moiety. These data indicated that a 4,6-dideoxyhexose moiety might be formed with transfer of hydrogen from the 4 to the 6 position of the glucose.

In connection with streptomycin biosynthesis (see Sect. B.I), the conversion of dTDP-glucose into dTDP-4-keto-6-deoxyglucose by the action of oxidoreductase has been described. In the present case, it is likely that the same pathway is involved

Table 7. Incorporation of doubly labeled glucose into spectinomycin. (FLOSS et al. 1978)

	[6-^{14}C,6-^{3}H]Glucose ^{3}H/^{14}C(^{3}H-retention)	[6-^{14}C,4-^{3}H]Glucose ^{3}H/^{14}C(^{3}H-retention)
Glucose fed	2.34 (100) [a]	2.34 (100) [a]
Spectinomycin	1.78 (76)	0.57 (24)
Actinamine	1.20 (49)	0.02 (1)
Acetic acid [b]	2.25 (96)	1.34 (57)

[a] Figures in brackets are percentages
[b] Corresponding to C-5′ and C-6′ of the actinospectose moiety

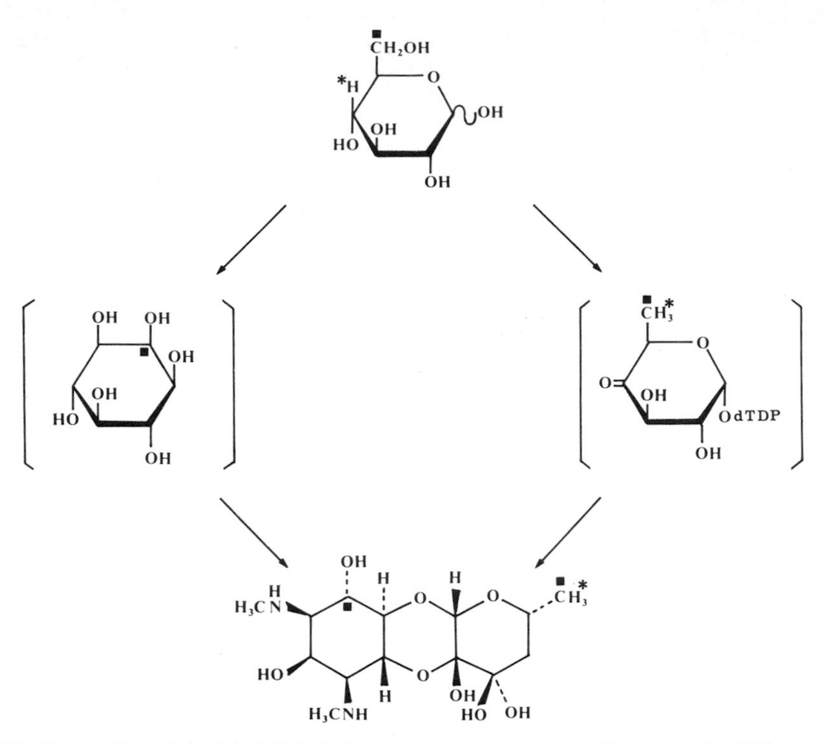

Fig. 27. Conversion of doubly labeled glucose to spectinomycin. (FLOSS et al. 1978)

and the resulting dTDP-4-keto-6-deoxyglucose is incorporated into spectinomycin. This scheme is illustrated in Fig. 27. The pathway, however, from dTDP-4-keto-6-deoxy-D-glucose to the actinospectose moiety (ring C) has not yet been clarified.

2. Subunit Assembly

MITSCHER et al. (1971) assumed a sequence in which the 3-ulose derivative (39) is bound to *N,N*-didemethylactinamine to form *N,N*-didemethylspectinomycin.

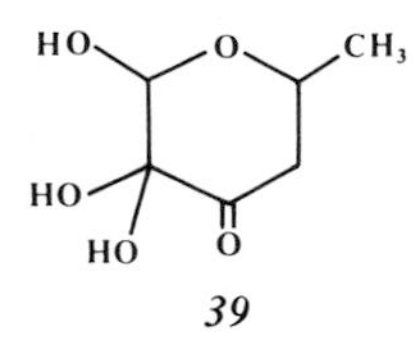

39

Later, HOEKSEMA and KNIGHT (1975) isolated an isomer of dihydrospectinomycin from the fermentation broth of *S. spectabilis* and determined it to be (35d) (see Fig. 25). Assuming that dihydrospectinomycin is a precursor of spectinomycin, they postulated the biosynthetic pathway shown in Fig. 28. As actinospectose itself was not directly incorporated into spectinomycin as indicated by MITSCHER et al. (1971), they considered compound (40) to be the precursor. Compound (40) was

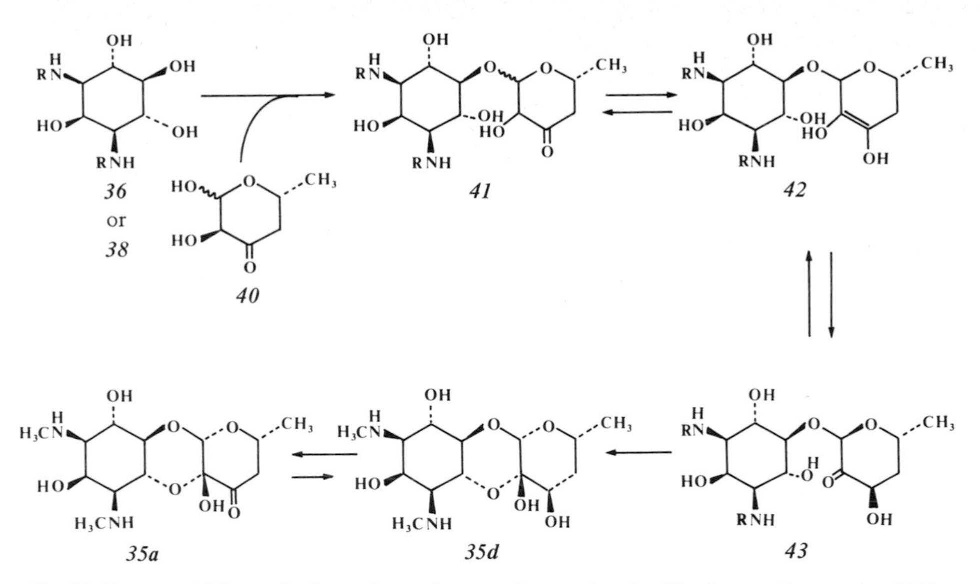

Fig. 28. Proposed biosynthetic pathway for spectinomycin via dihydrospectinomycin. *N,N*-didemethylactinamine (36) [R=H]; actinamine (38) [R=CH_3]. HOEKSEMA and KNIGHT (1975)

proposed as an intermediate from glucose to D-lankavose and D-desosamine, constitutional sugars of some macrolide antibiotics, by VANEK and MAJER (1967). Compound (40) combines with actinamine (38) or *N,N*-didemethylactinamine (36) to form the glycoside (41). Then compound (41), a 2-hydroxy-3-ulose derivative, is rearranged into the 3-hydroxy-2-ulose (43) via the endiol intermediate (42) and cyclized to dihydrospectinomycin (35d) which finally is oxidized to spectinomycin (35a). The role of dihydrospectinomycin as an intermediate is not proven, though the conversion of dihydrospectinomycin epimers into spectinomycin was attempted with an actinamine-requiring idiotroph of *S. spectabilis*.

Recently, objections were raised to the above pathway by FOLEY and WEIGELE (1978) who, as a result of chemical interconversion trials between dihydrospectinomycins and their derivatives, indicated that the presumed rearrangement of the thermodynamically stable compound (41) to the unstable compound (43) is irrational and contradictory to their experimental findings. They also suggested that a symmetrical cyclitol intermediate such as (43) will preferentially cyclize to form the spectinomycin skeleton. This suggestion was strengthened by HANESSIAN and ROY (1979) by their chemical synthesis of (+)-spectinomycin, in which a compound corresponding to (43) was readily cyclized to a dihydrospectinomycin derivative and oxidized to spectinomycin.

It is uncertain if this type of reaction is possible in the biologic system, so elucidation of the biosynthetic pathway of spectinomycin remains to be completed.

VII. Kasugamycin

Kasugamycin, produced by *S. kasugaensis* and other *Streptomyces* spp., is an *N*-carboxyformidoyl derivative of kasuganobiosamine (Fig. 29). Kasuganobiosamine

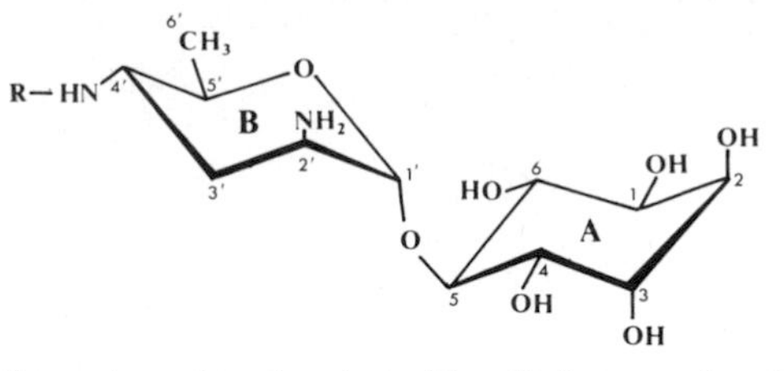

Fig. 29. Kasugamycin. *Ring A*, D-*chiro*-inositol; *Ring B*, kasugamine [R=H]; *Ring A+B*, kasugamycin [R=—C—COOH], kasuganobiosamine [R=H]. (Numbering of ring A is as
||
NH
proposed by FLETCHER et al. 1951)

is composed of kasugamine, 2,4-diamino-2,3,4,6-tetradeoxy-D-*arabino*-hexose, and D-*chiro*-inositol (formally called D-inositol). The biosynthesis of kasugamycin was reviewed by S. UMEZAWA and TSUCHIYA (1969).

1. Biosynthesis of Subunits

The biosynthesis of kasugamine and D-*chiro*-inositol, together with the origin of the carboxyformidoyl group, were studied in detail by FUKAGAWA et al. (1968 a–e) and SAWA et al. (1968), who examined the incorporation of labeled compounds into kasugamycin and its subunits by *S. kasugaensis*. Since kasugamycin is destroyed as the pH of the broth goes above 7.0, the labeled compounds were fed to the 70–90 h growing culture and 15–24 h later the fermentation was harvested. Incorporation of the test compounds into kasugamycin is shown in Table 8. D-Glucose, D-mannose, *myo*-inositol, and glycine were well incorporated into kasugamycin.

Table 8. Incorporation of labeled compounds into kasugamycin. (FUKAGAWA et al. 1968a)

[^{14}C]Compound	Incorporation (%)
[U-^{14}C]Maltose	1.9
[U-^{14}C]Glucose	10.7
[U-^{14}C]Mannose	10.0
[U-^{14}C]Ribose	3.5
[1-^{14}C]Glycerol	1.4
[U-^{14}C]Pyruvate	1.3
[1-^{14}C]Acetate	0.2
myo-[U-^{14}C]Inositol	71.6
D-[U-^{14}C]Inositol	0.5
[1-^{14}C]Glycine	17.9
[2-^{14}C]Glycine	23.0
[U-^{14}C]Glycine	13.0
[^{15}N]Glycine	13.9

a) Two-Carbon Side Chain

As expected, glycine was found to be incorporated mostly into the carboxyformidoyl group. Other plausible precursors for the two-carbon unit were also exam-

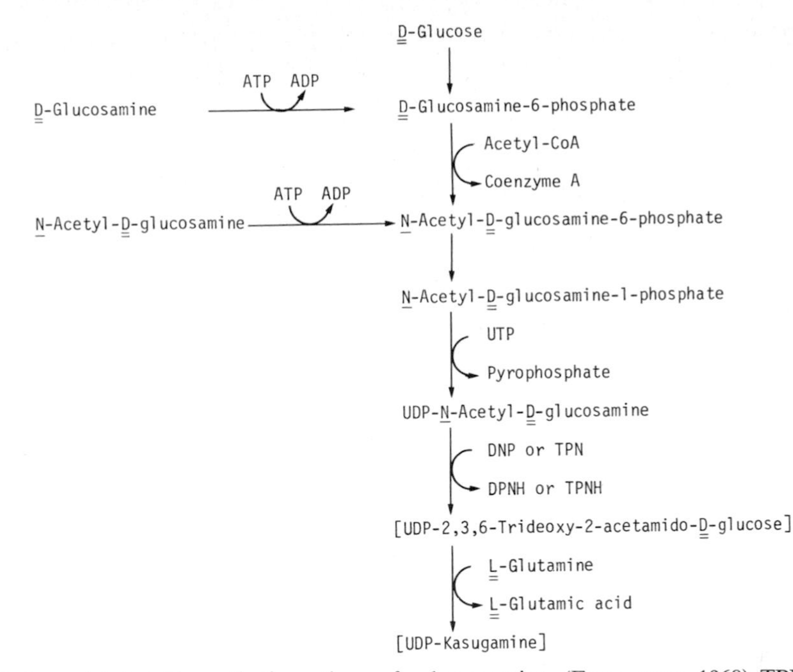

Fig. 30. A postulated biosynthetic pathway for kasugamine. (FUKAGAWA 1968) TPN, triphosphopyridine nucleotide; TPNH, reductive form of TPN; UDP, uridine 5′-diphosphate

ined. Acetate, pyruvate, lactate, glyoxylate, oxamate, and oxalate were not incorporated, but L-serine was incorporated, though only one-fourth to one-fifth as much as glycine. Finally, experiments with [^{15}N]-, [1-^{14}C]-, and [2-^{14}C]glycines demonstrated that glycine was incorporated into the carboxyformidoyl group without fragmentation as shown:

$$\rangle\!\!-NH_2 + H_2\overset{\triangle}{N}-\overset{*}{C}H_2-\overset{*}{C}OOH \rightarrow \rangle\!\!-NH-\underset{\underset{\underset{\triangle}{NH}}{\|}}{\overset{*}{C}}-\overset{*}{C}OOH$$

b) Kasugamine

D-[1-^{14}C]-, D-[2-^{14}C]-, and D-[6-^{14}C]Glucose were incorporated equally into kasugamycin (5.6%–7.9%). Label was found in the two subunits and the side chain. This indicated that D-glucose was, without fragmentation, utilized mainly for the two subunits, D-*chiro*-inositol (28%–34% of total incorporation) and kasugamine (64%–71%).

D-[1-^{14}C]Glucosamine was three times more efficiently incorporated than D-glucose with selective formation of the kasugamine moiety, indicating that D-glucosamine is a more direct precursor for kasugamine than D-glucose. Moreover, it was shown that *N*-acetyl-D-[1-^{14}C]glucosamine and UDP-*N*-acetyl-D-[1-^{14}C]glucosamine could be detected in the broth after feeding D-[1-^{14}C]glucosamine. *N*-Acetyl-D-[1-^{14}C]glucosamine was efficiently incorporated into the kasugamine moiety. From these observations, FUKAGAWA (1968) postulated the biosynthetic pathway of kasugamine shown in Fig. 30. In this pathway, the step from UDP-*N*-

acetyl-D-glucosamine to UDP-kasugamine involves epimerization and deacetylation at C-2, deoxygenation at C-3 and C-6, and amino substitution at C-4. Though the above reactions have not been demonstrated in *S. kasugaensis*, similar reactions have been observed in other microorganisms.

Transformation of D-glucose to dTDP-4-acetamido-4,6-dideoxy-D-glucose by *E. coli* (M. MATSUHASHI and STROMINGER 1964, 1966; GILBERT et al. 1965) and conversion of D-glucose to CDP-3,6-dideoxy-D-glucose by *Pasteurella pseudotuberculosis* (S. MATSUHASHI et al. 1966a, b; S. MATSUHASHI 1966) demonstrate deoxygenation at C-3, C-4, and C-6. The transformation of dTDP-D-glucose to dTDP-4-keto-6-deoxy-D-glucose by dTDP-D-glucose oxidoreductase from *E. coli* has already been discussed in connection with the biosynthesis of streptose.

Epimerizations at C-2 of *N*-acetyl-D-glucosamine, UDP-*N*-acetyl-D-glucosamine, and *N*-acetyl-D-glucosamine-6-phosphate are known (COMB and ROSEMAN 1958; GHOSH and ROSEMAN 1965a, b; ELBEIN and HEALTH 1965a, b). Epimerization at the C-2 center is found in the final step of tyvelose (3,6-dideoxy-D-mannose) biosynthesis (ELBEIN and HEALTH 1965a, b; S. MATSUHASHI 1966).

c) D-*Chiro*-Inositol [D- or (+)-Inositol]

As shown in Table 8, labeled *myo*-inositol was incorporated more efficiently than D-glucose into kasugamycin and was selectively distributed into the D-*chiro*-inositol moiety. D-*chiro*-Inositol is not incorporated and is not considered to be a direct precursor of kasugamycin. *myo*-Inositol was presumed to first bind with kasugamine with subsequent modification to the D-*chiro*-inositol configuration by an unknown mechanism.

The pathway from D-glucose to *myo*-inositol via D-glucose-6-phosphate has already been discussed (see Sect. B.I.1). Two possibilities were considered by FUKAGAWA et al. (1968e) for conversion of *myo*-inositol to D-*chiro*-inositol. *myo*-Inositol and D-*chiro*-inositol differ in configuration only at C-3. One possibility involves the oxidation of the equatorial hydroxyl group at C-3 of *myo*-inositol to a carbonyl group or removal of the hydroxyl group by degradation to form a double bond, followed by reduction of the carbonyl group or hydration of the double bond to give D-*chiro*-inositol. Another possibility is phosphorylation of the hydroxyl group at the epimeric center, followed by hydrolysis with fission between the C–O bond instead of the O–P bond to epimerize the carbon.

SCHOLDA et al. (1964a) showed that labeled *myo*-inositol is converted to labeled D-*chiro*-inositol[(+)-inositol], (+)-pinitol, and sequoyitol in leaves of crimson clover, *Trifolium incarnatum*. They also reported that the conversion to D-*chiro*-inositol probably takes place via *myo*-inosose-3 (SCHOLDA et al. 1964b). It is well known that axial hydroxyl groups of cyclitols are selectively oxidized chemically or by microbes such as *Aerobacter aerogenes* (MAGASANIK 1953) and *Acetobacter suboxydans* (POSTERNAK 1965). Therefore, direct oxidation of an equatorial group at C-3 of *myo*-inositol appears to be rather difficult.

The formation of *myo*-inosose-3 may also be possible according to the route proposed by MAGASANIK (1953) in the degradation process of *myo*-inositol by *Aerobacter aerogenes*. In this route, *myo*-inositol was first oxidized to *myo*-inosose-2 and then underwent interconversion to *myo*-inosose-3 through an endiol intermediate.

2. Subunit Assembly

In contrast with streptidine or 2-deoxystreptamine, the constitutional cyclitol, D-*chiro*-inositol, was not incorporated into kasugamycin but *myo*-inositol was utilized. FUKAGAWA et al. (1968e) suggested that kasugamine (more possibly nucleotidyl kasugamine) produced from glucose via UDP-*N*-acetyl-D-glucosamine first reacts with glycine or its activated derivative to give a nucleotide 4-*N*-carboxyformidoyl kasugamine which is then carried to the cell surface and combined with *myo*-inositol to form a pseudodisaccharide, "*myo*-kasugamycin," whose presence, however, has not yet been proven.

On the other hand, the fact that *N*-acetyl-D-glucosamine was detected in the fermentation broth of *S. kasugaensis* and could be effectively incorporated into kasugamycin resembles the situation with gentamicin, sisomicin, and butirosin, where glucosamine (probably Nuc-glucosamine) is first bound to aminocyclitols yielding pseudodisaccharide intermediates. If this is the case, the synthesis of kasugamycin from this pseudodisaccharide requires epimerization of the hydroxyl group at C-3 of the *myo*-inositol moiety and modification of the *N*-acetyl-D-glucosamine part to kasugamine as well as attachment of the carboxyformidoyl group to the amino group of kasugamine. Glycosidation of aminocyclitols with a simpler sugar is more common than with a highly modified sugar as the first step in the biosynthesis of aminoglycosides. The exact sequence of subunit assembly remains unknown.

3. Plasmid Involvement

When the kasugamycin-producing strain *S. kasugaensis* was incubated at 27 °C in medium containing 30 µg/ml of acriflavine, a plasmid-curing agent, 54.5% of the colonies isolated were deficient in antibiotic production. Further, when the strain was cultured at 35 °C, 5.3%–6.2% of the colonies isolated were unable to produce kasugamycin, whereas none of the colonies from broth cultivated at 27 °C were devoid of antibiotic production ability. Mutation in chromosomal DNA was unlikely in both cases, because none of the nonproducing strains showed differences from the parent strain in sugar utilization pattern. These phenomena strongly suggested the involvement of plasmids in kasugamycin biosynthesis (OKANISHI et al. 1970).

Later, three types of extrachromosomal closed circular DNA were discovered, one of which was assumed to be involved with kasugamycin production (OKANISHI 1977; OKANISHI and UMEZAWA 1978). The three types of DNA were, by electron microscopic analysis, found to be large (flower shaped), medium (supercoil), and small sized (open circular). Besides, *S. kasugaensis* and other strains often produce aureothricin, so that plasmid-curing of these strains was expected to give mutants producing no antibiotic, those producing only kasugamycin, and those producing only aureothricin. When the DNA of these mutants was studied, the results summarized in Table 9 were obtained.

It appears that the large flower-shaped DNA is involved in kasugamycin biosynthesis. The medium-sized DNA correlates well with aureothricin production and the small-sized DNA seems not to be related to antibiotic production.

Plasmids in *S. kasugaensis* MB 273, which produces kasugamycin and aureothricin, were reinvestigated recently by OKANISHI et al. (1980). One of the plasmids

Table 9. Electron microscopic analysis of plasmids in streptomycetes producing kasugamycin (KSM) and/or aureothricin (AT). (OKANISHI 1977; OKANISHI and UMEZAWA 1978)

Organisms	Antibiotic produced		Plasmid DNA detected		
	KSM	AT	Flower-shaped	Medium-sized	Small-sized
S. kasugaensis					
M 338 (At-536)[a, b]	+	+	+ (15 μm)[c]	+ (3.35 μm)[c]	+(0.59 μm, rare)
70-5	+	−	+ (15 μm)	−	+(0.59 μm, rare)
A-2	+	−	+	−	ND[d]
158-1	−	−	−	+ (3.12 μm)	+(0.59 μm, rare)
158-2	−	+	−	+ (3.35 μm)	ND
C	−	+	−	+ (3.35 μm)	ND
K-1	−	−	−	−	ND
MB 273[a, b]	+	+	+	+ (3.7 μm)	ND
S. kasugaspinus[a]					
MA 350	+	−	+	−	ND

[a] Parental kasugamycin-producing strain
[b] Modified according to OKANISHI et al. (1980)
[c] Errors of the measured contour length were in the range of ±0.05 μm in the middle-size plasmid and ±0.5 μm in 15 μm open circular DNA
[d] ND = not detected

(pSH1) was characterized as supercoiled DNA with a molecular weight of 6.7 megadaltons, but the physiologic functions were not described. Final conclusions on plasmid involvement await further experimentation.

VIII. Validamycin

Streptomyces hygroscopicus var. *limoneus* produces validamycin A, B, C, D, E, and F. Except for component B, all contain validoxylamine A (Fig. 31) which gives validamine, validatol, and deoxyvalidatol on hydrogenolysis. The validamycins

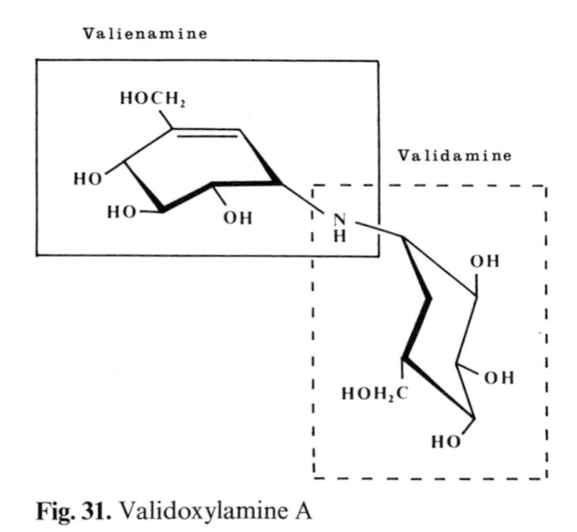

Fig. 31. Validoxylamine A

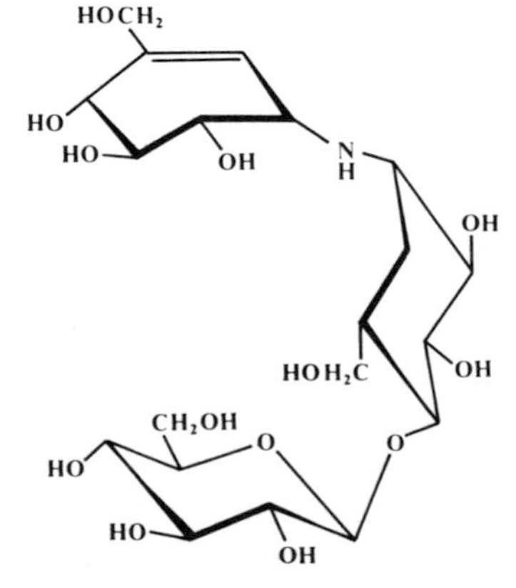

Fig. 32. Validamycin A

differ from one another in the number, the site, and the anomeric form of glucose residues glycosidically linked to validoxylamine A. The newly revised structure of validamycin A, a major component, is shown in Fig. 32 (SUAMI et al. 1980).

The biosynthetic pathway of validamycin A was partially elucidated by KAMEDA et al. (1975, 1978).

1. Biosynthesis of Subunits

All of the subunits of validamycin A are derived from glucose, since D-[U-^{14}C]glucose supplementation gave high incorporation ($\sim 10\%$) and approximately uniform distribution of the radioactivity into each of the three subunits (validamine, valienamine, and D-glucose). However, the pathways from glucose to validamine, valienamine, or validoxylamine A have not yet been reported.

2. Subunit Assembly

In a feeding experiment with [^{14}C]validoxylamine A, all the label was found in the validoxylamine A moiety (14.25% incorporation) and practically none in the D-glucose moiety. Therefore, it was assumed that the glycosidation of validoxylamine A is the final step of validamycin A biosynthesis. Also, microbial β-*O*-glucosidation of validoxylamine A to validamycin A was demonstrated with several strains of yeast, such as *Rhodotorula glutinis*, *R. lactosa*, etc., with cellobiose as a β-glucosyl donor. When lactose was supplied, it acted as a β-galactosyl donor to give β-galactosyl-validoxylamine A, di-β-D-galactosyl-validoxylamine A, and β-D-galactosyl-validamycin A.

KAMEDA et al. (1978) assumed that the following mechanism proposed by GORIN et al. (1964) for β-glucosidation is involved. GORIN et al. studied the microbial synthesis of β-galacto- and β-glucopyranosyl disaccharides by *Sporobomyces singularis* with lactose and cellobiose as glycosyl donors and proposed a reaction mechanism involving a "group transfer system" which can catalyze transfer as well as hydrolysis. At the active sites of the enzyme, lactose (or cellobiose) undergoes simultaneous protonation at the glycosidic oxygen and nucleophilic attack at C-1 to form the intermediate α-galactose- (or α-glucose-)enzyme complex which can react with an acceptor alcohol to give a new β-galactoside (or β-glucoside).

However, GRISEBACH (1978) pointed out that a nucleoside 5′-(α-*O*-D-glucosyl-diphosphate) is a more likely D-glucosyl donor in validamycin A biosynthesis.

IX. Miscellaneous Aminoglycosides

1. 1,4-Diaminocyclitol Aminoglycosides

Since the isolation of fortimicin from *Micromonospora*, a number of 1,4-diaminocyclitol-containing aminoglycosides (e.g., fortimicin minor components, isofortimicin, sporaricin, istamycin, sanamycin, KA-7038 I, II, and SF-2052, etc.) have been isolated from cultures of *Streptomyces*, *Micromonospora*, and other rare actinomycetes. The structures of some aminoglycosides of this group are depicted in Figs. 33 and 34.

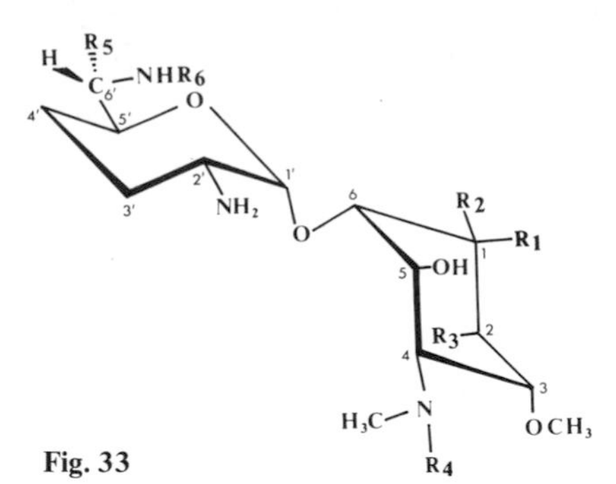

Fig. 33

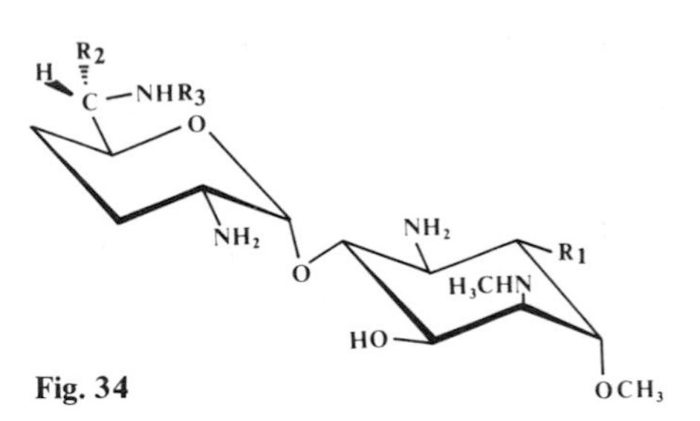

Fig. 34

Fig. 33. Fortimicin A and related antibiotics

	R_1	R_2	R_3	R_4	R_5	R_6
Fortimicin A	NH_2	H	OH	$COCH_2NH_2$	CH_3	H
Fortimicin C	NH_2	H	OH	$COCH_2NHCONH_2$	CH_3	H
Fortimicin D	NH_2	H	OH	$COCH_2NH_2$	H	H
Sanamycin A	NH_2	H	H	$COCH_2NH_2$	H	CH_3
Istamycin A	NH_2	H	H	$COCH_2NH_2$	H	CH_3
Istamycin B	H	NH_2	H	$COCH_2NH_2$	H	CH_3
Sporaricin A	H	NH_2	H	$COCH_2NH_2$	CH_3	H
Sporaricin B	H	NH_2	H	H	CH_3	H

Fig. 34. Fortimicin B and related antibiotics. Fortimicin B: $R_1 = OH$, $R_2 = CH_3$, $R_3 = H$; fortimicin KE: $R_1 = OH$, $R_2 = R_3 = H$; sanamycin B: $R_1 = H$, $R_2 = H$, $R_3 = CH_3$

These antibiotics contain both a 2,6-diaminosugar (purpurosamine) and a 1,4-diaminocyclitol. It is interesting that the purpurosamine A and B found in these antibiotics are C-6 epimers of purpurosamine A and B from gentamicin C_1 and C_2. Although there are no reports on the biosynthesis of 1,4-diaminocyclitols, RINEHART (1979) predicted that glucosamine would be a precursor of 1,4-diaminocyclitol with C-2 originating from C-6 of glucosamine and N-4 arising from the nitrogen of glucosamine.

Plasmid involvement in istamycin formation by *Streptomyces tenjimariensis*, a marine actinomycete, was assumed by OKAMI (1979).

Recently, NAKAYAMA et al. (1979f) isolated FU-10 (Fig. 35) from fermentation broth of *Micromonospora olivoasterospora*, a fortimicin-producing microorganism, and demonstrated that FU-10 was converted into fortimicin A and B by a washed cell suspension of the culture.

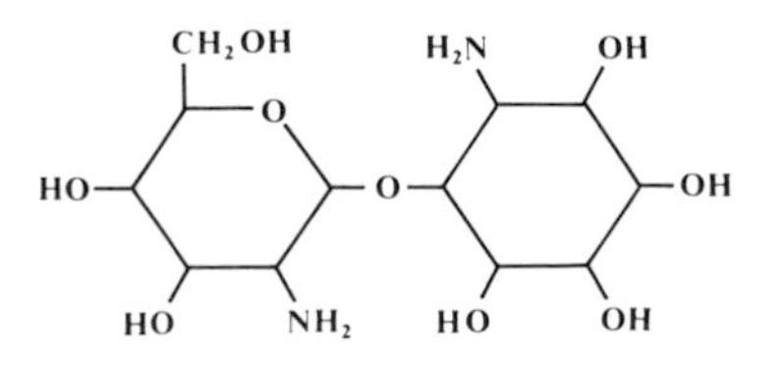

Fig. 35. FU-10

2. Monoaminocyclitol Aminoglycosides

Four monoaminocyclitol-containing aminoglycosides, SU-1, SU-2, SUM-3, and SUM-4 (Fig. 36), were reported recently by the Kyowa Hakko group (NAKAYAMA et al. 1979a–c, e). These antibiotics were produced by 2-deoxystreptamine-requiring idiotrophs (KY 11509, NRRL 11182) of gentamicin–sagamicin-producing *M. sagamiensis*. SU-1 and SU-2 are 1-deamino-1-hydroxy derivatives of gentamicin C_2 and C_{1a}, respectively; SUM-3 is 1-deamino-1-hydroxy-sagamicin, while SUM-4 was assumed to be a 3′- or 4′-hydroxy derivative of SU-2 (KASE et al. 1980).

As discussed earlier, 2-deoxystreptamine may be synthesized from D-glucose via 2-deoxy-*scyllo*-inosose (27a), 2-deoxy-*scyllo*-inosamine (28a), and monoamino-deoxy-*scyllo*-inosose (29a) (see Sect. B.II, Fig. 15). Antibiotic cosynthesis by mutant KY 11509 with other 2-deoxystreptamine-requiring idiotrophs revealed that this idiotroph was blocked between 2-deoxy-*scyllo*-inosamine (28a), which accumulated in the broth, and monoamino-deoxy-*scyllo*-inosose (29a). This mutant also produced 1-deamino-1-hydroxy derivatives of gentamicin A_2, A, and X together with 1-deamino-1-hydroxy G-418.

From the fermentation of a 2-deoxystreptamine-requiring idiotroph (strain S-11) of xylostasin-producing *B. circulans*, FUJIWARA et al. (1980b) isolated a new antibiotic S-11-A, together with inactive S-11-P, and identified them as 1-deamino-1-hydroxy-xylostasin (Fig. 37) and [(1L)-1,3,5/2,4-5-aminocyclohexanetetrol], respectively.

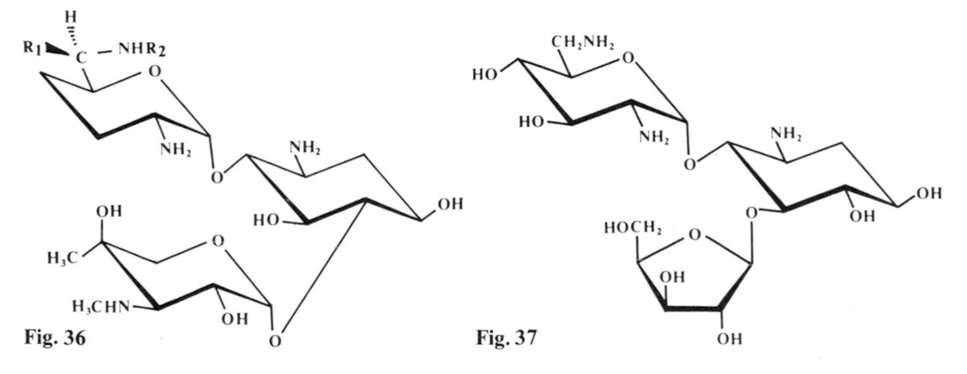

Fig. 36. Monoaminocyclitol-containing aminoglycosides. SU-1: $R_1 = CH_3$, $R_2 = CH_3$; SU-2: $R_1 = R_2 = H$; SUM-3: $R_1 = H$, $R_2 = CH_3$

Fig. 37. S-11-A

3. Apramycin

Apramycin (Fig. 38), a member of the nebramycin complex, produced by *S. tenebrarius* is unique in the C_8-aminosugar to which 2-deoxystreptamine and 4-amino-4-deoxyglucose are linked. According to the unpublished work of C. PEARCE and K. RINEHART cited by RINEHART (1979), glucose is incorporated into all units of apramycin, including C-1 through C-6 of the C_8-aminosugar moiety. C-7 and C-8 may come from C-2 and C-3 of pyruvate as do similar carbons of lincosamine. It

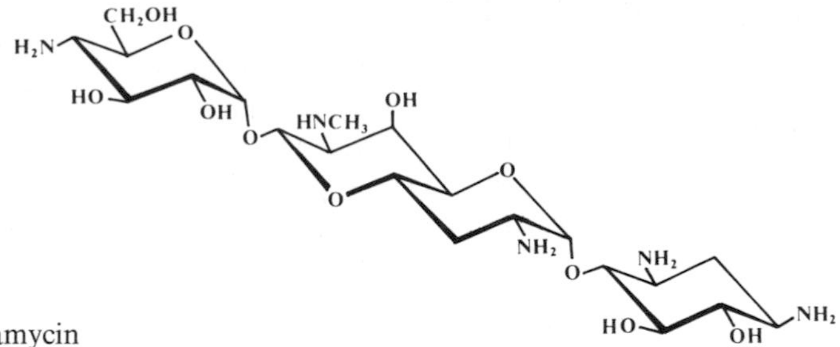

Fig. 38. Apramycin

is possible that 4-amino-4-deoxy-D-glucose is derived from D-glucose via 4-keto-D-glucose. UDP-4-keto-glucose was suggested to be present during conversion of UDP-galactose to UDP-glucose by *E. coli* UDP-galactose 4-epimerase (WEE and FREY 1973).

X. Comprehensive Discussion on the Biosynthesis of Aminoglycosides

When RINEHART reviewed the biosynthesis of aminoglycosides in 1976, each antibiotic was considered independently with few correlations between different groups. Since then, some general principles have emerged and, as with other secondary metabolites, a metabolic network (or grid) which correlates the biosynthetic pathway of many aminoglycosides has been developed. For example, the biosynthetic pathways for the 4,5-disubstituted 2-deoxystreptamine-containing aminoglycosides such as paromomycin, neomycin, ribostamycin, xylostasin, butirosin, and related antibiotics are summarized in Fig. 39 (NARA 1978).

This correlation came from the following findings: (1) The main route, 2-deoxystreptamine→paromamine→neamine→ribostamycin, was demonstrated in butirosin production by *B. circulans*. (2) One of the mutants derived from *B. circulans* produced both ribostamycin and xylostasin, while the other accumulated ribostamycin only. (3) A 2-deoxystreptamine-requiring idiotroph of *S. rimosus* forma *paromomycinus* converted neamine to neomycin. (4) A mutant of neomycin-producing *S. fradiae* accumulated ribostamycin instead of neomycin, suggesting that ribostamycin is an intermediate to neomycin. (5) Coproduction of ribosylparomamine (DAH-ribostamycin) by a paromomycin-producing strain indicates that this compound may be an intermediate between paromamine and paromomycin. (6) Paromomycin was detected as a minor component from a neomycin-producing strain.

In this scheme, solid and dotted lines show the pathway for *Bacillus* spp. and *Streptomyces* spp., respectively. Neomycin production by *Micromonospora* (WAGMAN et al. 1973) suggests that the above pathways exist in *Micromonospora* as well.

Ribose binds with paromamine or neamine to form ribosylparomamine or ribostamycin. Xylose may also bind with neamine to form xylostasin. However, xylostasin is also formed from ribostamycin by isomerization, as it seems likely that ribose plays a central role in the biosynthesis of these antibiotics.

Gentamicin and sisomicin are synthesized by the following sequence (see Fig. 23, Sect. B.V).

1. Combination of 2-deoxystreptamine with D-glucosamine to yield paromamine.
2. Addition of a second sugar to paromamine to form a pseudotrisaccharide.

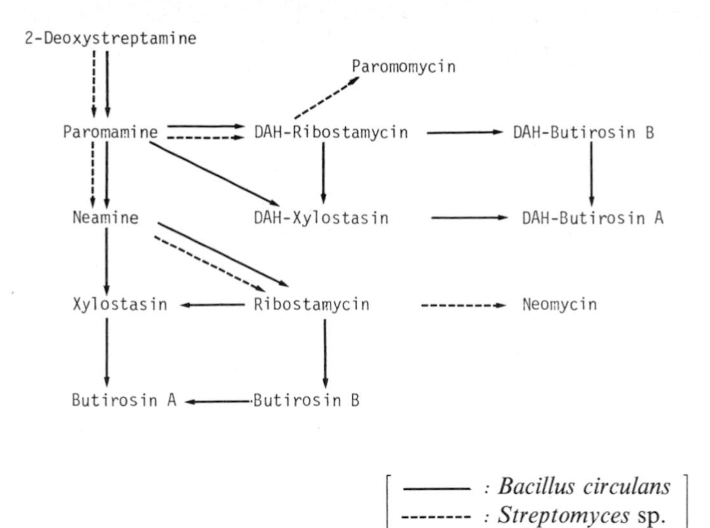

Fig. 39. Correlation between biosynthesis of paromomycin, ribostamycin, neomycin, butirosin, and related antibiotics. DAH, 6′-deamino-6′-hydroxy; ——, *Bacillus circulans*; – – – –, *Streptomyces* sp.

3. Modification of the glucosamine moiety and/or the second sugar moiety in the pseudotrisaccharide.

The second sugar involved in the biosynthesis of gentamicin and sisomicin is xylose in most cases, and from gentamicin A_2 a series of gentamicin–sisomicin aminoglycosides are derived by modification of the glucosamine or xylose moiety. Modification involves epimerization, amino substitution of the hydroxyl group, *C*- and *N*-methylation, deoxygenation, α,β-unsaturation, hydrogenation, etc.

A series of 3″-*N*- and 4″-*C*-demethyl derivatives of the gentamicin–sisomicin group are produced by strains of *Micromonospora* spp., probably by modification of the main gentamicin–sisomicin pathway. If 2-deoxystreptamine in the above sequence is replaced by 2-deoxy-*scyllo*-inosamine, a series of monoaminocyclitol-containing aminoglycosides, SU-1, SU-2, SUM-3, and SUM-4, are produced by a mutant of *M. sagamiensis* (see Sect. B.IX).

A total scheme for biosynthesis of gentamicin–sagamicin–sisomicin and related antibiotics is shown in Fig. 40.

Although kanamycin is similar to gentamicin, the biosynthetic pathways have not yet been fully elucidated. As shown in Fig. 19, the evidence supports a sequence similar to that for gentamicin. In this case, the second sugar which binds to neamine or paromamine is presumed to be glucose, which is then converted to kanosamine (3-amino-3-deoxy-D-glucose).

Isomerization and modification of the neutral sugar moiety of intermediates are important steps in aminoglycoside biosynthesis. Further investigation is required to clarify the mechanisms involved in most of these reactions.

At present, it is most likely that an unmodified sugar is used to form a pseudotrisaccharide, rather than a modified sugar such as NucDP-garosamine. In some cases the neutral sugar is converted to an aminosugar and then linked to the agly-

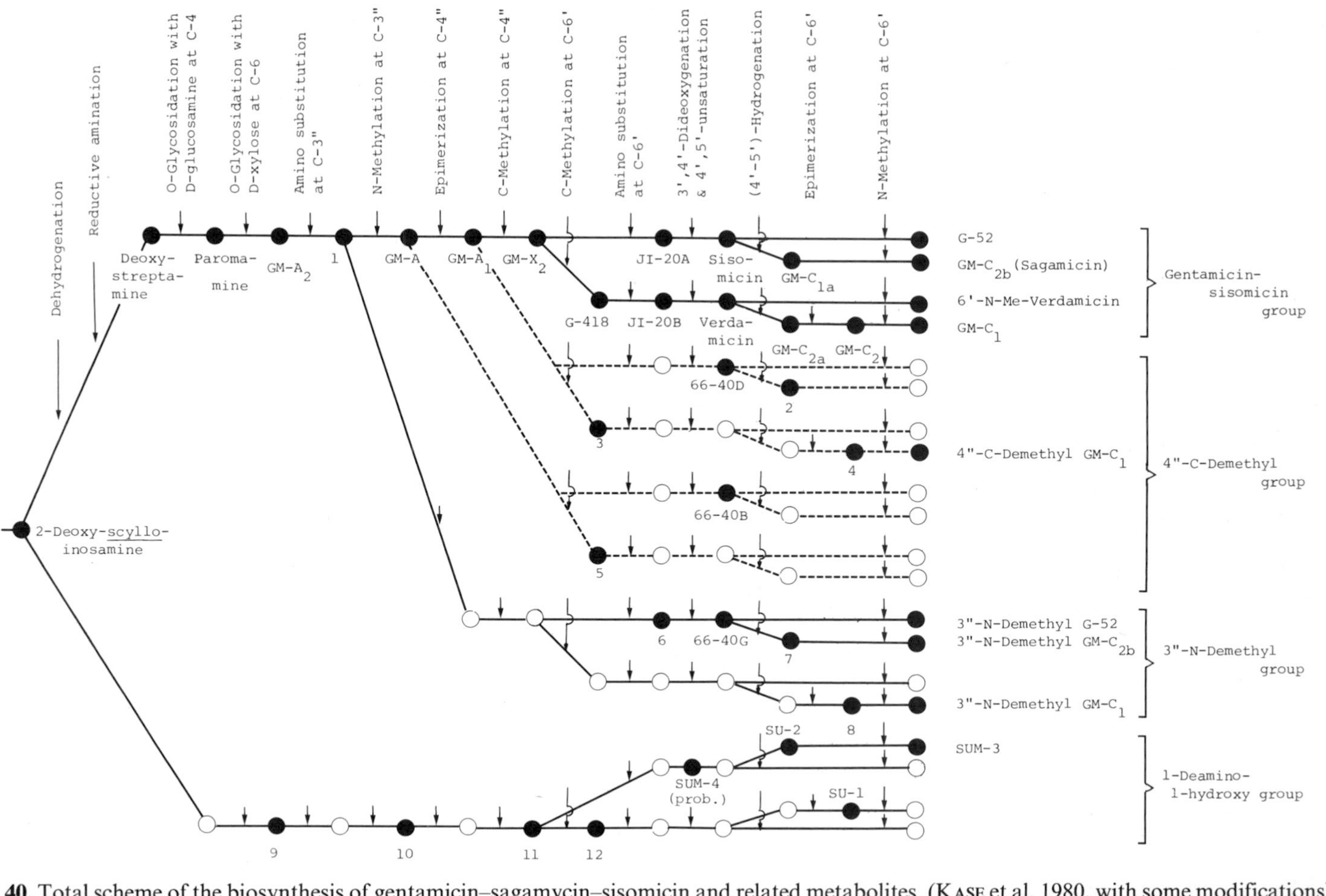

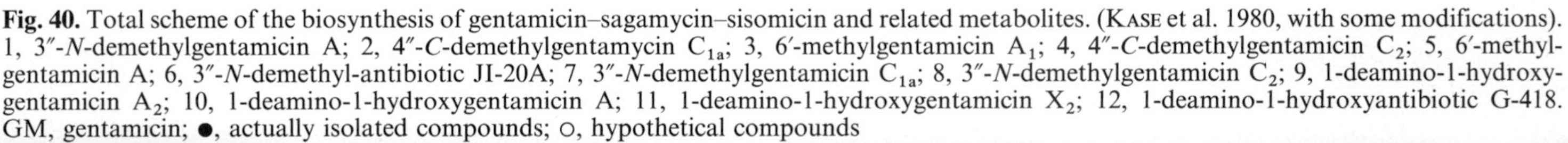

Fig. 40. Total scheme of the biosynthesis of gentamicin–sagamycin–sisomicin and related metabolites. (KASE et al. 1980, with some modifications). 1, 3″-*N*-demethylgentamicin A; 2, 4″-*C*-demethylgentamycin C_{1a}; 3, 6′-methylgentamicin A_1; 4, 4″-*C*-demethylgentamicin C_2; 5, 6′-methylgentamicin A; 6, 3″-*N*-demethyl-antibiotic JI-20A; 7, 3″-*N*-demethylgentamicin C_{1a}; 8, 3″-*N*-demethylgentamicin C_2; 9, 1-deamino-1-hydroxygentamicin A_2; 10, 1-deamino-1-hydroxygentamicin A; 11, 1-deamino-1-hydroxygentamicin X_2; 12, 1-deamino-1-hydroxyantibiotic G-418. GM, gentamicin; ●, actually isolated compounds; ○, hypothetical compounds

cone. For example, in streptomycin synthesis, dTDP-glucose is converted to dihydrostreptose and then bound to streptidine.

Paromamine formation from 2-deoxystreptamine and glucosamine is a key step in the biosynthesis of most aminoglycosides, but the details of this step are not known. Work in progress by RINEHART (1979) may help to answer these questions.

The aminocyclitol moiety is a characteristic subunit of aminoglycosides. Streptidine, bluensidine, actinamine, and 2-deoxystreptamine are all biosynthesized from D-glucose. The 1,4-diaminocyclitol in fortimicin and the monoaminocyclitol in the SU-2 series may originate from D-glucose as well. As already described, C-1 and C-6 of D-glucose become C-5 and C-6 of streptidine and bluensidine (Fig. 5) and C-1 and C-2 of 2-deoxystreptamine (Fig. 15). C-6 of D-glucose becomes C-6 of actinamine (Fig. 26).

The pathway from D-glucose to streptidine, bluensidine, and actinamine via *myo*-inositol has been determined (Sects. B.I.1, and B.VI.1). On the other hand, RINEHART has postulated two routes from D-glucose to 2-deoxystreptamine in neomycin biosynthesis as shown in Fig. 15. A part of route A was later proved in gentamicin and butirosin biosynthesis (Sects. B.V.1 and B.III.1) as follows: D-Glucose → *scyllo*-inositol derivative (26) → 2-deoxy-*scyllo*-inosose (27a) → 2-deoxy-*scyllo*-inosamine (28a) → monoamino-deoxy-*scyllo*-inosone (29a) → 2-deoxystreptamine (30). In 2-deoxystreptamine formation, the monoaminocyclitol undergoes amination to a diaminocyclitol in a clockwise direction. In streptidine or actinamine formation, the second amination or amidination probably goes anticlockwise.

The recent finding that 2-deoxy-*scyllo*-inosamine identified as (1L)-1,3,5/2,4-5-aminocyclohexanetetrol (FUJIWARA et al. 1980a; IGARASHI et al. 1980) is produced by a 2-deoxystreptamine-requiring idiotroph (S-11) of xylostasin-producing *B. circulans* strongly supports the route A in the above pathway (Fig. 15).

DAUM et al. (1977b) reported the conversion of DL-vivo-quercitol to 2-deoxystreptamine by a mutant of *M. inyoensis*. More data were needed to decide if vivo-quercitol is an intermediate in 2-deoxystreptamine formation. Since *scyllo*-inositol was not incorporated into 2-deoxystreptamine by a neamine-requiring idiotroph of *B. circulans* (FURUMAI et al. 1979), 2-deoxy-*scyllo*-inosose, which was converted into 2-deoxystreptamine, remains the first cyclic intermediate beyond D-glucose at present.

The following problems of 2-deoxystreptamine biosynthesis now remain: (1) Is deoxy-*scyllo*-inositol the first cyclitol intermediate as postulated by RINEHART et al? (2) What is the mechanism for conversion of D-glucose to deoxy-*scyllo*-inositol or 2-deoxy-*scyllo*-inosose?

The present authors speculate that 2-deoxy-*scyllo*-inosose may be formed from D-glucose by the steps shown in Fig. 41. This speculation was supported by the recent experimental facts found by KAKINUMA et al. (1981). Chemically, it is not irrational to consider that 2-deoxy-*scyllo*-inosose (27a) is synthesized by intramolecular aldol condensation of a keto-aldehyde compound (44) which is equivalent to compound (45) or (46). Compounds (45) and (46) may be obtained by hydrolysis of compounds (47) and (48), respectively. Compound (47) corresponds to the Δ^5-dehydrated glucose and may be derived from D-glucose biologically. Compound (48) is 4-keto-6-deoxyglucose which was shown to be derived from D-glucose by

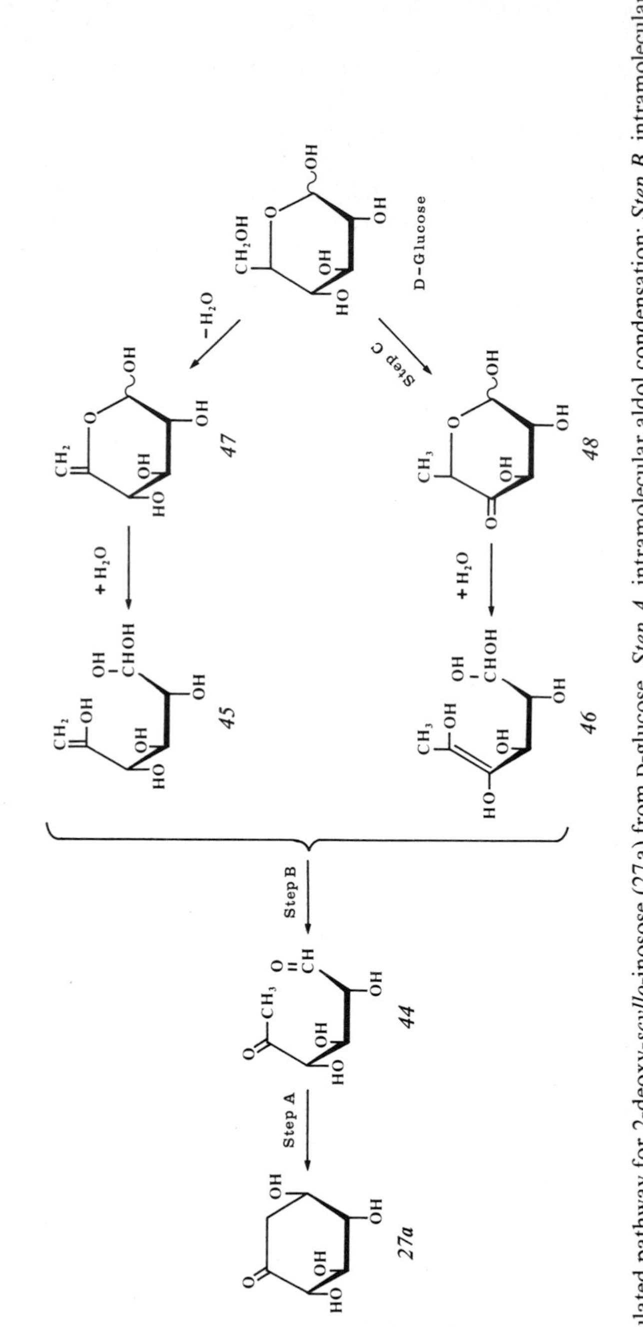

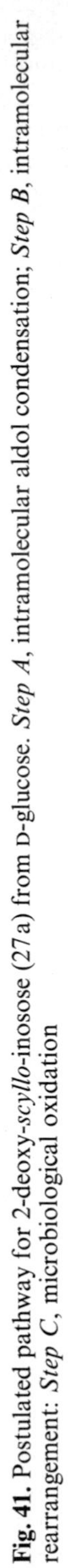

Fig. 41. Postulated pathway for 2-deoxy-*scyllo*-inosose (27a) from D-glucose. *Step A*, intramolecular aldol condensation; *Step B*, intramolecular rearrangement: *Step C*, microbiological oxidation

S. fradiae. It will be interesting to determine if compound (48) or its derivatives are incorporated into-2-deoxystreptamine by a 2-deoxystreptamine-requiring idiotroph of an aminoglycoside-producing microorganism.

C. Mutational Biosynthesis (Mutasynthesis)

We have seen in Sect. B that idiotrophs from antibiotic-producing strains often play an important role in elucidating the biosynthetic pathway of the parent antibiotic. Here we will discuss the use of idiotrophs for creating new antibiotics.

The enzymes involved in secondary metabolism are broad in substrate specificity and able to synthesize new antibiotics by incorporating precursor analogs.

This possibility was first proposed by BIRCH (1963) and demonstrated by SHIER et al. (1969) in the preparation of new neomycin analogs called hybrimycins by a 2-deoxystreptamine-requiring idiotroph of *S. fradiae*. This technique has been termed "mutational biosynthesis" (NAGAOKA and DEMAIN 1975) or "mutasynthesis" (RINEHART 1977). RINEHART (1977) has also proposed the term "mutasynthone" for the precursor used in mutasynthesis.

More than 40 mutasynthetic antibiotics have been prepared. Most of them are discussed in the reviews of RINEHART (1977), COX et al. (1977), QUEENER et al. (1978), DAUM and LEMKE (1979), and SEPULCHRE et al. (1980). Table 10 lists the mutasynthetic antibiotics with their producing idiotrophs, parent antibiotics, and mutasynthones.

This technique, however, does not always give the expected antibiotic, but occasionally produces an antibiotic with unexpected structure due to further modification. Also, the product is not necessarily bioactive. For instance, an actinamine-requiring idiotroph of *S. spectabilis* gave *epi*-spectinomycin when fed 2-*epi*-actinamine in place of actinamine, but this product was devoid of antibiotic activity (SLECHTA and COATS 1974). Most of the mutasynthesized antibiotics listed in Table 10 show no superiority to the parent antibiotic. The following are those mutasynthesized antibiotics which are considered to be the most interesting.

MU-1, MU-2, etc. (originally called mutamicin) were mutasynthesized by a 2-deoxystreptamine-requiring idiotroph of *M. inyoensis* (DANIELS 1978; DANIELS and RANE 1979). MU-1 (2-hydroxysisomicin) and MU-2 (5-deoxysisomicin) from streptamine and 2,5-dideoxystreptamine exhibited similar or slightly less activity than sisomicin against most bacteria. However, MU-1 was more active than sisomicin against sisomicin-resistant bacteria producing 2″-*O*-adenylating enzyme [ANT(2″)], and MU-2 was superior against those with a 3-*N*-acetylating enzyme [AAC(3)] (TESTA et al. 1974). MU-2 was superior to sisomicin in nephrotoxicity and ototoxicity in cats (DANIELS and RANE 1979). MU-6 (5-*epi*-sisomicin) derived from 5-*epi*-2-deoxystreptamine showed improved activity against gentamicin–sisomicin-resistant organisms containing the 2′-*N*-acetylating enzyme [AAC(2′)], ANT(2″), and AAC(3). Against *Pseudomonas*, it was more active than sisomicin. The acute toxicity in mice was slightly greater than that of sisomicin (WAITZ et al. 1978).

2-Hydroxygentamicin mutasynthesized from streptamine by a 2-deoxystreptamine-requiring idiotroph of *M. purpurea* has the same spectrum of activity as

Table 10. Idiotrophs and mutasynthetic antibiotics

Producing idiotroph [a]	Parent antibiotics	Precursors (mutasynthones)	Mutasynthetic antibiotics	Ref.
1. Neomycin analogs				
S. fradiae-DOS$^{\ominus}$ (ATCC 21401)	Neomycin B and C	Streptamine	2-Hydroxyneomycin B (Hybrimycin A_1) 2-Hydroxyneomycin C (Hybrimycin A_2)	[a–c]
	Neomycin B and C	2-*epi*-Streptamine	2-*epi*-Hydroxyneomycin B (Hybrimycin B_1) 2-*epi*-Hydroxyneomycin C (Hybrimycin B_2)	[a–c]
S. fradiae-DOS$^{\ominus}$ (ATCC 21401)	Neomycin B and C	2,6-Dideoxystreptamine	6-Deoxyneomycin B and C	[d, e]
S. fradiae-DOS$^{\ominus}$	Neomycin	2,5-Dideoxystreptamine	5-Deoxyneamine (prob.)	[f]
		6-*O*-Methyl-deoxystreptamine 3-*N*-Methyl-deoxystreptamine 2-Bromo-2-deoxystreptamine 6-Bromo-6-deoxystreptamine Streptidine	Converted to bioactive antibiotics but not isolated	[f]
S. rimosus forma *paromomycinus*-DOS$^{\ominus}$ (ATCC 21484)	Paromomycin I and II	Gentamine complex (C_1, C_2, and C_{1a})	3′, 4′-Dideoxyneomycin B and C	[e]
2. Paromomycin analogs				
S. rimosus forma *paromomycinus*-DOS$^{\ominus}$ (ATCC 14827) (ATCC 21485)	Paromomycin	Streptamine	2-Hydroxyparomomycin I (Hybrimycin C_1) 2-Hydroxyparomomycin II (Hybrimycin C_2)	[c, g]
S. rimosus forma *paromomycinus*-DOS$^{\ominus}$ (ATCC 21484)	Paromomycin I	2,6-Dideoxystreptamine	6-Deoxyparomomycin I and II	[d, e]

Table 10 (continued)

Producing idiotroph [a]	Parent antibiotics	Precursors (mutasynthones)	Mutasynthetic antibiotics	Ref.
3. Ribostamycin analogs				
S. ribosidificus-DOS$^{\ominus}$ (AF-1)	Ribostamycin	1-*N*-Methyl-deoxystreptamine	1-*N*-Methylribostamycin	[h, z]
		Streptamine	2-Hydroxyribostamycin	
		2-*epi*-Streptamine	2-*epi*-Hydroxyribostamycin	
		3′,4′-Dideoxyneamine	3′,4′-Dideoxyribostamycin	
4. Kanamycin analogs				
S. kanamyceticus-DOS$^{\ominus}$ (KN-4,FERM-P 2130)	Kanamycin	1-*N*-Methyl-deoxystreptamine	6′-Deamino-6′-hydroxy-1-*N*-methylkanamycin A	[h, z]
		2-*epi*-Streptamine	6′-Deamino-6′-hydroxy-2-*epi*-hydroxykanamycin A	
S. kanamyceticus-DOS$^{\ominus}$ (ATCC 21480)	Kanamycin	2-*epi*-Streptamine	Antibiotic compound not characterized	[c]
S. kanamyceticus-DOS$^{\ominus}$ (KN-4,FERM-P 2130)	Kanamycin	2,5-Dideoxystreptamine	5-Deoxykanamycin A	[i]
5. Gentamicin–sisomicin analogs				
Micromonospora inyoensis-DOS$^{\ominus}$ (1550F)	Sisomicin	Streptamine	2-Hydroxysisomicin (Mu-1)	[j]
			3″-*N*-Demethyl-3″-*N*-acetyl-2-hydroxysisomicin(Mu-1a)	
			3″-*N*-Demethyl-2-hydroxysisomicin(Mu-1b)	
		2,5-Dideoxystreptamine	5-Deoxysisomicin(Mu-2)	
			5-Deoxygentamicin A(Mu-2a)	
		2-*epi*-Streptamine	2-*epi*-Hydroxysisomicin(Mu-4)	[k, l]
		5-Amino-2,5-dideoxystreptamine	5-Amino-5-deoxysisomicin (Mu-5)	
		5-*epi*-2-Deoxystreptamine	5-*epi*-Sisomicin (Mu-6)	[k–m]
		3-*N*-Methyl-2-deoxystreptamine	3-*N*-Methylsisomicin (Mu-7)	
		1-*N*-Methyl-2,5-dideoxystreptamine	1-*N*-Methyl-5-deoxysisomicin (Mu-8)	

Table 10 (continued)

Producing idiotroph [a]	Parent antibiotics	Precursors (mutasynthones)	Mutasynthetic antibiotics	Ref.
		5-Fluoro-2,5-dideoxystreptamine	5-Fluoro-5-deoxysisomicin	[k, l]
		5-*epi*-Fluoro-2,5-dideoxystreptamine	5-*epi*-Fluoro-5-deoxysisomicin (Mu-X)	
Micromonospora purpurea-DOS⊖ (VI b)	Gentamicin	Streptamine		
		2,4,6/3,5-Pentahydroxycyclohexanone and its pentaacetate	2-Hydroxygentamicin C_1 and C_2 (trace C_{1a})	[n. o]
		scyllo-Inosamine		
		2,5-Dideoxystreptamine	5-Deoxygentamicin C_1, C_2, and C_{1a}	
		4,6-Hydrazino-1,3-cyclohexanediol		
		1,3-Di-*N*-benzylidene-2,5-dideoxystreptamine		[n]
		2-*epi*-Streptamine	2-*epi*-Hydroxygentamicin C_1, C_{1a}, and C_2	
6. Streptomycin analog				
S. griseus-streptidine⊖ (MIT-A5)	Streptomycin	2-Deoxystreptidine	Streptomutin A	[p, q, y]
7. Butirosin analogs				
Bacillus circulans-DOS⊖ (61 a and 79 d)	Butirosin	Streptamine	2-Hydroxybutirosin	[r, s]
		2,5-Dideoxystreptamine	5-Deoxystreptamine	
Bacillus circulans-DOS⊖ (MCRL 5004) or	Butirosin	6′-*N*-Methylneamine	6′-*N*-Methylbutirosin	
		3′,4′-Dideoxyneamine	3′,4′-Dideoxybutirosin	[t–w]
Bacillus circulans-neamine⊖ (MCRL 5003)		3′,4′-Dideoxyribostamycin		
		3′,4′-Dideoxy-6′-*N*-methylneamine	3′,4′-Dideoxy-6′-*N*-methylbutirosin	
		3′,4′-Dideoxy-6′-*C*-methylneamine	3′,4′-Dideoxy-6′-*C*-methylbutirosin	

Table 10 (continued)

Producing idiotroph[a]	Parent antibiotics	Precursors (mutasynthones)	Mutasynthetic antibiotics	Ref.
Bacillus vitellinus-neamine$^{\ominus}$ (GD-72) or	Butirosin	3′-Chloro-3′-deoxyneamine 3′-Chloro-3′-deoxyxylostasin	3′-Chloro-3′-deoxybutirosin A	[x]
Bacillus circulans-neamine$^{\ominus}$ (GD-205)		3′-Deoxyneamine 3′-deoxyxylostasin	3′-Deoxybutirosin A	

[a] DOS$^{\ominus}$ = 2-deoxystreptamine-requiring idiotroph; Neamine$^{\ominus}$ = neamine-requiring idiotroph; Streptidine$^{\ominus}$ = streptidine-requiring idiotroph
[a] SHIER et al. (1969); [b] SHIER et al. (1972); (c) SHIER et al. (1973); [d] CLEOPHAX et al. (1976); [e] GERO and MERCIER (1977); [f] RINEHART (1977); [g] SHIER et al. (1974); [h] KOJIMA and SATOH (1973); [i] YASUDA et al. (1978); [j] TESTA et al. (1974); [k] DAUM and LEMKE (1979); [l] TESTA (1979); [m] WAITZ et al. (1978); [n] ROSI et al. (1977); [o] DAUM et al. (1977b); [p] NAGAOKA and DEMAIN (1975); [q] LEMKE and DEMAIN (1976); [r] CLARIDGE et al. (1974); [s] TAYLOR and SCHMITZ (1976); [t] TAKEDA et al. (1978a); [u] TAKEDA et al. (1978c); [v] TAKEDA et al. (1978d); [w] TAKEDA et al. (1978e); [x] NOGAMI et al. (1976); [y] DEMAIN and NAGAOKA (1976); [z] YASUDA et al. (1975)

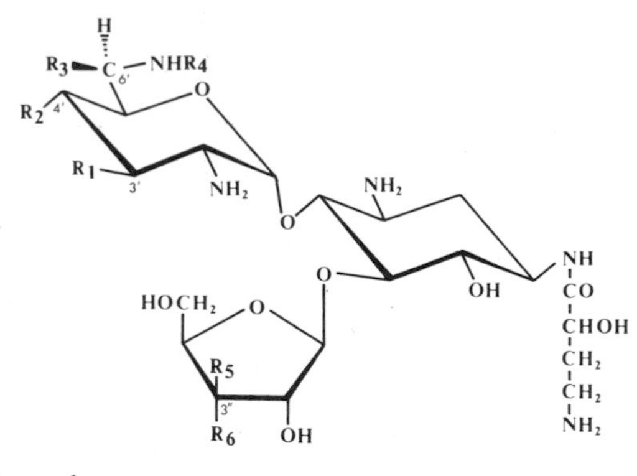

Fig. 42. New butirosin analogs

	R_1	R_2	R_3	R_4	R_5	R_6
NMB-A	OH	OH	H	CH_3	OH	H
NMB-B	OH	OH	H	CH_3	H	OH
DMB-A	H	H	H	CH_3	OH	H
DMB-B	H	H	H	CH_3	H	OH
DCB-A	H	H	CH_3	H	OH	H
DCB-B	H	H	CH_3	H	H	OH
DDB-A	H	H	H	H	OH	H
DDB-B	H	H	H	H	H	OH
Butirosin A	OH	OH	H	H	OH	H
Butirosin B	OH	OH	H	H	H	OH

gentamicin. The antimicrobial potency against gentamicin-sensitive strains is two to two and a half times less than that of gentamicin, but is improved against strains with ANT(2″). Moreover, the acute intravenous toxicity in mice was approximately one-half and the vestibular- and nephrotoxicity were one-fourth and one-sixth that of gentamicin. 2-Hydroxygentamicin is now under clinical investigation (DAUM et al. 1977b; DAUM 1979).

5-Deoxygentamicin derived from 2,5-dideoxystreptamine exhibited increased activity, especially against strains containing AAC(3), but the acute intravenous toxicity in mice and the nephrotoxicity in rats were two and a half and two times greater, respectively, than for gentamicin (ROSI et al. 1977; DAUM 1979). KOJIMA and SATOH (1973) prepared 3′,4′-dideoxyribostamycin from 3′,4′-dideoxyneamine (gentamine C_{1a}) with a 2-deoxystreptamine-requiring idiotroph of *S. ribosidificus*. This compound showed stronger activity than ribostamycin against *Pseudomonas aeruginosa* and kanamycin–ribostamycin-resistant *E. coli*.

TAKEDA et al. (1978a, c–e) prepared 6′-*N*-methylbutirosin (NMB), 3′,4′-dideoxybutirosin (DDB), 3′,4′-dideoxy-6′-*N*-methylbutirosin (DMB), and 3′,4′-dideoxy-6′-*C*-methylbutirosin (DCB) (Fig. 42) from the corresponding neamine analogs, 6′-*N*-methylneamine, 3′,4′-dideoxyneamine, 3′,4′-dideoxy-6′-*N*-methylneamine, and 3′,4′-dideoxy-6′-*C*-methylneamine by using 2-deoxystreptamine- or neamine-requiring idiotrophs of *B. circulans*. As expected from the resistance mechanism (H. UMEZAWA 1974), these analogs exhibited interesting antimicrobial activity. DMB and DCB were superior to butirosin against resistant strains with a 3′-*O*-phosphorylating enzyme [APH(3′)-II] and 6′-*N*-acetylating enzyme [AAC(6′)]. DMB and DCB showed activity as well against some clinical isolates resistant to gentamicin and/or dibekacin. Furthermore, DMB showed slightly less acute intravenous toxicity in mice than butirosin A.

D. Conclusion

Rapid development of the field of biosynthetic research in recent years is due mainly to the ^{13}C-isotope technique and use of blocked mutants of producing strains. The importance of mutants in biosynthetic research is demonstrated by the fact that the glycosidation of streptidine by streptose derivatives was the only pathway elucidated without the aid of a mutant. However, it should be kept in mind that the incorporation behavior shown by mutants is not always the same, probably due to differences of cell wall permeability of the mutants. Protoplasts may give better results (RINEHART 1979).

Once a biosynthetic pathway is outlined, it should be confirmed by isolated enzyme studies as was done for streptidine. However, this method has been applied in only a few cases.

Although great progress in understanding the biosynthesis of aminoglycosides has been made, it must be emphasized that many points are still speculative, as pointed out throughout this chapter. Much work remains to be done in order to complete our understanding of these processes.

Acknowledgment. The authors are grateful to Prof. K. L. Rinehart, Jr., University of Illinois, for permission to use his ^{13}C-*NMR* chart and to Dr. M. Okanishi, National Institute of Health, and Dr. Y. Okami, Institute of Microbial Chemistry, for discussions concerning plasmid involvement in biosynthesis. They also sincerely thank past and present colleagues in the Microbiological Research Laboratory, especially Dr. T. Furumai and Dr. K. Takeda, for their help in the preparation of the manuscript and for stimulating discussion.

References

Akamatsu N (1968) Biosynthesis of streptomycin (in Japanese). Kagaku no Ryoiki 22:375–381

Anisova LN, Kovolenko IV, Kornitskaya EYa, Krasilnikova OL, Soifer VS, Tovarova II, Khokhlov AS (1976) Mutant *Actinomyces streptomycini* blocked in streptidine biosynthesis (in Russian). Antibiotiki 21:6–10

Arima K, Okazaki H, Ono H, Yamada K, Beppu T (1973) Effect of exogenous fatty acids on the cellular fatty acid composition and neomycin formation in a mutant strain of *Streptomyces fradiae*. Agric Biol Chem 37:2313–2317

Axelrod B (1960) Other pathways of carbohydrate metabolism. In: Greenberg DM (ed) Metabolic pathways, vol I. Academic Press, New York London, pp 205–249

Baddiley J, Blumson NL, DiGirolamo A, DiGirolamo M (1961) Thymidine diphosphate sugar derivatives and their transformation in *Streptomyces griseus*. Biochim Biophys Acta 50:391–393

Barabás GY, Szabó G (1977) Effect of penicillin on streptomycin production by *Streptomyces griseus*. Antimicrob Agents Chemother 11:392–395

Basak K, Majumdar SK (1978) Enzymatic studies on kanamycin biosynthesis. Indian J Exp Biol 16:57–61 (cf Microbiol Abstr 9270-B 14)

Baud H, Betencourt A, Peyre M, Penasse L (1977) Ribostamycin, as an intermediate in the biosynthesis of neomycin. J Antibiot (Tokyo) 30:720–723

Benveniste R, Davies J (1973) Aminoglycoside antibiotic-inactivating enzymes in actinomycetes similar to those present in clinical isolate of antibiotic-resistant bacteria. Proc Natl Acad Sci USA 70:2276–2280

Bérdy J, Pauncz JK, Vajna ZM, Horváth GY, Gyimesi J, Koczka I (1977) Metabolites of gentamicin-producing *Micromonospora* species I. Isolation and identification of metabolites. J Antibiot (Tokyo) 30:945–954

Birch AJ (1963) The biosynthesis of antibiotics. Pure Appl Chem 7:527–537

Blumson NL, Baddiley J (1961) Thymidine diphosphate mannose and thymidine diphosphate rhamnose in *Streptomyces griseus*. Biochem J 81:114–124

Borisova LN, Ivkina NS (1968) Mutants of *Actinomyces streptomycini* (*Streptomyces griseus*) with altered biosynthesis of antibiotics (in Russian). Spetsifichnost Khim Mutageneza Mater Vses Simp 138–146 (cf. Chem Abstr 71:36586a)

Bruce RM, Ragheb HS, Weiner H (1968) Biosynthesis of streptomycin. Origin of streptidine from D-glucose. Biochim Biophys Acta 158:499–500

Bruton J, Horner WH (1966) Biosynthesis of streptomycin. III. Origin of the carbon atoms of streptose. J Biol Chem 241:3142–3146

Bruton J, Horner WH (1969) Biosynthesis of streptomycin. V. Origin of the formyl carbon atom of streptose. Biochim Biophys Acta 184:641–642

Bruton J, Horner WH, Russ GA (1967) Biosynthesis of streptomycin. IV. Further studies on the biosynthesis of streptidine and *N*-methyl-L-glucosamine. J Biol Chem 242:813–818

Bu'Lock JD (1965) The biosynthesis of natural products. An introduction to secondary metabolism. McGraw-Hill, London

Bu'Lock JD (1967) Essays in biosynthesis and microbial development. Wiley & Sons Chichester

Candy DJ, Baddiley J (1965) The biosynthesis of streptomycin. The origin of the *C*-formyl group of streptose. Biochem J 96:526–529

Candy DJ, Blumson NL, Baddiley J (1964) The biosynthesis of streptomycin. Incorporation of ^{14}C-labeled compounds into streptose and *N*-methyl-L-glucosamine. Biochem J 91:31–35

Chang LT, Behr DA, Elander RP (1978) Effects of plasmid-curing agents on cultural characteristics and kanamycin formation in a production strain of *Streptomyces kanamyceticus*. Abstr 73 of the 3rd International Symposium on the Genetics of Industrial Microorganisms, University of Wisconsin, Madison June 4–9. Available from: Publication office, American Society for Microbiology, 1913 I St., NW, Washington DC 20006

Chen IW, Charalampous FC (1965a) Inositol 1-phosphate as intermediate in the conversion of glucose 6-phosphate to inositol. Biochem Biophys Res Commun 19:144–149

Chen IW, Charalampous FC (1965b) Biochemical studies on inositol. VIII. Purification and properties of the enzyme system which converts glucose 6-phosphate to inositol. J Biol Chem 240:3507–3512

Chen IW, Charalampous FC (1966a) Biochemical studies on inositol. IX. D-Inositol 1-phosphate as intermediate in the biosynthesis of inositol from glucose 6-phosphate, and characteristics of two reactions in this biosynthesis. J Biol Chem 241:2194–2199

Chen IW, Charalampous FC (1966b) Biochemical studies on inositol. X. Partial purification of yeast inositol 1-phosphatase and its separation from glucose 6-phosphate cyclase. Arch Biochem Biophys 117:154–157

Chen IW, Charalampous FC (1967) Studies on the mechanism of cyclization of glucose 6-phosphate to D-inositol 1-phosphate. Biochim Biophys Acta 136:568–570

Chen Y-M, Walker JB (1977) Transaminations involving keto- and amino-inositols and glutamine in actinomycetes which produce gentamicin and neomycin. Biochem Biophys Res Commun 77:688–692

Chung S-T, Morris RL (1978) Isolation and characterization of plasmid deoxyribonucleic acid from *Streptomyces fradiae*. Abstr 78 of the 3rd International Symposium on the Genetics of Industrial Microorganisms, University of Wisconsin, Madison, June 4–9. Available from: Publication Office, American Society for Microbiology, 1913 I St., NW, Washington DC 20006

Claes PJ, Compernolle F, Vanderhaeghe H (1974) Chromatographic analysis of neomycin. Isolation and identification of minor components. J Antibiot (Tokyo) 27:931–942

Claridge CA, Bush JA, Defuria MD, Price KE (1974) Fermentation and mutation studies with a butirosin-producing strain of *Bacillus circulans*. Dev Indust Microbiol 15:101–113

Cleophax J, Gero SD, Leboul J, Akhtar M, Barnett JEG, Pearce CJ (1976) A chiral synthesis of D-(+)-2,6-dideoxystreptamine and its microbial incorporation into novel antibiotics. J Am Chem Soc 98:7110–7112

Comb DG, Roseman S (1958) Enzymic synthesis of *N*-acetyl-D-mannosamine. Biochim Biophys Acta 29:653–654

Cox DA, Richardson K, Ross BC (1977) The aminoglycosides. Top Antibiot Chem 1:2–90

Daniels PJL (1978) Synthetic and mutasynthetic antibiotics related to sisomicin. 18th Interscience Conference on Antimicrobial Agents and Chemotherapy, Session 51, Atlanta, Georgia, Oct. 1–4 (cf. Daum and Lemke 1979). Available from: Publications Office, American Society for Microbiology, 1913 I St., NW, Washington DC 20006

Daniels PJL, Rane DF (1979) Synthetic and mutasynthetic antibiotics related to sisomicin. In: Schlessinger D (ed) Microbiology-1979. American Society for Microbiology, Washington, DC, pp 314–317

Daniels PJL, Yehaskel A, Morton JB (1976) The biosynthetic origin of the methyl groups of the gentamicin antibiotics. 16th Interscience Conference on Antimicrobial Agents and Chemotherapy, No. 45, Chicago, Oct 27–29. Available from: Publications Office, American Society for Microbiology, 1913 I St., NW, Washington DC 20006

Daum SJ, (1979) New gentamicin-type antibiotics produced by mutasynthesis. In: Schlessinger D (ed) Microbiology-1979. American Society for Microbiology, Washington, DC, pp 312–313

Daum SJ, Lemke JR (1979) Mutational biosynthesis of new antibiotics. Annu Rev Microbiol 33:241–265

Daum SJ, Rosi D, Goss WA (1977a) Production of antibiotics by biotransformation of 2,4,6/3,5-pentahydroxycyclohexanone and 2,4/3,5-tetrahydroxycyclohexanone by a deoxystreptamine-negative mutant of *Micromonospora purpurea*. J Am Chem Soc 99:283–284

Daum SJ, Rosi D, Goss WA (1977b) Mutational biosynthesis by idiotrophs of *Micromonospora purpurea*. II. Conversion of non-amino containing cyclitols to aminoglycoside antibiotics. J Antibiot (Tokyo) 30:98–105

Davies J, Houk C, Yagisawa M, White TJ (1979) Occurrence and function of aminoglycoside-modifying enzymes. In: Sebek OK, Laskin AL (eds) Genetics of industrial microorganisms. American Society for Microbiology, Washington, DC, pp 166–169

Deguchi T, Okumura S, Ishii A, Tanaka M (1977) Synthesis of carbon-14 and tritium labeled sagamicin. J Antibiot (Tokyo) 30:993–998

Delic V, Pigac J, Sermonti G (1969) Detection and study of cosynthesis of tetracycline antibiotics by an agar method. J Gen Microbiol 55:103–108

Demain AL, Inamine E (1970) Biochemistry and regulation of streptomycin and mannosidostreptomycinase (α-D-mannosidase) formation. Bacteriol Rev 34:1–19

Demain AL, Nagaoka K (1976) Derivatives of streptomycin and production of streptomycin derivatives by mutational biosynthesis. US patent 3,956,275; US patent 3,993,544; Japan Kokai 51–118, 748

Dolak LA, Castle TM, Dietz A, Laborde AL (1980) 3-Amino-3-deoxyglucose produced by a *Streptomyces* sp. J Antibiot (Tokyo) 33:900–901

Elbein AD, Health EC (1965a) The biosynthesis of cell wall lipopolysaccharide in *Escherichia coli*. I. The biochemical properties of a uridine diphosphate galactose 4-epimeraseless mutant. J Biol Chem 240:1919–1925

Elbein AD, Health EC (1965b) The biosynthesis of cell wall lipopolysaccharide in *Escherichia coli*. II. Guanosine diphosphate 4-keto-6-deoxy-D-mannose, an intermediate in the biosynthesis of guanosine diphosphate colitose. J Biol Chem 240:1926–1931

Fletcher HG Jr, Anderson L, Lardy H (1951) The nomenclature of the cyclohexitols and their derivatives. J Org Chem 16:1238–1246

Floss HG, Chang C-J, Mascaretti O, Shimada K (1978) Studies on the biosynthesis of antibiotics. Planta Med 34:345–380

Foley L, Weigele M (1978) Spectinomycin chemistry. 1. Characterization of a 5a,9a-*epi*-4(R)-dihydrospectinomycin derivative. J Org Chem 43:4355–4359

Fujiwara T, Tanimoto T, Matsumoto K, Kondo E (1978) Ribostamycin production by a mutant of butirosin producing bacteria. J Antibiot (Tokyo) 31:966–969

Fujiwara T, Takahashi Y, Matsumoto K, Kondo E (1980a) Isolation of an intermediate of 2-deoxystreptamine biosynthesis from a mutant of *Bacillus circulans*. J Antibiot (Tokyo) 33:824–829

Fujiwara T, Takahashi Y, Matsumoto K, Kondo E (1980b) Production of a new aminoglycoside antibiotic by a mutant of *Bacillus circulans*. J Antibiot (Tokyo) 33:836–841

Fukagawa Y (1968) Studies on biosynthesis of kasugamycin. PhD thesis, Kyushu University, Fukuoka, Japan (cf. Umezawa S and Tsuchiya T 1969)

Fukagawa Y, Sawa T, Homma I, Takeuchi T, Umezawa H (1968a) Studies on biosynthesis of kasugamycin. IV. Biosynthesis of the kasugamine moiety from [1-^{14}C]-glucosamine and [1,2 or 6-^{14}C]-glucose. J Antibiot (Tokyo) 21:358–360

Fukagawa Y, Sawa T, Homma I, Takeuchi T, Umezawa H (1968b) Studies on biosynthesis of kasugamycin. V. Biosynthesis of the amidine group. J Antibiot (Tokyo) 21:410–412

Fukagawa Y, Sawa T, Takeuchi T, Umezawa H (1968c) Studies on biosynthesis of kasugamycin. I. Biosynthesis of kasugamycin and the kasugamine moiety. J Antibiot (Tokyo) 21:50–54

Fukagawa Y, Sawa T, Takeuchi T, Umezawa H (1968d) Biosynthesis of kasugamycin. II. Biosynthesis of the two-carbon side chain of kasugamycin. J Antibiot (Tokyo) 21:182–184

Fukagawa Y, Sawa T, Takeuchi T, Umezawa H (1968e) Studies on biosynthesis of kasugamycin. III. Biosynthesis of the D-inositol moiety. J Antibiot (Tokyo) 21:185–188

Furumai T, Takeda K, Kinumaki A, Ito Y, Okuda T (1979) Biosynthesis of butirosins. II. Biosynthetic pathway of butirosins elucidated from cosynthesis and feeding experiments. J Antibiot (Tokyo) 32:891–899

Gabriel O, Lindquist LC (1968) Biological mechanisms involved in the formation of deoxy sugars. IV. Enzymatic conversion of thymidine diphosphoglucose-4T to thymidine diphospho-4-keto-6-deoxyglucose-6T. J Biol Chem 243:1479–1484

Galanina LA, Agatov PA (1959) Effect of some chemical compounds on formation of streptomycin by LS1 strain of *Actinomyces streptomycini* (in Russian). Doklady Akad Nauk SSSR 127:450–452 (cf. Chem Abstr 54:2586i)

Ganelin VL, Demina AS, Petyushenko RM, Sazykin YO, Navashin SM (1979) Aminoglycoside-3′-phosphotransferase from *Actinomyces fradiae*. Isolation, purification and properties (in Russian). Antibiotiki 24:424–430

Gero SD, Mercier D (1977) Neomycin and paromomycin analogues for use as broad-spectrum antibiotics prepared by fermentation (in Japanese). Japan Kokai 52-142044

Ghosh S, Roseman S (1965a) The sialic acids. IV. *N*-acyl-D-glucosamine 6-phosphate 2-epimerase. J Biol Chem 240:1525–1530

Ghosh S, Roseman S (1965b) The sialic acids. V. *N*-acyl-D-glucosamine 2-epimerase. J Biol Chem 240:1531–1536

Gilbert JM, Matsuhashi M, Strominger JL (1965) Thymidine diphosphate 4-acetamido-4,6-dideoxyhexoses. II. Purification and properties of thymidine diphosphate D-glucose oxidoreductase. J Biol Chem 240:1305–1308

Gorin PAJ, Spencer JFT, Phaff HJ (1964) The synthesis of β-galacto- and β-glucopyranosyl disaccharides by *Sporobolomyces singularis*. Can J Chem 42:2307–2317

Grisebach H (1978) Biosynthesis of sugar components of antibiotic substances. Adv Carbohydr Chem Biochem 35:81–126

Hanessian S, Roy R (1979) Synthesis of (+)-spectinomycin. J Am Chem Soc 101:5839–5841

Hayakawa T, Otake N, Yonehara H, Tanaka T, Sakaguchi K (1979) Isolation and characterization of plasmids from *Streptomyces*. J Antibiot (Tokyo) 32:1348–1350

Heding H (1964) Radioactive myoinositol incorporation into streptomycin. Science 143:953–954

Heding H (1968) *N*-Demethyl-streptomycin. I. Microbiological formation and isolation. Acta Chim Scand 22:1649–1654

Heding H, Bajpai K (1973) Last step in the biosynthesis of streptomycin: *N*-methylation of *N*-demethylstreptomycin. J Antibiot (Tokyo) 26:725–727

Hessler EJ, Jahnke HK, Robertson JH, Tsuji K, Rinehart KL Jr, Shier WT (1970) Neomycins D, E and F: identity with paromamine, paromomycin I and paromomycin II. J Antibiot (Tokyo) 23:464–466

Heyes WF (1978) The biosynthesis and commercial production of neomycin – a review. Process Biochem 13(12):10–12

Hockenhull DJD (1960) The biochemistry of streptomycin production. Prog Ind Microbiol 2:132–165

Hoeksema H, Knight JC (1975) The production of dihydrospectinomycin by *Streptomyces spectabilis*. J Antibiot (Tokyo) 28:240–241

Hopwood DA (1978) Extrachromosomally determined antibiotic production. Annu Rev Microbiol 32:373–392

Horner WH (1964a) Biosynthesis of streptomycin. I. Origin of the guanidine group. J Biol Chem 239:578–581

Horner WH (1964b) Biosynthesis of streptomycin. II. Myoinositol, a precursor of the streptidine moiety. J Biol Chem 239:2256–2258

Horner WH (1967) Streptomycin. In: Gottlieb D, Shaw PD (eds) Biosynthesis. Springer, Berlin Heidelberg New York Antibiotics, vol 2, pp 373–399

Horner WH, Russ GA (1969) Biosynthesis of streptomycin. VI. *Myo*-inosose-2, an intermediate in streptidine biosynthesis. Biochem Biophys Acta 192:352–354

Horner WH, Russ GA (1971) Biosynthesis of streptomycin. VII. Stereospecificity of the enzymatic dehydrogenation of 1-guanidino-1-deoxy-*scyllo*-inositol. Biochem Biophys Acta 237:123–127

Horner WH, Thaker IH (1968) The metabolism of *scyllo*-inositol in *Streptomyces griseus*. Biochem Biophys Acta 165:306–308

Hotta K, Okami Y, Umezawa H (1977) Elimination of the ability of a kanamycin-producing strain to biosynthesize deoxystreptamine moiety by acriflavine. J Antibiot (Tokyo) 30:1146–1149

Hunter GD, Hockenhull DJD (1955) Actinomycete metabolism. Incorporation of ^{14}C-labelled compounds into streptomycin. Biochem J 59:268–272

Igarashi K, Honma T, Fujiwara T, Kondo E (1980) Structure elucidation of an intermediate of 2-deoxystreptamine biosynthesis. J Antibiot (Tokyo) 33:830–835

Ikeda A, Kokan A, Yoshimura Y, Nimi O, Nomi R (1977) Correlation between streptomycin biosynthesis and cell wall formation (in Japanese). Abstr 306 of the Annual Meeting of the Society of Fermentation Technology, Japan, Osaka, Nov 10–12. Available from: Business Office, The Society of Fermentation Technology, Japan, Faculty of Engineering, Osaka University, Suita-shi, Osaka 565, Japan

Kakinuma K, Ogawa Y, Sasaki T, Seto H, Otake N (1981) Stereochemistry of the ribostamycin biosynthesis studied by ^{2}H-NMR spectroscopy. Symposium paper 70 of the 24th Symposium on the Chemistry of Natural Products, Midokaikan, Osaka, Oct 13–16. Available from: Organizing Committee, Faculty of Pharmaceutical Sciences, Osaka University, Suita-shi, Osaka 565, Japan

Kameda Y, Horii S, Yamano T (1975) Microbial transformation of validamycins. J Antibiot (Tokyo) 28:298–306

Kameda Y, Asano N, Hashimoto T (1978) Microbial glycosidation of validamycins. J Antibiot (Tokyo) 31:936–938

Karow EO, Peck RL, Rosenblum C, Woodbury DT (1952) Microbiological synthesis of ^{14}C-labeled streptomycin. J Am Chem Soc 74:3056–3059

Kase H, Odakura Y, Nakayama K (1980) Sagamicin biosynthesis and fermentation by *Micromonospora sagamiensis* (in Japanese). Abstr 4 of the Symposium on Recent Topics on Biosynthesis, Tokyo, Jan 25. Available from: Agricultural Chemical Society of Japan, Japan Academic Societies Center, 4–16 Yayoi 2-chome, Bunkyo-ku, Tokyo 113, Japan

Kawamura T, Ichihara N, Ishimoto N, Ito E (1975) Biosynthesis of uridine diphosphate *N*-acetyl-D-mannosaminuronic acid from uridine diphosphate *N*-acetyl-D-glucosamine in *Escherichia coli*. Separation of enzymes responsible for epimerization and dehydrogenation. Biochem Biophys Res Commun 66:1506–1512

Khokhlov AS, Tovarova II, Borisova LN, Pliner SA, Shévchenko LN, Kornitskaya EYa, Ivkina NS, Rapoport IA (1967) The A-factor responsible for the biosynthesis of streptomycin in mutant strains of *Actinomyces streptomycini* (in Russian). Dokl Akad Nauk SSSR 117:232–235

Khokhlov AS, Anisova LN, Tovarova II, Kleiner EM, Kovalenko IV, Krasilnikova OI, Kornitskaya EYa, Pliner SA (1973) Effect of A-factor on asporogenous and non-streptomycin producing mutants of *Streptomyces griseus*. Z Allg Mikrobiol 13:647–655

Kindle H, Biedl-Neubacher J, Hoffmann-Ostenhop O (1965) Untersuchungen über die Biosynthese der Cyclite. IX. Überführung von D-Glucose und D-Glucose-6-phosphate in *meso*-Inosit durch einen zellfreien Extrakt aus *Candida utilis*. Biochem Z 341:157–167

Kirby R, Wright LF, Hopwood DA (1975) Plasmid-determined antibiotic synthesis and resistance in *Streptomyces coelicolor*. Nature 254:265–267

Kirby JP, Borders DB, Van Lear GE (1977) Structure of LL-BM408, an aminocyclitol antibiotic. J Antibiot (Tokyo) 30:175–177

Kleiner EM, Pliner SA, Soifer VS, Onoprienko VV, Balashova TA, Rozynov BV, Khokhlov AS (1976) Structure of the A-factor, a bioregulator from *Streptomyces griseus* (in Russian). Bioorg Khim 2:1142–1147

Kleiner EM, Onoprienko VV, Pliner SA, Soifer VS, Khokhlov AS (1977) Synthesis of A-factor racemate – A biological regulator from *Streptomyces griseus* (in Russian). Bioorg Khim 3:424–426

Kniep B, Grisebach H (1976) Enzymic synthesis of streptomycin. Transfer of L-dihydrostreptose from dTDP-L-dihydrostreptose to streptidine-6-phosphate. FEBS Lett 65:44–46

Kniep B, Grisebach H (1980a) Biosynthesis of streptomycin. Purification and properties of dTDP-L-dihydrostreptose: streptidine-6-phosphate dihydrostreptosyltransferase from *Streptomyces griseus*. Eur J Biochem 105:139–144

Kniep B, Grisebach H (1980b) Biosynthesis of streptomycin. Enzymatic formation of dihydrostreptomycin 6-phosphate from dihydrostreptosyl streptidine 6-phosphate. J Antibiot (Tokyo) 33:416–419

Kojima M (1974) Studies on bioconversion of ribostamycin (SF-733). PhD thesis. Tokyo University, Tokyo

Kojima M, Satoh A (1973) Microbial semi-synthesis of aminoglycosidic antibiotics by mutants of *S. ribosidificus* and *S. kanamyceticus*. J Antibiot (Tokyo) 26:784–786

Kojima M, Yamada Y, Umezawa H (1968) Studies on the biosynthesis of kanamycins. Part I. Incorporation of ^{14}C-glucose or ^{14}C-glucosamine into kanamycins and kanamycin-related compounds. Agric Biol Chem 32:467–473

Kojima M, Yamada Y, Umezawa H (1969) Studies on the biosynthesis of kanamycins. Part II. Incorporation of the radioactive degradation products of kanamycin A or related metabolites into kanamycin A. Agric Biol Chem 33:1181–1185

Kojima M, Inouye S, Niida T (1973) Bioconversion of ribostamycin (SF-733). I. Isolation and structure of 3 (or 1)-*N*-carboxymethylribostamycin. J Antibiot (Tokyo) 26:246–248

Kojima M, Ezaki N, Amano S, Inouye S, Niida T (1975a) Bioconversion of ribostamycin (SF-733). II. Isolation and structure of 3-*N*-acetylribostamycin, a microbiologically inactive product of ribostamycin produced by *Streptomyces ribosidificus*. J Antibiot (Tokyo) 28:42–47

Kojima M, Inouye S, Niida T (1975b) Bioconversion of ribostamycin (SF-733). III. Formation, structure and synthesis of 3-*N*-carboxymethyl ribostamycin. J Antibiot (Tokyo) 28:48–55

Kornitskaya EYa, Tovarova II, Khokhlov AS (1975) The peculiarity of A-factor interaction with mutant 1439 of *Act. streptomycini* during biosynthesis of streptomycin (in Russian). Antibiotiki 20:978–982

Kornitskaya EYa, Tovarova II, Soifer VS, Khokhlov AS (1976a) Investigation on the streptomycin biosynthesis regulation with the use of a blocked mutant *Act. streptomycini* (in Russian). Antibiotiki 21:10–14

Kornitskaya EYa, Tovarova II, Khokhlov AS (1976b) Formation of A factor by various actinomycetes. Microbiology (Engl Transl Mikrobiologiya) 45:264–267

Köster H, Liebermann B, Reuter G (1975) Physiologie und Biochemie der Streptomyceten. III. Einbau von D-Glucose-U-^{14}C in Paromomycin als Indikator für die Antibioticabildung durch *Streptomyces albus var metamycinus* nov. var. Z Allg Mikrobiol 15:437–445

Köster H, Liebermann B, Reuter G (1977) Physiologie und Biochemie der Streptomyceten. XI. Unterschiedlicher Einbau von D-Glucose-U-^{14}C in die Paromomycin-isomere und in die Bausteine von Paromomycin I. Z Allg Mikrobiol 17:433–436

Krasilnikova OL, Anisova LN, Khokholov AS (1978a) Mutants of *Actinomyces streptomycini* blocked with respect to biosynthesis of streptobiosamine moiety of streptomycin molecule (in Russian). Antibiotiki 23:135–138

Krasilnikova OL, Anisova LN, Khokhlov AS (1978b) Low active mutants of *Actinomyces streptomycini* (*Streptomyces griseus*) with protein in biosynthesis of streptidine part of streptomycin molecule (in Russian). Antibiotiki 23:204–207

Kugelman M, Jaret RS, Mittelman S (1978) The structure of aminoglycoside antibiotic 66-40G produced by *Micromonospora inyoensis*. J Antibiot (Tokyo) 31:643–645

Kumagai AH, Akamatsu N (1977) Biosynthesis of *N*-methyl-L-glucosamine from D-glucose by *Streptomyces griseus*. Biochim Biophys Acta 499:447–449

Lee BK, Testa RT, Wagman GH, Liu CM, McDaniel L, Schaffner C (1973) Incorporation of L-methionine-methyl-^{14}C into gentamicins. J Antibiot (Tokyo) 26:728–731

Lee BK, Condon RG, Marawski A, Wagman GH (1975) Incorporation of L-methionine-methyl-^{14}C into gentamicins. III. Chromatographic separation and degradation of components of methyl-^{14}C-gentamicin complex. J Antibiot (Tokyo) 28:163–166

Lee BK, Condon RG, Wagman GH, Katz E (1976) *Micromonospora*-produced gentamicin components. Antimicrob Agents Chemother 9:151–159

Lee BK, Bailey JV, Condon RG, Marquez JA, Wagman GH, Weinstein MJ (1977) Biotransformation of sisomicin to gentamicin C_{2b}. Antimicrob Agents Chemother 12:335–338

Lee BK, Nagabhushan TL, Condon RG, Cooper AB, Waitz JA (1978) Antibiotic biosynthesis by cofermentation of blocked mutants of two *Micromonospora* species. Antimicro Agents Chemother 14:73–77

Lee BK, Nagabhushan TL, Condon RG, Shimonaski G, Kalyanpur MG, Patel M, Waitz JA (1979) Biosynthetic pathway leading to gentamicin C_{2b}. Antimicrob Agents Chemother 16:589–591

Lemieux RU, Wolfrom ML (1948) The chemistry of streptomycin. Adv Carbohydr Chem 3:337–384

Lemke JR, Demain AL (1976) Preliminary studies on streptomutin A. Eur J Appl Microbiol 2:91–94

Lowther DA, Rogers HJ (1956) The role of glutamine in the biosynthesis of hyaluronate by Streptococcal suspensions. Biochem J 62:304–314

Magasanik B (1953) Enzymatic adaptation in the metabolism of cyclitols in *Aerobacter aerogenes*. J Biol Chem 205:1007–1018

Maier S, Grisebach H (1979) Biosynthesis of streptomycin. Enzymic oxidation of dihydrostreptomycin (6-phosphate) to streptomycin (6-phosphate) with a particulate fraction of *Streptomyces griseus*. Biochim Biophys Acta 586:231–241

Maier S, Matern U, Grisebach H (1975) On the role of dihydrostreptomycin in streptomycin biosynthesis. FEBS Lett 49:317–319

Majumdar MK, Majumdar SK (1969) Amino sugar antibiotic as phosphoamide from *Streptomyces fradiae*. J Antibiot (Tokyo) 22:174–175

Majumdar MK, Majumdar SK (1970) Isolation and characterization of three phosphoamido-neomycins and their conversion into neomycin by *Streptomyces fradiae*. Biochem J 120:271–278

Majumdar MK, Majumdar SK (1971) Relationship between alkaline phosphatase and neomycin formation in *Streptomyces fradiae*. Biochem J 122:397–404

Majumdar SK, Kutzner HJ (1962) Studies on the biosynthesis of streptomycin. Appl Microbiol 10:157–168

Matsuhashi M, Strominger JL (1964) Thymidine diphosphate 4-acetamido-4,6-dideoxyhexoses. I. Enzymatic synthesis by strains of *Escherichia coli*. J Biol Chem 239:2454–2463

Matsuhashi M, Strominger JL (1966) Thymidine diphosphate 4-acetamido-4,6-dideoxyhexoses. III. Purification and properties of thymidine diphosphate 4-keto-6-deoxy-D-glucose transaminase from *Escherichia coli* strain B. J Biol Chem 241:4738–4744
Matsuhashi S (1966) Enzymatic synthesis of cytidine diphosphate 3,6-dideoxyhexoses. II. Reversible 2-epimerization of cytidine diphosphate paratose. J Biol Chem 241:4275–4282
Matsuhashi S, Matsuhashi M, Brown JG, Strominger JL (1966a) Enzymatic synthesis of cytidine diphosphate 3,6-dideoxyhexoses. III. Cytidine diphosphate D-glucose oxidoreductase. J Biol Chem 241:4283–4287
Matsuhashi S, Matsuhashi M, Strominger JL (1966b) Enzymatic synthesis of cytidine diphosphate 3,6-dideoxyhexoses. I. Over-all reactions. J Biol Chem 241:4267–4274
Matsuhashi Y, Sawa T, Kondo S, Takeuchi T (1977) Aminoglycoside 3′-phosphotransferase in *Bacillus circulans* producing butirosins. J Antibiot (Tokyo) 30:435–437
Matsumura S, Shirafuji H, Nogami I (1978) Formation of butirosin A by washed cell suspensions of *Bacillus vitellinus* (in Japanese). J Takeda Res Lab 37:278–285
Melo A, Elliott WH, Glaser L (1968) The machanism of 6-deoxyhexose synthesis. I. Intramolecular hydrogen transfer catalyzed by deoxythymidine diphosphate D-glucose oxidoreductase. J Biol Chem 243:1467–1474
Mendicino J, Picken JM (1966) Biosynthesis of streptomycin. In: Snell JF (ed) Biosynthesis of antibiotics, vol I. Academic Press, New York London,pp 121–140
Miller AL, Walker JB (1969) Enzymatic phosphorylation of streptomycin by extracts of streptomycin-producing strains of *Streptomyces*. J Bacteriol 99:401–405
Miller AL, Walker JB (1970) Accumulation of streptomycin-phosphate in cultures of streptomycin producers grown on a high-phosphate medium. J Bacteriol 104:8–12
Mitscher LA, Martin LL, Feller DR (1971) The biosynthesis of spectinomycin. J Chem Soc Chem Commun 1971:1541–1542
Munro MHG, Taniguchi M, Rinehart KL Jr, Gottlieb D, Stoudt TH, Rogers TO (1975) Carbon-13 evidence for the stereochemistry of streptomycin biosynthesis from glucose. J Am Chem Soc 97:4782–4783
Murase M, Ito T, Fukatsu S, Umezawa H (1970) Studies on kanamycin related compounds produced during fermentation by mutants of *Streptomyces kanamyceticus*. Isolation and properties. Progr Antimicrob Anticancer Chemother 2:1098–1110
Nagaoka K, Demain AL (1975) Mutational biosynthesis of a new antibiotic, streptomutin A, by an idiotroph of *Streptomyces griseus*. J Antibiot (Tokyo) 28:627–635
Nakahama K, Shirafuji H, Nogami I, Kida M, Yoneda M (1977) Butirosin 3′-phosphotransferase from *Bacillus vitellinus*, a butirosin-producing organism. Agric Biol Chem 41:2437–2445
Nakayama K, Kase H, Kitamura S, Shirahata K, Iida T (1979a) New substance SUM-4 and production thereof (in Japanese). Japan Kokai 54-135,704
Nakayama K, Kase H, Kitamura S, Shirahata K, Iida T (1979b) Antibiotic SU-1 and production thereof (in Japanese). Japan Kokai 54-135,705
Nakayama K, Kase H, Odakura Y, Iida T, Shirahata K (1979c) Antibiotic SU-2 and production thereof (in Japanese). Japan Kokai 54-59,202
Nakayama K, Kase H, Shimura H (1979d) Production of gentamicin Cs (in Japanese). Japan Kokai 54-160,796
Nakayama K, Kase H, Shirahata K, Iida T, Mori Y, Mochida K (1979e) Antibiotic SUM-3 and production thereof (in Japanese). Japan Kokai 54-117,477
Nakayama K, Ito S, Odakura Y, Shirahata K, Takahashi K (1979f) A new compound FU-10 and production thereof (in Japanese). Japan Kokai 54-128,547
Nara T (1977) Aminoglycoside antibiotics. In: Perlman D, Tsao GT (eds) Annual reports on fermentation process. Vol 1. Academic Press, New York San Francisco London, pp 299–326
Nara T (1978) Aminoglycoside antibiotics. In: Perlman D, Tsao GT (eds) Annual reports on fermentation process. Vol 2. Academic Press, New York San Francisco London, pp 223–266
Neuss N (1975) The use of ^{13}C labeling in the study of antibiotic biosynthesis. Methods Enzymol 43:404–425

Nimi O, Kiyohara H, Mizoguchi T, Ohata Y, Nomi R (1970) Biosynthesis of streptomycin Part VII. A specific enzyme responsible for dephosphorylation of phosphorylated streptomycin. Agric Biol Chem 34:1150–1156

Nimi O, Ito G, Ohata Y, Funayama S, Nomi R (1971 a) Streptomycin-phosphorylating enzyme produced by *Streptomyces griseus*. Agric Biol Chem 35:856–861

Nimi O, Ito G, Sueda S, Nomi R (1971 b) Phosphorylation of streptomycin at C_6-OH of streptidine moiety by an intracellular enzyme of *Streptomyces griseus*. Agric Biol Chem 35:848–855

Nimi O, Norimoto Y, Nomi R (1971 c) Incorporation of streptidine-C_6-phosphate into phosphorylated streptomycin by resting cell of *Streptomyces griseus*. Agric Biol Chem 35:1819–1821

Nimi O, Kokan A, Manabe K, Maehara K, Nomi R (1976) Correlation between streptomycin formation and mucopeptide biosynthesis. J Ferment Technol 54:587–595

Nogami I, Arai Y, Horii S, Yoneda M (1974) Production of antibiotics (in Japanese). Japan Kokai 49-117,685

Nogami I, Arai Y, Kida M, Hiraga K (1976) Butirosin A or its derivatives (in Japanese). Japan Kokai 51-1,694

Nojiri C, Watabe H, Katsumata K, Yamada Y, Murakami T, Kumata Y (1980) Isolation and characterization of plasmids from parent and variant strains of *Streptomyces ribosidificus*. J Antibiot (Tokyo) 33:118–121

Nomi R (1978) Biosynthesis of aminoglycoside antibiotics – a review (in Japanese). Hakkokogaku Kaishi 5:479–493

Nomi R, Nimi O (1969) Biosynthesis of streptomycin. Part VI. Chemical structure of a streptomycin precursor. Agric Biol Chem 33:1459–1463

Nomi R, Nimi O, Kado T (1968) Biosynthesis of streptomycin. Part IV. Accumulation of a streptomycin precursor in the culture broth and partial purification of the precursor. Agric Biol Chem 32:1256–1260

Nomi R, Nimi O, Kado T (1969) Biosynthesis of streptomycin. Part V. Purification and properties of a streptomycin precursor. Agric Biol Chem 33:1454–1458

Oka Y, Ishida H, Morioka M, Numazaki Y, Yamafugi T, Ozono T, Umezawa H (1979) New antibiotics and production thereof (in Japanese). Japan Kokai 54-98,741

Okami Y (1979) Antibiotics from marine microorganisms with reference to plasmid involvement. J Nat Prod 42:583–595

Okanishi M (1977) Secondary metabolite production and plasmid (in Japanese). Amino Acid Nucleic Acid 35:15–30

Okanishi M (1978) Plasmids and their functions involved in antibiotic production (in Japanese). Hakkokogaku Kaishi 56:468–478

Okanishi M (1979) Antibiotic production and episomic factors (in Japanese). Ferment Industry 37:33–40

Okanishi M (1980) Role of plasmid genes in antibiotic production. In: Umezawa H, Tanaka N (eds) Advances in antibiotic research. Japan Scientific Societies Press, Tokyo, pp 35–52.

Okanishi M, Umezawa H (1978) Plasmids involved in antibiotic production in *Streptomycetes*. In: Freerksen E, Tarnok I, Thumin JH (eds) Genetics of the actinomycetales. Fischer, Stuttgart New York, pp 19–38

Okanishi M, Ohta T, Umezawa H (1970) Possible control of formation of aerial mycelium and antibiotic production in *Streptomyces* by episomic factors. J Antibiot (Tokyo) 23:45–47

Okanishi M, Manome T, Umezawa H (1980) Isolation and characterization of plasmid DNAs in actinomycetes. J Antibiot (Tokyo) 33:88–91

Okazaki H, Ono H, Yamada K, Beppu T, Arima K (1973) Relationship among cellular fatty acid composition, amino acid uptake and neomycin formation in a mutant strain of *Streptomyces fradiae*. Agric Biol Chem 37:2319–2325

Okazaki H, Beppu T, Arima K (1974) Induction of antibiotic formation in *Streptomyces* sp. No. 362 by the change of cellular fatty acid spectrum. Agric Biol Chem 38:1455–1461

Ortmann R, Matern U, Grisebach H, Stadler P, Sinnwell V, Paulsen H (1974) NADPH-dependent formation of thymidine diphosphodihydrostreptose from thymidine diphospho-D-glucose in a cell-free system from *S. griseus* and its correlation with streptomycin biosynthesis. Eur J Biochem 43:265–271

Pearce CJ, Barnett JEG, Anthony C, Akhtar M, Gero SD (1976) The role of the pseudo-disaccharide neamine as an intermediate in the biosynthesis of neomycin. Biochem J 159:601–606

Pearce CJ, Akhtar M, Barnett JEG, Mercier D, Sepulchre A-M, Gero SD (1978) Sub-unit assembly in the biosynthesis of neomycin. The synthesis of 5-*O*-β-D-ribofuranosyl and 4-*O*-β-D-ribofuranosyl-2,6-dideoxystreptamines. J Antibiot (Tokyo) 31:74–81

Petyushenko RM, Ganelin VL, Chernyshev AI, Denaina AS, Esipov SE, Sazykin YuO, Navashin SM (1979) Aminoglycoside-3′-phosphotransferase from *Actinomyces fradiae*. Identification of inactivation product (in Russian). Antibiotiki 24:430–436

Piwowarski JM, Shaw PD (1979) Streptomycin resistance in a streptomycin-producing microorganism. Antimicrob Agents Chemother 16:176–182

Posternak T (1965) The cyclitols. In: Lederer E (ed) Chemistry of natural products. Holden-Day, San Francisco, pp 152–156

Queener SW, Sebek OK, Vézina C (1978) Mutants blocked in antibiotic synthesis. Annu Rev Microbiol 32:593–636

Reuter G, Köster H, Liebermann (1977) Physiologie und Biochemie der Streptomyceten. XIII. Biosynthese von Paromomycin unter Einsatz von ^{14}C-Glucose, -Glucosamin, -2-Desoxystreptamin und -Ribose durch *Streptomyces albus var. metamycinus nov. var.* Z Allg Mikrobiol 17:543–547

Rinehart KL Jr (1961) The neomycins and related antibiotics. Wiley & Sons, New York London Sydney, pp 93–94

Rinehart KL Jr (1977) Mutasynthesis of new antibiotics. Pure Appl Chem 49:1361–1384

Rinehart KL Jr (1979) Biosynthesis and mutasynthesis of aminocyclitol antibiotics. Jpn J Antibiot 32:S-32–S-46

Rinehart KL Jr, Schimbor RF (1967) Neomycins. In: Gottlieb D, Shaw PD (eds) Biosynthesis. Springer, Berlin Heidelberg New York (Antibiotics, vol 2, pp 359–372)

Rinehart KL Jr, Stroshane RM (1976) Biosynthesis of aminocyclitol antibiotics. J Antibiot (Tokyo) 29:319–353

Rinehart KL Jr, Malik JM, Nystrom RS, Stroshane RM, Truitt ST, Taniguchi M, Rolls JP, Haak WJ, Buff BA (1974) Biosynthetic incorporation of [1-^{13}C]glucosamine and [6-^{13}C]glucose into neomycin. J Am Chem Soc 96:2263–2265

Rolls JP, Ruff BD, Haak WJ, Rinehart KL Jr, Stroshane RM (1975) The use of precursors labeled with stable isotopes to study the biosynthesis of neomycin. Abstr 75th Annu Meet Am Soc Microbiol

Rosi D, Goss WA, Daum SJ (1977) Mutational biosynthesis by idiotrophs of *Micromonospora purpurea*. I. Conversion of aminocyclitols to new aminoglycoside antibiotics. J Antibiot (Tokyo) 30:88–97

Russ GA (1975) Studies on the biosynthesis of streptomycin and its streptidine moiety by *Streptomyces griseus*. Diss Abstr Int B Sci Eng 35:4810–4811

Satoh A, Ogawa H, Satomura Y (1975a) Effect of sclerin on production of aminoglycoside antibiotics accompanied by salvage function in *Streptomyces*. Agric Biol Chem 39:1593–1598

Satoh A, Ogawa H, Satomura Y (1975b) Role and regulation mechanism of kanamycin acetyltransferase in kanamycin biosynthesis. Agric Biol Chem 39:2331–2336

Satoh A, Ogawa H, Satomura Y (1976) Regulation of *n*-acetylkanamycin amidohydrolase in the idiophase in kanamycin fermentation. Agric Biol Chem 40:191–196

Sawa T, Fukagawa Y, Homma I, Takeuchi T, Umezawa H (1968) Studies on biosynthesis of kasugamycin. VI. Some relationships between the incorporation of ^{14}C-compounds and the production of kasugamycin. J Antibiot (Tokyo) 21:413–420

Scholda R, Billek G, Hoffmann-Ostenhof O (1964a) Untersuchungen über die Biosynthese der Cyclite. I. Bildung von D-Pinit, D-Inosit und Sequoyit aus *meso*-Inosit in Blättchen von *Trifolium incarnatum*. Z Physiol Chem 335:180–186

Scholda R, Billek G, Hoffmann-Ostenhof O (1964b) Untersuchungen über die Biosynthese der Cyclite. VIII. Der Mechanismus der Umwandlung von *meso*-Inosit in D-Pinit und D-Inosit in *Trifolium incarnatum*. Monatsh Chem 95:1311–1317

Sepulchre A-M, Quiclet B, Gero SD (1980) Bioconversion dans le domaine des antibiotiques aminocyclitolglycosidiques. Bull Soc Chim Fr II-56–II-65

Shaw PD, Piwowarski J (1977) Effects of ethidium bromide and acriflavine on streptomycin production by *Streptomyces bikiniensis*. J Antibiot (Tokyo) 30:404–408

Shevchenko LA, Popova IS, Tovarova II, Kovalenko IV, Anisova LN, Khokhlov AS (1977) Relation of two *Actinomyces streptomycini* mutants in streptomycin biosynthesis (in Russian). Izw Akad Nauk SSSR Ser Biol 1977:551–557 (Chem Abstr 87:116377d)

Shier WT, Rinehart KL Jr, Gottlieb D (1969) Preparation of four new antibiotics from a mutant of *Streptomyces fradiae*. Proc Natl Acad Sci USA 63:198–204

Shier WT, Rinehart KL Jr, Gottlieb D (1972) Antibiotics containing the aminocyclitol subunit. US 3,669,838

Shier WT, Ogawa S, Hichens M, Rinehart KL Jr (1973) Chemistry and biochemistry of the neomycins. XVII. Bioconversion of aminocyclitols to aminocyclitol antibiotics. J Antibiot (Tokyo) 26:551–561

Shier WT, Schaefer PC, Gottlieb D, Rinehart KL Jr (1974) Use of mutants in the study of aminocyclitol antibiotic biosynthesis and the preparation of the hybrimycin C complex. Biochemistry 13:5073–5078

Shirafuji H, Nakahama K, Nogami I, Kida M, Yoneda M (1977) Accumulation of 6′-*N*-pyrophosphoamide butirosin A by phosphatase deficient mutants (in Japanese). Abstr Ann Meet Agric Chem Soc Jpn:156

Silverman M, Rieder SV (1960) The formation of *N*-methyl-L-glucosamine from D-glucose by *Streptomyces griseus*. J Biol Chem 235:1251–1254

Slechta L, Coats JH (1974) Studies of the biosynthesis of spectinomycin. Abstr 294 of the 14th Interscience Conference on Antimicrobial Agents and Chemotherapy, San Francisco, Calif., Sept 11–13. Available from: Publications Office, American Society for Microbiology, 1913 I St., NW, Washington DC 20006

Snipes CE, Brillinger G-U, Sellers L, Mascaro L, Floss HG (1977) Stereochemistry of the dTDP-glucose oxidoreductase reaction. J Biol Chem 252:8113–8117

Stepnov VP, Garaev MM, Fedotov AR, Golub EI (1978) Plasmids in Actinomycetes producing oxytetracyline and neomycin (in Russian). Antibiotiki 23:892–895

Stroshane RM (1976) Biosynthetic studies on the aminocyclitol antibiotics neomycin and spectinomycin. PhD thesis, University of Illinois, Urbana. Xerox Univ. Microfilm, 76-16202 (cf. Heyes WF 1978)

Stroshane RM, Taniguchi M, Rinehart KL Jr, Rolls JP, Haak WJ, Ruff BA (1976) Spectinomycin biosynthesis studied by carbon magnetic resonance spectroscopy. J Am Chem Soc 98:3025–3027

Suami T, Ogawa S, Chida N (1980) The revised structure of validamycin A. J Antibiot (Tokyo) 33:98–99

Takeda K, Kinumaki A, Furumai T, Yamaguchi T, Ohshima S, Ito Y (1978a) Mutational biosynthesis of butirosin analogs. J Antibiot (Tokyo) 31:247–249

Takeda K, Aihara K, Furumai T, Ito Y (1978b) An approach to the biosynthetic pathway of butirosins and the related antibiotics. J Antibiot (Tokyo) 31:250–253

Takeda K, Okuno S, Ohashi Y, Furumai T (1978c) Mutational biosynthesis of butirosin analogs. I. Conversion of neamine analogs into butirosin analogs by mutants of *Bacillus circulans*. J Antibiot (Tokyo) 31:1023–1030

Takeda K, Kinumaki A, Okuno S, Matsushita T, Ito Y (1978d) Mutational biosynthesis of butirosin analogs. III. 6′-*N*-Methylbutirosins and 3′,4′-dideoxy-6′-*C*-methylbutirosins, new semisynthetic aminoglycosides. J Antibiot (Tokyo) 31:1039–1045

Takeda K, Kinumaki A, Hayasaka H, Yamaguchi T, Ito Y (1978e) Mutational biosynthesis of butirosin analogs. II. 3′,4′-Dideoxy-6′-*N*-methylbutirosins, new semisynthetic aminoglycosides. J Antibiot (Tokyo) 31:1031–1038

Takeda K, Aihara K, Furumai T, Ito Y (1979) Biosynthesis of butirosins I. Biosynthetic pathways of butirosins and related antibiotics. J Antibiot (Tokyo) 32:18–28

Taylor HD, Schmitz H (1976) Antibiotics derived from a mutant of *Bacillus circulans*. J Antibiot (Tokyo) 29:532–535
Testa TR, Tilley BC (1975) Biotransformation, a new approach to aminoglycoside biosynthesis. I. Sisomicin. J Antibiot (Tokyo) 28:573–579
Testa RT, Tilley BC (1976) Biotransformation, a new approach to aminoglycoside biosynthesis. II. Gentamicin. J Antibiot (Tokyo) 29:140–146
Testa RT, Tilley BC (1979) Biosynthesis of sisomicin and gentamicin. Jpn J Antibiot 32:S-47–S-59
Testa RT, Wagman GH, Daniels PJL, Weinstein MJ (1974) Mutamicins. Biosynthetically created new sisomicin analogs. J Antibiot (Tokyo) 27:917–921
Tsukiura H, Saito K, Kobaru S, Konishi M, Kawaguchi H (1973) Aminoglycoside antibiotics. IV. BU-1709 E_1 and E_2, new aminoglycoside antibiotics related to the butirosins. J Antibiot (Tokyo) 26:386–388
Turner WB (1971) Fungal metabolites. Academic Press, London New York
Umbarger E, Davis BD (1962) Pathways of amino acid biosynthesis. In: Gunsalus IC, Stanier RY (eds) Biosynthesis. Academic Press, New York London (The bacteria, a treatise on structure and function, vol III, pp 167–251)
Umezawa H (1967) Advances in fundamental research on kanamycin. I. Structure and biosynthesis (in Japanese). J Jpn Med Assoc 58:1328–1334
Umezawa H (1974) Biochemical mechanism of resistance to aminoglycosidic antibiotics. Adv Carbohydr Chem Biochem 30:183–225
Umezawa H (1976) Secondary metabolites of microorganisms – plasmids and biologically active products (in Japanese). Kagaku 46:130–134
Umezawa H (1977) Recent advances in bioactive microbial secondary metabolites. Jpn J Antibiot 30:S-138–S-163
Umezawa S, Tsuchiya T (1969) Fermentation production of aminosugars and biosynthetic mechanism (in Japanese). J Chem Soc Jpn, Industr Chem Sect 72:425–431
Umezawa S, Umino K, Shibahara S, Hamada M, Omoto S (1967) Fermentation of 3-amino-3-deoxy-D-glucose. J Antibiot (Tokyo) Ser A 20:355–360
Umezawa S, Shibahara S, Omoto S, Takeuchi T, Umezawa H (1968) Studies on biosynthesis of 3-amino-3-deoxy-D-glucose. J Antibiot (Tokyo) 21:485–491
Vaněk Z, Majer J (1967) Macrolide antibiotics. In: Gottlieb D, Shaw D (eds) Biosynthesis. Springer, Berlin Heidelberg New York (Antibiotics, vol II, pp 154–188)
Virtanen AI, Hietala PK (1955) Enzymic decarboxylation of γ-hydroxyglutamic acid to α-hydroxy-γ-amino-butyric acid. Acta Chem Scand 9:549–550
Vitális S, Szabó G, Vályi-Nagy T (1963) Comparison of the morphology of streptomycin-producing and nonproducing strains of *Streptomyces griseus*. Acta Biol Acad Sci Hung 14:1–15
Volk WA (1959) The enzymatic formation of D-arabinose 5-phosphate from L-arabinose and adenosine triphosphate by *Propionibacterium pentosaceum*. J Biol Chem 234:1931–1936
Wagman GH, Marquez JA, Watkins PD, Bailey JV, Gentile F, Weinstein MJ (1973) Neomycin production by *Micromonospora* species 69-683. J Antibiot (Tokyo) 26:732–736
Wahl HP, Grisebach H (1979) Biosynthesis of streptomycin dTDP-dihydrostreptose synthase from *Streptomyces griseus* and dTDP-4-keto-L-rhamnose 3,5-epimerase from *S. griseus* and *Escherichia coli* Y10. Biochim Biophys Acta 568:243–252
Wahl HP, Matern U, Grisebach H (1975) Two enzymes in *Streptomyces griseus* for the synthesis of dTDP-L-dihydrostreptose from dTDP-6-deoxy-D-*xylo*-4-hexosulose. Biochem Biophys Res Commun 64:1041–1045
Waitz JA, Miller GH, Moss E Jr, Chiu PJS (1978) Chemotherapeutic evaluation of 5-episisomicin (Sch 22591), a new semisynthetic aminoglycoside. Antimicrob Agents Chemother 13:41–48
Walker JB (1958) Further studies on the mechanism of transamidinase action: Transamidination in Streptomyces griseus. J Biol Chem 231:1–9
Walker JB (1971) Enzymatic reactions involved in streptomycin biosynthesis and metabolism. Lloydia (Cinci) 34:363–371
Walker JB (1974) Biosynthesis of the monoguanidinated inositol moiety of bluensomycin, a possible evolutionary precursor of streptomycin. J Biol Chem 249:2397–2404

Walker JB (1975) Pathways of the guanidinated inositol moieties of streptomycin and bluensomycin. Methods Enzymol 43:429–470

Walker JB (1978) Biosynthesis of aminocyclitols and guanidinocyclitols. In: Wells WW, Elsenberg F Jr (eds) Cyclitols and phosphoinositides. Academic Press, New York, pp 423–438

Walker JB, Skorvaga M (1973a) Phosphorylation of streptomycin and dihydrostreptomycin by *Streptomyces*. Enzymatic synthesis of different diphosphorylated derivatives. J Biol Chem 248:2435–2440

Walker JB, Skorvaga M (1973b) Streptomycin biosynthesis and metabolism. Phosphate transfer from dihydrostreptomycin 6-phosphate to inosamines, streptamine and 2-deoxy-streptamine. J Biol Chem 248:2441–2446

Walker JB, Walker MS (1967a) Enzymatic synthesis of streptidine from *scyllo*-inosamine. Biochemistry 6:3821–3829

Walker JB, Walker MS (1967b) Streptomycin biosynthesis. Enzymatic synthesis of *O*-phosphorylstreptidine from streptidine and adenosinetriphosphate. Biochem Biophys Acta 148:335–341

Walker JB, Walker MS (1967c) Streptomycin biosynthesis. Participation of a phosphatase, aminating enzyme, and kinase in cell-free synthesis of streptidine-*P* from inosamine-*P*. Biochem Biophys Res Commun 26:278–283

Walker JB, Walker MS (1968) Streptomycin biosynthesis. Enzymatic synthesis of *scyllo*-inosamine from *scyllo*-inosose and L-glutamine. Biochim Biophys Acta 170:219–220

Walker JB, Walker MS (1969) Streptomycin biosynthesis. Transamination reactions involving inosamines and inosadiamines. Biochemistry 8:763–770

Walker MS, Walker JB (1964) Biosynthesis of streptomycin. Cell-free transamidination in *Streptomyces griseus*. Biochim Biophys Acta 93:201–203

Walker MS, Walker JB (1965) Evidence for participation of a phosphorylated derivative of streptidine in streptomycin biosynthesis. Biochim Biophys Acta 97:397–398

Walker MS, Walker JB (1966) Enzymic studies on the biosynthesis of streptomycin. Transamidination of inosamine and streptamine derivatives. J Biol Chem 241:1262–1270

Walker MS, Walker JB (1967) Streptomycin biosynthesis. Conversion of *myo*-inositol to *O*-phosphorylstreptidine. Biochim Biophys Acta 136:272–278

Walker MS, Walker JB (1971) Streptomycin biosynthesis. Separation and substrate specificities of phosphatases acting on guanidino-deoxy-*scyllo*-inositol phosphate and streptomycin-(*streptidino*)phosphate. J Biol Chem 246:7034–7040

Wee TG, Frey PA (1973) Studies on the mechanism of action of uridine diphosphate galactose 4-epimerase. II. Substrate-dependent reduction by sodium borohydride. J Biol Chem 248:33–40

White TJ, Davies J (1978) Possible involvement of plasmids in the biosynthesis of paromomycin. Abstr 79 of the 3rd International Symposium on the Genetics of Industrial Microorganisms, University of Wisconsin, Madison, June 4–9. Available from: Publication Office, American Society for Microbiology, 1913 I St., NW, Washington DC 20006

Wright LF, Hopwood DA (1976) Identification of the antibiotic determined by the SCP, plasmid of *Streptomyces coelicolor* A_3-2. J Gen Microbiol 95:96–106

Xue Y-G, Dong K-N, Li M, Zhu Y-F, Yang N-Q (1978) Genetic evidence of the presence of plasmid in *Streptomyces griseus* and its relation to the biosynthesis of streptomycin (in Chinese). Wei Sheng Wu Hsueh Pao 18:195–201 (Chem Abstr 89:193699d)

Yagisawa M, Huang T-S R, Davies JE (1978) Possible involvement of plasmids in biosynthesis of neomycin. J Antibiot (Tokyo) 31:809–813

Yasuda H, Suami T, Ishikawa T, Umezawa S (1975) Preparation of aminocyclitol derivatives (in Japanese). Japan Kokai 50-25,793

Yasuda H, Suami T, Ishikawa T, Umezawa S, Umezawa H (1978) Aminocyclitol derivatives and production thereof (in Japanese). Japan Kokai 53-34,988

Yoshikawa H, Takiguchi H (1976) Effect of alanine in the fermentation of butirosins (in Japanese). Abstr 324 of the 28th Meeting of the Society of Fermentation Technology, Osaka, Oct 25–27. Available from: Business Office, The Society of Fermentation Technology, Japan, Faculty of Engineering, Osaka University, Suita-shi, Osaka 565, Japan

CHAPTER 4

Antibacterial Activity of Aminoglycoside Antibiotics

S. MITSUHASHI

A. Introduction

The discovery of chemotherapeutic agents was a great moment in the long history of medicine. Yet we are now faced with the problems of drug resistance in bacteria only 50 years after the real start of chemotherapy. The presence of resistance (R) factors and their worldwide spread have caused many problems in medicine, stock farming, and the fish breeding industry. In addition, the prevalence of R factors has broadened our perspective on the role that genetic exchange plays in the natural history of bacterial species.

B. Drug Resistance Plasmids

Despite improved sanitation and prophylactic inoculation, the incidence of infections caused by *Shigella* strains did not significantly decrease until 1970 in Japan. Bacillary dysentery was therefore an important problem, and many research committees were organized to study the disease and related bacterial drug resistance.

Soon after the discovery of sulfanilamide (SA), it was found that derivatives of SA were effective against bacillary dysentery as well as infectious diseases caused by gram-positive bacteria, and as a result, a large amount of SA was used in Japan after 1940. But its effectiveness lasted only about 10 years because SA-resistant *Shigella* strains soon appeared and reached a maximum of 80%–90% of all *Shigella* isolates. At about the same time, production started on antibiotics such as streptomycin (SM), tetracycline (TC), and chloramphenicol (CM) which were also quite effective against bacillary dysentery. Soon after the introduction into practical use of these antibiotics, however, *Shigella* strains resistant to TC or SM were isolated in 1952. The first isolation of a multiply resistant *Shigella* strain from a patient with bacillary dysentery occurred in 1952; the strain carried resistance to TC, SM, and SA. In 1955 a *Shigella* strain showing quadruple resistance to TC, SM, SA, and CM was isolated from another patient with bacillary dysentery.

In 1957 our laboratory reported the first isolation in our area of multiply resistant *Shigella* and *Escherichia coli* strains; they were found in specimens obtained during an epidemic in a tuberculosis sanatorium. In 1958 we again isolated *E. coli* and *S. flexneri* 3a strains resistant to TC, CM, SM, and SA in both specimens from two patients infected with *S. flexneri* 3a. In 1959 we isolated *S. flexneri* and *E. coli* strains resistant to (CM, SM, SA) from a patient. From a patient with dysentery we also isolated (TC, CM, SM, SA)-resistant strains of *Citrobacter freundii* and *E. coli*. These observations indicated that multiple resistance was a problem not restricted to *Shigella*; it evidently involved all the enteric bacteria.

I. The Discovery of R Factors

In 1959 independent reports by OCHIAI et al. and by AKIBA et al. (see review by MITSUHASHI 1977) indicated that multiple resistance was transferable by mixed cultivation of *Shigella* and *E. coli*. Their findings were discussed extensively at a meeting held in November 1959, but the processes involved in the transmission of resistance remained a mystery. We used a U-shaped tube fitted with ultrafine fritted glass that was devised by DAVIS (1950), who used it to prove the conjugal transmission of the F factor by cell-to-cell contact. With this method we discovered that the transfer of multiple resistance was not mediated by filtrable agents such as bacteriophages and deoxyribonucleic acids (MITSUHASHI et al. 1960a). Drug resistance was transmitted by mixed cultivation between drug-resistant *E. coli* K 12 F^+ (or Hfr) and drug-sensitive *Shigella*, and between substrains of *E. coli* K 12, regardless of the polarity of the F agent (MITSUHASHI et al. 1960a).

These facts indicated to us that transferable drug resistance was transmitted independently of the donor strain chromosome and that the agent was different from the F factor. Furthermore, we found by chance that the transferable drug resistance agent was spontaneously lost from resistant strains of *Shigella* or *E. coli* during storage in a cooked-meat medium (MITSUHASHI et al. 1060b, c). Similarly, the property of transferable drug resistance was artificially lost from resistant strains of *Shigella* or *E. coli* following treatment with acriflavine (MITSUHASHI et al. 1960c, 1961). These observations favor the view that transmissible drug resistance is carried by an agent which exists extrachromosomally in the bacterial cell. Thus the term "R (resistance) factor" was proposed for the property of transmissible drug resistance (MITSUHASHI 1960).

It was found that R factors are transferable among all species of the family *Enterobacteriaceae*, the *Vibrio* group, *Pasteurella pestis*, *Aeromonas*, and *Bordetella bronchiseptica*. Because the R factor can replicate autonomously and can be transmitted to a wide range of enteric bacteria, it plays an extremely important role in public health and animal husbandry.

II. The Discovery of Nonconjugative Resistance (r) Plasmids

The nonconjugative resistance (r) plasmids are small in size and are nontransferable by conjugation. They confer usually single or double resistance on their host bacteria (INOUE and MITSUHASHI 1980).

Strains of *Staphylococcus aureus* are frequently isolated from clinical sources and play an important role in pathologic lesions. We have collected *S. aureus* strains since 1961 and studied the reasons for the prevalence of drug-resistant strains and for the acquisition of multiple resistance in staphylococci from the epidemiologic and genetic standpoints.

In 1963 we found that cross-resistance to macrolide (Mac) antibiotics in staphylococci was irreversibly eliminated by treatment with acriflavine and was jointly transduced with typing phages 80 and 81, indicating that the determinants governing cross-resistance to Mac antibiotics were located on a single genetic element different from the chromosome, that is, on a plasmid (MITSUHASHI et al. 1963). It was subsequently found that penicillin (PC) resistance was eliminated by treatment with acriflavine (HASHIMOTO et al. 1964; MITSUHASHI et al. 1965, 1973, 1976).

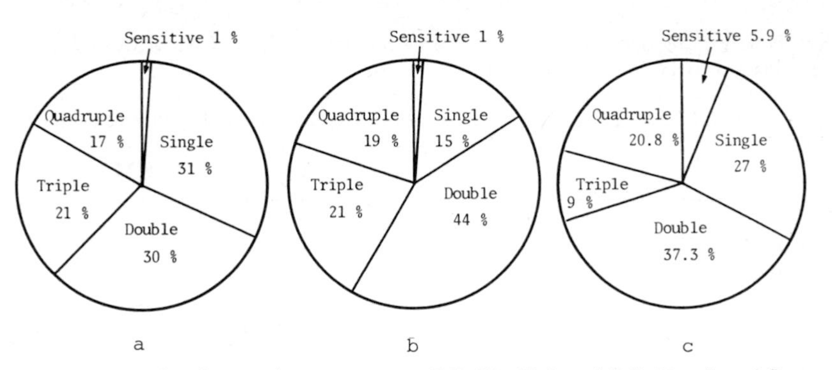

Fig. 1 a–c. Patterns of resistance in *S. aureus* to TC, SA, SM, and PC. (Bracketed figures are percentages.) **a** Summary of results from 2,099 strains isolated between 1961 and 1965. **b** Summary of results from 4,293 strains isolated between 1966 and 1972. **c** Summary of results from 1,948 strains isolated between 1974 and 1976

NOVICK (1963) also proposed the possibility that PC resistance in *S. aureus* is associated with a plasmid and is thus inherited extrachromosomally. As evidence against the possibility of a PC plasmid, however, he reported that no increase in the number of PC-sensitive mutants resulted from propagation in the presence of acriflavine.

We now have various methods to confirm the presence of r plasmids in bacteria, i.e., transformation through DNA isolated from drug-resistant bacteria and transduction to a recombination-deficient (rec^-) recipient from drug-resistant bacteria, indicating that r plasmids exist in many strains of both gram-positive and gram-negative bacteria (MITSUHASHI 1979, 1980).

C. Resistance Patterns of Bacteria

In every species of bacteria there are specific resistance patterns that result from the following factors: (1) the clinical use of drugs, which causes the selection of resistant bacteria, and (2) genetic mechanisms that confer resistance, such as plasmids, transposons, and easily combinable resistance determinants (MITSUHASHI 1977a, 1980).

Staphylococci exhibit resistance to TC, SM, SA, and PC. Strains showing double resistance were isolated most frequently, followed by those with quadruple, triple, and single resistance (Fig. 1). Staphylococci resistant to other drugs, such as Mac antibiotics and kanamycin (KM), were frequently found among those carrying quadruple and triple resistance, indicating that multiply resistant strains easily acquired resistance to other drugs when new drugs were introduced for clinical use (Table 1).

Streptococcus pyogenes strains demonstrate resistance primarily to Mac antibiotics, TC, and CM. Most Mac-resistant strains were found to be additionally resistant to lincomycin (LC). Strains resistant to (Mac, TC, CM) were isolated most frequently, followed by those resistant to double combinations of Mac, TC, and CM, and by those showing single resistance. It was observed that most *S. pyogenes* strains are still sensitive to PC and aminoglycoside antibiotics (Fig. 2).

Table 1. Isolation frequency of *S. aureus* strains resistant to Mac, CM, KM, and SM among strains resistant to TC, SA, SM, and PC

Patterns of resistance to TC, SA, SM, and PC		Isolation frequency (%) of strains resistant to			
		Mac	CM	KM	SM
Single					
1961–1965	(31)[a]	9.6	11.8	8.3	1.0
1966–1969	(15)	9.9	11.0	14.1	1.5
1972	(18)	6.0	8.0	10.0	0
1976	(35)	11.0	8.8	2.4	0
Double					
1961–1965	(30)	21.2	27.4	24.9	13.2
1966–1969	(42)	21.4	27.6	36.1	14.5
1972	(44)	18.0	19.0	18.0	12.8
1976	(28)	20.0	14.7	12.0	11.6
Triple and quadruple					
1961–1965	(38)	69.2	60.8	66.8	85.8
1966–1969	(43)	68.7	61.4	49.8	84.0
1972	(25)	76.0	71.0	74.0	87.2
1976	(37)	69.0	76.5	85.6	88.4

The results are based on surveys of 6,930 strains of clinical isolates. The isolation frequency indicates the distribution of strains resistant to each drug among strains carrying single, double, triple, and quadruple resistance to TC, SA, SM, and PC during the survey period

[a] Figures in brackets indicate total isolation frequency (%) for each resistance pattern during the survey period

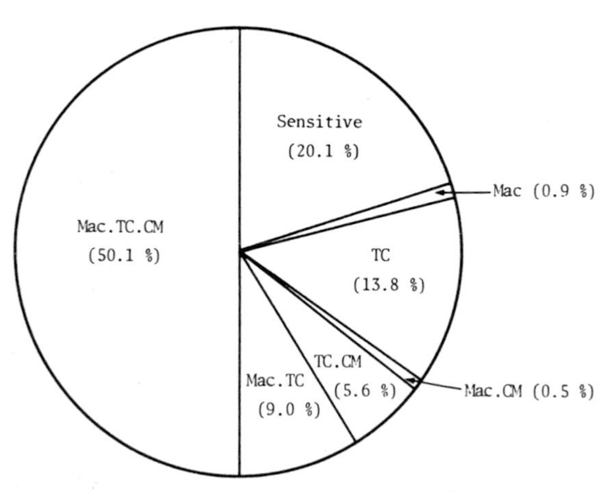

Fig. 2. Resistance patterns of *S. pyogenes* strains. (Bracketed figures are percentages.) Results based on surveys of 2,001 strains isolated between 1970 and 1975

Gram-negative bacteria frequently show specific patterns of resistance to TC, CM, SM, and SA. In the pattern known as the *E. coli–Shigella* type, strains with quadruple resistance were isolated most frequently, followed by those with single, double, and triple resistance. Among strains of *Serratia marcescens*, those with double resistance were isolated most frequently, followed by those showing quad-

Table 2. Bacterial resistance patterns (%) to TC, CM, SM, and SA

Resistance pattern	Organism							
	Shigella	*E. coli*	*K. pneumoniae*	*Salmonella*	*Proteus*		*E. cloacae*	*S. marcescens*
					(indol−)	(indol+)		
Quadruple	91.1	61.6	67.2	13.8	12.7	48.3	26.3	29.5
Triple	6.2	16.4	22.1	57.8	11.6	17.7	28.9	18.9
Double	2.7	20.7	8.8	25.9	12.8	16.9	21.0	33.9
Single	0.1	1.3	1.8	2.4	62.8	16.9	23.8	17.6

The results are based on surveys of 21, 800 strains isolated between 1970 and 1979

ruple and triple resistance, in that order. Among strains of indol(−) *Proteus*, those with single resistance were isolated most frequently and those with quadruple, triple, and double resistance were not isolated frequently (Table 2). In singly resistant strains of *Shigella*, *E. coli*, *Salmonella*, and *Klebsiella*, resistance to SA was most common, followed by resistance to TC, SM, and CM. Characteristically, there are few singly CM- or SM-resistant strains. In the *Proteus* group, 92.6% of all singly resistant strains were TC-resistant; SA-, CM-, and SM-resistant strains were rarely observed in single resistance. Double resistance in *Shigella*, *E. coli*, *Salmonella*, *K. Pneumoniae*, and *S. marcescens* was most frequently seen as (SM, SA) resistance. We also found strains resistant to (TC, SA) and (TC, CM), but we rarely observed resistance to other double combinations of the drugs, indicating that the frequency of resistance to each of the four drugs is not the same in these bacteria. In the *Proteus* group, (TC, CM)-resistant strains were isolated most frequently, followed by those resistant to (TC, SA), (TC, SM), and (SM, SA). In strains of *S. marcescens*, most double resistance appeared as resistance to (TC, SA). Triple resistance was seen most frequently as (TC, SM, SA) or (CM, SM, SA) resistance; we rarely found strains resistant to other triple combinations of the drugs. These results can be explained by the presence of easily combinable resistance determinants, SA, SM, (SM, SA), (CM, SM, SA), (TC, SM, SA), and (TC, CM, SM, SA).

Epidemiologic studies of *Shigella* and *S. aureus* strains disclosed that singly SA-resistant strains quickly appeared and that more than 95% of the strains became SA-resistant 10 years after the introduction into practical use of SA. Singly SA-resistant strains are isolated with a high frequency and most SA resistance is found to be due to the presence of the nonconjugative r(SA) plasmid. According to these results, it can be estimated that the r(SA) plasmid appeared soon after the real start of chemotherapy.

Recent studies have also shown that there are two types of mechanism of SA resistance, i.e., a decrease in the permeability of SA through the cell membrane (type 1) and formation of SA-resistant dihydropteroate synthetase (DHPS) (type 2) (Mitsuhashi et al. 1977a; Mitsuhashi 1979). The mechanism of SA resistance mediated by r(SA), R(SA), r(SM, SA), and R(SM, SA) plasmids is mainly the formation of SA-resistant DHPS. But SA resistance mediated by R plasmids encoding triple and quadruple resistance is due to a decrease in the permeability of

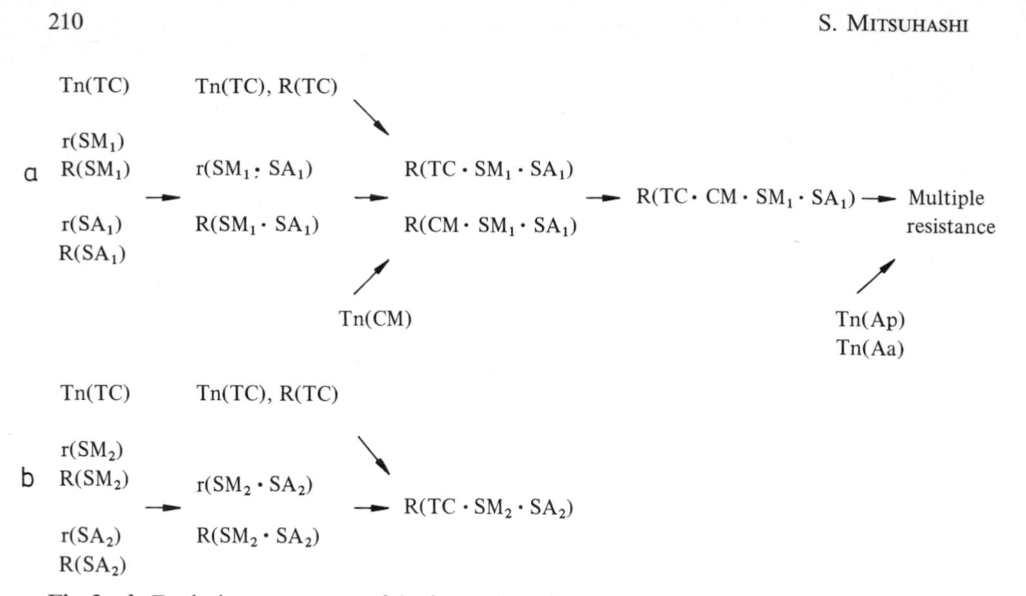

Fig. 3a, b. Evolutionary process of the formation of R plasmids. **a** Main path to the formation of R plasmids carrying multiple resistance. **b** Path to the formation of plasmids carrying resistance to SM_2, SA_2, or both. SM_1, adenylylation of SM; SM_2, phosphorylation of SM; SA_1, decrease in the permeation of SA; SA_2, formation of SA-resistant DHPS; Tn, transposon; Aa, aminoglycoside antibiotics; r, nonconjugative resistance plasmid; R, conjugative resistance plasmid; Ap, ampicillin

the drug through the cell membrane. These results indicate that there are at least two evolutionary routes for the formation of R plasmids encoding multiple resistance: one with a group consisting of plasmids encoding SA, SM, and (SM, SA) resistance, and the other with a group consisting of R(TC, CM, SM, SA), R(TC, SM, SA), and R(CM, SM, SA) plasmids.

There are two types of plasmid-mediated SM resistance, i.e., phosphorylation and adenylylation (see Chap. 6). SM resistance mediated by R(SM), r(SM), R(SM, SA), and r(SM, SA) is mainly due to phosphorylation of the drug (type 2). By contrast, SM resistance mediated by R(CM, TC, SM, SA), R(CM, SM, SA), and R(TC, SM, SA), is mainly due to adenylylation of the drug (type 1). Accordingly, the (SM, SA) resistance mediated by R plasmids encoding triple and quadruple resistance to TC, CM, SM, and SA involves mechanisms of type 1 SA and type 1 SM resistance. By contrast, the SM and SA resistance mediated by plasmids encoding single or double resistance to SA and SM is mostly due to type 2 SM and type 2 SA resistance. Therefore, the evolutionary process of R plasmids to multiple resistance can be accounted for by the following factors: (1) selective force by drugs used, (2) the presence of easily combinable resistance determinants such as SA_1 and SM_1, SA_2 and SM_2, and (3) the presence of transposons. A possible process of the R plasmid evolution is shown in Fig. 3.

We can demonstrate both r and R plasmids encoding SA_2, SM_2, or (SM_2, SA_2) resistance from bacteria of both human and livestock origin, but very few plasmids showing single SA_1 and SM_1 and double (SM_1, SA_1) resistance. By contrast, we can isolate R plasmids carrying multiple resistance including SM_1 and SA_1 resistance at a high frequency. Few R(CM) plasmids are isolated from bacteria of live-

Table 3. Isolation frequency (%) of SM-, KM-, and GM-resistant strains

Strains resistant to	Bacteria										
	S. aureus	*S. pyogenes*	*E. coli*	*Shigella*	*Salmonella*	*Proteus* (indol−)	*Proteus* (indol+)	*Klebsiella*	*E. cloacae*	*S. marcescens*	*P. aeruginosa*
SM	32.0	0	52.0	70.8	37.1	23.0	46.0	41.7	73.7	45.0	97.1
KM	28.0	0	5.9	0.6	10.2	10.0	16.9	12.0	68.4	37.2	99.3
GM	0.1	0	0.2	0	0	0.7	4.2	1.4	47.3	26.1	42.0

The results are based on surveys of 25, 700 strains isolated between 1968 and 1979

stock origin but R(TC,SA), R(SM_1,SA_2), and R(SM_2,SA_1) plasmids were not found from bacteria of either human or livestock origin. These facts indicate that the plasmids encoding SM_1 or SA_1 resistance have been pushed to the formation of R(SM_1,SA_1) and from there to the R plasmids carrying multiple resistance by picking up the CM and TC transposons. The reason why the TC and CM resistance determinants are easily transposed to the R plasmids encoding both SM_1 and SA_1 resistance, resulting in the formation of R(CM, SM_1, SA_1), R(TC, SM_1, SA_1), and R(TC, CM, SM_1, SA_1), still remains to be elucidated.

D. Bacterial Strains Resistant to Aminoglycoside Antibiotics

The isolation frequencies of strains resistant to aminoglycoside antibiotics such as KM, SM, and gentamicin (GM) are shown in Table 3. It should be noted that aminoglycoside- and PC-resistant strains have not been isolated so far from *Streptococcus pyogenes* strains. The isolation frequency of GM-resistant strains is rather low in Japan, except for *Enterobacter cloacae*, *Serratia marcescens*, and *Pseudomonas aeruginosa* strains. The strains resistant to SM and KM are often seen in *E. cloacae*, *S. marcescens*, and *P. aeruginosa*. About 20%–50% of other species of bacterial strains are resistant to SM and the isolation frequency of SM-resistant strains is much higher than that of KM-resistant ones.

Bacterial strains resistant to TC, CM, SM, and SA and to combinations thereof are often seen in gram-negative bacteria, with the relation between SM resistance and the patterns of resistance to TC, CM, SM, and SA in Table 4. Strains resistant to SM are most often seen in quadruply resistant strains to TC, CM, SM, and SA, followed by triply, doubly, and singly resistant ones. Similarly, KM-resistant strains are most often observed among strains carrying quadruple or triple resistance to the four drugs (Table 5).

About 60%–80% of the strains resistant to SM, KM, or GM in gram-negative bacteria were found to bear conjugative R plasmids. In relation to bacterial patterns of resistance to TC, CM, SM, and SA, R plasmids encoding resistance to (TC, CM, SM, SA), (CM, SM, SA), and (TC, SM, SA) are most often seen in clinical isolates, and these plasmids often carry resistance to β-lactam and aminoglycoside antibiotics in addition to SM resistance. The isolation frequency of R plasmids encoding resistance to aminoglycoside antibiotics is rather low in *P. aeruginosa*

Table 4. Relation between SM resistance and resistance patterns to TC, CM, SM, and SA

Resistance[a] patterns	Isolation frequency of SM-resistant strains (%)						
	E. coli	*Shigella*	*Salmonella*	*Proteus*	*Klebsiella*	*S. marcescens*	*E. cloacae*
Quadruple	61.6	91.1	13.8	62.2	67.2	59.7	35.8
Triple	16.4	6.2	57.8	27.1	22.1	27.2	39.3
Double	20.7	2.7	25.9	9.3	8.8	1.3	17.8
Single	1.3	0.1	2.4	1.3	1.8	0	7.1

[a] Resistance patterns to TC, CM, SM, and SA

Table 5. Relation between KM resistance and resistance patterns to TC, CM, SM and SA

Resistance[a] patterns	Isolation frequency of KM-resistant strains (%)						
	E. coli	*Shigella*	*Salmonella*	*Proteus*	*Klebsiella*	*E. cloacae*	*S. marcescens*
Quadruple	64.2	75.9	15.5	75.4	66.7	26.9	65.7
Triple	22.6	8.6	59.9	21.3	20.5	34.6	16.4
Double	7.5	10.3	20.9	3.3	6.4	19.2	16.4
Single	5.7	1.7	3.7	0	1.3	0	1.5
Sensitive	0	3.4	0	0	5.1	19.2	0

[a] Resistance patterns to TC, CM, SM, and SA

Table 6. Isolation frequency (%) of R plasmids carrying SM, KM, or GM resistance from drug-resistant strains

Bacteria resistant to	*E. coli*	*Shigella*	*Salmonella*	*Proteus*	*K. pneumoniae*	*E. cloacae*	*P. aeruginosa*	*S. marcescens*
SM	61.0	85.3	57.3	53.1	60.0	52.0	23.0	65.4
KM	69.0	78.5	62.5	54.5	58.3	58.3	14.0	64.2
GM	89.0	0	0	35.4	66.0	78.6	26.0	66.0

strains compared with that of other species of gram-negative bacteria. By contrast, the nonconjugative resistance (r) plasmids encoding resistance to aminoglycoside antibiotics are often seen in *P. aeruginosa* (Table 6).

I. Drug Resistance Mediated by R Plasmids

Bacterial patterns of resistance to TC, CM, SM, and SA are often seen in gram-negative bacteria, which are mostly mediated by R, r, or both plasmids. R plasmid resistance to TC, CM, SM, and SA or to combinations thereof is shown in Fig. 4. R plasmid-mediated quadruple resistance to TC, CM, SM, and SA is often seen

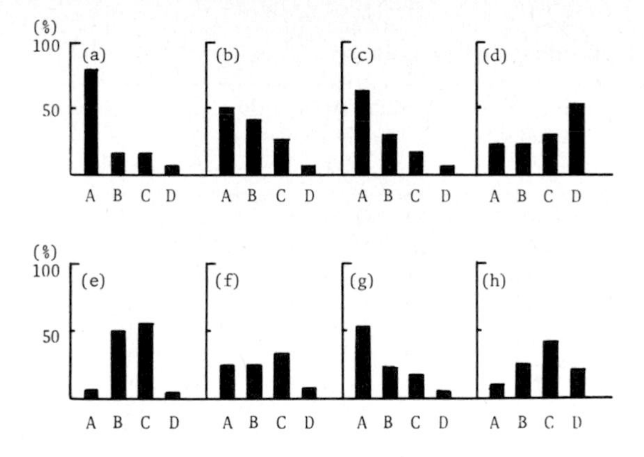

Fig. 4a–h. Patterns of resistance of R plasmids to TC, CM, SM, and SA. *A*, quadruple resistance to TC, CM, SM, and SA; *B*, triple resistance; *C*, double resistance; *D*, single resistance. **a** 1,890 R plasmids from *Shigella;* **b** 680 R plasmids from *E. coli*; **c** 535 R plasmids from *K.* pneumoniae; **d** 970 R plasmids from *Salmonella*; **e** 475 R plasmids from *Proteus*; **f** 145 R plasmids from *P. aeruginosa*; **g** 120 R plasmids from *E. cloacae*; **h** 160 R plasmids from *S. marcescens*

Table 7. Resistance patterns of R plasmids carrying KM resistance

Resistance pattern	No. of R plasmids (%)
TC, CM, SM, SA, APC, KM	18.4
Quintuple resistance	16.5
Quadruple resistance	19.2
Triple resistance	28.9
Double resistance	12.5
Single KM resistance	4.4

The R plasmids (473) carrying KM resistance were isolated from 19,984 strains of gram-negative bacteria including *E. coli*, *Shigella*, *Salmonella*, *K. pneumoniae*, *Proteus*, and *S. marcescens*

in *Shigella*, *E. coli*, *K. Pneumoniae*, and *E. cloacae* strains, followed by triple, double, and single resistance, in that order. In *Proteus* and *S. marcescens*, triple and double resistance are most often observed, followed by quadruple and single resistance. This fact can be accounted for by the low frequency of isolation of R plasmids encoding resistance to CM and TC, which are mostly due to the presence of nonconjugative r(TC) and r(CM) plasmids. It is characteristic that TC-resistant strains, due to the presence of r(TC) plasmids, are often isolated from *Proteus* strains which are mostly nonconjugative.

The resistance patterns of R plasmids carrying KM resistance are shown in Table 7. The R plasmids encoding triple resistance, including resistance to KM, are most often seen, followed by those carrying quadruple, sexituple, and double resistance, in that order.

Table 8. R plasmids encoding single resistance

Organism	No. of plasmids	R plasmids encoding single resistance to							
		TC	CM	SM	SA	KM	APC	GM	Mercury
Shigella	747	49	0	0	0	4	11	0	0
E. coli	247	20	0	0	1	4	9	0	0
Salmonella	330	61	0	1	1	0	5	0	0
K. pneumoniae	360	14	0	0	0	3	7	0	0
Proteus	303	0	0	0	5	0	13	0	0
P. aeruginosa	318	0	0	4	4	0	0	0	95
S. marcescens	304	0	0	0	0	10	1	0	0
Total	2,609	144	0	5	11	21	46	0	95

Table 9. R plasmids encoding double resistance to TC, CM, SM, and SA

Organism	No. of plasmids	R plasmids encoding double resistance to				
		SM SA	TC SM	CM SA	CM TC	TC SA
Shigella	747	79	1	8	0	0
E. coli	247	15	3	1	0	0
Salmonella	330	27	11	0	0	0
K. pneumoniae	360	22	6	1	0	0
Proteus	303	63	3	1	1	0
S. marcescens	304	181	0	0	0	0
Total	2,291	387	24	11	1	0

As shown in Table 8, R plasmids encoding single resistance to aminoglycoside antibiotics are rarely seen among clinical isolates in contrast to the high isolation frequency of R plasmids governing multiple resistance, including resistance to aminoglycoside antibiotics. It should be noted that R(SM, SA) plasmids are most often seen among the R plasmids encoding double resistance, resulting in the evolutionary formation of R plasmids carrying multiple resistance, i.e., R(TC, SM, SA), R(CM, SM, SA), R(CM, TC, SM, SA), and R plasmids encoding resistance to β-lactam and aminoglycoside antibiotics in addition to the four drugs (Table 9).

Nonconjugative resistance (r) plasmids are often isolated from *S. aureus* (MITSUHASHI et al. 1961, 1973, 1976) and from *S. pyogenes* (NAKAE et al. 1975) which carry mostly single resistance to TC, SA, CM, PC, Mac, etc. Ampicillin (APC) resistance in *Haemophilus influenzae* and *Neisseria gonorrhoeae* is mediated by r plasmids and the isolation frequency of r plasmids from gram-negative rods carrying nonconjugative resistance is rather high (Table 10). The plasmid-mediated resistance patterns of natural isolates are summarized in Fig. 5. Plasmid-mediated resistance in *H. influenzae*, *N. gonorrhoeae*, and *S. pyogenes* is type 1 and multiple resistance of *S. aureus* strains is due to the presence of various r plasmids in a cell (type 2). In gram-negative rods, types 5 and 6 are most often seen in natural isolates from humans and livestock.

1.	r	3.	R	5.	R + r
2.	$r_1 + r_2 + r_3$	4.	$R_1 + R_2$	6.	$R + r_1 + r_2$

Fig. 5. The type of resistance mediated by plasmids. R, conjugative resistance plasmid; r, nonconjugative resistance plasmid

Table 10. Isolation frequency of nontransferable resistance (r) plasmids from bacteria carrying nontransferable resistance

Bacteria	Isolation frequency of r plasmids (%)
S. aureus	85.0
S. pyogenes	95.0
H. influenzae	56.0
E. coli	96.0
Shigella	98.0
Salmonella	96.2
P. mirabilis	89.6
E. cloacae	87.5
S. marcescens	89.5
P. aeruginosa	95.3

The presence of r plasmids was examined from 740 clinical isolates carrying nontransferable resistance

Table 11. Resistance patterns of r plasmids

Organism	Resistance pattern(s) of r plasmids
S. aureus	TC, CM, SM, SA, PC, Mac, (PC, Mac)
S. pyogenes	APC
H. influenzae	APC
N. gonorrhoeae	APC
Enterobacteriaceae	TC, SA, APC, SM, CM, KM, (SM, SA), (SM, SA, Aa), (SM, SA, APC)[a]
P. aeruginosa	(SM, SA), (SA, Aa), (SA, APC), (SM, SA, Hg), (SM, SA, Aa), (SM, SA, APC)
S. marcescens	TC, CM, (SM, SA), (SA, Aa), (SA, APC), (SM, SA, Aa), (SM, SA, APC)

[a] Aa = aminoglycoside antibiotics

The resistance patterns mediated by r plasmids are shown in Table 11. The r plasmids mediating double resistance are often seen as r(SM, SA), r(SA, Aa), and r(SA, APC), and the plasmids encoding triple resistance are often found as r(SM, SA, Aa) and r(SM, SA, APC) plasmids.

II. Antibacterial Activity of Aminoglycoside Antibiotics

The chemical structures of aminoglycoside antibiotics are summarized in Fig. 6, and the sites of inactivation of these drugs are indicated (see also Chap. 6).

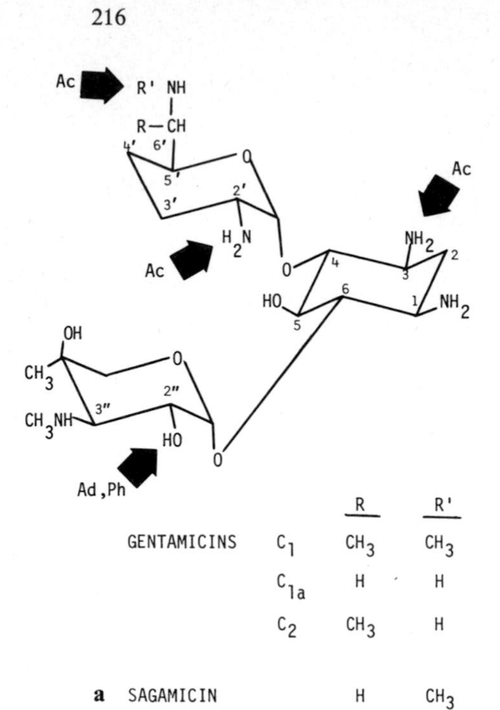

		R	R'
GENTAMICINS	C_1	CH_3	CH_3
	C_{1a}	H	H
	C_2	CH_3	H
a SAGAMICIN		H	CH_3

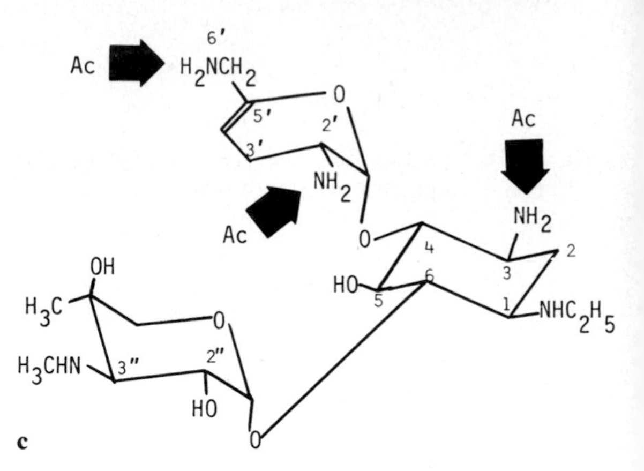

c

Ac

6'

R_1CH_2

Ad R_3 4' 5' O Ac

R_4 3' 2' R_2 NH_2

Ph Ac O 4 3 2 2-Deoxystreptamine

$HOCH_2$ HO 6 1 NHR_5

HO O 5

H_2N 3" 2" Kanosamine

HO O

Ad,Ph

	R_1	R_2	R_3	R_4	R_5
Kanamycin A	NH_2	OH	OH	OH	H
Kanamycin B	NH_2	NH_2	OH	OH	H
Kanamycin C	OH	NH_2	OH	OH	H
Amikacin	NH_2	OH	OH	OH	$CO-CH(OH)-CH_2CH_2NH_2$
Dibekacin	NH_2	NH_2	H	H	H
b Tobramycin	NH_2	NH_2	OH	H	H

Fig. 6a, b

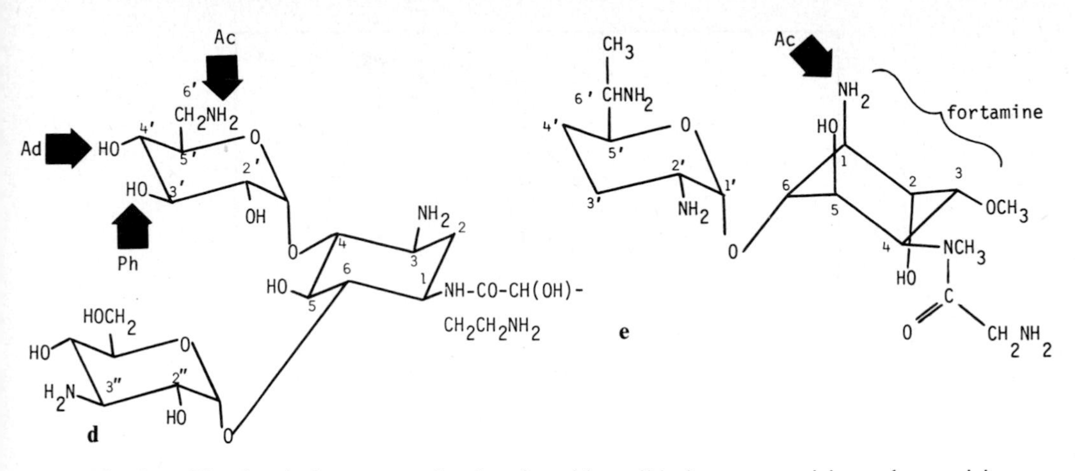

Fig. 6a–e. The chemical structure of aminoglycoside antibiotics. **a** gentamicins and sagamicin; **b** kanamycins; **c** netilmicin; **d** amikacin; **e** fortimicin. *Arrows* indicate the site of inactivation. Ac, acetylation; Ad, adenylylation; Ph, phosphorylation

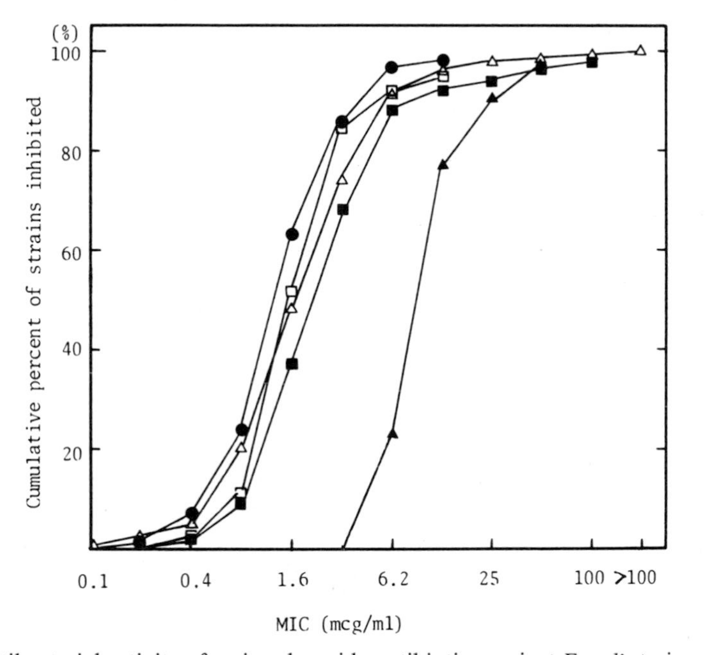

Fig. 7. Antibacterial activity of aminoglycoside antibiotics against *E. coli* strains. ▲, amikacin (AK); ●, gentamicin (GM); △, sagamicin (SG); □, tobramycin (TB); ■, 3′,4′-dideoxykanamycin B (DKB)

The antibacterial activity of aminoglycoside antibiotics against clinical isolates was examined using *E. coli*, *P. aeruginosa*, and *S. marcescens* strains. As shown in Fig. 7, GM, tobramycin (TB), sagamicin (SG), and dibekacin (DKB) exhibited almost the same activity against *E. coli* strains, and amikacin (AK) was slightly less active toward the organism. The antibacterial activity of TB against *P. aeruginosa*

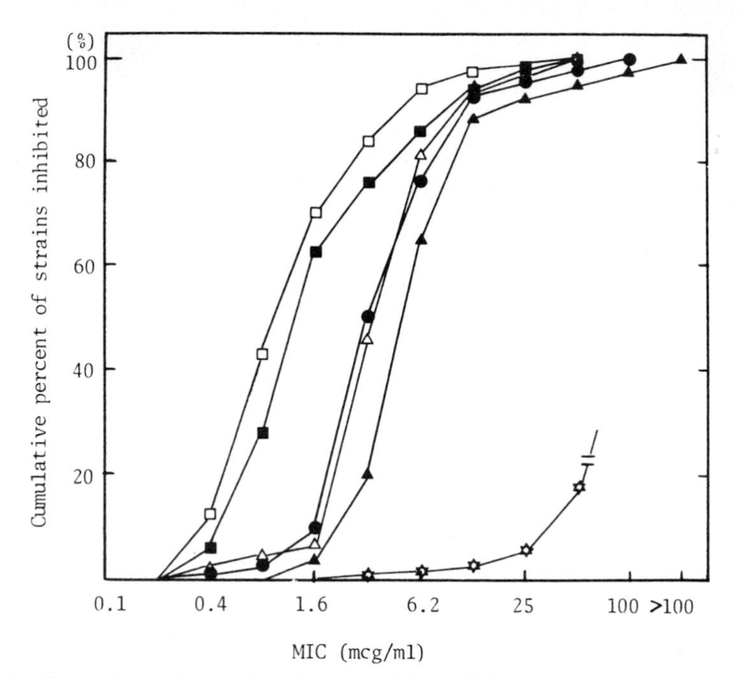

Fig. 8. Antibacterial activity of aminoglycoside antibiotics against *P. aeruginosa* strains. For symbols, see the legend to Fig. 6. ✡, kanamycin (KM)

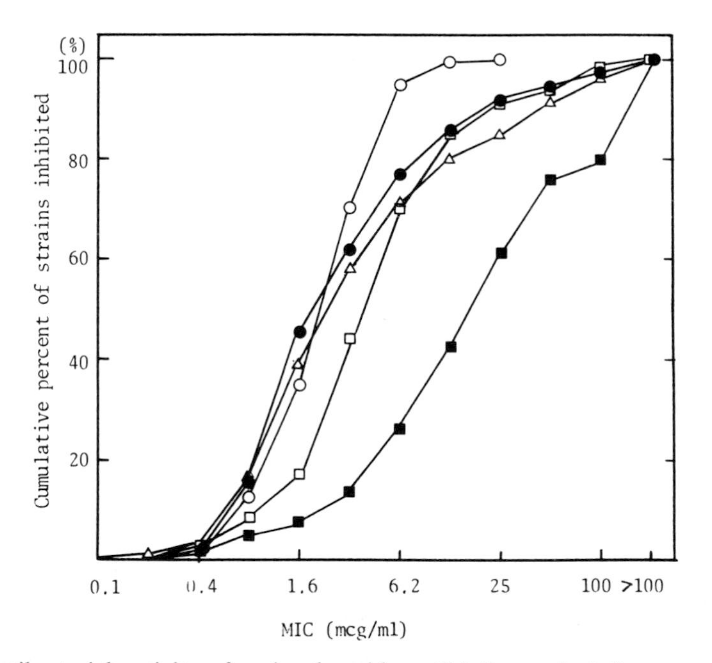

Fig. 9. Antibacterial activity of aminoglycoside antibiotics against *S. marcescens* strains. For symbols, see the legend to Fig. 6. o, fortimicin (FT)

Table 12. Inactivation of aminoglycoside antibiotics by aminoglycoside-inactivating enzymes

Drug	Inactivating enzyme														
	APH(3′)-I	APH(3′)-II	APH(3′)-III	AAC(2′)	AAC(6′)-I	AAC(6′)-II	AAC(6′)-III	AAC(6′)-IV	AAC(3)-I	AAC(3)-II	AAC(3)-III	AAC(3)-IV	AAD(4′)	AAD(2″)	APH(2″)
KM	+	+	+	−	+	+	+	+	−	+	+	+	+	+	+
FT	−	−	−	−	−	−	−	−	+	−	−	−	−	−	−
AK	−	−	−	−	−	−	−	+	−	−	−	−	+	−	+
NT	−	−	−	+	−	+	+	+	−	+	+	+	−	−	−(or +)

strains was the highest, followed by that of DKB, GM, SG, and AK (Fig. 8). Against *S. marcescens* strains, the antibacterial activity of fortimicin (FT) was the highest, with a sharp slope of the cumulative percentage curve of inhibited strains, followed by that of GM, SG, TB, and DKB (Fig. 9).

The stability of aminoglycoside antibiotics to aminoglycoside-inactivating enzymes is summarized in Table 12. FT is inactivated only by AAC(3)-I. AK is inactivated by AAC(6′)-IV, AAD(4′), and APH(2″), resulting in a low isolation frequency of strains resistant to FT or AK. By contrast, the isolation frequencies of strains resistant to KM, GM, SG, netilmicin (NT), etc., have already increased in number due to the spread of plasmids mediating the production of enzymes capable of inactivating the drugs.

E. Conclusion

Aminoglycoside antibiotics are some of the most active agents against various species of bacteria, except anaerobic ones. Parallel to the increase in the amount of the drugs used, bacterial strains multiply resistant to the drugs have often been found in clinical isolates. It should be noted that bacterial resistance to aminoglycoside antibiotics is mostly due to the presence of drug resistance plasmids. Plasmids encoding single resistance to aminoglycoside antibiotics are rarely found in clinical isolates and plasmids carrying resistance to aminoglycoside antibiotics are capable of conferring multiple resistance to TC, CM, SM, SA, and β-lactam antibiotics. Because the inactivation sites of the drugs are the amino and hydroxy groups, plasmid-mediated resistance often results in cross-resistance to several aminoglycoside antibiotics.

References

Davis BD (1950) Nonfiltrability of the agents of genetic recombination in *Escherichia coli*. J Bacteriol 60:507–508

Hashimoto H, Kono K, Mitsuhashi S (1964) Elimination of penicillin resistance of *Staphylococcus aureus* by treatment with acriflavine. J Bacteriol 88:261–262

Inoue M, Mitsuhashi S (1980) The discovery of non-transferable drug resistance (r) plasmids. In: Mitsuhashi S (ed) Bacterial drug resistance. Kodansha, Tokyo, p 19

Mitsuhashi S (1960) Drug-resistance of enteric bacteria (in Japanese). Science (Tokyo) 30:628–633
Mitsuhashi S (1977) Epidemiology of bacterial drug resistance. In: Mitsuhashi S (ed) R factor-drug resistance plasmid. Japan Scientific Societies Press, University Park Press, Tokyo Baltimore, p 3
Mitsuhashi S (1979) Drug resistance plasmids. Molecular Cellular Biochem 26:135–181
Mitsuhashi S (1980) The epidemiology of bacterial resistance. In: Mitsuhashi S (ed) Bacterial drug resistance-R plasmids. Kodansha, Tokyo, p 6
Mitsuhashi S, Harada K, Hashimoto H (1960a) Multiple resistance of enteric bacteria and transmission of drug-resistance to other strains by mixed cultivation. Jpn J Exp Med 30:179–184
Mitsuhashi S, Hashimoto H, Harada K, Suzuki M, Kameda M, Matsuyama T (1960b) Multiple resistance of *S. flexneri* 3a and *E. coli* isolated from the epidemy in Gunma Prefecture (in Japanese). Jpn J Bacteriol 15:844–848
Mitsuhashi S, Harada K, Kameda M (1960c) Elimination of transmissible drug-resistance by treatment with acriflavine (in Japanese). Tokyo Iji Shinshi 77:462
Mitsuhashi S, Harada K, Kameda M (1961) Elimination of transmissible drug-resistance by treatment with acriflavine. Nature 189:947
Mitsuhashi S, Morimura M, Kono K, Oshima H (1963) Elimination of drug resistance of *Staphylococcus aureus* by treatment with acriflavine. J Bacteriol 86:162–163
Mitsuhashi S, Hashimoto H, Kono M, Morimura M (1965) Joint elimination and joint transduction of the determinants of penicillinase production and resistance to macrolide antibiotics. J Bacteriol 89:988–992
Mitsuhashi S, Inoue M, Kawabe H, Oshima H, Okubo T (1973) Genetic and biochemical studies of drug resistance in staphylococci. In: Jeljaszewicz J (ed) Staphylococci and staphylococcal infections. Karger, Basel, p 144
Mitsuhashi S, Inoue M, Oshima H, Okubo T, Saito T (1976) Epidemiologic and genetic studies of drug resistance in staphylococci. In: Jeljaszewicz J (ed) Staphylococci and staphylococcal diseases. Fischer, Stuttgart New York, p 255
Mitsuhashi S, Kawabe H, Nagate T, Inoue K (1977a) Evolutionary process of the formation of multiple resistance plasmid. In: Drews J, Hoegenauer G (eds) Topics in infectious diseases, vol 2, Springer, Berlin Heidelberg New York, p 165
Nakae M, Inoue M, Mitsuhashi S (1975) Artificial elimination of drug resistance from group A beta-hemolytics streptococci. Antimicrob Agents Chemother 7:719–720
Novick RP (1963) Analysis by transduction of mutation affecting penicillinase formation in *Staphylococcus aureus*. J Gen Microbiol 33:121–136

CHAPTER 5

Mechanism of Action of Aminoglycoside Antibiotics

N. TANAKA

A. The Effects on Bacterial Cells and Their Components

I. In vivo Effects on Bacteria in Relation to Mode of Action

Aminoglycoside antibiotics are, in general, bactericidal, showing a broad antimicrobial spectrum, and are active against mycobacteria, staphylococci, and gram-negative bacteria. Spectinomycin and kasugamycin are bateriostatic. Since the early finding that streptomycin affects protein synthesis in susceptible cells (FITZGERALD et al. 1948), extensive studies have been carried out on the effects of aminoglycosides on sensitive bacteria. Eukaryotic cells are resistant to most aminoglycosides.

The lethal action of streptomycin or kanamycin is reversed by various inhibitors of protein synthesis such as chloramphenicol, erythromycin, mikamycin A, blasticidin S, and tetracycline, but it is stimulated by puromycin (ANAND and DAVIS 1960; YAMAKI and TANAKA 1963; WHITE and WHITE 1964). These effects of protein synthesis inhibitors favor the assumption that killing depends on ribosomal activity in protein synthesis or the normal ribosomal cycle must be in operation for the aminoglycosides to exert a bactericidal action.

HERZOG (1964) found that cells treated with streptomycin contain an abnormally high content of "stuck" monoribosomes, which are resistant to dissociation in low concentrations of Mg^{2+}. This observation suggests that the antibiotic interferes with chain termination or with initiation and freezes the ribosomes as 70 S particles. The polysome level decreases in cells treated with streptomycin, resulting in accumulation of monoribosomes, bearing mRNA and fMet-tRNA, which are incapable of protein synthesis in vivo and in vitro (LUZZATTO et al. 1968, 1969 a, b; KOGUT and PRIZANT 1970), and which show impaired responsiveness to initiation factor 3 (IF-3) (WALLACE and DAVIS 1973; WALLACE et al. 1973 b). These findings also suggest that the antibiotic acts on peptide chain initiation, and the accumulated monoribosomes are ribosomes blocked in aberrant initiation complexes. Unlike streptomycin, the antibiotics neomycin, spectinomycin, chloramphenicol, and tetracycline accumulate polysomes, suggesting that these drugs may act on peptide elongation (GURGO et al. 1969).

Most aminoglycoside antibiotics, except kasugamycin and spectinomycin, cause phenotypic suppression or in vivo codon misreading (see Sect. A.V.2).

In addition to interfering with protein synthesis, aminoglycosides induce membrane damage (ANAND and DAVIS 1960; DUBIN et al. 1963), impairment of respiration (DUBIN et al. 1963), RNA accumulation (STERN et al. 1966), and cell death in susceptible cells. Electron microscopic studies (IIDA and KOIKE 1974) have revealed that aminoglycoside antibiotics promote the formation of blebs of the cell envelope.

The most distinct in vivo effects of aminoglycoside antibiotics on bacterial cells are inhibition of protein synthesis and membrane damage. Mutation of ribosomes or addition of protein synthesis inhibitors eliminates the membrane damage, suggesting that the target or receptor of aminoglycosides is the ribosome, and the membrane damage is a secondary effect, resulting from the interference with ribosomal functions. However, the mode of action of aminoglycoside antibiotics may be different from that of chloramphenicol, tetracyclines, macrolides, and other inhibitors of ribosomal functions, because most aminoglycosides promote codon misreading in vivo and in vitro, and cause membrane damage. Moreover, most of the aminoglycosides are bactericidal drugs; but chloramphenicol, tetracyclines, and macrolides are bacteriostatic.

II. Interference with Protein Synthesis in vitro

The inhibitory effects of streptomycin on initiation, elongation, and termination of protein synthesis are pleiotropic effects due to the same interaction of the antibiotic with the ribosome. Of the aminoglycoside group of antibiotics, the mechanism of action of streptomycin has been studied most extensively and all the other aminoglycosides were considered to have a similar mode of action. However, considerable evidence has recently accumulated, showing that the details of the method by which aminoglycosides prevent ribosomal functions differ with different antibiotics. Most of the aminoglycosides (streptomycin, kanamycin, gentamicin, neomycin, etc.) strongly stimulate codon misreading, but kasugamycin and spectinomycin do so only slightly. Initiation of protein synthesis is affected by various aminoglycosides in diverse ways (see Sect. A.V.1). Recently, the translocation of peptidyl-tRNA on the ribosome has been observed to be inhibited by kanamycin, gentamicin, neomycin, and related antibiotics, but not by streptomycin (MISUMI et al. 1978 b; CABAÑAS et al. 1978 a, b; MISUMI and TANAKA 1980). The two groups of aminoglycosides also differ from each other in their interaction with the ribosome and ribosomal subunits (see Sect. A.IV). The detailed mechanism of protein synthesis inhibition or interaction with the ribosome will be described in subsequent sections. Several reviews on the subject have appeared lately: SCHLESSINGER and MEDOFF (1975), TANAKA (1975 a), PESTKA (1977), WALLACE et al. (1979), and VÁZQUEZ (1979).

III. Localization of Drug Sensitivity, Resistance, and Dependence on the Ribosome

The bacterial or prokaryotic ribosome has a molecular weight of 2.7×10^6 daltons and a sedimentation constant of 70 S; it consists of large (50 S) and small (30 S) subunits. The 50 S subunit is made up of 34 proteins (L 1–L 34) and 2 species of RNA (23 S and 5 S); the 30 S subunit is composed of 21 proteins (S 1–S 21) and a single kind of RNA (16 S). S 20 protein of the small subunit is identical with L 26 protein of the large subunit.

The inhibition by streptomycin of protein synthesis is attributed to bacterial ribosomes (SPOTTS and STANIER 1961; FLAKS et al. 1962; MAGER et al. 1962; SPEYER et al. 1962). Furthermore, sensitivity and resistance to, and dependence on, streptomycin are determined by the 30 S ribosomal subunit (COX et al. 1964; DAVIES et al. 1964; LIKOVER and KURLAND 1967). Reconstitution experiments have shown that ribosomal protein S 12, in *Escherichia coli*, is responsible for streptomycin sensitivity and resistance, which is coded for by the *strA* gene (OZAKI et al. 1969). The 30 S ribosomal particle reconstituted with S 12 from a streptomycin-resistant mutant and all other proteins from a susceptible strain, is resistant to the antibiotic. Conversely, the particle reconstituted with S 12 from sensitive cells and all other proteins from a resistant mutant, is sensitive to the drug. Moreover, the source of 16 S RNA (from either sensitive or resistant ribosomes) does not influence the ability of the 30 S particle to bind dihydrostreptomycin. Resistant mutants show diverse point alterations in S 12 protein. In some mutants, lysine at position 42 is replaced by asparagine, threonine, or arginine, and in others lysine at position 87 is replaced by arginine (FUNATSU and WITTMANN 1972; FUNATSU et al. 1972 b). A different type of mutant has been reported, in which one tyrosine is replaced by phenylalanine and one valine by alanine (BRAKIER-GINGRAS et al. 1974). Streptomycin dependence is due to alteration of S 12. The reversion from streptomycin dependence to independence is sometimes associated with mutations of S 4 or S 5 protein (BIRGE and KURLAND 1970; HASENBANK et al. 1973; OLSSON et al. 1974). There are some streptomycin-resistant or -dependent mutants, in which S 4, S 5, and S 12 proteins are altered (WITTMANN and APIRION 1975).

By reconstitution methods similar to those employed for streptomycin, sensitivity and resistance to other aminoglycoside antibiotics have been studied. Thus ribosomal protein S 5 is responsible for spectinomycin sensitivity and resistance (BOLLEN et al. 1969; FUNATSU et al. 1972 a). The mutational alteration for neamine resistance is linked to S 17 protein (BOLLEN et al. 1975), in which histidine at position 30 is replaced by proline (YAGUCHI and WITTMANN 1976). In a kanamycin-resistant mutant, the resistance is located in the 23 S core of the 30 S ribosomal subunit (MASUKAWA et al. 1968 b), in which S 12 protein is altered (MASUKAWA 1969). Protein L 6 of the 50 S ribosomal subunit is changed in gentamicin-resistant mutants, which show cross-resistance to kanamycin, neomycin, and streptomycin, and reduced codon misreading activity in the presence of aminoglycosides (BUCKEL et al. 1977; KÜHBERGER et al. 1979). Recently we have isolated kanamycin-resistant mutants of *E. coli*, showing various degrees of cross-resistance to gentamicin, neomycin, and streptomycin. Resistance is linked to the 30 S ribosomal subunit in some of the mutants and to the 50 S ribosomal subunit in the others (CHOI et al. 1980).

The kasugamycin resistance of *E. coli* is associated with 16 S RNA, but not with proteins, of the 30 S ribosomal subunit. Resistance is attributed to lack of methylation of 16 S RNA. The 16 S RNA from the resistant mutant differs from the sensitive one in that it lacks methylation of two adjacent adenine residues near the 3′ end of the molecule. The sensitive strain contains an RNA methylase which is able to methylate the 16 S RNA from the resistant mutant. The 21 S core particle is a substrate for the methylase, but the isolated 16 S RNA is not. Methylation converts resistant 16 S RNA into sensitive material. This methylase is lacking or inactive in the resistant cells (HELSER et al. 1971, 1972). The mutation maps near the leucine region and far from the *strA* gene (SPARLING 1970). Another type of kasugamycin resistance is attributed to an alteration of ribosomal protein S 2 (OKUYAMA et al. 1974).

IV. Interaction with Ribosomes and Ribosomal Components

Since the binding of aminoglycoside antibiotics to ribosomes and ribosomal proteins is weak or reversible, it is usually studied by equilibrium dialysis and/or nitrocellulose filtration methods using radioactive antibiotics, but not by centrifugation or gel filtration.

1. Binding of Streptomycin to the Ribosome and Ribosomal Subunits

The binding of streptomycin or dihydrostreptomycin to 70 S ribosomes and the 30 S subunit from susceptible bacteria is well established (LEON and BROCK 1967; WOLFGANG and LAWRENCE 1967; KAJI and TANAKA 1968; OZAKI et al. 1969); a single binding site (CHANG and FLAKS 1972a, b; SCHREINER and NIERHAUS 1973) or two binding sites (KAJI and TANAKA 1968; BISWAS and GORINI 1972) have been postulated. The contradictory reports on the amount of dihydrostreptomycin binding to the 30 S subunit (0.3–2 molecules) seem to be due to ionic conditions, particularly monovalent ion (NH_4^+) concentrations, and the condition of the ribosomes, i.e., amounts of bound initiation factors, mRNA and tRNA.

CHANG and FLAKS (1972a, b) have reported that *E. coli* 70 S ribosomes bind one molecule of dihydrostreptomycin at concentrations up to 10 μM; Ka is 10^7 M^{-1} for 70 S ribosomes and 10^6 M^{-1} for the 30 S subunit. The binding is independent of temperature and requires Mg^{2+}.

2. Binding Site of Streptomycin on the Ribosome

Reconstitution experiments have shown that streptomycin resistance and dependency are attributed to alteration of ribosomal protein S 12 (OZAKI et al. 1969; BIRGE and KURLAND 1969). The S 12 protein controls the binding of the antibiotic to the ribosome, but itself neither binds streptomycin nor forms a part of the binding site. None of the separated ribosomal proteins binds streptomycin, and the conformation of the 30 S ribosomal subunit seems to be needed for drug binding.

CHANG and FLAKS (1970) have found, by successive treatment of the 30 S ribosomal subunit with trypsin, that the removal of S 9 and S 14 results in a loss of dihydrostreptomycin binding. SCHREINER and NIERHAUS (1973) have observed that the 30 S subunit loses the capacity to bind dihydrostreptomycin by washing in 1.15–2.0 *M* LiCl. Of proteins eliminated, S 3 and S 5 can restore binding by the nonbinding core, and the ability of S 3 + S 5 is increased by the addition of S 9, S 10, and S 14; but the binding is independent of the presence of S 12 protein.

By treating ribosomes with graded concentrations of *N*-ethylmaleimide, a blocker of the sulfhydryl group, GINZBURG et al. (1973) have assigned S 1, S 14, and S 21 to the streptomycin binding site.

Two groups of investigators have obtained different results concerning the streptomycin binding site by affinity labeling of ribosomes with different photoactive analogs of streptomycin; i.e., PONGS and ERDMANN (1973) have labeled S 3 and S 4 proteins, and GIRSHOVICH et al. (1976) S 7, S 14 , and S 16/S 17.

LELONG et al. (1974) have studied the binding site of streptomycin, using specific immunoglobulin fragments (Fab) for 30 S ribosomal proteins, and found that antibodies directed against S 1, S 10, S 11, S 18, S 19, S 20, and S 21 interfere with the binding of dihydrostreptomycin to 30 S or 70 S ribosomes. Monovalent antibody against S 12 protein does not appreciably impair the binding.

As described above, the diverse results presented by a number of investigators using different methods make it impossible to specify any ribosomal protein(s) for the binding site of streptomycin. BISWAS and GORINI (1972) and GARVIN et al. (1974) have presented evidence that 16 S RNA is the attachment site of streptomycin to the 30 S ribosomal subunit and binds two molecules of the antibiotic per RNA molecule. 16 S RNA derived from either streptomycin-sensitive or -resistant ribosomes, but not 23 S RNA, shows the same capability of binding the drug; S 12 protein may control the availability of streptomycin binding sites of 16 S RNA.

Although the precise binding site of streptomycin is not well established, WALLACE et al. (1979) have suggested that the binding site is present in the region between the platform and cleft in the 30 S ribosomal subunit (LAKE 1976) or the similar region between the head and neck (STÖFFLER and WITTMANN 1977), where S 4, S 12, and the 3′ terminus of 16 S RNA are located. They maintain that this assumption can explain the inhibition of various ribosomal functions by the antibiotic.

3. Binding of Kanamycin to the Ribosome and Ribosomal Subunits

We have found that viomycin, a peptide antibiotic, inhibits initiation of protein synthesis and translocation of peptidyl-tRNA on ribosomes, and binds to both 30 S and 50 S subunits of ribosomes (LIOU and TANAKA 1976; MISUMI et al. 1978 a). During the studies on the mechanism of action of viomycin, we employed kanamycin as a control drug, and observed that kanamycin also blocks translocation (MISUMI et al. 1978 b) as well as initiation (OKUYAMA et al. 1972; OKUYAMA and TANAKA 1972). The similarity of the effects on ribosomal functions of kanamycin and viomycin suggests that kanamycin may interact with both ribosomal subunits, as does viomycin; the assumption has been tested by studying the binding of [^{3}H]kanamycin (6.3 Ci/mol) to the ribosome and ribosomal subunits of *E. coli*, using equilibrium dialysis and nitrocellulose (Millipore) filtration methods (MISUMI et al. 1978 b).

The binding of kanamycin to the ribosome reaches an equilibrium within 5 min and is relatively temperature-independent in the range 0°–37 °C. Optimal binding requires 10 m*M* Mg^{2+}. Equilibrium dialysis experiments have been carried out over a range of [^{3}H]kanamycin concentrations; the concentration dependence on kanamycin for binding is presented in Fig. 1. Using 1 μ*M* *E. coli* ribosomes or ribosomal subunits and a drug concentration range of 0.3–10 μ*M*, there is a progressive increase of binding up to 2.2 molecules per ribosome, with more kanamycin binding to the ribosome at higher antibiotic concentrations, indicating that the ribosome has more than two binding sites for the antibiotic. In the binding curve with the small ribosomal subunit, over a [^{3}H]kanamycin concentration range of 0.3–8 μ*M* the binding increases with increasing drug concentrations up to a plateau

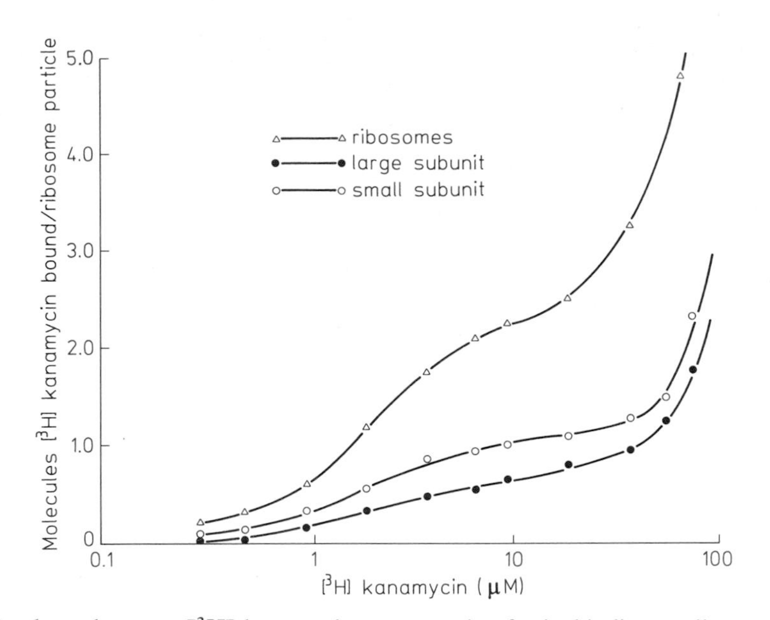

Fig. 1. The dependence on [^{3}H] kanamycin concentration for its binding to ribosomes and ribosomal subunits (MISUMI et al. 1978b). △—△, ribosomes; ●—●, large subunit; ○—○, small subunit

level of approximately one molecule per subunit, and additional molecules are attached to the subunit over an antibiotic concentration of 40 μ*M*. With the large ribosomal subunit, a similar tendency is observed. Binding reaches a plateau of ~0.8 molecule per subunit at drug concentrations from 8 to 40 μ*M* and more kanamycin binds to the subunit at concentrations above 60 μ*M*. The results indicate that the affinity of kanamycin for the small ribosomal subunit is similar to that for the large subunit.

The Scatchard plot of data for equilibrium binding of kanamycin to ribosomes and ribosomal subunits is shown in Fig. 2. There appears to be a linear relationship between r and r/A, where r is the number of molecules of bound [^{3}H]kanamycin per ribosome or subunit, and A is the molar concentration of free [^{3}H]kanamycin. The 70 S ribosome seems to possess two major binding sites with an apparent association constant of approximately 7.4×10^5 M^{-1}, and more binding sites with lower association constants. The binding sites on each ribosomal subunit include one with stronger affinity (association constant 4.0×10^5 M^{-1} for the 50 S subunit and 5.5×10^5 M^{-1} for the 30 S subunit), and more with less affinity. The results indicate that kanamycin binds not only to the 30 S ribosomal subunit but also to the 50 S ribosomal subunit, and each subunit possesses one major binding site. The effects of some antibiotics on the binding of [^{3}H]kanamycin to ribosomes and ribosomal subunits have been examined by the equilibrium dialysis technique (Table 1). The binding of radioactive material to the ribosome and its subunits is decreased to approximately one-tenth by the addition of a tenfold higher concentration of unlabeled kanamycin. The results indicate that the observed binding is specific for kanamycin. Neomycin reverses the binding of [^{3}H]kanamycin to ribo-

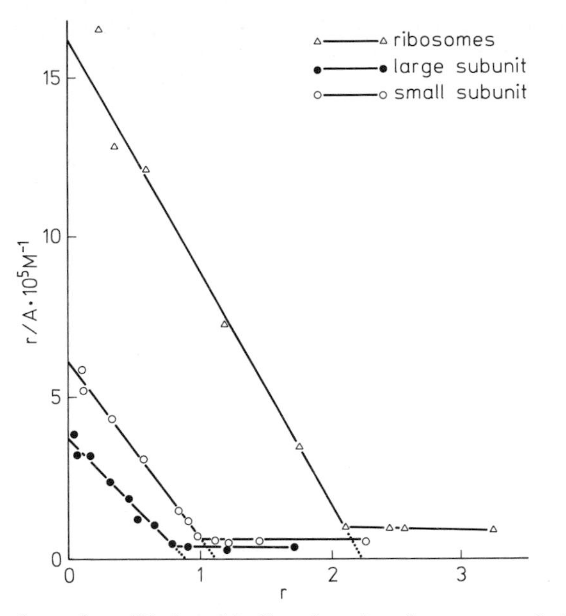

Fig. 2. Scatchard plots of equilibrium binding data for ribosomes and ribosomal subunits (MISUMI et al. 1978b). △—△, ribosomes; ●—●, large subunit; ○—○, small subunit

Table 1. Effects of some antibiotics on the binding of [^{3}H]kanamycin to ribosomes and ribosomal subunits. (MISUMI et al. 1978b)

Addition of antibiotic	Ribosomes	Ribosomal subunits	
	70S	30S	50S
None	228 [a]	97	95
Kanamycin	23	10	12
Neomycin	22	9	11
Gentamicin	30	12	26
Streptomycin	207	87	90
Viomycin	125	71	57
Chloramphenicol	225	89	90

[a] The results are expressed as pmol of [^{3}H]kanamycin bound to 100 pmol of the ribosome or ribosomal subunit

somes and ribosomal subunits at the same level as unlabeled kanamycin, suggesting that both antibiotics interact with the same binding sites on the ribosome. A similar tendency, with somewhat less inhibition, is found with gentamicin. Less interference is observed with viomycin. Streptomycin and chloramphenicol do not significantly affect the interaction of [^{3}H]kanamycin and ribosomes.

The effects of aminoglycoside antibiotics on the binding of [^{14}C]tuberactinomycin O (MISUMI et al. 1978a), an antibiotic closely related to viomycin, have also been studied (Table 2). Kanamycin, neomycin, and gentamicin reverse the binding

Table 2. Effects of aminoglycoside antibiotics on the binding of [^{14}C] tuberactinomycin 0. (MISUMI et al. 1978b)

Addition of antibiotic	Ribosomes	Ribosomal subunits	
	70S	30S	50S
None	89 [a]	58	79
Kanamycin	28	7.8	24
Neomycin	30	9.6	29
Gentamicin	32	10	32

[a] The results are expressed as pmol of [^{14}C]tuberactinomycin 0 bound per 100 pmol of the ribosome or ribosomal subunit

to ribosomes and both ribosomal subunits, indicating that these aminoglycosides interact with the 50 S ribosomal subunit as well as with the 30 S ribosomal subunit.

The ribosomes of kanamycin-resistant *E. coli* mutants exhibit less affinity for [^{3}H]kanamycin than the sensitive parental ribosomes. In some mutants, the binding of [^{3}H]kanamycin to the 30 S subunit is reduced but that to the 50 S subunit is not significantly affected. In others, binding to the 50 S ribosomal subunit is reduced but that to the 30 S subunit is not reduced. Mutational alterations of either large or small ribosomal subunits result in reduced affinity for the antibiotic by the 70 S ribosomes (CHOI et al. 1980).

4. Binding of Other Aminoglycosides to the Ribosome and Ribosomal Subunits

LANDO et al. (1976) have observed that [^{14}C]paromomycin binds specifically to a single site on the *E. coli* ribosome. Streptomycin, gentamicin, kanamycin, kasugamycin, and spectinomycin do not compete. Both 30 S and 50 S ribosomal subunits do not specifically bind paromomycin but exhibit marked nonspecific binding at high antibiotic: ribosome ratios. Their definition of specific and nonspecific binding is not completely clear, but it apparently means strong and weak binding. LE GOFFIC et al. (1979) synthesized [^{3}H]tobramycin and studied binding to *E. coli* ribosomes by the equilibrium dialysis method. It has been shown that tobramycin has two types of selective binding sites on the ribosome itself as well as on the 50 S ribosomal subunit, while it has only one type of binding site on the 30 S subunit. Of the two types of binding sites, the primary one may be responsible for the inhibition of protein synthesis, whereas the secondary one is probably related to codon misreading and reading-through of the termination codon.

The interaction of neomycin, kanamycin, gentamicin, and related antibiotics with ribosomal subunits has also been suggested by the effects on ribosomal functions (CAMPUZANO et al. 1979). The GDP-EF-G-50 S subunit–fusidic acid complex (where GDP is guanosine-5′ diphosphate and EF-G is elongation factor G) is stabilized by kanamycin, gentamicin, and neomycin, but not by streptomycin. Treatment of the 30 S ribosomal subunit, but not of the 50 S subunit, with neomycin B or kanamycin B, followed by removal of unbound drug and supplementation with untreated pair subunit, enhances translation errors. A similar treatment of either subunit with neomycin B blocks translocation. CAMPUZANO et al. suggested that the interaction of neomycin and related antibiotics with the 30 S ribosomal subunit causes codon misreading and prevents translocation; the interaction with the 50 S subunit stabilizes EF-G on the ribosome and also inhibits translocation.

OKUYAMA et al. (1975) have demonstrated by equilibrium dialysis that [^{3}H]kasugamycin stoichiometrically binds to *E. coli* ribosomes as well as to the 30 S ribosomal subunit, but only slightly to the 50 S subunit. A single binding site is present on the ribosome. Streptomycin, kanamycin, and gentamicin do not compete.

The binding of [^{3}H]dihydrospectinomycin to *E. coli* ribosomes is reversible and is dependent upon time and temperature, but is independent of Mg^{2+} concentration. At low drug concentration, the 70 S ribosome and 30 S ribosomal subunit from spectinomycin-sensitive cells bind more antibiotic than those from spectinomycin-resistant organisms, but the selectivity disappears at high drug concentrations (BOLLEN et al. 1969).

More than one binding site of the ribosome for gentamicin is also suggested by the triphasic concentration effects on translation: at low concentrations elongation is markedly inhibited; at higher concentrations the inhibition diminishes, while misreading is enhanced and synthesis is prolonged; at still higher concentrations inhibition increases again (TAI and DAVIS 1979). Contrary to the results with gentamicin, streptomycin shows a monophasic effect, suggesting that streptomycin has a single binding site on the ribosome.

V. Interference with Ribosomal Functions

The function of ribosomes is protein synthesis, which consists of three steps: initiation, elongation, and termination (Fig. 3). Some protein factors and guanosine-5′-triphosphate (GTP) are required for each process, i.e., initiation factors (IF-1, 2, and 3) and GTP for initiation, elongation factors (EF-Tu, -Ts, and -G) and GTP for elongation, and releasing factors (RF-1, 2, and 3) for termination. The messenger RNA, transcripted from the genetic code of DNA, guides the translation as a template, which contains an initiation codon (AUG or GUG), codons corresponding to sequential amino acids, and a termination codon (UAA, UGA, or UAG). The process of peptide chain elongation is carried out by a cyclic reaction, consisting of: (1) aminoacyl-tRNA-GTP-EF-Tu complex binding to the acceptor site (A-site) of ribosomes, (2) peptidyl transferase reaction or peptide bond formation between the C end of peptide moiety of peptidyl-tRNA on the donor site (D-site) and the N end of aminoacyl-tRNA on the A-site, and (3) translocation of peptidyl-tRNA from the A-site to the D-site with one codon movement of mRNA.

1. Inhibition of Initiation of Protein Synthesis

a) Kasugamycin

We have found that kasugamycin selectively inhibits initiation of protein synthesis by blocking formation of the 30 S initiation complex, fMet-tRNA$_F$-mRNA-30 S ribosomal subunit, but does not significantly affect elongation of the peptide chain

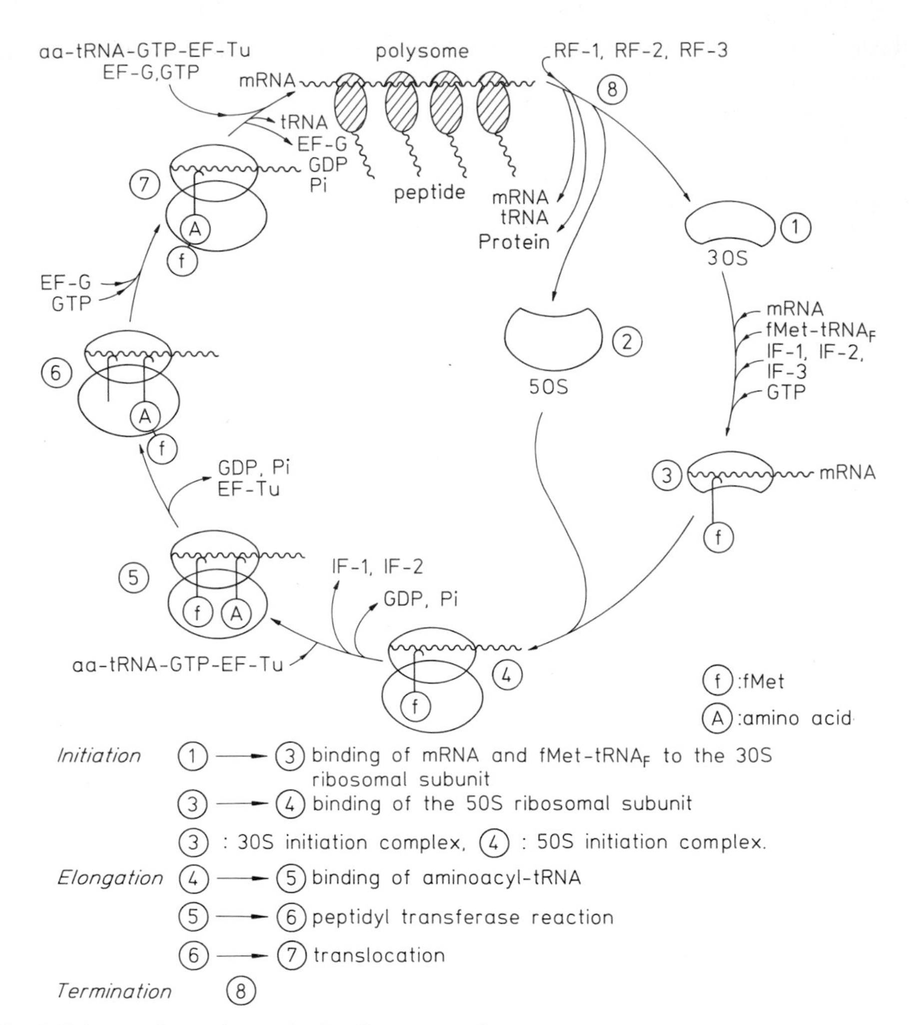

Fig. 3. Scheme of protein synthesis–ribosome cycle

(OKUYAMA et al. 1971, 1972). Kasugamycin prevents protein synthesis, but does not cause codon misreading (TANAKA et al. 1965, 1966a, b). The binding of fMet-$tRNA_F$ to the 30S ribosomal subunit with mRNA is markedly inhibited by kasugamycin, but not significantly by streptomycin, kanamycin, or gentamicin (Table 3). With f2 phage RNA, kasugamycin blocks initiation of translation of the maturation protein cistron more markedly than that of the coat protein cistron, while kanamycin and gentamicin inhibit the latter more strongly than the former. Streptomycin affects both at the same level (OKUYAMA and TANAKA 1972; KOZAK and NATHANS 1972). Comparative studies of several phage cistron sequences have suggested that there may be cistron-specific sequences for ribosomal binding, pairing with the 3′ terminus of 16S tRNA, at the 5′ side of the initiator AUG codon (STEITZ 1969; SHINE and DALGARNO 1975). It has been indicated that there may be

Table 3. Effects of kasugamycin on binding of fMet-tRNA to ribosomes. (OKUYAMA et al. 1971)

Ribosomes	mRNA	Addition	fMet-tRNA bound (pmol/tube)	% Inhibition
70 S	f2 RNA	–	4.44	
		ksg 2×10^{-5} *M*	2.01	55
		2×10^{-4}	0.09	98
		str 2×10^{-5}	0	100
70 S	AUG	–	6.30	
		ksg 2×10^{-4} *M*	0	100
70 S	f2 RNA	GMPPCP	1.21	
		+ksg 2×10^{-4} *M*	0	100
		+str 2×10^{-5}	1.11	8
30 S	polyAUG	–	4.45	
		ksg 2×10^{-4} *M*	2.14	62
		str 2×10^{-5}	4.42	1
		kan 2×10^{-5}	4.48	–
		gen 2×10^{-5}	4.59	–

Abbreviations: ksg = kasugamycin, str = streptomycin, kan = kanamycin, gen = gentamicin

cistron-specific initiation sequences which can be competed differentially with polynucleotides (REVEL et al. 1970; OKUYAMA and TANAKA 1973). Thus, kasugamycin may affect the initiation signal for maturation protein cistron more markedly than that for coat protein cistron.

b) Streptomycin

Streptomycin affects initiation as well as elongation and termination of protein synthesis. The antibiotic prevents initiation-dependent translation of viral and bacterial mRNA more strongly than that of endogenous mRNA (MODOLELL and DAVIS 1968; LUZZATTO et al. 1968, 1969 a, b). Formation of the initiation complex of fMet-$tRNA_F$-mRNA-30 S ribosomal subunit is not significantly affected by streptomycin (OKUYAMA et al. 1971, 1972; OKUYAMA and TANAKA 1972). The joining of the 50 S subunit to the 30 S initiation complex in the presence of streptomycin causes breakdown of the 70 S initiation complex, resulting in the release of fMet-$tRNA_F$ (MODOLELL and DAVIS 1970; LELONG et al. 1971). The breakdown occurs very rapidly (the half-life is 5 min), and is apparently correlated with GTP hydrolysis; fMet-$tRNA_F$ is released from the puromycin-reactive donor site.

In contrast, it has been reported that fMet-$tRNA_F$ accumulates on ribosomes in cells treated with streptomycin (LENNETTE and APIRION 1970). The discrepancy of the results in vivo and in vitro may be explained by the fact that streptomycin inhibits initiation complex formation with washed 70 S ribosomes but not with unwashed ribosomes, indicating that the effect of streptomycin on initiation depends on the conformation of ribosomes (OKUYAMA et al. 1972).

Ribosomal dissociation, induced in vitro by IF-3, is blocked by streptomycin (GARCIA-PATRONE et al. 1971; HERZOG et al. 1971; WALLACE et al. 1973 a, b); the equilibrium is shifted to the 70 S ribosome (CHANG and FLAKS 1972a; WALLACE et al. 1973b).

Abortive unstable initiation complexes and polysomes with impaired responsiveness to IF-3 are formed by the treatment of *E. coli* cells with streptomycin. Streptomycin-damaged ribosomes are released from the initiation complexes and polysomes and are then engaged in the cyclic abortive reinitiation (LUZZATTO et al. 1968, 1969a, b; WALLACE and DAVIS 1973; WALLACE et al. 1973b).

c) Other Aminoglycoside Antibiotics

We have found that kanamycin and gentamicin somewhat affect initiation, as well as elongation, of f2 phage RNA translation. The antibiotics block initiation of coat protein synthesis, but do not significantly affect initiation of maturation protein synthesis. The drugs inhibit slightly the 30 S initiation complex formation and release fMet-$tRNA_F$ from the 70 S initiation complex, although to a much lesser degree than streptomycin (OKUYAMA and TANAKA 1972; OKUYAMA et al. 1972). Inhibition of initiation by gentamicin is also confirmed by the finding that the antibiotic shows greater inhibition with an initiating system (with R 17 phage RNA as messenger) than with pure chain elongation on purified endogenous polysomes (TAI and DAVIS 1979). On the other hand, it has been reported that gentamicin has less effect on initiation complex formation with late T4 phage mRNA or AUG triplet (LELONG et al. 1971; LANDO et al. 1973). These results suggest that the effects of gentamicin and kanamycin on initiation depend upon the conformation of RNA around the initiation sites.

Kanamycin, neomycin B, and paromomycin prevent the dissociation of free ribosomes into 30 S and 50 S subunits by IF-3 (GARCIA-PATRONE et al. 1971).

Spectinomycin selectively blocks initiating ribosomes, but does not inhibit initiation; the initial dipeptide formation is not affected by the antibiotic (ANDERSON et al. 1967; WALLACE et al. 1974). Spectinomycin may inhibit the first translocation (see a review by WALLACE et al. 1979).

2. Chain Elongation Processes Affected

As described above, aminoglycosides affect peptide chain initiation by blocking 30 S initiation complex formation, by causing breakdown of the 70 S initiation complex, and/or by inhibiting ribosomal dissociation. However, aminoglycoside antibiotics also affect peptide chain elongation, i.e., they cause codon misreading, interfere with aminoacyl-tRNA binding, and/or inhibit translocation of peptidyl-tRNA.

a) Codon Misreading

Streptomycin, kanamycin, gentamicin, neomycin, and other aminoglycosides with a streptamine or 2-deoxystreptamine moiety provoke codon misreading or induce the uptake of incorrect amino acids which do not correspond to the codon (coding nucleotides) in vivo (GORINI and KATAJA 1964, 1965) and in vitro (DAVIES et al. 1964, 1965). In contrast, kasugamycin (TANAKA et al. 1966a, b, 1967) and spectinomycin (ANDERSON et al. 1967) do not stimulate ambiguity of translation.

GORINI and KATAJA (1964, 1965) have observed that streptomycin, kanamycin, neomycin, and paromomycin disturb the fidelity of translation of the genetic codon in vivo, and a similar effect has been demonstrated in vitro by DAVIES et al. (1965) with these antibiotics as well as with hygromycin B and gentamicin.

The range and type of translation errors differ with the kind of antibiotics and are influenced by different polynucleotide templates and conditions. The coding changes caused by neomycin, kanamycin, gentamicin, and hygromycin B are more pronounced than those induced by streptomycin. This is in accord with the assumption that streptomycin acts on a single site of the ribosome but the other aminoglycosides possess multiple sites of action (see Sect. A.IV) (DAVIES et al. 1965, 1966; DAVIES and DAVIS 1968).

Although the miscoding activity of aminoglycosides has been extensively studied with synthetic polynucleotide messengers, the work of DAVIS and collaborators provides evidence that streptomycin induces codon misreading with natural (endogenous or viral) messenger. In a protein-synthesizing system containing 15 or 20 amino acids, streptomycin enhances incorporation with initiation-free polysomes (DAVIS et al. 1974). Moreover, under conditions where deprivation of an aminoacyl-tRNA is achieved more completely by using the extract of a mutant with a temperature-sensitive synthetase for Glu-tRNA or Val-tRNA, streptomycin strongly stimulates peptide synthesis on polysomes over a wide range of concentrations (TAI et al. 1978). A higher concentration is needed, with natural messenger, for gentamicin to cause misreading than to inhibit total protein synthesis or initiation. Gentamicin causes slowing and a decrease in total synthesis but little translation error at a drug concentration of 2 μM. Stimulated codon misreading is observed at a higher concentration (TAI and DAVIS 1979).

The miscoding effect of aminoglycosides was originally suggested as the basis for phenotypic repair or suppression, i.e., some auxotrophs are able to grow without an essential amino acid in the presence of sublethal levels of streptomycin, kanamycin, neomycin, or paromomycin (GORINI and KATAJA 1964, 1965). Although the demonstration of translation errors in vivo is generally difficult, *E. coli* has been found to produce altered β-galactosidase in the presence of low concentrations of streptomycin or neomycin (BISSEL 1965; PINKETT and BROWNSTEIN 1974; BRANSCOMB and GALAS 1975).

b) Interference with Aminoacyl-tRNA Binding

Both EF-Tu- and GTP-dependent and -independent binding of aminoacyl-tRNA are blocked by streptomycin (KAJI et al. 1966; OKUYAMA et al. 1972). Streptomycin also enhances the binding of noncognate aminoacyl-tRNA (Ile-, Leu-, or Ser-tRNA with poly[U]), which seems to be consistent with the codon misreading effect on translation (KAJI and KAJI 1965; PESTKA et al. 1965).

Kanamycin, neomycin, gentamicin, and related antibiotics are weaker inhibitors of the GTP- and EF-Tu-dependent binding of [^{3}H]Phe-tRNA to ribosomes than streptomycin. Moreover, when purified [^{14}C]Phe-tRNA is used in binding experiments the inhibition disappears, indicating that the effect of the aminoglycosides may be due to stimulated competition between [^{3}H]Phe-tRNA and other tRNAs caused by increased misreading, rather than to direct inhibition of the binding process (CABAÑAS et al. 1978a, b).

c) Inhibition of Translocation of Peptidyl-tRNA on Ribosomes

During translocation, deacylated tRNA is ejected from the donor site of ribosomes, peptidyl-tRNA moves from the acceptor (puromycin-unreactive) site to the donor (puromycin-reactive) site, and the ribosome moves precisely one codon closer to the 3′ end of mRNA. The translocation, therefore, can be assayed by peptidylpuromycin synthesis, enhanced by EF-G and GTP, or by release of deacylated tRNA from the ribosome.

EF-G- and GTP-dependent translocation is inhibited by kanamycin, gentamicin, neomycin, hygromycin B, apramycin, and related antibiotics, but not by streptomycin. The peptidyl transferase reaction is not significantly affected by the aminoglycoside antibiotics (MISUMI et al. 1978 b; CABAÑAS et al. 1978 a, b; PERZYNSKI et al. 1979; MISUMI and TANAKA 1980).

First we observed that viomycin, a peptide antibiotic, inhibits initiation and translocation (LIOU and TANAKA 1976), and interacts with both 30 S and 50 S ribosomal subunits (MISUMI et al. 1978 a); then we found that kanamycin, gentamicin, and neomycin also interact with both ribosomal subunits. These results suggest that kanamycin and viomycin possess a similar mechanism of action, although their chemical structures are distinctly different. These findings indicate that kanamycin and related antibiotics may inhibit translocation.

N-Acetylphenylalanyl-puromycin formation by the ribosome with *N*-acetyl-[^{14}C]phenylalanyl-tRNA and puromycin in the absence of EF-G and GTP can be used as a model system for studying the peptidyl transferase reaction; the effects of aminoglycoside antibiotics are presented in Table 4. The puromycin reaction is not significantly affected by kanamycin, neomycin, gentamicin, or streptomycin up to concentrations of 10 μM. Slight inhibition by kanamycin, neomycin, or gentamicin is observed at a concentration of 100 μM. Translocation of *N*-acetylphenylalanyl-tRNA from the acceptor site to the donor site can be assayed by the puromycin reaction enhanced by the addition of EF-G and GTP (TANAKA et al. 1968; TANAKA 1975 b). The stimulated reaction is profoundly prevented by kanamycin, neomycin, or gentamicin but not significantly by streptomycin (Table 4). The results indicate that translocation is inhibited by the former group of aminoglycosides but not by streptomycin.

The translocation of peptidyl-tRNA in a crude, complete polypeptide-synthesizing system, containing endogenous *E. coli* polysomes, is also blocked by hygromycin B, neomycin, kanamycin, gentamicin, and related antibiotics (CABAÑAS et al. 1978a, b).

The mechanism of inhibition by aminoglycosides of translocation has been not well established. Fusidic acid, a steroidal antibiotic, interacts with EF-G, stabilizes the EF-G-GDP-ribosome complex, and blocks overall translocation without affecting the first cycle of translocation [cf. review by TANAKA (1975 b)]. Contrary to the action of fusidic acid, kanamycin, as well as viomycin, inhibits a single cycle of translocation. Therefore, kanamycin may be a direct inhibitor of translocation, but fusidic acid an indirect inhibitor (MISUMI and TANAKA 1980). GTP hydrolysis, catalyzed by EF-G and ribosomes, or the interaction of EF-G, GTP, and ribosomes, is inhibited by fusidic acid, but not by kanamycin and hygromycin B. These aminoglycosides may interfere with translocation by fixing peptidyl-tRNA to the

Table 4. Effects of aminoglycoside antibiotics on *N*-acetylphenylalanyl-puromycin synthesis in the absence or presence of EF-G and GTP. (MISUMI et al. 1978b)

Antibiotic		*N*-Ac-[^{14}C]Phe-puromycin formed	
		Without EF-G and GTP	Enhanced by EF-G and GTP
None		100% (637 cpm)	100% (1714 cpm)
Kanamycin	0.1 μ*M*	97	72
	1	95	32
	10	95	17
	100	85	3
Neomycin	0.1	95	68
	1	93	27
	10	90	12
	100	86	2
Gentamicin	0.1	97	74
	1	95	34
	10	94	15
	100	88	2
Streptomycin	0.1	102	97
	1	97	95
	10	96	92
	100	93	81
Blasticidin S	100	16	6

The assay for peptidyltransferase reaction and translocation of peptidyl-tRNA was carried out by acetylphenylalanyl-puromycin synthesis

acceptor site but not to the donor site (CABAÑAS et al. 1978b; MISUMI and TANAKA 1980).

A single cycle of translocation can be assayed by GMPP(NH)P- and EF-G-dependent *N*-acetyl-diphenylalanyl-puromycin synthesis on the ribosome possessing *N*-acetyl-diPhe-tRNA at the acceptor site and deacylated tRNA^{Phe} at the donor site. The translocation is promoted by the presence of a stoichiometric amount of EF-G, when GMPP(NH)P is substituted for GTP. The single cycle of translocation is markedly inhibited by kanamycin and viomycin, but not by fusidic acid, when a substrate amount of EF-G is employed (Fig. 4). In a simultaneous experiment, the translocation with GTP and a catalytic amount of EF-G is prevented by all three antibiotics (overall translocation).

The exit of deacylated tRNA^{Phe} from the donor site with concomitant translocation of *N*-acetyl-diPhe-tRNA from the acceptor site to the donor site can be assayed by the following two procedures. In the first method, the release of deacylated tRNA^{Phe} is determined by aminoacylation with [^{14}C]phenylalanine by Phe-tRNA synthetase. In the second, the amount of [^{3}H]tRNA bound to ribosomes is measured by a nitrocellulose (Millipore) filter technique. The effects of kanamycin, in comparison with viomycin and fusidic acid, are presented in Table 5. In experiment I, using the first assay, the exit of deacylated tRNA^{Phe} from the donor site occurs in the presence of a substrate amount of EF-G with GTP or guanyl-imido-

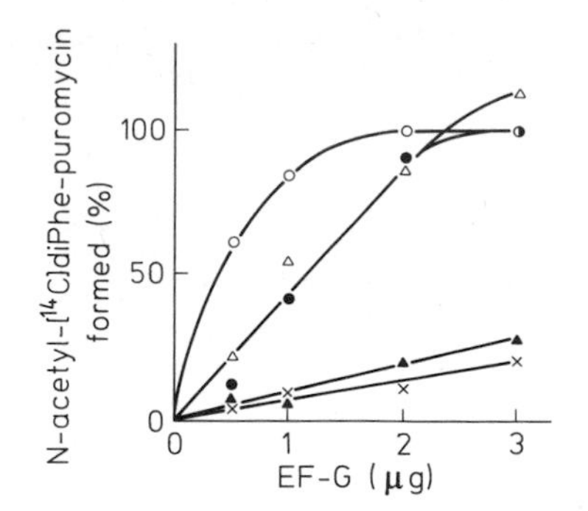

Fig. 4. The effects of antibiotics on the translocation of *N*-acetyl-[^{14}C]-diPhe-tRNA in the presence of GMPP(NH)P: Dependence upon EF-G concentration (MISUMI and TANAKA 1980). The assay for the translocation was performed by the procedure of INOUE-YOKOSAWA et al. (1974). ○, GTP; ●, GMPP(NH)P; ×, GMPP(NH)P+0.1 m*M* kanamycin; ▲, GMPP(NH)P+0.1 m*M* viomycin; △, GMPP(NH)P+1 m*M* fusidic acid

Table 5. The effects of antibiotics on the release of deacylated tRNA^{Phe} and translocation of *N*-acetyl-diPhe-tRNA on the ribosome with *N*-acetyl-diPhe-tRNA at the acceptor site and deacylated tRNA^{Phe} at the donor site. (MISUMI and TANAKA 1980)

Addition	Exp. I	Exp. II	
	tRNA^{Phe} released	[^{3}H]tRNA bound	*N*-Ac-[^{14}C] diePhe-puromycin formed
None	0.7[a]	9.4	0.8
EF-G	1.1	9.3	0.4
EF-G, GTP	9.3	4.6	9.7
EF-G, GTP, fusidic acid 1 m*M*	10.4	4.4	9.6
EF-G, GTP, viomycin 0.1 m*M*	2.2	9.0	1.7
EF-G, GTP, kanamycin 0.1 m*M*	2.7	8.6	2.0
EF-G, GMPP(NH)P	7.1	5.2	7.1
EF-G, GMPP(NH)P, fusidic acid 1 m*M*	7.6	4.3	7.8
EF-G, GMPP(NH)P, viomycin 0.1 m*M*	2.4	8.3	1.4
EF-G, GMPP(NH)P, kanamycin 0.1 m*M*	2.0	8.0	1.6

[a] Results are expressed as pmol/per 0.1 ml of the reaction mixture

diphosphate [GMPP(NH)P]. It is profoundly blocked by kanamycin as well as viomycin, but not by fusidic acid. In experiment II, using the second procedure, the release of [^{3}H]tRNA and simultaneous translocation of *N*-acetyl-[^{14}C]diPhe-tRNA, induced by a substrate amount of EF-G with GTP or GMPP(NH)P, are also inhibited by kanamycin and viomycin, but not significantly by fusidic acid.

Since *N*-acetyl-Phe-tRNA bound to the acceptor site is released by decreasing the NH_4^+ concentration (WATANABE 1972), the effects of antibiotics on the *N*-acetyl-Phe-tRNA were studied by this procedure. As illustrated in Fig. 5, kanamycin and viomycin block the release of *N*-acetyl-Phe-tRNA, indicating that the antibiotics fix *N*-acetyl-Phe-tRNA to the acceptor site.

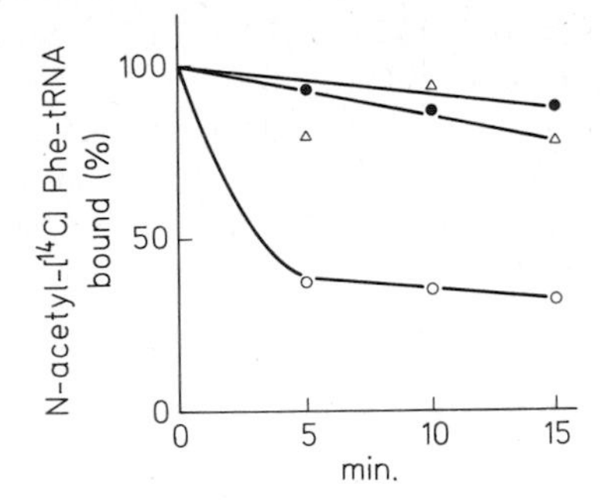

Fig. 5. Kinetics of protection by antibiotics against the release of *N*-acetyl-[^{14}C]Phe-tRNA from the ribosomal acceptor site, induced by NH_4^+ depletion (MISUMI and TANAKA 1980). ○, no antibiotic; ●, 0.1 m*M* kanamycin; △, 0.1 m*M* viomycin

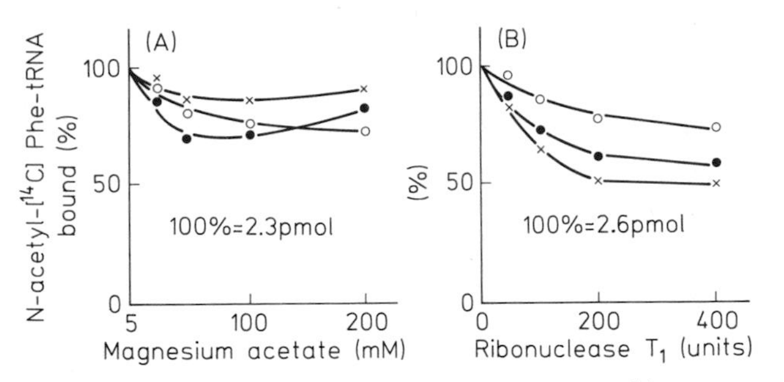

Fig. 6A, B. The effects of antibiotics on the release of *N*-acetyl-[^{14}C]-Phe-tRNA from the ribosomal donor site, caused by increasing Mg^{2+} concentration **A** and by digestion with ribonuclease T_1 **B** (MISUMI and TANAKA 1980). ○, no antibiotic; ●, kanamycin 0.1 m*M*; ×, viomycin 0.1 m*M*

Table 6. The effect of antibiotics on ribosome-dependent GTPase reaction of EF-G. (MISUMI and TANAKA 1980)

Additions		[^{14}C]GTP hydrolyzed
None		100% (21 pmol)
Viomycin	0.02 m*M*	94
	0.2	77
Kanamycin	0.02 m*M*	91
	0.2	72
Fusidic acid	0.1 m*M*	16

N-Acetyl-Phe-tRNA bound to the donor site is released by increasing Mg^{2+} concentration or by digestion with ribonuclease T_1 (ČERNÁ et al. 1973). These methods reveal that kanamycin and viomycin do not significantly affect the release of *N*-acetyl-Phe-tRNA from the donor site (Fig. 6).

The hydrolysis of GTP to GDP by EF-G and ribosomes is not significantly affected by kanamycin or viomycin, although a slight inhibition is observed at high antibiotic concentrations of 0.2 mM (Table 6). In a parallel experiment, fusidic acid blocks the GTPase reaction. The formation of EF-G-[^{14}C]GDP-ribosome complex with or without fusidic acid is not significantly affected by kanamycin or viomycin. These results indicate that kanamycin, as well as viomycin, does not interfere with the interaction of EF-G, GTP, and ribosomes.

3. Interference with Termination

Streptomycin inhibits chain termination by blocking release factor-dependent codon recognition (Caskey et al. 1969).

Codon misreading, stimulated by aminoglycoside antibiotics, favors reading-through of termination codons, and the synthesis of longer than normal peptides is promoted due to termination errors (Tai and Davis 1979; Zierhut et al. 1979).

VI. Interaction with Bacterial Cell Envelope

1. Membrane Damage

Streptomycin induces damage to the bacterial membrane or envelope. It is demonstrated by excretion of nucleotides and other low molecular weight materials from intracellular pools (Anand and Davis 1960), leakage of ions from cells, and crypticity of β-galactosidase (Dubin and Davis 1961; Dubin et al. 1963). The rapid efflux of K^+ from cells remains the earliest event to be detected after treatment with streptomycin. Membrane damage appears as soon as protein synthesis is affected.

The drug resistance mutation of ribosomes or addition of chloramphenicol, an inhibitor of ribosomes, eliminates the membrane damage, suggesting that the effect on cell envelope is a secondary consequence, derived from the ribosomal changes induced by the aminoglycoside. In this connection, it is of interest that the ribosome is resistant to spectinomycin, and a major cytoplasmic membrane protein, I-19, is lacking in sucrose-dependent and spectinomycin-resistant mutants of *E. coli* (Miyoshi and Yamagata 1975; Mizuno et al. 1975). In addition, the treatment of sensitive cells with spectinomycin results in the same deficiency of I-19 (Mizuno et al. 1977).

Cell envelope alteration has also been demonstrated by electron microscopic observations with *E. coli* and *Pseudomonas aeruginosa* (Iida and Koike 1974). Dibekacin, streptomycin, spectinomycin, and kasugamycin stimulate formation of blebs (small extrusions) on the cell envelope. This effect requires cell growth and is blocked by ribosomal inhibitors (chloramphenicol, tetracycline, and erythromycin), suggesting that bleb formation is related to ribosomal alterations. However, the relationship between the bleb formation and membrane damage remains to be determined. It has been also demonstrated by a countercurrent distribution method that a streptomycin-resistant change of ribosomal protein S 12 results in altered surface properties or charge of *E. coli* cells (Pestka et al. 1977).

However, the mechanism by which the binding of the aminoglycoside antibiotics to the ribosome and the consequent ribosomal alterations result in membrane damage remains to be determined. Bermingham et al. (1970) suggested that streptomycin at sublethal concentrations induces changes in lipid composition of the cell membrane of *Serratia marcescens*, i.e., the phospholipid content increases and that of cyclic depsipeptides decreases. This effect is considered to be unrelated to protein synthesis inhibition and may account for the ion efflux because cyclic depsipeptides act as ion carriers across the membrane. The direct interaction of aminoglycoside antibiotics with phospholipid has been also reported by ALEXANDER et al. (1979) (see Sect. B.IV).

We have observed by the electrophoretic analysis method of SPRATT (1977) that [^{14}C]streptomycin does not covalently bind to membrane proteins of *E. coli* (N. TANAKA, unpublished work).

2. Uptake of Streptomycin by Bacterial Cells

The entry of streptomycin into *E. coli* cells occurs in two phases (ANAND et al. 1960; HURWITZ and ROSANO 1962; ANDRY and BOCKRATH 1974; BRYAN and VAN DEN ELZEN 1976). The initial uptake, which takes place even at 0 °C and is reversed by salts (ANAND et al. 1960; PLOTZ et al. 1963; RAMIREZ-RONDA et al. 1975; BEGGS and ANDREWS 1976), may be due to ionic binding of the drug to the cell surface. A lag phase or a slow accumulation of the antibiotic follows the binding to the cell surface (ANAND et al. 1960; BRYAN and VAN DEN ELZEN 1976).

Then the second phase of streptomycin uptake occurs. The uptake rate of the drug rapidly increases and simultaneously the permeability of the cell envelope changes (ANAND et al. 1960; DUBIN et al. 1963; WYATT et al. 1972). The second phase of antibiotic uptake requires energy and may represent an active transport process. The uptake occurs in aerobic conditions, and is blocked by anaerobiosis (HANCOCK 1962a; KOGUT et al. 1965). This may explain one aspect of the antibacterial spectrum of aminoglycoside antibiotics: strongly active against aerobic bacteria but not against anaerobic bacteria. Electron transport inhibitors or uncouplers of oxidative phosphorylation (HANCOCK 1962a, b; TSENG et al. 1972; ANDRY and BOCKRATH 1974; BRYAN and VAN DEN ELZEN 1976) and chloramphenicol (ANAND et al. 1960; HURWITZ and ROSANO 1962; BRYAN and VAN DEN ELZEN 1976) prevent the second phase uptake. In addition, in cells whose permeability has already been changed by dihydrostreptomycin, electron transport inhibitors block further uptake of labeled streptomycin (BRYAN and VAN DEN ELZEN 1976). Moreover, a heme-deficient mutant and two mutants with other defects in the electron transport system show decreased uptake of the antibiotic and increased resistance to its action (BRYAN and VAN DEN ELZEN 1977). These results suggest that drug transport is energy dependent. A streptomycin-hypersensitive mutant has been found to exhibit an impaired Mg^{2+}-ATPase and no oxidative phosphorylation activity (TURNOCK 1970; TURNOCK et al. 1972).

Other aminoglycoside antibiotics may also enter the bacterial cells by an active, carrier-mediated transport process, similar to streptomycin. The membrane damage caused by aminoglycosides may stimulate or modify the entry of the antibiotics into the cells and the efflux from them.

3. Drug Resistance Due to Transport Barriers

The resistance of bacteria to aminoglycoside antibiotics is mostly attributed to production of drug-modifying enzymes or to ribosomal alterations. In addition, the drug resistance of some organisms is due to decreased permeability of antibiotics

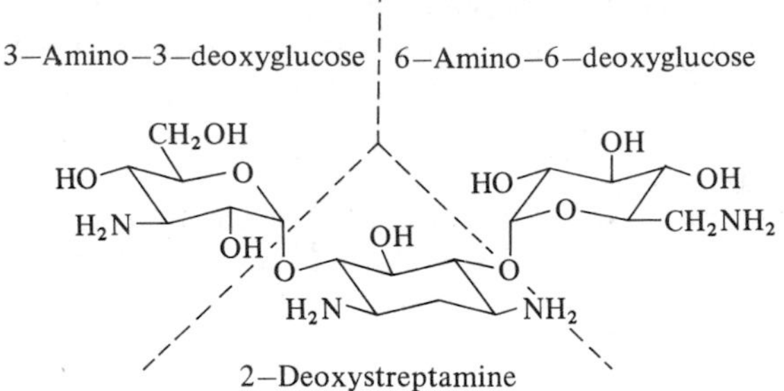

Fig. 7. Structure of kanamycin

into bacterial cells, based on alterations of the cell envelope (KONO and O'HARA 1976; BRYAN et al. 1976). BRYAN et al. (1976) have examined three clinical isolates of *P. aeruginosa* possessing nontransferable plasmids and showing broad aminoglycoside resistance (gentamicin, sisomicin, kanamycin, amikacin, tobramycin, and streptomycin). The resistant strains exhibit a marked reduction in energy-dependent accumulation of gentamicin compared to a susceptible strain, but do not contain gentamicin-modifying enzymes; gentamicin inhibits protein synthesis equally well with ribosomes obtained from either resistant or sensitive cells. KONO and O'HARA (1977) have found that a strain of *P. aeruginosa* with R plasmid, showing multiple drug resistance to tetracycline, chloramphenicol, sulfonamides, streptomycin, and kanamycin, neither accumulates kanamycin nor produces kanamycin-modifying enzymes, and its ribosome is sensitive to kanamycin. By comparison with the same organism without R plasmid, they have presented evidence suggesting that the presence of R plasmid directly affects the cell envelope.

The drug-resistant changes of ribosomes and transport systems and production of modifying enzymes may take place separately or independently, or may simultaneously occur in a single strain.

VII. Structure–Activity Relationships

1. Structure Required for Codon Misreading Activity

All the aminoglycosides capable of causing codon misreading contain a 2-deoxystreptamine or streptamine moiety in the molecule (streptomycin, kanamycin, gentamicin, neomycin, paromomycin, hygromycin B, etc.), and those lacking such a residue cannot stimulate misreading (kasugamycin and spectinomycin). We have proposed that the 2-deoxystreptamine moiety is responsible for the misreading activity of aminoglycoside antibiotics (TANAKA et al. 1967).

Since kasugamycin fails to promote codon misreading (TANAKA et al. 1965, 1966a, b), TANAKA et al. (1967) studied the structural features of kanamycin involved in misreading activity and showed that of the three sugar components of kanamycin, 2-deoxystreptamine has a weak ability to provoke translation errors, but 6-amino-6-deoxyglucose and 3-amino-3-deoxyglucose lack misreading activity, though the whole structure is required for full activity in promoting misreading (Fig. 7).

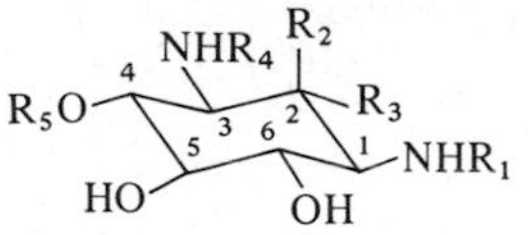

NHR_4 R_2 R_3 R_5O NHR_1 HO OH

	R_1	R_2	R_3	R_4	R_5
Deoxystreptamine	H	H	H	H	H
Streptamine	H	OH	H	H	H
N–methyldeoxy–streptamine	CH_3	H	H	H	H
Actinamine	CH_3	H	OH	CH_3	H
Paromamine	H	H	H	H	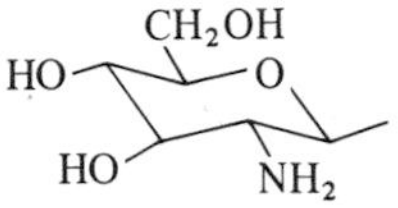 CH_2OH, O, HO, HO, NH_2
Neamine	H	H	H	H	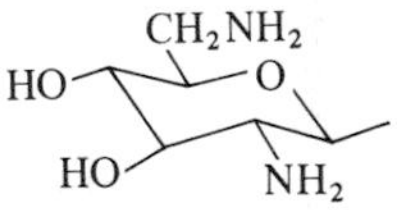 CH_2NH_2, O, HO, HO, NH_2

Fig. 8. 2-Deoxystreptamine and related compounds (MASUKAWA and TANAKA 1968)

Neamine and paromamine also possess misreading activity; the potency is lower than that of kanamycin but higher than that of 2-deoxystreptamine. *N*-methyldeoxystreptamine exhibits less misreading activity than deoxystreptamine. The activity of streptamine is similar to that of 2-deoxystreptamine. Actinamine lacks the ability to stimulating codon misreading (Fig. 8). The stereochemistry of the 2 position and free amino groups at the 1 and 3 positions of aminocyclitol are essential for misreading activity (MASUKAWA and TANAKA 1968). A marked loss of misreading ability is noted in the neomycin–hybrimycin group if the deoxystreptamine moiety is replaced by an epi-streptamine residue (DAVIES 1970). This also supports the importance of the stereochemistry in the 2 position of aminocyclitol antibiotics.

Negamycin, a basic peptide antibiotic, has been shown to promote codon misreading (MIZUNO et al. 1970; UEHARA et al. 1972). A possible similarity in the three-dimensional structures of negamycin and the aminocyclitol antibiotics is indicated by the use of a Corey, Pauling, and Koltun (CPK) molecular model. As illustrated in Fig. 9, the position of the hydrazid and β-amino groups in negamycin coincides with that of the 1- and 3-amino groups in the 2-deoxystreptamine moiety; the ε-amino group can be placed in a position similar to that of the 2′-hydroxyl group in kanamycin. The basic groups in one possible conformation of negamycin can be superimposed upon those of paromamine. For this conformation of negamycin, the presence of the carbonyl and *N*-methyl groups and the stereochemistry of the

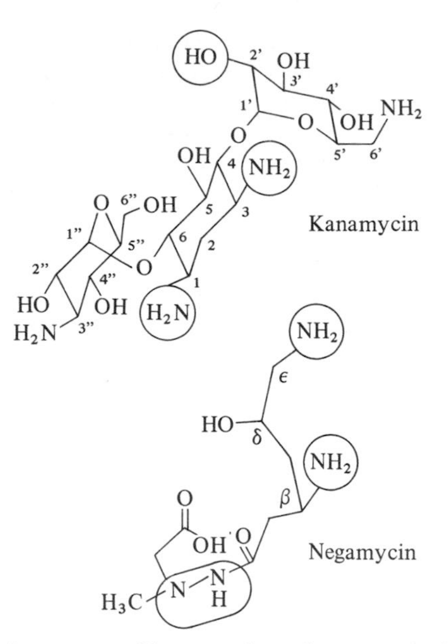

Fig. 9. Three-dimensional structure of kanamycin and negamycin (UEHARA et al. 1972)

β-amino and δ-hydroxyl groups are critical (UEHARA et al. 1972). In support of this view, an antipode of negamycin, synthesized from 3-amino-3-deoxy-D-glucose, has been demonstrated to show much weaker misreading activity than negamycin (SHIBAHARA et al. 1972). The studies on negamycin seem to support the hypothesis that the 2-deoxystreptamine moiety is essential for the misreading activity of aminocyclitol antibiotics.

2. Structure Needed for the Inhibition of Translocation

The EF-G- and GTP-dependent translocation of peptidyl-tRNA from the acceptor site to the donor site on ribosomes is inhibited by kanamycin, gentamicin, neomycin, hygromycin B, apramycin, and related aminoglycosides, but not by streptomycin (MISUMI et al. 1978 b; CABAÑAS et al. 1978 a, b; MISUMI and TANAKA 1980). Structural difference between streptomycin and the other aminoglycosides must be responsible for the inhibitory activity on translocation. In addition, viomycin, a basic peptide antibiotic with a unique structure, blocks translocation in a similar manner (LIOU and TANAKA 1976; MODOLELL and VAZQUEZ 1977; MISUMI and TANAKA 1980). These findings suggest some aspects of the structure–activity relationships for inhibition of translocation but clarification must await further experiments.

B. Effects on Mammalian or Eukaryotic Cells and Their Components

The aminoglycoside group of antibiotics may cause certain side effects: nephrotoxicity, ototoxicity, and neuromuscular blockade. These side effects are dose dependent and are considered to be a direct toxic action on mammalian cells rather than an allergic reaction. Aminoglycosides have been reported to interact with various mammalian cell components, including ribosomes, tubulin, actin, phospholipid, and nucleic acids. However, the biochemical basis for the side effects remains to be determined. In addition, some cases of allergic shock are also reported (HALL 1977).

I. Interaction with Ribosomes and Interference with Ribosomal Functions

Although all the aminoglycoside antibiotics interfere with prokaryotic ribosomes, eukaryotic cytoplasmic ribosomes are also affected by some aminoglycosides such as hygromycin B and paromomycin, but not significantly by the other aminoglycosides. Hygromycin B and paromomycin are active against both prokaryotic and eukaryotic cells. The sensitivity of eukaryotic mitochondrial ribosomes to the antibiotics seems to be similar to that of bacterial ribosomes.

WILHELM et al. (1978a, b) observed in *Tetrahymena*, wheat germ, and human cultured cell (KB) systems that paromomycin, kanamycin C, and lividomycin B strongly promote translation errors, but neomycin and kanamycin B show much lower activity. They suggest that the activity is related to the structure of paromamine or 3′-deoxyparomamine, which contains a 6′-hydroxyl group. Evidence has been also presented that paromomycin may cause the insertion of methionine into a particular protein which normally contains little or no methionine. The results suggest that paromomycin can provoke codon misreading of natural messenger in a human cell system.

Streptomycin and neomycin do not significantly stimulate translation errors with ribosomes from rat liver or rabbit spleen and reticulocytes (WEINSTEIN et al. 1966; FRIEDMAN et al. 1968; STAVY 1968). In addition, kanamycin, neomycin, and streptomycin exhibit greater inhibition of protein synthesis and higher levels of codon misreading with mitochondrial ribosomes than with cytoplasmic ribosomes of the chicken embryo (KURZ 1974).

Streptomycin and neomycin do not stimulate ambiguity of translation in an extract from *Saccharomyces cerevisiae* (SCHLANGER and FRIEDMAN 1973). Phenotypic suppression or in vivo misreading as well as in vitro misreading in the yeast is caused by hygromycin B, paromomycin, and lividomycin B, but not by streptomycin. Kanamycin B is more active than kanamycin C. The misreading activity is not confined to paromamine-containing antibiotics (SINGH et al. 1979). Phenotypic suppression of the methionine requirement of nonsense mutants of the yeast is strongly induced by paromomycin but not by streptomycin. Neomycin shows limited activity (PALMER et al. 1979).

Poly[U]-directed polyphenylalanine synthesis is inhibited by kasugamycin in a fungal (*Piricularia oryzae*) ribosomal system at a level similar to that active in the bacterial system (MASUKAWA et al. 1968a).

Polypeptide synthesis in cell-free extracts from rabbit reticulocytes, wheat germ, and yeast is strongly inhibited by hygromycin B. The antibiotic blocks peptide chain elongation by yeast polysomes by preventing EF-2-dependent translocation, although it affects neither the formation of EF-2-GTP-ribosome complex nor

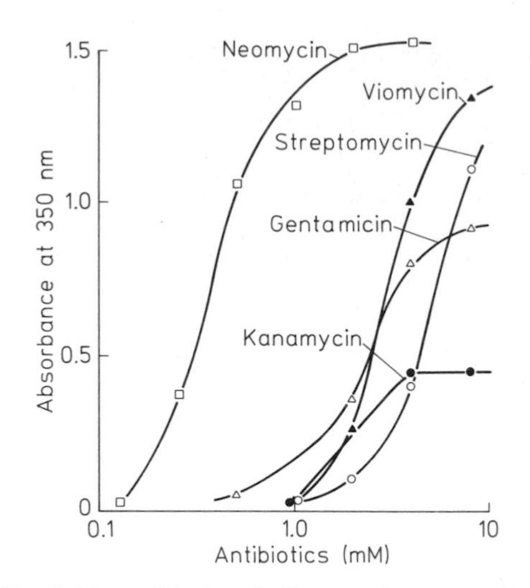

Fig. 10. Formation of insoluble antibiotic–tubulin complex, assayed by turbidimetry (AKIYAMA et al. 1978)

EF-2- and ribosome-dependent GTP hydrolysis. The peptidyl transferase reaction and nonenzymic translocation are not affected by hygromycin B (GONZALEZ et al. 1978).

The mammalian or eukaryotic ribosome has a molecular weight of 4.5×10^6 daltons, a sedimentation constant of 80 S, and consists of a large (60 S) and a small (40 S) subunit. The ribosome is made up of more than 70 proteins and 4 kinds of RNA (18 S, 28 S, 5.8 S, and 5 S).

The difference in size between bacterial and mammalian ribosomes and ribosomal components indicates a difference in structure, which may be the basis for the selective toxicity of antibacterial agents, including aminoglycoside antibiotics. Also, transport mechanisms participate in the selective toxicity of aminoglycosides.

II. Interaction with Tubulin and Microtubules

AKIYAMA et al. (1978) have observed that addition of neomycin, streptomycin, kanamycin, gentamicin, or viomycin to porcine brain tubulin, purified by the polymerization–depolymerization method of SHELANSKI et al. (1973), causes an increase in turbidity due to formation of an insoluble complex, reaching a maximum in 5 min at 18 °C. The final turbidity attained is dependent upon the antibiotic concentration at a constant concentration of tubulin (Fig. 10). Neomycin is more active in inducing formation of the insoluble complex than streptomycin, gentamicin, and kanamycin.

Electron microscopic analysis reveals a new type of tubulin assembly from interaction with the antibiotic, that shows a characteristic ordered structure. The structure is different from natural microtubules or vinblastine-induced microtubular crystals, but resembles the tubulin assembly induced by polycations. It possesses double walls with a diameter of 25 nm at the outer edge of the inner wall and 38 nm at the outer wall. Both walls show the same axial periodicity of 5 nm each

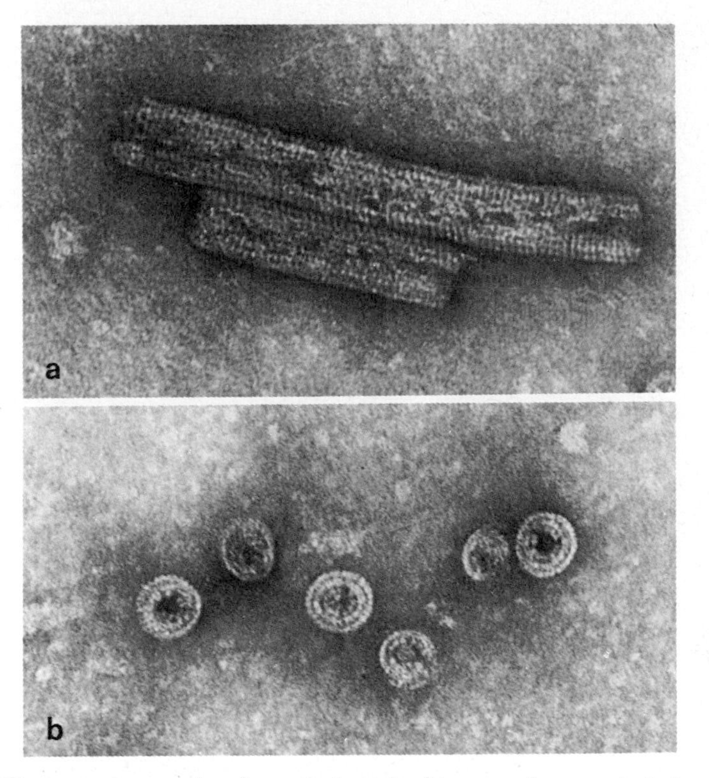

Fig. 11a, b. Electron micrographs of negatively stained images of neomycin-induced tubulin assembly. Samples were stained with 4% uranyl acetate. **a** lateral views; **b** end-on views (AKIYAMA et al. 1978)

(Fig. 11). Its optical diffraction pattern exhibits relatively strong 5-nm meridional and off-meridional reflections. Off-meridional reflections of 4 nm, obtained in natural microtubule assembly, as described later, are not recognized (Fig. 12).

Addition of the antibiotic to microtubules, normally assembled in vitro at 37 °C, induces reassembly of microtubules and laterally attached bundle formation (Fig. 13). At an early stage the microtubules with 4-nm axial periodicity are surrounded by an outer wall of 5-nm periodicity with a diameter of 38 nm (Fig. 14). Finally, the newly assembled structure possesses double walls, accompanied by lateral association or bundle formation, as shown in Fig. 13b. The optical diffraction pattern shows clear 5-nm meridional reflections and both 4- and 5-nm off-meridional reflections (Fig. 12b).

Various agents which block natural microtubule assembly do not affect formation of the tubulin–antibiotic complex, suggesting that they are produced by different mechanisms. Low temperature (4 °C), 1–10 m*M* colchicine, and 5 m*M* *N*-ethylmaleimide, which prevent natural microtubule assembly, do not significantly affect the formation of the antibiotic–tubulin complex. Other inhibitors of natural microtubule assembly, 4 m*M* $CaCl_2$ and 3.2 m*M* EDTA, exhibit weak inhibitory effects on the antibiotic–tubulin interaction.

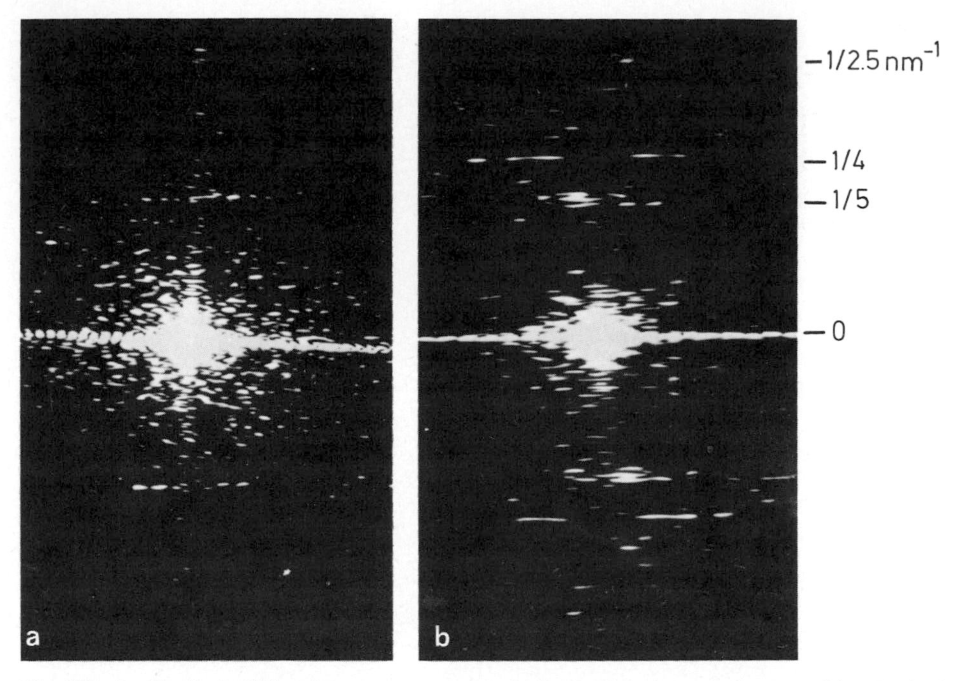

Fig. 12 a, b. Optical diffraction patterns of tubulin and microtubule assembly. Optical diffraction patterns were obtained by an optical diffractometer with He-Ne laser similar to KLUG and BERGER's lens system. **a** The pattern obtained from the negative of electron micrograph of neomycin-induced tubulin assembly with two walls of 5-nm periodicity. **b** The pattern obtained from the negative of electron micrograph of a part of neomycin-induced microtubule assembly with duplex crystalline form (AKIYAMA et al. 1978)

Since tubulin is an acidic protein and the antibiotics are basic substances, the complex formation may be due to ionic interaction. However, complex formation with tubulin or microtubules seems to be characteristic of the aminoglycoside and viomycin groups of antibiotics. Addition of some other basic antibiotics, such as bleomycin and anthracycline antibiotics, to tubulin solutions does not cause an increase in turbidity.

III. Interaction with Actin

It has been found by centrifugation, turbidity, and viscosity measurements that aminoglycoside antibiotics (neomycin, gentamicin, kanamycin, and streptomycin), viomycin, polymyxin B, and tetracycline interact with skeletal muscle actin to form insoluble complexes (Fig. 15) (SOMEYA and TANAKA 1979). A linear relationship is observed between the amount of actin polymerization and the number of primary amino groups of the aminoglycoside antibiotics, except for kanamycin (Fig. 16). Of the antibiotics tested, neomycin is most efficient in actin polymerization. Polymerization of actin is not significantly induced by kasugamycin, chloramphenicol, erythromycin, benzylpenicillin, angustmycin A, formycin A, actinomycin D, and mitomycin C. The aminoglycosides and viomycin block the acto-HMM Mg^{2+}-

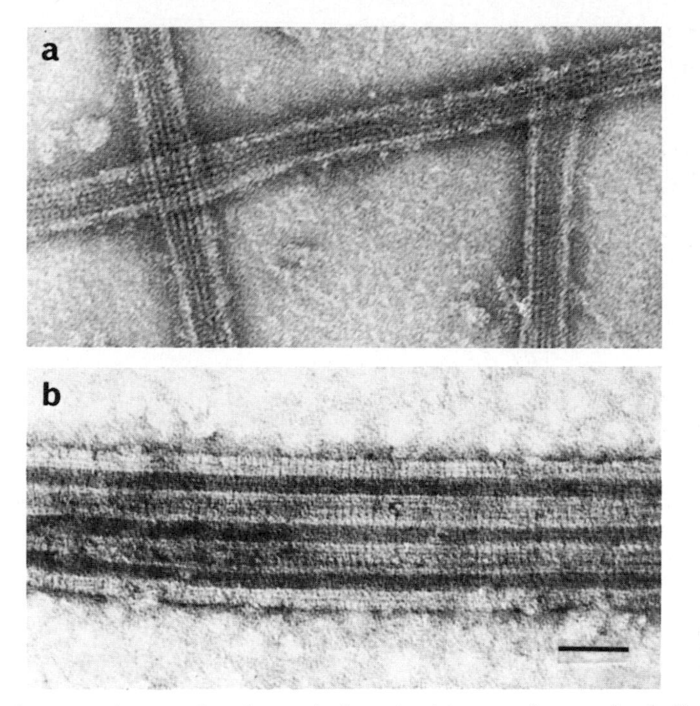

Fig. 13a, b. Electron micrographs of negatively stained image of natural tubulin assembly and neomycin-induced microtubule assembly. Negatively stained by the same procedure as Fig. 11. Inserted scales are 50 nm. **a** Natural microtubules assembled at 37 °C; **b** crystalline-like structure of neomycin-induced microtubule assembly (AKIYAMA et al. 1978)

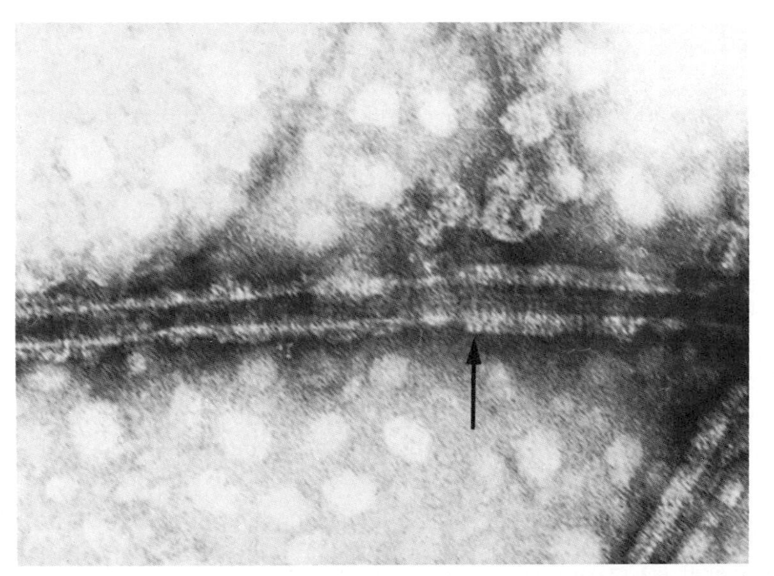

Fig. 14. Electron micrograph of negatively stained image of natural microtubules, partly surrounded by a neomycin-induced outer wall. *Arrow* shows a growing point of the duplex outer wall (AKIYAMA et al. 1978)

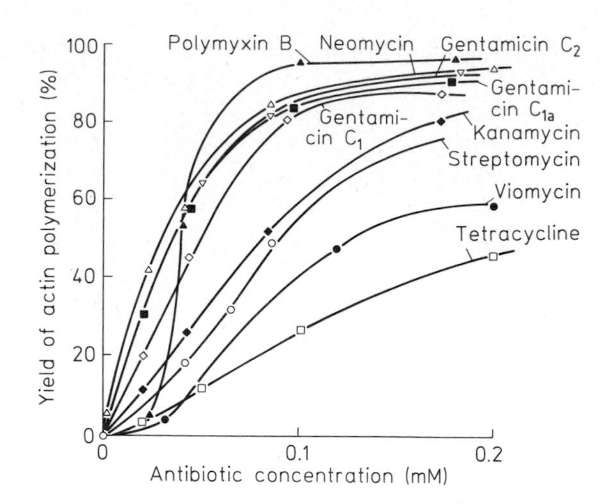

Fig. 15. Percentage of actin polymerization as a function of antibiotic concentration (SOMEYA and TANAKA 1979)

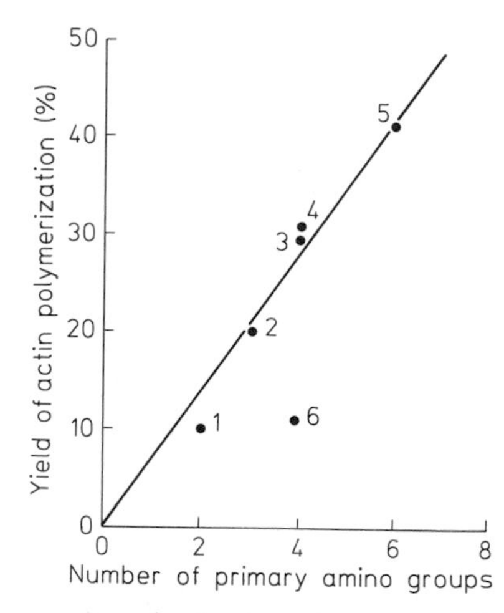

Fig. 16. Relationship of the number of primary amino groups of aminoglycoside antibiotics to the yield of actin polymerization (SOMEYA and TANAKA 1979). *1*, streptomycin; *2*, gentamicin C_1; *3*, gentamicin C_{1a}; *4*, gentamicin C_2; *5*, neomycin; *6*, kanamycin

ATPase reaction but do not significantly affect HMM Mg^{2+}-ATPase activity, indicating that the inhibition results from the interaction with actin. It is observed by equilibrium dialysis that [^{3}H]dihydrostreptomycin binds to actin.

IV. Interaction with Membrane or Phospholipid

CARRADO et al. (1975) observed that aminoglycosides inhibit the phospholipid-mediated diffusion of cations across a model membrane, presumably by binding to the acidic groups of the phospholipids with a higher affinity than the inorganic cations. Among the phospholipids present in the model membrane, phosphatidyl inositol is most active in binding calcium ions. ORSULAKOVA et al. (1976) reported competitive binding of neomycin and calcium to inner ear tissue homogenates and suggested that a complex is formed between the drug and polyphosphoinositides. STOCKHORST and SCHACHAT (1977) have found that neomycin increases the turbidity of polyphosphoinositides at low ionic strength. ALEXANDER et al. (1979) have demonstrated interaction with phospholipid liposomes by microelectrophoresis.

C. Peptide Antibiotics Showing Similar Mechanisms of Inhibition of Ribosomal Functions

I. Viomycin

Viomycin is a peptide antibiotic, active against mycobacteria. Capreomycin and tuberactinomycin are similar to viomycin in chemical structure and biologic properties. The viomycin group of antibiotics causes nephrotoxicity and ototoxicity. Therefore, the biologic activities (effects and side effects) are similar to those of aminoglycoside antibiotics. Concerning the mechanism of action, viomycin binds to, or interacts with, the ribosome and inhibits initiation and translocation in protein synthesis. In this respect, viomycin shows a similar mechanism of action to that of the aminoglycoside antibiotics.

1. Inhibition of Protein Synthesis

Viomycin inhibits protein synthesis but does not cause codon misreading, in spite of biologic activity similar to that of aminoglycoside antibiotics in an *E. coli* ribosomal system (DAVIES et al. 1965; TANAKA and IGUSA 1968). LIOU and TANAKA (1976) have found that viomycin blocks natural or viral messenger-directed protein synthesis more markedly than poly[U]-dependent polyphenylalanine synthesis, suggesting the inhibition of initiation of protein synthesis. Initiation complex formation on both the 30 S ribosomal subunit and the 70 S ribosome (fMet-$tRNA_F$ binding) is prevented by the antibiotic. In the peptide chain elongation process, viomycin does not significantly affect aminoacyl-tRNA binding to ribosomes and the peptidyl transferase reaction, but strongly inhibits translocation of peptidyl-tRNA from the acceptor site to the donor site.

2. Binding to Ribosomes and Ribosomal Subunits

MISUMI et al. (1978a) prepared [^{14}C]tuberactinomycin O (15.0 Ci/mol), an antibiotic closely related to viomycin, by incubating the antibiotic with an equal amount of [^{14}C]urea in 3 *N* HCl for 40 days at room temperature, and then purifying it by Sephadex G 10 column chromatography (Fig. 17). It has been demonstrated by equilibrium dialysis and the Millipore filter method that [^{14}C]tuberactinomycin O reversibly binds to the 70 S ribosome and to both 30 S and 50 S ribosomal subunits. As illustrated in Fig. 18, at saturation levels of the antibiotic approximately 2 mol of the drug are bound per mol of ribosomes. The shape of the binding curve also suggests that there may be at least two binding sites with

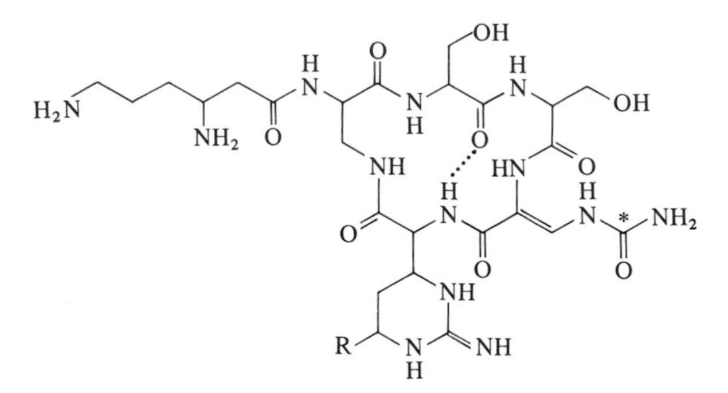

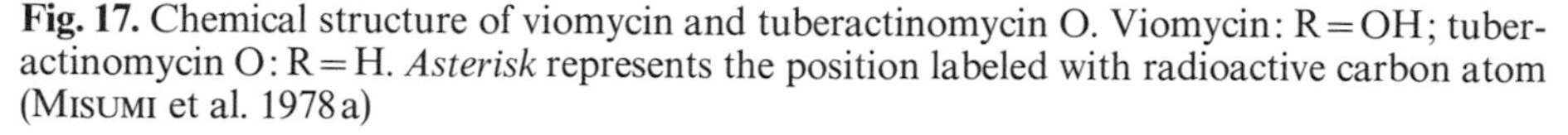
Fig. 17. Chemical structure of viomycin and tuberactinomycin O. Viomycin: R=OH; tuberactinomycin O: R=H. *Asterisk* represents the position labeled with radioactive carbon atom (MISUMI et al. 1978a)

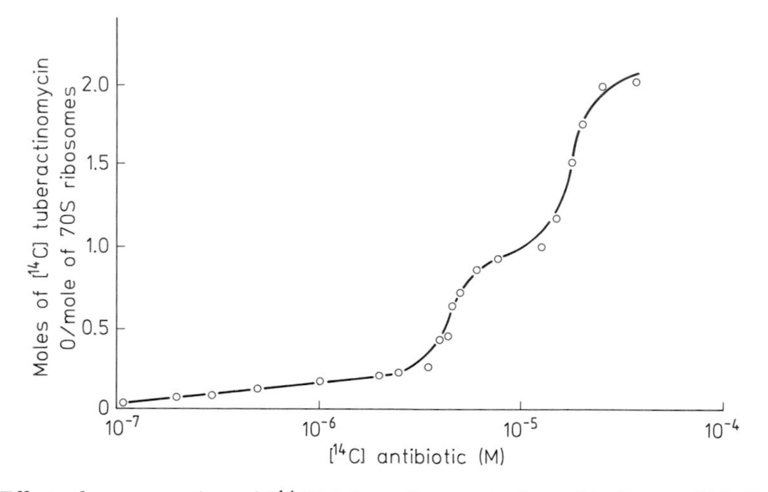

Fig. 18. Effect of concentration of [^{14}C] tuberactinomycin O on binding to 70S ribosomes (MISUMI et al. 1978a)

different association constants. Binding is dependent upon temperatures; for example, the antibiotic binds to the ribosome in a molar ratio of 0.2:1 at 4 °C (Fig. 18) and 0.5:1 at 37 °C at an antibiotic concentration of 1 μ*M*, which causes approximately 50% inhibition of polyphenylalanine synthesis. Figures 19 and 20 show Scatchard plots for the equilibrium binding of the antibiotic to the ribosome and ribosomal subunits. There appears to be a linear relationship between r and r/A, where r represents moles of bound [^{14}C]tuberactinomycin O per mol of ribosomes or subunits, and A represents molar concentration of the free [^{14}C]antibiotic. The 70 S ribosome seems to possess one binding site with an association constant of approximately 6.0×10^5 M^{-1}, and another site with a lower binding constant. The number of binding sites on the 30 S ribosomal subunit is one (r=0.95) with an association constant of 2.3×10^5 M^{-1}, and that of the 50 S subunit is one (r=0.85) with a binding constant of 7.2×10^5 M^{-1}. Thus, each ribosomal subunit possesses one binding site for tuberactinomycin O, and the large subunit shows higher affin-

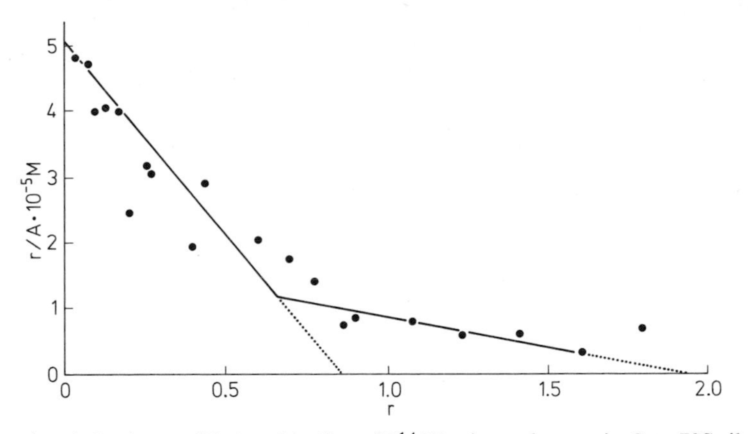

Fig. 19. Scatchard plot for equilibrium binding of [^{14}C] tuberactinomycin O to 70S ribosomes (MISUMI et al. 1978a)

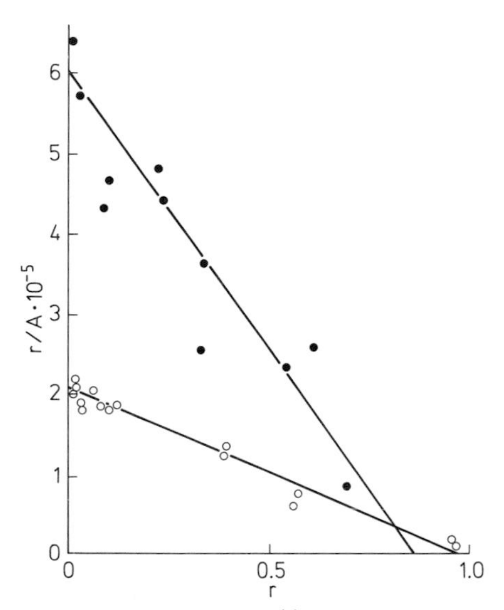

Fig. 20. Scatchard plot for equilibrium binding of [^{14}C] tuberactinomycin O to the ribosomal subunits (MISUMI et al. 1978a). —○—○—, 30S subunit; —●—●—, 50S subunit

ity than the small subunit. The binding of [^{14}C]tuberactinomycin O is decreased by the presence of unlabeled tuberactinomycin O and viomycin at the same level, indicating that binding is specific for the antibiotic and both drugs possess the same binding site on the ribosome and ribosomal subunits. However, it remains to be determined whether a single molecule of the antibiotic binds to both ribosomal subunits or separate molecules bind to each subunit.

3. Localization of Drug Resistance in the Ribosome

YAMADA et al. (1972, 1976) have observed by the inhibition of polyphenylalanine synthesis that resistance to viomycin is due to alteration of the 30 S ribosomal sub-

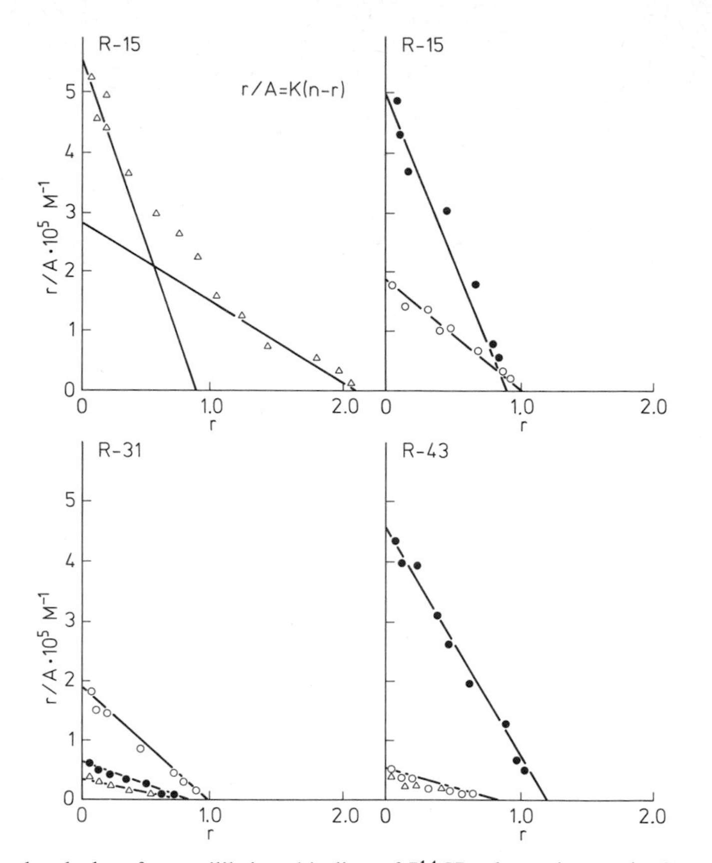

Fig. 21. Scatchard plots for equilibrium binding of [^{14}C] tuberactinomycin O to ribosomal particles, derived from viomycin-sensitive (R-15) and -resistant (R-31 and R-43) strains of *Mycobacterium smegmatis* (N. TANAKA and M. MISUMI, unpublished work). The assay was carried out by the method of CHOI et al. (1979). △, ribosomes; ○, 30S subunit; ●, 50S subunit

unit in some resistant mutants of *Mycobacterium smegmatis*, and to alteration of the 50 S ribosomal subunit in other mutants. YAMADA et al. (1978) have studied the detailed localization of viomycin resistance by the drug-induced 70 S couple formation of reconstituted ribosomal subunits, and found that resistance is conferred by RNA but not by proteins of either large or small ribosomal subunit.

CHOI et al. (1979) have prepared ribosomes and ribosomal subunits from viomycin-sensitive and -resistant strains of *M. smegmatis*. They studied the effects of viomycin on polypeptide synthesis, translocation of peptidyl-tRNA on hybrid ribosomes, and interaction of [^{14}C]tuberactinomycin O with ribosomes and ribosomal subunits. Viomycin inhibits polyphenylalanine synthesis and translocation of peptidyl-tRNA on ribosomes derived from a sensitive strain (R-15), but not with ribosomes from viomycin-resistant mutants (R-31 and R-43). The binding of [^{14}C]tuberactinomycin O, an analog of viomycin, to ribosomal particles has been studied by the Millipore filter method and the association constants have been ob-

Table 7. Association constants (Ka) obtained from the Scatchard plots of data for binding of [^{14}C] tuberactinomycin O to the ribosomes and ribosomal subunits. (N. TANAKA and M. MISUMI, unpublished work)

Ribosomal particles	*Mycobacterium smegmatis strains*		
	R-15 [a]	R-31 [b]	R-43 [b]
Ribosome	$5\times10^5\ M^{-1}$ 2×10^5	3×10^4	3×10^4
Large subunit	4×10^5	3×10^4	4×10^5
Small subunit	2×10^5	2×10^5	3×10^4

[a] R-15, viomycin-sensitive strain
[b] R-31 and R-43, viomycin-resistant mutants

tained by Scatchard plots for equilibrium binding. We repeated the binding experiments and the results are presented in Fig. 21 and Table 7 (N. TANAKA and M. Misumi, unpublished work). The viomycin-sensitive R-15 ribosome appears to possess two major binding sites with association constants (Ka) of approximately $5\times10^5\ M^{-1}$ and $2\times10^5\ M^{-1}$. The viomycin-resistant ribosomes of R-31 or R-43 seem to possess one major binding site with Ka $3\times10^4\ M^{-1}$, which is about $^1/_{17}$ the Ka of R-15 ribosomes. The results show that the resistant ribosomes (R-31 and R-43) interact with the antibiotic more weakly than the sensitive ribosome (R-15). The R-31 large ribosomal subunit shows lower affinity for the drug (Ka $3\times10^4\ M^{-1}$) than the R-15 and R-43 large subunits (Ka $4\times10^5\ M^{-1}$), indicating that the former one is resistant to, and the latter two are sensitive to, the antibiotic. The R-15 and R-31 small subunits exhibit higher affinity (Ka $2\times10^5\ M^{-1}$) than the R-43 small subunits (Ka $3\times10^4\ M^{-1}$), showing that the former two are sensitive and the latter is resistant. The results indicate that drug resistance can be attributed to poor affinity of the ribosomal subunit for the antibiotics, i.e., the 50 S subunit of R-31 and the 30 S subunit of R-43 are resistant to viomycin. The binding of the drug to the sensitive ribosomal subunit is markedly reduced by combination with the resistant pair subunit which renders the entire ribosome resistant to the antibiotic.

4. Mechanism of Translocation Inhibition

The mechanism of inhibition by viomycin of translocation is similar to that by kanamycin (MISUMI and TANAKA 1980). Viomycin blocks a single cycle of translocation on the poly[U]-ribosome, carrying *N*-acetyl-diPhe-tRNA on the acceptor site and deacylated tRNA at the donor site. Inhibition of translocation has been demonstrated by enhanced puromycin reactivity of *N*-acetyl-diPhe-tRNA and by release of deacylated tRNA. The GTPase reaction, catalyzed by EF-G and ribosomes, is not significantly affected by the antibiotic. Viomycin may interfere with translocation by fixing *N*-acetyl-Phe-tRNA to the acceptor site, but not to the donor site (see Sect. A.V.2).

II. Negamycin

Negamycin is a dipeptide antibiotic, containing a hydrazide group and unusual amino acids (Kondo et al. 1971). The structure is presented in Fig. 9. The antibiotic shows a broad antibacterial spectrum, including activity against *Pseudomonas*. The drug inhibits protein synthesis in vivo and in vitro, and promotes codon misreading (Mizuno et al. 1970; Uehara et al. 1972). In this respect, the mechanism of action of negamycin is similar to that of the aminoglycoside antibiotics. A possible structural basis for codon misreading is discussed in Sect. A.VII.1. Negamycin selectively inhibits the termination process of protein synthesis (Uehara et al. 1974; 1976a, b). Viral (f2 phage) RNA-directed protein synthesis is not totally blocked by negamycin even at high drug concentrations, and a long polypeptide accumulates on the ribosome. The molecular weight of accumulated polypeptide is close to that of the coat protein with higher histidine content. Negamycin may, therefore, inhibit the termination mechanism. A higher concentration of the drug is required for promoting codon misreading. Unlike inhibitors of initiation, negamycin prevents polysome breakdown. Contrary to aminoglycoside antibiotics, negamycin shows bactericidal action even in the presence of chloramphenicol.

D. Discussion

Of the molecular events in bacteria altered by the aminoglycoside antibiotics, the inhibition of ribosomal functions and membrane damage are the most prominent phenomena. Therefore, the drugs seem to act on the ribosome or cell membrane. It remains to be determined which is the chemoreceptor or primary site of action.

Aminoglycoside-resistant alterations of ribosomes result in resistance of the cell membrane to the antibiotics and the cells are not killed by the drugs. Chloramphenicol and other ribosomal inhibitors reverse the lethal action of aminoglycoside antibiotics. These and other results with aminoglycosides accumulated to date indicate that the receptor is the ribosome of bacteria. However, the detailed site of action on the ribosome needs further clarification.

Studies on the mechanism of action of antibiotics aim at the elucidation of unknown biologic events, using antibiotics as tools in molecular biology, as well as elucidating receptors, selective toxicity, and chemical reactions between the drug and receptor(s).

The investigations with aminoglycoside antibiotics have contributed to the progress of molecular biology. The streptomycin resistance gene (*rps 12*) is the first genetic locus determined among the ribosomal protein genes. Similarly, the spectinomycin resistance gene (*rps 5*) has been assigned. The kasugamycin resistance gene, involving 16S RNA, has also been determined. The genetic and biochemical aspects of resistance to kanamycin, neomycin, and gentamicin seem to be more complicated and have yet to be determined.

Phenotypic suppression or codon misreading provoked by aminoglycosides have helped elucidate the translation fidelity mechanism. The aminoglycoside antibiotics can be used as inhibitors of protein synthesis, particularly kasugamycin as a selective inhibitor of initiation.

The lethal action of streptomycin and kanamycin is reversed by chloramphenicol or other protein synthesis inhibitors, suggesting that the events are related to ribosomal function in protein synthesis. It is of interest that kasugamycin and spectinomycin, which are incapable of stimulating translation errors, are bacteriostatic, but misreading-promoting aminoglycosides (streptomycin, kanamycin, gentamicin, neomycin, etc.) are bactericidal. WALLACE et al. (1979) have discussed the lethality of streptomycin, and insist that accumulation of faulty proteins due to the drug-induced codon misreading cannot explain the rapid killing effect of the antibiotic. An understanding of the mechanism by which interference with ribosomal functions results in killing the cells awaits further experiments. The alteration of ribosomes induced by aminoglycosides may result in membrane damage, which may lead to cell death. However, the precise relationship between membrane damage and lethality is not clear. Blebs are observed by electron microscopy in the cell surface in the presence of aminoglycosides. The relationship between bleb formation and membrane damage or leakage has not yet been elucidated. It is noteworthy that the blebs are formed not only by bactericidal drugs (dibekacin and streptomycin), but also by bacteriostatic ones (spectinomycin and kasugamycin).

The aminoglycoside antibiotics affect initiation, elongation (translocation), and termination of protein synthesis, and promote translation errors. The pleiotropic effects of aminoglycosides, especially interference with the codon–anticodon interaction, may be explained by distortion of the A-site. It is consistent with the finding that the inhibition of translocation by kanamycin, gentamicin, neomycin, hygromycin B, etc. is caused by fixation of aminoacyl- or peptidyl-tRNA to the A-site. However, the inhibition of initiation, particularly breakdown of the initiation complex, may be caused by the distortion of the D-site (MODOLELL and DAVIS 1970).

The aminoglycosides inhibit growth of mycobacteria, staphylococci, and gram-negative bacteria, but do not significantly inhibit that of streptococci, anaerobic bacteria, and fungi. The antibacterial spectrum can be explained by the transport mechanism; i.e., the energy-dependent, second-phase uptake of the antibiotics which occurs only in aerobic conditions, and is prevented by anaerobiosis.

The selective toxicity of aminoglycoside antibiotics depends upon the transport mechanism as well as the drug sensitivity of the receptor, i.e., the ribosome.

E. Summary

The mechanism by which the aminoglycosides kill bacterial cells remains mysterious. However, the evidence accumulated to date shows that the primary site of action or receptor of the aminoglycoside antibiotics may be the ribosome, the protein-synthesizing machinery. The pleiotropic effects of the antibiotics on bacteria can be attributed to interaction with the ribosome. However, the detailed mechanism of action differs with each drug. Concerning the mode of action, the aminoglycosides clinically used as antibacterial agents may belong to the following three groups: (1) streptomycin, (2) kanamycin–gentamicin–neomycin, and (3) spectinomycin. The mechanism of action of kasugamycin differs from those of these antibiotics.

Most aminoglycoside antibiotics are bactericidal, but kasugamycin and spectinomycin are bacteriostatic. The lethal action of streptomycin or kanamycin is reversed by chloramphenicol and other inhibitors of ribosomes, suggesting that the killing depends upon ribosomal activity. The polysome level decreases in cells treated with streptomycin, resulting in accumulation of monoribosomes incapable of protein synthesis. Unlike streptomycin, neomycin and spectinomycin accumulate polysomes.

Most aminoglycosides, except kasugamycin and spectinomycin, stimulate codon misreading in vitro and in vivo or phenotypic suppression.

In addition to the interference with protein synthesis, aminoglycosides induce membrane damage, impairment of respiration, RNA accumulation, and cell death. Electron microscopic studies have revealed that the antibiotics promote the formation of blebs of the cell envelope.

The most distinct in vivo effects of aminoglycoside antibiotics on bacterial cells are the inhibition of protein synthesis and membrane damage. The mutation of ribosomes or additon of ribosomal inhibitors eliminates the membrane damage, suggesting that the target or receptor of aminoglycosides is the ribosome, and the membrane damage is a secondary effect, resulting from the inhibition of ribosomal functions. However, the mode of action of aminoglycosides may be different from those of chloramphenicol, tetracyclines, macrolides, and other ribosomal inhibitors, because most aminoglycosides promote codon misreading and cause membrane damage. Moreover, most aminoglycosides are bactericidal, but chloramphenicol, tetracyclines, and macrolides are bacteriostatic.

Of the aminoglycoside antibiotics, the mechanism of action of streptomycin has been most studied and all the other aminoglycosides were considered to show a similar mode of action. However, considerable evidence has recently accumulated showing that the detailed mechanisms by which aminoglycosides prevent ribosomal functions differ from each other. The interaction with ribosomal subunits differs with each drug. Initiation of protein synthesis is affected by various aminoglycosides in diverse ways. The translocation of peptidyl-tRNA is inhibited by kanamycin, gentamicin, and neomycin, but not by streptomycin.

I. Localization of Drug Sensitivity, Resistance, and Dependence on the Ribosome

Reconstitution experiments have shown that ribosomal protein S 12, in *E. coli*, is responsible for streptomycin sensitivity, resistance, and dependence, which is conferred by the *strA* gene. In some resistant mutants, lysine at position 42 of S 12 is replaced by asparagine, threonine, or arginine; in others lysine at position 87 is replaced by arginine. The reversion from streptomycin dependence to independence is sometimes associated with mutation of S 4 or S 5 protein. There are some streptomycin-resistant or -dependent mutants, in which S 4, S 5, and S 12 proteins are altered.

Similarly, it has been demonstrated that ribosomal protein S 5 is responsible for spectinomycin sensitivity and resistance, and S 17 for neamine resistance. In a kanamycin-resistant mutant, resistance is linked to the 23 S core of the 30 S ribosomal subunit, in which S 12 is altered. Protein L 6 is changed in gentamicin-resistant mutants. Kanamycin resistance is linked to the 30 S ribosomal subunit in some mutants of *E. coli*, and to the 50 S subunit in the others. Kasugamycin resistance is associated with 16 S RNA of the 30 S ribosomal subunit. The RNA methylase is lacking in the mutant. In another kasugamycin-resistant mutant, protein S 2 is altered.

II. Binding of Aminoglycosides to the Ribosome

Streptomycin or dihydrostreptomycin binds to the 70 S ribosome or 30 S subunit. There are one or two specific binding sites on the ribosome. Ribosomal protein S 12 controls the binding of the antibiotic to the ribosome, but does not itself bind streptomycin. Contradictory results have been obtained concerning the drug-binding ribosomal component(s) by a number of investigators, using different approaches.

It has been observed that [^{3}H]kanamycin binds to the 70 S ribosome and to both subunits. The 70 S ribosome binds approximately 2 molecules of the antibiotic up to a drug concentration of 10 μM, and more at higher concentrations. Each ribosomal subunit has a single major binding site. The binding of [^{3}H]kanamycin to ribosomes and ribosomal subunits is reversed by neomycin or gentamicin, but not by streptomycin, showing that kanamycin, gentamicin, and neomycin possess the same or similar binding sites on the ribosome, differing from the streptomycin site.

[^{14}C]Paromomycin has been shown to bind specifically to a single site on the ribosome. Streptomycin, gentamicin, kanamycin, kasugamycin, and spectinomycin do not compete for binding. [^{3}H]Tobramycin has been observed to possess two types of selective binding sites on the ribosome and on the 50 S subunit, while it has only one type of binding site on the 30 S subunit.

[^{3}H]Kasugamycin stoichiometrically binds to the ribosome and to the 30 S subunit. A single binding site is present on the ribosome. Streptomycin, kanamycin, and gentamicin do not compete. [^{3}H]Spectinomycin reversibly binds to the ribosome and to the 30 S ribosomal subunit.

III. Inhibition of Initiation of Protein Synthesis

Kasugamycin selectively inhibits initiation of protein synthesis by blocking formation of the 30 S initiation complex, fMet-tRNA$_F$-mRNA-30 S ribosomal subunit, but does not significantly affect elongation of the peptide chain.

Streptomycin affects initiation as well as elongation and termination of protein synthesis. The antibiotic causes breakdown of the 70 S initiation complex, resulting in the release of fMet-tRNA$_F$. The ribosomal dissociation, induced by IF-3, is blocked by streptomycin and other aminoglycosides.

Kanamycin, gentamicin, and neomycin interfere with initiation of protein synthesis. However, the antibiotics affect elongation of the peptide chain more markedly than initiation.

IV. Stimulation of Codon Misreading

Streptomycin, kanamycin, gentamicin, neomycin, and other aminoglycosides with a streptamine or 2-deoxystreptamine moiety provoke codon misreading or induce the uptake of incorrect amino acids which do not correspond to the codon (coding nucleotides) in vivo and in vitro. In contrast, kasugamycin and spectinomycin do not stimulate translation errors. GORINI and KATAJA (1964, 1965) first observed that streptomycin, kanamycin, neomycin, and paromomycin disturb the fidelity of translation in vivo, i.e., phenotypic repair or suppression. A similar effect has been demonstrated in vitro by DAVIES et al. (1965).

V. Interference with Aminoacyl-tRNA Binding

Both EF-Tu- and GTP-dependent and -independent binding of aminoacyl-tRNA to ribosomes are blocked by streptomycin, kanamycin, or gentamicin. Streptomycin also stimulates the binding of noncognate aminoacyl-tRNA, which seems to be consistent with the codon misreading effect.

VI. Inhibition of Translocation of Peptidyl-tRNA

The EF-G- and GTP-dependent translocation is inhibited by kanamycin, gentamicin, neomycin, hygromycin B, apramycin, and related antibiotics, but not by streptomycin. Peptidyl transferase reaction is not significantly affected by the aminoglycoside antibiotics. GTP hydrolysis, catalyzed by EF-G and ribosomes, or the interaction of EF-G, GTP, and ribosomes, is not blocked by kanamycin and hygromycin B. These aminoglycosides may interfere with translocation by fixing peptidyl-tRNA to the A-site but not to the D-site. The single cycle of translocation as well as the overall translocation are inhibited by kanamycin.

VII. Interference with Termination of Protein Synthesis

Streptomycin inhibits chain termination by blocking release factor-dependent codon recognition. Codon misreading, caused by aminoglycosides, favors reading-through of termination codons and the synthesis of longer than normal peptides due to termination errors.

VIII. The Effects on Cell Membrane

Streptomycin induces damage to the bacterial membrane or envelope, resulting in excretion of nucleotides and other low molecular weight materials. The rapid efflux of K^+ remains the earliest event to be detected after treatment with streptomycin. The drug resistance mutation of ribosomes or addition of chloramphenicol eliminates the membrane damage, suggesting that the effect on the cell envelope is a secondary consequence, derived from the ribosomal change induced by the aminoglycoside.

Dibekacin, streptomycin, spectinomycin, and kasugamycin have been observed by electron microscopy to stimulate the formation of blebs of the cell envelope.

IX. Uptake of Aminoglycosides by Bacterial Cells

The entry of streptomycin into *E. coli* cells occurs in two phases. The initial uptake may be due to ionic binding of the antibiotic to the cell surface. After a lag phase, the second phase of uptake occurs. The uptake rate rapidly increases and simultaneously the permeability of the cell envelope changes. The second phase of drug uptake requires energy and may represent an active transport process. Other aminoglycoside antibiotics may also enter the bacterial cells by an active, carrier-mediated transport, similar to streptomycin. The uptake of aminoglycosides occurs in aerobic conditions, and is blocked by anaerobiosis. This may explain the antibacterial spectrum: strongly active against aerobic bacteria, but not against anaerobic bacteria.

In some drug-resistant mutants and clinical isolates, resistance to aminoglycosides is attributed to transport barriers.

X. Effects on Mammalian or Eukaryotic Cell Components

The aminoglycoside antibiotics interact with eukaryotic ribosomes, RNA, tubulin or microtubules, actin, phospholipid, and membrane. However, the biologic significance of these effects or the relationship to the side effects remains to be determined.

The selective toxicity of aminoglycoside antibiotics depends upon the transport mechanism and the sensitivity of the ribosome.

References

Akiyama T, Tanaka K, Tanaka N, Nonomura Y (1978) Interaction of viomycin and aminoglycoside antibiotics with tubulin and microtubules. J Antibiot (Tokyo) 31:1306–1309

Alexander AM, Gonda I, Harpur ES, Kayes JB (1979) Interaction of aminoglycoside antibiotics with phospholipid liposomes studied by microelectrophoresis. J Antibiot (Tokyo) 32:504–510

Anand N, Davis BD (1960) Effect of streptomycin on *Escherichia coli*. Nature 185:22–23

Anand N, Davis BD, Armitage AK (1960) Uptake of streptomycin by *Escherichia coli*. Nature 185:23–24

Anderson P, Davies J, Davis BD (1967) Effect of spectinomycin on polypeptide synthesis in extracts of *Escherichia coli*. J Mol Biol 29:203–215

Andry K, Bockrath RC (1974) Dihydrostreptomycin accumulation in *E. coli*. Nature 251:534–536

Beggs WH, Andrews FA (1976) Inhibition of dihydrostreptomycin binding to *Mycobacterium smegmatis* by monovalent and divalent cation salts. Antimicrob Agents Chemother 9:393–396

Bermingham MAC, Deol BS, Still JL (1970) Effect of streptomycin on lipid composition with particular reference to cyclic depsipeptide biosynthesis in *Serratia marcescens* and other micro-organisms. Biochem J 119:861–869

Birge EA, Kurland CG (1969) Altered ribosomal protein in streptomycin-dependent *Escherichia coli*. Science 166:1282–1284

Birge EA, Kurland CG (1970) Reversion of streptomycin dependent strain of *Escherichia coli*. Mol Gen Genet 109:356–369

Bissel DM (1965) Formation of an altered enzyme in *E. coli* in the presence of neomycin. J Mol Biol 14:619–622

Biswas DK, Gorini L (1972) The attachment site of streptomycin to the 30 S ribosomal subunit. Proc Natl Acad Sci USA 69:2141–2144

Bollen A, Davies J, Ozaki M, Mizushima S (1969) Ribosomal protein conferring sensitivity to the antibiotic spectinomycin in *Escherichia coli*. Science 165:85–86

Bollen A, Cabezon T, Wilde MDE, Villarroel R, Herzog A (1975) Alteration of ribosomal protein S 17 by mutation linked to neamine resistance in *Escherichia coli*. J Mol Biol 99:795–806

Brakier-Gingras L, Lacoste L, Boileau G (1974) Streptomycin resistance and ribosomal proteins: amino acid substitution in the str protein of one streptomycin-resistant mutant of *Escherichia coli* K 12 after mutagenesis with ethylmethanesulfonate. Can J Biochem 52:304–309

Branscomb EW, Galas DJ (1975) Progressive decrease in protein synthesis accuracy induced by streptomycin in *Escherichia coli*. Nature 254:161–163

Bryan LE, van den Elzen HM (1976) Streptomycin accumulation in susceptible and resistant strains of *Escherichia coli* and *Pseudomonas aeruginosa*. Antimicrob Agents Chemother 9:928–938

Bryan LE, van den Elzen HM (1977) Effects of membrane-energy mutations and cations on streptomycin and gentamicin accumulation by bacteria: A model for entry of streptomycin and gentamicin in susceptible and resistant bacteria. Antimicrob Agents Chemother 12:163–177

Bryan LE, Haraphonge R, van den Elzen HM (1976) Gentamicin resistance in clinical isolates of *Pseudomonas aeruginosa* associated with diminished gentamicin accumulation and no detectable enzymatic modification. J Antibiot (Tokyo) 29:743–753

Buckel P, Buchberger A, Böck A, Wittmann HG (1977) Alteration of ribosomal protein L 6 in mutants of *Escherichia coli* resistant to gentamicin. Mol Gen Genet 158:47–54

Cabañas MJ, Vázquez D, Modolell J (1978 a) Dual interference of hygromycin B with ribosomal translocation and with aminoacyl-tRNA recognition. Eur J Biochem 87:21–27

Cabañas MJ, Vázquez D, Modolell J (1978 b) Inhibition of ribosomal translocation by aminoglycoside antibiotics. Biochem Biophys Res Commun 83:991–997

Campuzano S, Vázquez D, Modolell J (1979) Functional interaction of neomycin B and related antibiotics with 30 S and 50 S ribosomal subunits. Biochem Biophys Res Commun 87:960–966

Carrado AP, Prado WA, Pimenta de Morais I (1975) Competitive antagonism between calcium and aminoglycoside antibiotics in skeletal and smooth muscles. In: Rocha e Silva M, Suarez-Kurts G (eds) Concepts of membranes in regulation and excitation. Raven, New York, p 212

Caskey T, Scolnick E, Tompkins R, Goldstein J, Milman G (1969) Peptide chain termination, codon, protein factor and ribosomal requirements. Cold Spring Harbor Symp Quant Biol 34:479–488

Černá J, Rychlík I, Jonák J (1973) Peptidyl-transferase activity of *Escherichia coli* ribosomes digested by ribonuclease T_1. Eur J Biochem 34:551–556

Chang FN, Flaks JG (1970) Topography of the *Escherichia coli* 30 S ribosomal subunit and streptomycin binding. Proc Natl Acad Sci USA 67:1321–1328

Chang FN, Flaks JG (1972 a) The binding of dihydrostreptomycin to *E. coli* ribosomes: characteristics and equilibrium of the reaction. Antimicrob Agents Chemother 2:294–307

Chang FN, Flaks JG (1972 b) The binding of dihydrostreptomycin to *E. coli* ribosomes: kinetics of the reaction. Antimicrob Agents Chemother 2:308–319

Choi EC, Misumi M, Nishimura T, Tanaka N, Nomoto S, Teshima T, Shiba T (1979) Viomycin resistance: alterations of either ribosomal subunit affect the binding of the antibiotic to the pair subunit and the entire ribosome becomes resistant to the drug. Biochem Biophys Res Commun 87:904–910

Choi EC, Nishimura T, Tanaka N (1980) Mutational alterations of either large or small ribosomal subunit for the kanamycin resistance. Biochem Biophys Res Commun 94:755–762

Cox EC, White JR, Flaks JG (1964) Streptomycin action and the ribosome. Proc Natl Acad Sci USA 51:703–709

Davies J (1970) Structure-activity relationships among aminoglycoside antibiotics: comparison of the neomycins and hybrimycins. Biochim Biophys Acta 222:674–676

Davies J, Davis BD (1968) Misreading of RNA code words induced by aminoglycoside antibiotics: The effect of drug concentration. J Biol Chem 243:3312–3316

Davies J, Gilbert W, Gorini L (1964) Streptomycin, suppression and the code. Proc Natl Acad Sci USA 51:883–890

Davies J, Gorini L, Davis BD (1965) Misreading of RNA code words induced by aminoglycoside antibiotics. Mol Pharmacol 1:93–106

Davies J, Jones DS, Khorana HG (1966) A further study of misreading of codons induced by streptomycin and neomycin using ribopolynucleotides containing two nucleotides in alternating sequence as templates. J Mol Biol 18:48–57

Davis BD, Tai P-C, Wallace BJ (1974) Complex interactions of antibiotics with the ribosome. In: Nomura M, Tissieres A, Langyel P (eds) Ribosomes. Cold Spring Harbor Laboratory, Cold Spring Harber, New York, p 771–789

Dubin DT, Davis BD (1961) The effect of streptomycin on potassium flux in *Escherichia coli*. Biochim Biophys Acta 52:400–402

Dubin DT, Hancock R, Davis BD (1963) The sequence of some effects of streptomycin in *Escherichia coli*. Biochim Biophys Acta 74:476–489

Fitzgerald RJ, Bernheim F, Fitzgerald DB (1948) The inhibition by streptomycin of adaptive enzyme formation in Mycobacteria. J Biol Chem 175:195–200

Flaks JG, Cox EC, Witting ML, White JR (1962) Polypeptide synthesis with ribosomes from streptomycin-resistant and dependent *E. coli*. Biochem Biophys Res Commun 7:390–393

Friedman SM, Berezney R, Weinstein IB (1968) Fidelity in protein synthesis – The role of the ribosome. J Biol Chem 243:5044–5048

Funatsu G, Wittmann HG (1972) Ribosomal proteins. XXXIII. Location of amino-acid replacements in protein S 12 isolated from *Escherichia coli* mutants resistant to streptomycin. J Mol Biol 68:547–550

Funatsu G, Nierhaus K, Wittmann-Liebold B (1972a) Ribosomal proteins. XXII. Studies on the altered protein S 5 from a spectinomycin-resistant mutant of *Escherichia coli*. J Mol Biol 64:201–209

Funatsu G, Nierhaus K, Wittmann HG (1972b) Ribosomal proteins. XXXVII. Determination of allele types and amino acid exchanges in proteins S 12 of three streptomycin-resistant mutants of *Escherichia coli*. Biochim Biophys Acta 287:282–291

Garcia-Patrone M, Perazzolo CA, Baralle F, Gonzalez NS, Algranati ID (1971) Studies on dissociation factor of bacterial ribosomes: effect of antibiotics. Biochim Biophys Acta 246:291–299

Garvin RT, Biswas DK, Gorini L (1974) The effects of streptomycin or dihydrostreptomycin binding to 16S RNA or to 30S ribosomal subunits. Proc Natl Acad Sci USA 71:3814–3818

Ginzburg I, Miskin R, Zamir A (1973) N-Ethyl maleimide as a probe for the study of functional sites and conformations of 30S ribosomal subunits. J Mol Biol 79:481–494

Girshovich AS, Bochkareva ES, Ouchinnikov YA (1976) Identification of components of the streptomycin-binding center of *E. coli* MRE 600 ribosomes by photo-affinity labelling. Mol Gen Genet 144:205–212

González A, Jiménez A, Vázquez D, Davies JE, Schindler D (1978) Studies on the mode of action of hygromycin B, an inhibitor of translocation in eukaryotes. Biochim Biophys Acta 521:459–469

Gorini L, Kataja E (1964) Phenotypic repair by streptomycin of defective genotypes in *E. coli*. Proc Natl Acad Sci USA 51:487–493

Gorini L, Kataja E (1965) Suppression activated by streptomycin and related antibiotics in drug-sensitive strains. Biochem Biophys Res Commun 18:656–663

Gurgo C, Apirion D, Schlessinger D (1969) Polyribosome metabolism in *Escherichia coli* treated with chloramphenicol, neomycin, spectinomycin or tetracycline. J Mol Biol 45:205–220

Hall FJ (1977) Anaphylaxis after gentamicin. Lancet II:455

Hancock R (1962a) Uptake of ^{14}C-streptomycin by *Bacillus megaterium*. J Gen Microbiol 28:503–516

Hancock R (1962b) Uptake of ^{14}C-streptomycin by some microorganisms and its relation to their streptomycin sensitivity. J Gen Microbiol 28:493–501

Hasenbank R, Guthrie C, Stöffler G, Wittmann HG, Rosen L, Apirion D (1973) Electrophoretic and immunological studies on ribosomal proteins of 100 *Escherichia coli* revertants from streptomycin dependence. Mol Gen Genet 127:1–18
Helser TL, Davies JE, Dahlberg JE (1971) Change in methylation of 16S ribosomal RNA associated with mutation to kasugamycin resistance in *Escherichia coli*. Nature New Biol 233:12–14
Helser TL, Davies JE, Dahlberg JE (1972) Mechanism of kasugamycin resistance in *Escherichia coli*. Nature New Biol 235:6–9
Herzog A (1964) An effect of streptomycin on the dissociation of *Escherichia coli* 70S ribosomes. Biochem Biophys Res Commun 15:172–176
Herzog A, Ghysen A, Bollen A (1971) Sensitivity and resistance to streptomycin in relation with factor-mediated dissociation of ribosomes. FEBS Lett 15:291–294
Hurwitz C, Rosano CL (1962) Accumulation of label from ^{14}C-streptomycin by *Escherichia coli*. J Bacteriol 83:1193–1201
Iida K, Koike M (1974) Cell wall alterations of Gram-negative bacteria by aminoglycoside antibiotics. Antimicrob Agents Chemother 5:95–97
Inoue-Yokosawa N, Ishikawa C, Kaziro Y (1974) The role of guanosine triphosphate in translation reaction catalyzed by elongation factor G. J Biol Chem 249:4321–4323
Kaji H, Kaji A (1965) Specific binding of sRNA to ribosomes: Effect of streptomycin. Proc Natl Acad Sci USA 54: 213–219
Kaji H, Tanaka Y (1968) Binding of dihydrostreptomycin to ribosomal subunits. J Mol Biol 32:221–230
Kaji H, Suzuka I, Kaji A (1966) Binding of specific soluble ribonucleic acid to ribosomes: Binding of soluble ribonucleic acid to the template-30S subunits complex. J Biol Chem 241:1251–1256
Kogut M, Prizant E (1970) Effects of dihydrostreptomycin treatment *in vivo* on the ribosome cycle in *Escherichia coli*. FEBS Lett 12:17–20
Kogut M, Lightbown JW, Isaacson P (1965) Streptomycin action and anaerobiosis. J Gen Microbiol 39:155–164
Kondo S, Shibahara S, Takahashi K, Maeda K, Umezawa H (1971) Negamycin, a novel hydrazide antibiotic. J Am Chem Soc 93:6305–6306
Kono M, O'Hara K (1976) Mechanism of streptomycin(SM)-resistance of highly SM-resistant *Pseudomonas aeruginosa* strains. J Antibiot (Tokyo) 29:169–175
Kono M, O'Hara K (1977) Kanamycin-resistance mechanism of *Pseudomonas aeruginosa* governed by an R-plasmid independently of inactivating enzymes. J Antibiot (Tokyo) 30:688–690
Kozak M, Nathans D (1972) Differential inhibition of coliphage MS2 protein synthesis by ribosomal-directed antibiotics. J Mol Biol 70:41–55
Kühberger R, Piepersberg W, Petzet A, Buckel P, Böck A (1979) Alteration of ribosomal protein L6 in gentamicin-resistant strains of *Escherichia coli*. Effects on fidelity of protein synthesis. Biochemistry 18:187–193
Kurz DI (1974) Fidelity of protein synthesis with chicken embryo mitochondrial and cytoplasmic ribosomes. Biochemistry 13:572–577
Lake JA (1976) Ribosome structure determined by electron microscopy of *Escherichia coli* small subunits, large subunits and monomeric ribosomes. J Mol Biol 105:131–159
Lando D, Cousin MA, Privat de Garilhe M (1973) Misreading, a fundamental aspect of the mechanism of action of several aminoglycosides. Biochemistry 12:4528–4533
Lando D, Cousin MA, Ojasoo T, Raynaud J-P (1976) Paromomycin and dihydrostreptomycin binding to *Escherichia coli* ribosomes. Eur J Biochem 66:597–606
Le Goffic F, Tangy F, Moreau B, Capmau M-L (1979) Binding of tobramycin to *Escherichia coli* ribosomes: characteristics and equilibrium of the reaction. J Antibiot (Tokyo) 32:1288–1292
Lelong JC, Cousin MA, Gros D, Grunberg-Manago M, Gros F (1971) Streptomycin induced release of fMet-$tRNA_F$ from the ribosomal initiation complex. Biochem Biophys Res Commun 42:530–537
Lelong JC, Gros D, Gros F, Bollen A, Maschler R, Stöffler G (1974) Function of individual 30S subunit proteins of *Escherichia coli*. Effect of specific immunoglobulin fragments (Fab) on activities of ribosomal decoding sites. Proc Natl Acad Sci USA 71:248–252

Lennette ET, Apirion D (1970) The level of fMet-tRNA on ribosomes from streptomycin treated cells. Biochem Biophys Res Commun 41:804–811
Leon SA, Brock TD (1967) Effect of streptomycin and neomycin on physical properties of the ribosome. J Mol Biol 24:391–404
Likover TE, Kurland CG (1967) Ribosomes from a streptomycin-dependent strain of *Escherichia coli.* J Mol Biol 25:497–504
Liou Y-F, Tanaka N (1976) Dual actions of viomycin on the ribosomal functions. Biochem Biophys Res Commun 71:477–483
Luzzatto L, Apirion D, Schlessinger D (1968) Mechanism of action of streptomycin in *E. coli.* Interruption of the ribosome cycle at the initiation of protein synthesis. Proc Natl Acad Sci USA 60:873–880
Luzzatto L, Apirion D, Schlessinger D (1969a) Streptomycin action: greater inhibition of *Escherichia coli* ribosome function with exogenous than with endogenous messenger ribonucleic acid. J Bacteriol 99:206–209
Luzzatto L, Apirion D, Schlessinger D (1969b) Polyribosome depletion and blockage of the ribosome cycle by streptomycin in *Escherichia coli.* J Mol Biol 42:315–335
Mager J, Benedict M, Artman M (1962) A common site of action for polyamines and streptomycin. Biochim Biophys Acta 62:202–204
Masukawa H (1969) Localization of sensitivity to kanamycin and streptomycin in 30S ribosomal proteins of *Escherichia coli.* J Antibiot (Tokyo) 22:612–623
Masukawa H, Tanaka N (1968) Miscoding activity of aminosugars. J Antibiot (Tokyo) 21:70–72
Masukawa H, Tanaka N, Umezawa H (1968a) Inhibition by kasugamycin of protein synthesis in *Piricularia oryzae.* J Antibiot 21:73–74
Masukawa H, Tanaka N, Umezawa H (1968b) Localization of kanamycin sensitivity in the 23S core of 30S ribosomes of *E. coli.* J Antibiot 21:517–518
Misumi M, Tanaka N (1980) Mechanism of inhibition of translocation by kanamycin and viomycin: a comparative study with fusidic acid. Biochem Biophys Res Commun 92:647–654
Misumi M, Tanaka N, Shiba T (1978a) Binding of [^{14}C]tuberactinomycin O, an antibiotic closely related to viomycin to the bacterial ribosome. Biochem Biophys Res Commun 82:971–976
Misumi M, Nishimura T, Komai T, Tanaka N (1978b) Interaction of kanamycin and related antibiotics with the large ribosomal subunit of ribosomes and the inhibition of translocation. Biochem Biophys Res Commun 84:358–365
Miyoshi Y, Yamagata H (1975) Sucrose-dependent spectinomycin resistant mutants of *Escherichia coli.* J Bacteriol 125:142–148
Mizuno S, Nitta K, Umezawa H (1970) Mechanism of action of negamycin in *E. coli* K 12. II. Miscoding activity in polypeptide synthesis directed by synthetic polynucleotide. J Antibiot (Tokyo) 23:589–594
Mizuno T, Yamada H, Yamagata H, Mizushima S (1975) Coordinated alterations in ribosomes and cytoplasmic membrane in sucrose-dependent, spectinomycin-resistant mutants of *Escherichia coli.* J Bacteriol 125:524–530
Mizuno T, Yamagata H, Mizushima S (1977) Interaction of cytoplasmic membrane and ribosomes in *Escherichia coli.* Spectinomycin-induced disappearance of membrane protein I-19. J Bacteriol 129:326–332
Modolell J, Davis BD (1968) Rapid inhibition of polypeptide chain extension by streptomycin. Proc Natl Acad Sci USA 61:1279–1286
Modolell J, Davis BD (1970) Breakdown by streptomycin of initiation complexes formed on ribosomes of *Escherichia coli.* Proc Natl Acad Sci USA 67:1148–1155
Modolell J, Vazquez D (1977) The inhibition of ribosomal translocation by viomycin. Eur J Biochem 81:491–497
Okuyama A, Tanaka N (1972) Differential effects of aminoglycosides on cistron-specific initiation of protein synthesis. Biochem Biophys Res Commun 49:951–957
Okuyama A, Tanaka N (1973) Studies on the ribosomal binding sites of natural messenger RNA. Biochem Biophys Res Commun 52:1463–1469

Okuyama A, Machiyama N, Kinoshita T, Tanaka N (1971) Inhibition by kasugamycin of initiation complex formation on 30 S ribosomes. Biochem Biophys Res Commun 43:196–199

Okuyama A, Watanabe T, Tanaka N (1972) Effects of aminoglycoside antibiotics on initiation of viral RNA-directed protein synthesis. J Antibiot (Tokyo) 25:212–218

Okuyama A, Yoshikawa M, Tanaka N (1974) Alteration of ribosomal protein S 2 in kasugamycin-resistant mutant derived from *Escherichia coli* AB 312. Biochem Biophys Res Commun 60:1163–1169

Okuyama A, Tanaka N, Komai T (1975) The binding of kasugamycin to the *Escherichia coli* ribosomes. J Antibiot (Tokyo) 28:903–905

Olsson M, Isaksson L, Kurland CG (1974) Pleiotropic effects of ribosomal protein S 4 studied in *Escherichia coli* mutants. Mol Gen Genet 135:191–202

Orsulakova A, Stockhorst E, Schacht J (1976) Effect of neomycin on phosphoinositide labelling and calcium binding in guinea-pig inner ear tissues *in vivo* and *in vitro*. J Neurochem 26:285–290

Ozaki M, Mizushima S, Nomura M (1969) Identification and functional characterization of the protein controlled by the streptomycin-resistant locus in *E. coli*. Nature 222:333–339

Palmer E, Wilhelm JM, Sherman F (1979) Phenotypic suppression of nonsense mutants in yeast by aminoglycoside antibiotics. Nature 277:148–150

Perzynski S, Cannon M, Cundliffe E, Chahwala SB, Davies J (1979) Effects of apramycin, a novel aminoglycoside antibiotic, on bacterial protein synthesis. Eur J Biochem 99:623–628

Pestka S (1977) Inhibitors of protein synthesis. In: Weissbach H, Pestka S (eds) Molecular mechanisms of protein biosynthesis. Academic Press, New York, pp 467–553

Pestka S, Marshall R, Nirenberg M (1965) RNA codewords and protein synthesis. V. Effect of streptomycin on the formation of ribosome-sRNA complexes. Proc Natl Acad Sci USA 53:639–646

Pestka S, Walter H, Wayne LG (1977) Altered surface properties of *Escherichia coli* associated with a specific amino acid change in the S 12 ribosomal protein of streptomycin-resistant mutants. Antimicrob Agents Chemother 11:978–983

Pinkett MO, Brownstein BL (1974) Streptomycin-induced synthesis of abnormal protein in an *Escherichia coli* mutant. J Bacteriol 119:345–350

Plotz PH, Dubin DT, Davis BD (1963) Influence of salts on the uptake of streptomycin by *Escherichia coli*. Nature 191:1324–1325

Pongs O, Erdmann VA (1973) Affinity labeling of *E. coli* ribosomes with a streptomycin-analogue. FEBS Lett 37:47–50

Ramirez-Ronda CH, Holmes RK, Sanford JP (1975) Effect of divalent cations on binding of aminoglycoside antibiotics to human serum proteins and to bacteria. Antimicrob Agents Chemother 7:238–245

Revel M, Greenshpan H, Herzberg M (1970) Specificity in the binding of *Escherichia coli* ribosomes to natural messenger RNA. Eur J Biochem 16:117–122

Schlanger G, Friedman SM (1973) Ambiguity in a polypeptide-synthesizing extract from *Saccharomyces cerevisiae*. J Bacteriol 115:129–138

Schlessinger D, Medoff G (1975) Streptomycin, dihydrostreptomycin and the gentamicins. In: Corcoran JW, Hahn FE (eds) Antibiotics, vol III. Springer, Berlin Heidelberg New York, pp 535–549

Schreiner G, Nierhaus KH (1973) Protein involved in the binding of dihydrostreptomycin to ribosomes of *Escherichia coli*. J Mol Biol 81:71–82

Shelanski ML, Gaskin F, Cantor CR (1973) Microtubule assembly in the absence of added nucleotides. Proc Natl Acad Sci USA 70:765–786

Shibahara S, Kondo S, Maeda K, Umezawa H, Ohno M (1972) The total synthesis of negamycin and the antipode. J Am Chem Soc 94:4353–4354

Shine J, Dalgarno L (1975) Determinant of cistron specificity in bacterial ribosomes. Nature 254:34–36

Singh A, Ursic D, Davies J (1979) Phenotypic suppression and misreading in *Saccharomyces cerevisiae*. Nature 277:146–148

Someya A, Tanaka N (1979) Interaction of aminoglycosides and other antibiotics with actin. J Antibiot 32:156–160
Sparling PF (1970) Kasugamycin resistance: 30S ribosomal mutation with an unusual location on the *Escherichia coli* chromosome. Science 167:56–58
Speyer JF, Langyel P, Basillo C (1962) Ribosomal localization of streptomycin sensitivity. Proc Natl Acad Sci USA 48:684–686
Spotts CR, Stanier RY (1961) Mechanism of streptomycin action on bacteria: a unitary hypothesis. Nature 192:633–637
Spratt BG (1977) Properties of the penicillin-binding proteins of *Escherichia coli* K 12. Eur J Biochem 72:341–352
Stavy L (1968) Miscoding in a cell-free system from spleen. Proc Natl Acad Sci USA 61:347–353
Steitz JA (1969) Polypeptide chain initiation: Nucleotide sequence of the three ribosomal binding sites in bacteriophage R 17 RNA. Nature 224:957–964
Stern JL, Barner HD, Cohen SS (1966) The lethality of streptomycin and the stimulation of RNA synthesis in the absence of protein synthesis. J Mol Biol 17:188–217
Stockhorst E, Schachat J (1977) Radioactive labelling of phospholipids and proteins by cochlear perfusion in the guinea pig and the effect of neomycin. Acta Otolaryngol (Stockh) 83:401–409
Stöffler G, Wittmann HG (1977) Primary structure and three-dimensional arrangement of proteins within *Escherichia coli* ribosomes. In: Weissbach H, Pestka S (eds) Molecular mechanisms of protein biosynthesis. Academic Press, New York, pp 117–202
Tai P-C, Davis BD (1979) Triphasic concentration effects of gentamicin on activity and misreading in protein synthesis. Biochemistry 18:193–198
Tai P-C, Wallace BJ, Davis BD (1978) Streptomycin causes misreading of natural messenger by interacting with ribosomes after initiation. Proc Natl Acad Sci USA 75:275–279
Tanaka N (1975a) Aminoglycoside antibiotics. In: Corcoran JW, Hahn FE (eds) Antibiotics, vol III. Springer, Berlin Heidelberg New York, pp 340–364
Tanaka N (1975b) Fusidic acid. In: Corcoran JW, Hahn FE (eds) Antibiotics, vol III. Springer, Berlin Heidelberg New York, pp 436–447
Tanaka N, Igusa S (1968) Effects of viomycin and polymyxin B on protein synthesis *in vitro*. J Antibiot 21:239–240
Tanaka N, Nishimura T, Yamaguchi H, Yamamoto C, Yoshida Y, Sashikata K, Umezawa H (1965) Mechanism of action of kasugamycin. J Antibiot (Tokyo) 18:139–144
Tanaka N, Yoshida Y, Sashikata K, Yamaguchi H, Umezawa H (1966a) Inhibition of polypeptide synthesis by kasugamycin, an aminoglycosidic antibiotic. J Antibiot (Tokyo) 19:65–68
Tanaka N, Yamaguchi H, Umezawa H (1966b) Mechanism of kasugamycin action on polypeptide synthesis. J Biochem 60:429–434
Tanaka N, Masukawa H, Umezawa H (1967) Structural basis of kanamycin for miscoding activity. Biochem Biophys Res Commun 26:544–549
Tanaka N, Kinoshita T, Masukawa H (1968) Mechanism of protein synthesis inhibition by fusidic acid and related antibiotics. Biochem Biophys Res Commun 30:278–283
Tseng JT, Bryan LE, van den Elzen HM (1972) Mechanism and spectrum of streptomycin resistance in a natural population of *Pseudomonas aeruginosa*. Antimicrob Agents Chemother 2:136–141
Turnock G (1970) The action of streptomycin in a mutant of *Escherichia coli* with increased sensitivity to the antibiotic. Biochem J 118:659–666
Turnock G, Erickson SK, Ackrell BAC, Birch B (1972) A mutant of *Escherichia coli* with a defect in energy metabolism. J Gen Microbiol 70:507–515
Uehara Y, Kondo S, Umezawa H, Suzukake K, Hori M (1972) Negamycin, a miscoding antibiotic with a unique structure. J Antibiot (Tokyo) 25:685–688
Uehara Y, Hori M, Umezawa H (1974) Negamycin inhibits termination of protein synthesis directed by phage f2 RNA *in vitro*. Biochim Biophys Acta 374:82–95
Uehara Y, Hori M, Umezawa H (1976a) Specific inhibition of the termination process of protein synthesis by negamycin. Biochim Biophys Acta 442:251–262

Uehara Y, Hori M, Umezawa H (1976b) Inhibitory effect of negamycin on polysomal ribosomes of *Escherichia coli*. Biochim Biophys Acta 447:406–412
Vázquez D (1979) Inhibitors of protein biosynthesis. Springer, Berlin Heidelberg New York
Wallace BJ, Davis BD (1973) Cyclic blockade of initiation sites by streptomycin-damaged ribosomes in *Escherichia coli*. An explanation for dominance of sensitivity. J Mol Biol 75:377–390
Wallace BJ, Tai P-C, Davis BD (1973a) Effect of streptomycin on the response of *Escherichia coli* ribosomes to the dissociation factor. J Mol Biol 75:391–400
Wallace BJ, Tai P-C, Herzog EL, Davis BD (1973b) Partial inhibition of polysomal ribosomes of *Escherichia coli* by streptomycin. Proc Natl Acad Sci USA 70:1234–1237
Wallace BJ, Tai P-C, Davis BD (1974) Selective inhibition of initiating ribosomes by spectinomycin. Proc Natl Acad Sci USA 71:1634–1638
Wallace BJ, Tai P-C, Davis BD (1979) Streptomycin and related antibiotics. In: Hahn EF (ed) Antibiotics, vol V/1. Springer, Berlin Heidelberg New York, pp 272-303
Watanabe S (1972) Interaction of siomycin with the acceptor site of *Escherichia coli* ribosomes. J Mol Biol 67:443–457
Weinstein IB, Ochoa M Jr, Friedman SM (1966) Fidelity in the translation of messenger ribonucleic acids in mammalian subcellular systems. Biochemistry 5:3332–3339
White JR, White HL (1964) Streptomycinoid antibiotics: Synergism by puromycin. Science 146:772–774
Wilhelm JM, Pettitt SE, Jessop JJ (1978a) Aminoglycoside antibiotics and eukaryotic protein synthesis: Structure-function relationships in the stimulation of misreading with a wheat embryo system. Biochemistry 17:1143–1149
Wilhelm JM, Jessop JJ, Pettitt SE (1978b) Aminoglycoside antibiotics and eukaryotic protein synthesis: Stimulation errors in the translation of natural messengers in extracts of cultured human cells. Biochemistry 17:1149–1153
Wittmann HG, Apirion D (1975) Analysis of ribosomal proteins in streptomycin resistant and dependent mutants isolated from streptomycin independent *Escherichia coli* strains. Mol Gen Genet 141:331–341
Wolfgang RW, Lawrence NL (1967) Binding of streptomycin by ribosomes of sensitive, resistant and dependent *Bacillus megaterium*. J Mol Biol 29:531–535
Wyatt PJ, Berkman RM, Phillips DT (1972) Osmotic sensitivity in *Staphylococcus aureus* induced by streptomycin. J Bacteriol 110:523–528
Yaguchi M, Wittmann HG (1976) Alteration of ribosomal protein S17 by mutation linked to neamine resistance in *Escherichia coli*. II. Localization of the amino acid replacement in protein S17 from a nea A mutant. J Mol Biol 104:617–620
Yamada T, Masuda K, Shoji K, Hori M (1972) Analysis of ribosomes from viomycin-sensitive and -resistant strains of *Mycobacterium smegmatis*. J Bacteriol 112:1–6
Yamada T, Masuda K, Mizuguchi Y, Suga K (1976) Altered ribosomes in antibiotic-resistant mutants of *Mycobacterium smegmatis*. Antimicrob Agents Chemother 9:817–823
Yamada T, Mizuguchi Y, Nierhaus KH, Wittmann HG (1978) Resistance to viomycin conferred by RNA of either ribosomal subunit. Nature 275:460–461
Yamaki H, Tanaka N (1963) Effects of protein synthesis inhibitors on the lethal action of kanamycin and streptomycin. J Antibiot (Tokyo) 16:222–226
Zierhut G, Piepersberg W, Böck A (1979) Comparative analysis of the effect of aminoglycosides on bacterial protein synthesis *in vitro*. Eur J Biochem 98:577–583

CHAPTER 6

Mechanisms of Resistance to Aminoglycoside Antibiotics

H. UMEZAWA and S. KONDO

A. Introduction

During the early 1950s when strongly resistant organisms had not yet appeared, the chemotherapy of most bacterial infections was assumed to be possible. However, tubercle bacilli soon became resistant to streptomycin and new active agents were required for the treatment of tuberculosis. At that time, UMEZAWA discovered the aminoglycoside antibiotic, kanamycin, in the search for new water-soluble basic antibiotics (H. UMEZAWA et al. 1957). Kanamycin was evaluated as an effective agent for the treatment of infections with resistant staphylococci and streptomycin-resistant tuberculosis, and later for the treatment of infections with resistant gram-negative bacteria. However, after widespread use of the antibiotic, in 1965 kanamycin-resistant strains appeared in patients, although at a frequency of less than 5%. Therefore, UMEZAWA undertook studies on the biochemical mechanisms of resistance to aminoglycoside antibiotics (H. UMEZAWA et al. 1967a, b). The results of these studies suggested structures which would be active against resistant strains and many derivatives of aminoglycoside antibiotics were synthesized. Among these, 3′,4′-dideoxykanamycin B (dibekacin) (H. UMEZAWA et al. 1971) was useful in the treatment of infections with resistant gram-positive and -negative bacteria, including pseudomonas, and was marketed in 1975.

In this chapter, we will discuss the biochemical mechanisms of resistance to aminoglycoside antibiotics and the development of derivatives which are active against resistant strains.

The stereochemistry and absolute configuration of most aminoglycoside antibiotics were derived by chemical methods and ^{1}H nuclear magnetic resonance (^{1}H NMR) spectral correlations. The structures of kanamycin A monosulfate monohydrate (KOYAMA et al. 1968), streptomycin oxime sesquiselenate tetrahydrate (NEIDLE et al. 1968), spectinomycin dihydrobromide pentahydrate (COCHRAN and ABRAHAM 1972), apramycin hydroiodide (O'CONNOR et al. 1976), and fortimicin B hydrate (HIRAYAMA et al. 1978) were confirmed by X-ray studies. The stereostructures of all aminoglycoside antibiotics depicted in this chapter are based on these absolute structures.

B. Biochemical Mechanisms of Resistance

I. Discovery of Enzymes Involved in Resistance

OCHIAI and AKIBA found that the resistance of dysentery bacteria was transferred to *Escherichia coli* in mixed culture (OCHIAI et al. 1959; AKIBA et al. 1960). Their

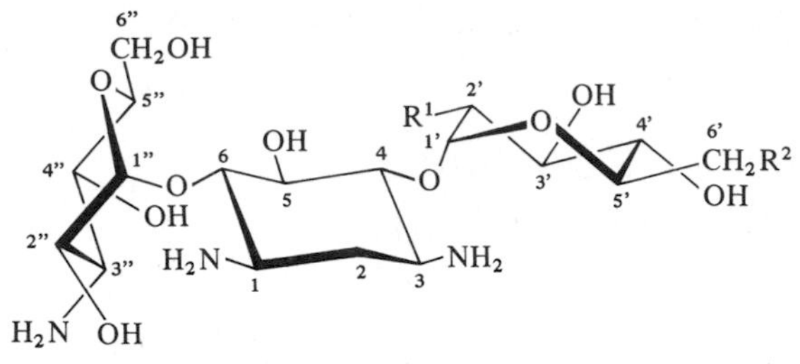

Fig. 1. Kanamycins. Kanamycin A: $R^1=OH$, $R^2=NH_2$; kanamycin B: $R^1=NH_2$, $R^2=NH_2$; kanamycin C: $R^1=NH_2$, $R^2=OH$

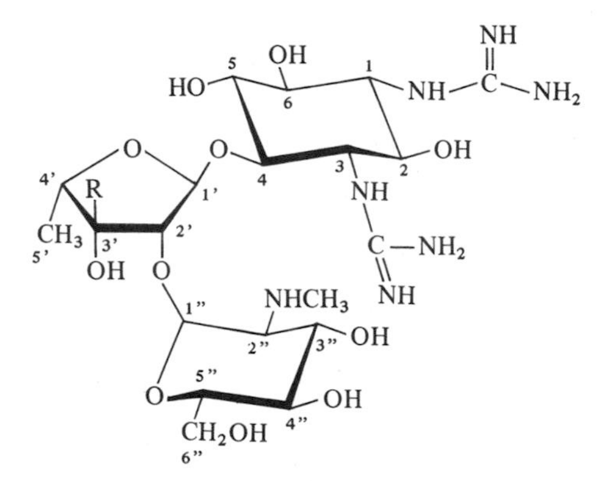

Fig. 2. Streptomycins. Streptomycin: $R=CHO$; dihydrostreptomycin: $R=CH_2OH$

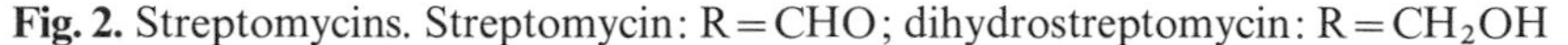

studies, and much subsequent work in microbial genetics, led to the realization that the resistance of gram-negative bacteria is due to extrachromosomal genetic material (plasmid) called R factor, which can be transferred by conjugation from resistant to sensitive strains of the same species and also between different species. Genes involved in the resistance of staphylococci also lie on plasmids and are transferred by transduction. Resistance of *Pseudomonas aeruginosa* is also due to plasmids which are transferred by conjugation from resistant to sensitive strains of the same species.

MIYAMURA found that resistant dysentery bacteria of clinical origin inactivated chloramphenicol (MIYAMURA 1961), and OKAMOTO and SUZUKI found that *E. coli* carrying R factor produced an intracellular enzyme which acetylated chloramphenicol in the presence of acetyl CoA (OKAMOTO and SUZUKI 1965). It was suggested that another enzyme which might transfer the acetyl group to kanamycin A from acetyl CoA was also produced by the strain. H. UMEZAWA et al. (1967a) isolated the reaction product of kanamycin A with the homogenate of *E. coli* K 12 R 5 and by chemical methods determined the structure of the reaction product to be 6′-*N*-acetylkanamycin A. This strain, which produces an enzyme modifying kanamycin A to 6′-*N*-acetylkanamycin A, is resistant to kanamycin A and B but sensitive to kanamycin C, which has a hydroxyl group in place of the 6′-amino group of kanamycin B. Resistant strains of this type which are inhibited by kanamycin C are rare.

Table 1. Aminoglycoside-modifying enzymes found in resistant strains

Enzymes		Substrate
ATP: aminoglycoside 3′-phosphotransferase I	APH(3′)-I	KM, KM-B, NM, PM, RM; LV(5″-OH)
ATP: aminoglycoside 3′-phosphotransferase II	APH(3′)-II	KM, KM-B, NM, PM, RM, BT
ATP: aminoglycoside 3′-phosphotransferase III	APH(3′)-III	KM, KM-B, RM, BT; LV(5″-OH)
ATP: aminoglycoside 5″-phosphotransferase	APH(5″)	RM
ATP: aminoglycoside 2″-phosphotransferase	APH(2″)	GM-C, KM, DKB
ATP: aminoglycoside 3″-phosphotransferase	APH(3″)	SM
ATP: aminoglycoside 6-phosphotransferase	APH(6)	SM
Nucleoside triphosphate: aminoglycoside 2″-nucleotidyltransferase	AAD(2″)	GM-C, KM, DKB
ATP: aminoglycoside 4′-adenylyltransferase	AAD(4′)	TB, KM, NM, PM, RM, BT, AK; DKB(4″-OH)
ATP: aminoglycoside 3″-adenylyltransferase	AAD(3″)	SM; SP(9-OH)
ATP: aminoglycoside 6-adenylyltransferase	AAD(6)	SM
Acetyl CoA: aminoglycoside 6′-acetyltransferase 1	AAC(6′)-1	KM, KM-B
Acetyl CoA: aminoglycoside 6′-acetyltransferase 2	AAC(6′)-2	KM, KM-B, GM-C_{1a}, GM-C_2
Acetyl CoA: aminoglycoside 6′-acetyltransferase 3	AAC(6′)-3	KM, KM-B, GM-C_{1a}, GM-C_2, DKB
Acetyl CoA: aminoglycoside 6′-acetyltransferase 4	AAC(6′)-4	KM, KM-B, GM-C_{1a}, GM-C_2, DKB, AK
Acetyl CoA: aminoglycoside 3-acetyltransferase I	AAC(3)-I	GM-C; FT(1-NH_2)
Acetyl CoA: aminoglycoside 3-acetyltransferase II	AAC(3)-II	GM-C, KM-B, TB
Acetyl CoA: aminoglycoside 3-acetyltransferase III	AAC(3)-III	GM-C, KM, KM-B, TB, NM, PM
Acetyl CoA: aminoglycoside 3-acetyltransferase IV	AAC(3)-IV	GM-C, KM, KM-B, TB, NM, PM, AP
Acetyl CoA: aminoglycoside 2′-acetyltransferase	AAC(2′)	GM-C, KM-B, KM-C, NM, RM, BT, LV, DKB

Abbreviations: KM, kanamycin; NM, neomycin; PM, paromomycin; RM, ribostamycin; LV, lividomycin; BT, butirosin; SM, streptomycin; GM, gentamicin; DKB, dibekacin; TB, tobramycin; AK, amikacin; SP, spectinomycin; AP, apramycin; FT, fortimicin

Most kanamycin-resistant strains isolated from patients were resistant to all kanamycins. Therefore, UMEZAWA studied the resistance mechanism of *E. coli* K 12 ML 1629 which was resistant to all kanamycins and neomycins, and found that the homogenate of the resistant strain catalyzed the transfer of the terminal phosphate group of ATP to the 3′-hydroxyl group of kanamycins and paromamine (H. UMEZAWA et al. 1967 b; OKANISHI et al. 1968; KONDO et al. 1968). The presence of a similar 3′-phosphotransferase was also found in resistant staphylococci (DOI et al. 1968 a) and *P. aeruginosa* (H. UMEZAWA et al. 1968 b; DOI et al. 1968 a; MAEDA et al. 1968).

An adenylyltransferase which transfers AMP from ATP to the 3-hydroxyl group of the *N*-methyl-L-glucosamine moiety of streptomycin has been also discovered (H. UMEZAWA et al. 1968a; TAKASAWA et al. 1968).

Thus, the method of clarifying the biochemical mechanism of plasmid-mediated resistance to aminoglycoside antibiotics by structural elucidation of the enzyme reaction products was established (H. UMEZAWA 1970, 1974, 1975). Besides 6′-acetyltransferase, 3′-phosphotransferase, and 3″-adenylyltransferase described above, other enzymes involved in resistance to aminoglycoside antibiotics have been found in resistant strains. As shown in Table 1, a classification with names and abbreviations of these aminoglycoside-modifying enzymes was proposed by UMEZAWA, DAVIES, and MITSUHASHI (MITSUHASHI 1975). Among these enzymes, APH(3′) emzymes are the most widely distributed in resistant bacteria.

II. Resistance to 2-Deoxystreptamine-Containing Antibiotics

1. 3′-Phosphotransferase [APH(3′)]

The enzyme which transfers the phosphate group to the 3-hydroxyl group of the 6-amino-6-deoxy-D-glucose, 2,6-diamino-2,6-dideoxy-D-glucose, or 2-amino-2-deoxy-D-glucose moiety in kanamycins, neomycins, ribostamycin, neamine, paromomycins, or paromamine was originally called kanamycin–neomycin phosphotransferase or neomycin–kanamycin phosphotransferase (H. UMEZAWA 1974). However, this is now termed aminoglycoside 3′-phosphotransferase. Depending on difference in substrate specificity, there are three kinds of phosphotransferases: APH(3′)-I, II, and III.

The APH(3′)-I was first found in the supernatant from 105,000 *g* centrifugation (105S fraction) of disrupted cells of *E. coli* K12 ML1629 (H. UMEZAWA et al. 1967b; OKANISHI et al. 1968). This strain was highly resistant to kanamycins and neomycins, and was obtained by transmission of R plasmid from a clinically isolated resistant strain of *E. coli* to *E. coli* K12 ML1410, which was resistant to nalidixic acid. The 105S fraction catalyzes the reaction of kanamycin A and paromamine with ATP, yielding kanamycin A 3′-phosphate and paromamine 3′-phosphate, respectively. These 3′-phosphates do not inhibit growth of sensitive strains or protein synthesis by ribosome systems (HORI and H. UMEZAWA 1967). Kanamycin A 3′-phosphate was isolated by column chromatography on Amberlite IRC-50, CG-50, and Dowex 1-X2 resin from the enzymatic reaction mixture and the structure was elucidated chemically (H. UMEZAWA et al. 1967b; KONDO et al. 1968). Paromamine 3′-phosphate was crystallized as the dihydrate from aqueous methanol. The structure was also determined by chemical methods and the configuration at C-3 was confirmed by the ^{1}H NMR spectrum (MAEDA et al. 1968). The NMR spectra of kanamycin A 3′-phosphate and paromamine 3′-phosphate were analyzed in detail (NAGANAWA et al. 1971a).

The 100S fractions containing APH(3′)-I which were obtained from *E. coli* K12 ML1629, K12 ML1410 R81, and K12 J5 R11-2, and *P. aeruginosa* TI-13 phosphorylated the 5″-hydroxyl group of lividomycin A in the presence of ATP (KONDO et al. 1972; H. UMEZAWA et al. 1973a). The structure of lividomycin A 5″-phosphate was elucidated by chemical degradation and ^{1}H NMR spectroscopy

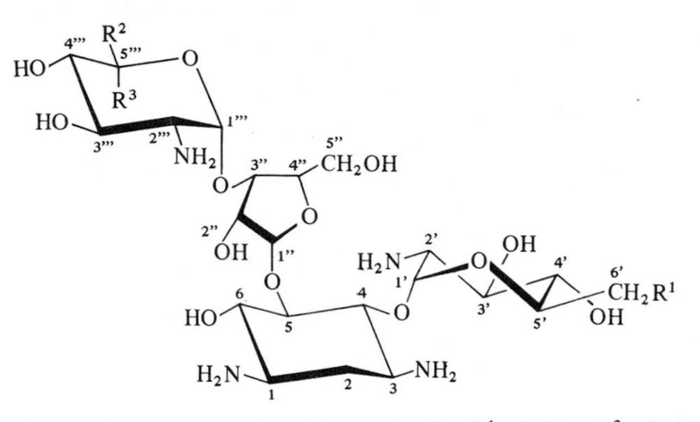

Fig. 3. Neomycins and paromomycins. Neomycin B: $R^1=NH_2$, $R^2=H$, $R^3=CH_2NH_2$; neomycin C: $R^1=NH_2$, $R^2=CH_2NH_2$, $R^3=H$; paromomycin I: $R^1=OH$, $R^2=H$, $R^3=CH_2NH_2$; paromomycin II: $R^1=OH$, $R^2=CH_2NH_2$, $R^3=H$

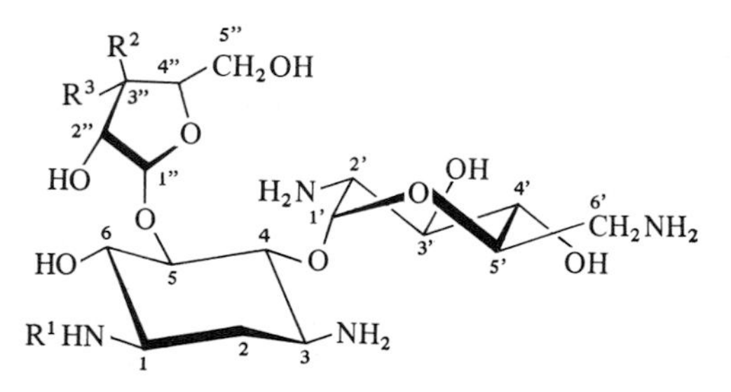

Fig. 4. Ribostamycin and butirosins. Ribostamycin: R^1, $R^2=H$, $R^3=OH$; xylostasin: R^1, $R^3=H$, $R^2=OH$; butirosin A: $R^1=NH_2CH_2CH_2CH(OH)CO$, $R^2=OH$, $R^3=H$; butirosin B: $R^1=NH_2CH_2CH_2CH(OH)CO$, $R^2=H$, $R^3=OH$

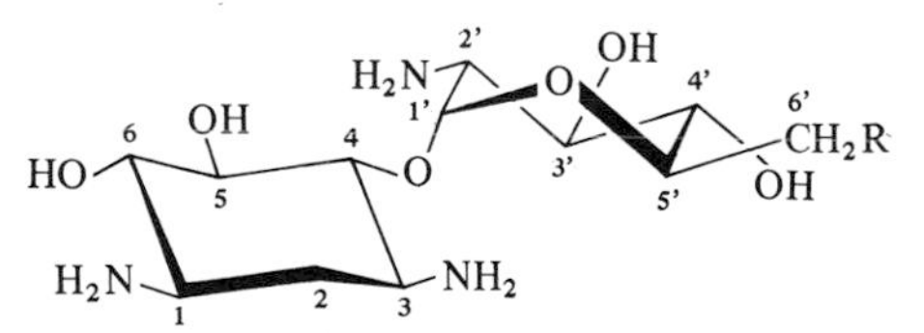

Fig. 5. Neamine and paromamine. Neamine: $R=NH_2$; paromamine: $R=OH$

and confirmed by chemical synthesis (YAMAMOTO et al. 1972a). The same enzyme is involved in phosphorylation of the 3′-hydroxyl group of the kanamycins and the 5″-hydroxyl group of the lividomycins. The APH(3′)-I was purified 25- to 40-fold in phosphorylating activity for both kanamycin A and lividomycin A by affinity chromatography using a lividomycin A–Sepharose 4B column. The kinetic data on this enzyme preparation showed competitive inhibition of lividomycin A phosphorylation by kanamycin A (H. UMEZAWA et al. 1973a). Ribostamycin has two hydroxyl groups which are phosphorylated by APH(3′)-I, the 3-hydroxyl group of the 2,6-diamino-2,6-dideoxy-D-glucose moiety and the 5-hydroxyl group of the ribose moiety. A molecular model in which these two hydroxyl groups are located

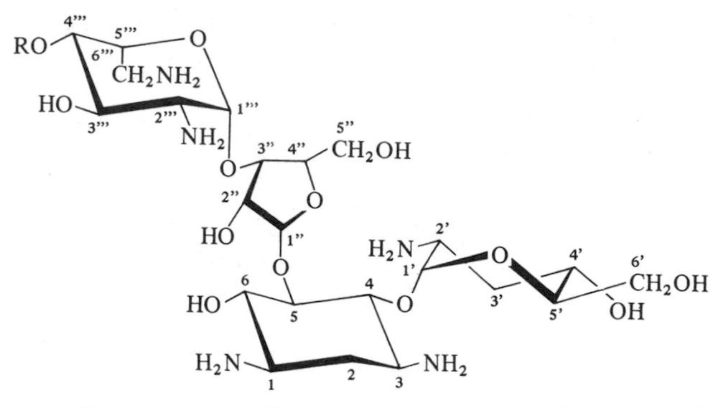

Fig. 6. Lividomycins. Lividomycin A: R = α-D-mannopyranosyl; lividomycin B: R = H

close to each other can be easily built. Therefore, in this enzyme reaction the terminal phosphate group of ATP is thought to be located close to both hydroxyl groups. It appears to be closer to the 3′-hydroxyl group because the reaction product of ribostamycin is ribostamycin 3′-phosphate. However, the enzyme reaction with 3′,4′-dideoxyribostamycin gives the 5″-phosphate (H. UMEZAWA et al. 1973a). APH(3′)-I cannot phosphorylate the 3′-hydroxyl group of the butirosins, which have a 4-amino-2-hydroxybutyryl group on the 1-amino group.

Another phosphotransferase, APH(3′)-II, which phosphorylates the 3′-hydroxyl group of butirosins but not the 5″-hydroxyl group of lividomycins, was found in *E. coli* JR 66/W 677 independently by two research groups (YAGISAWA et al. 1972c; BRZEZINSKA and DAVIES 1973). The structure of butirosin A 3′-phosphate was elucidated chemically and by ^{1}H NMR spectroscopy (YAGISAWA et al. 1972c).

The APH(3′) found in *P. aeruginosa* H-9 also phosphorylated kanamycin A and paromamine (H. UMEZAWA et al. 1968b; MAEDA et al. 1968). The APH(3′) in three strains of *P. aeruginosa* and in two strains of *E. coli* was studied by MATSUHASHI et al. (1975). *P. aeruginosa* TI-13 and H-9 produced APH(3′)-I and II, respectively. Strain B-13 produced both enzymes. The APH(3′)-I enzymes which were isolated and purified by affinity chromatography from *P. aeruginosa* TI-13, B-13, and *E. coli* K 12 J 5 R 11-2 were different from each other in chromatographic behavior, molecular weight, optimum pH, and Ki. However, the APH(3′)-II enzymes in *P. aeruginosa* H-9 and *E. coli* JR 66/W 677 showed similar behavior. The molecular weight of APH(3′)-II was about 27,000 by the gel filtration method. Using the partially purified APH(3′)-II of *P. aeruginosa* H-9, the following reaction was demonstrated (DOI et al. 1969):

$$\text{Kanamycin} + \text{ATP} \xrightarrow[\text{Mg}^{2+}]{\text{APH(3')}} \text{Kanamycin 3'-phosphate} + \text{ADP}$$

ATP could not be replaced by the other nucleoside triphosphates. Magnesium was required but could be replaced by manganese, zinc, and cobalt divalent cations. The substrate specificity of this enzyme indicated a requirement for a 4-*O*-(aminoglycosyl)-2-deoxystreptamine moiety such as that found in neamine, paromamine, and 4-*O*-(6-amino-6-deoxy-α-D-glucopyranosyl)-2-deoxystreptamine. Methyl 3-amino-3-deoxy-α-D-glucopyranoside and kanamycin A 3′-phos-

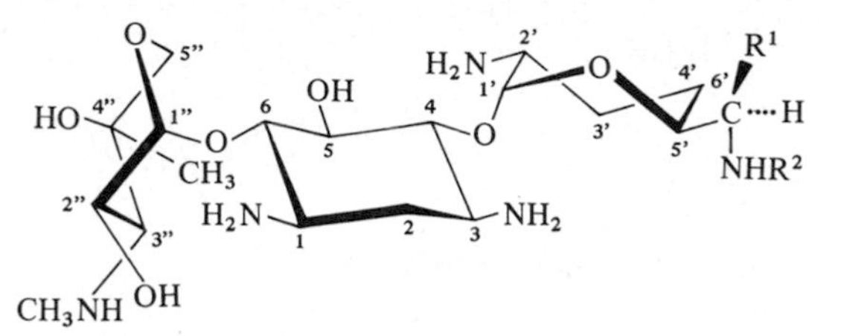

Fig. 7. Gentamicin C components. Gentamicin C_1: R^1, $R^2=CH_3$; gentamicin C_2: $R^1=CH_3$, $R^2=H$; gentamicin C_{1a}: R^1, $R^2=H$

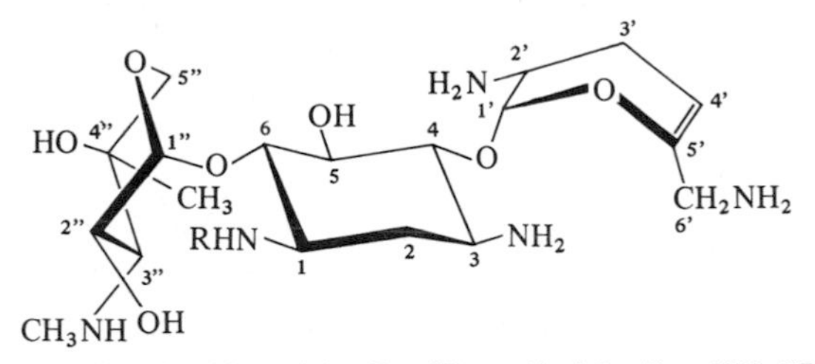

Fig. 8. Sisomicin and netilmicin. Sisomicin: R=H; netilmicin: $R=CH_2CH_3$

phate showed relatively strong inhibition of the enzyme reaction. Inhibition by the methyl glycoside was competitive with kanamycin A.

In two clinical isolates (B294 and B295) of drug-resistant *Staphylococcus aureus*, APH(3′) phosphorylating the 3′-hydroxyl group of kanamycin A was also found (DOI et al. 1968b). Kanamycin–lividomycin cross-resistance in staphylococci suggested the presence of APH(3′)-I. An enzyme which phosphorylates the 5″-hydroxyl group of lividomycins was found in resistant *S. aureus* and *S. epidermidis* (KOBAYASHI et al. 1973). Recently, the APH(3′)-II-type enzyme was also found in clinical isolates of *Acinetobacter calcoaceticus* (MURRAY and MOELLERING 1979).

The APH(3′)-II from *E. coli* JR66/W677 was completely purified by repeated column chromatography and affinity chromatography on kanamycin–Sepharose 4B (MATSUHASHI et al. 1976a). Rabbit antiserum prepared against the purified enzyme was useful for identification of the enzyme (MATSUHASHI et al. 1976b). By immunodiffusion, a precipitin line was observed between the antiserum and APH(3′)-II prepared from *E. coli* JR66/W677 or *P. aeruginosa* H9, but not between the antiserum and APH(3′)-I or APH(3′)-III. Localization of APH(3′)-II on the cellular surface of *E. coli* JR66/W677 was shown by an immunofluorescent method using the antiserum (MATSUHASHI et al. 1976c).

The APH(3′)-III obtained from *P. aeruginosa* 21-75 phosphorylated both the 3′-hydroxyl group of butirosins and the 5″-hydroxyl group of lividomycins (Y. UMEZAWA et al. 1975).

2. 5″-Phosphotransferase [APH(5″)]

The APH(5″) found in *P. aeruginosa* GN573 transferred the phosphate group of ATP preferentially to the 5″-hydroxyl group of ribostamycin (KIDA et al. 1974). In this reaction the terminal phosphate group of ATP is thought to be located closer to the 5″-hydroxyl group than to the 3′-hydroxyl group.

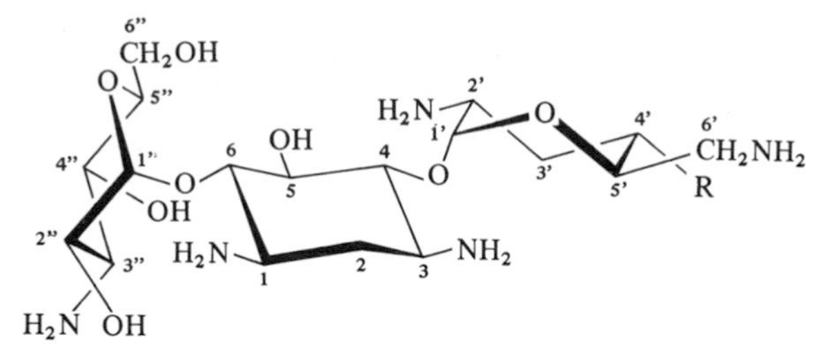

Fig. 9. Dibekacin and tobramycin. Dibekacin: R=H; tobramycin: R=OH

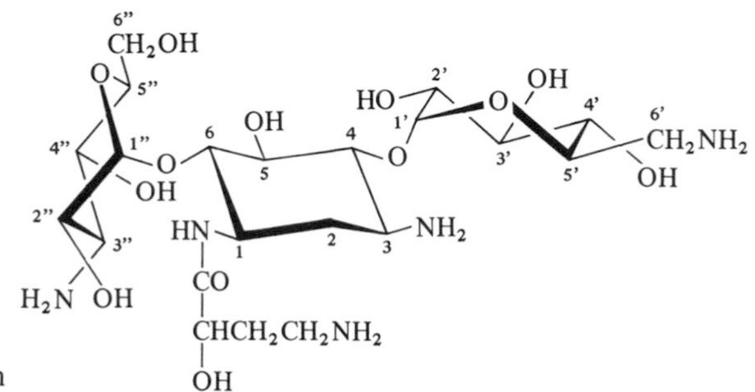

Fig. 10. Amikacin

3. 2″-Phosphotransferase [APH(2″)]

An enzyme, APH(2″), found in *S. aureus* R. Palm and JF 75-21 transferred the phosphate group of ATP to the 2″-hydroxyl group of sisomicin (LEGOFFIC et al. 1977) and gentamicin C_1 (KAWABE et al. 1978). This enzyme also had AAC(6′) activity as described later (LEGOFFIC 1977) (see Sect. B.II.6).

4. 2″-Adenylyltransferase [AAD(2″)]

BENVENISTE and DAVIES transferred the R plasmid of a resistant strain of *Klebsiella pneumoniae* to *E. coli* W 677 and obtained a resistant strain designated *E. coli* JR 66/W 677. An enzyme which catalyzes adenylylation of gentamicin C_1, C_{1a}, C_2, and kanamycins was found in this resistant strain (BENVENISTE and DAVIES 1971 a). The structure of the adenylylated product of dibekacin was determined to be the 2″-adenylate by chemical methods and by ^1H NMR spectroscopy (YAGISAWA et al. 1971; NAGANAWA et al. 1971 b). The enzyme, which was named AAD(2″), also transferred the guanylyl and inosinyl groups from GTP and ITP, respectively, to the 2″-hydroxyl group of dibekacin (YAGISAWA et al. 1972 a). Similar enzymes were found in *E. coli* carrying an R plasmid of *K. pneumoniae* origin (LEGOFFIC and CHEVEREAU 1972; KOBAYASHI et al. 1971).

5. 4′-Adenylyltransferase [AAD(4′)]

The AAD(4′) found in *S. epidermidis* 109 (SANTANAM and KAYSER 1976) and *S. aureus* Ap 01 (LEGOFFIC et al. 1976) adenylylated the 4′-hydroxyl group of tobramycin and kanamycins. The AAD(4′) also adenylylated the 4″-hydroxyl group of dibekacin. It has been suggested that this is due to the similar shape of the tobramycin molecule and the 180°-rotated dibekacin molecule (LeGoffic 1977). Adenylylation of amikacin with AAD(4′) gives the 4′-adenylate (Toda et al. 1978).

6. 6′-Acetyltransferase [AAC(6′)]

Among the enzymes involved in resistance to aminoglycoside antibiotics, AAC(6′) was first found by Umezawa et al. (H. Umezawa et al. 1967a; Okanishi et al. 1967) in *E. coli* K 12 R 5 obtained by transmission of R plasmid from naturally isolated drug-resistant dysentery bacteria. The 100S fraction of this strain inactivated kanamycin A in the presence of acetyl CoA. The structure of this reaction product was shown by chemical degradation to be 6′-*N*-acetylkanamycin A (H. Umezawa et al. 1967a). AAC(6′) similar to Umezawa's enzyme was obtained by Benveniste and Davies from *E. coli* W 677 carrying either R plasmid R 5, NR 79, or NR 79-5. This enzyme, which acetylates kanamycins A and B, neomycin B, and gentamicin C_{1a}, was purified approximately tenfold from an osmotic shockate of strain NR 79/W 677 by precipitation of nucleic acids, ammonium sulfate fractionation, and DEAE-cellulose column chromatography. It required magnesium ions for both activity and stability. The position of acetylation was not determined, but the substrate specificity suggested that the 6′-amino group was acetylated (Benveniste and Davies 1971b).

AAC(6′) was also found in *P. aeruginosa* GN 315 which is resistant to kanamycin A and B, dibekacin, neomycins, and ribostamycin (Yagisawa et al. 1972b). The structures of 6′-*N*-acetylkanamycin A, 6′-*N*-acetylribostamycin (Yamamoto et al. 1972c), and 6′-*N*-acetyldibekacin (Yagisawa et al. 1972b) were confirmed by the ^{1}H NMR spectra.

The AAC(6′) was divided into 4 groups (Kawabe et al. 1975): AAC(6′)-1 found in *E. coli* K 12 R 5 acetylated kanamycin A and B and neomycins, but not gentamicin C_{1a}, dibekacin, and amikacin; AAC(6′)-2 found in *Moraxella* (LeGoffic and Martel 1974) acetylated kanamycin A and B, neomycins, and gentamicin C_{1a}, but not dibekacin and amikacin; AAC(6′)-3 found in *P. aeruginosa* GN 4925 and GN 5462 acetylated kanamycin A and B, neomycins, gentamicin C_{1a}, dibekacin, and 6′-*N*-methyldibekacin, but not amikacin; AAC(6′)-4 found in *P. aeruginosa* GN 315 acetylated kanamycin A and B, gentamicin C_{1a}, dibekacin, and amikacin, but not 6′-*N*-methyldibekacin. An enzyme similar to AAC(6′)-3 was also found in *P. aeruginosa* (Haas et al. 1976).

An enzyme was extracted and purified by affinity chromatography from *S. aureus* R. Palm resistant to tobramycin, gentamicins, and sisomicin, and showed both APH(2″) and AAC(6′) activity (LeGoffic et al. 1977; LeGoffic 1977). Gentamicin C components were more sensitive to 2″-*O*-phosphorylation than to 6′-*N*-acetylation. The presence of both APH(2″) and AAC(6′) activity in a single enzyme was explained by binding of the adenine moiety of acetyl CoA and ATP to the same part of the enzyme (LeGoffic 1977).

Gentamicin C_1 and 6′-*N*-ethylamikacin showed a low affinity (Km $> 2 \times 10^{-3}$ *M*) for AAC(6′)-4 prepared from *P. aeruginosa* GN 315 and were barely acetylated (Yagisawa et al. 1975).

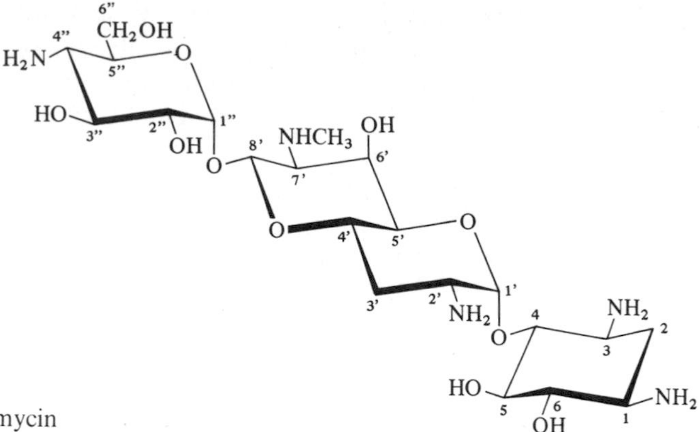

Fig. 11. Apramycin

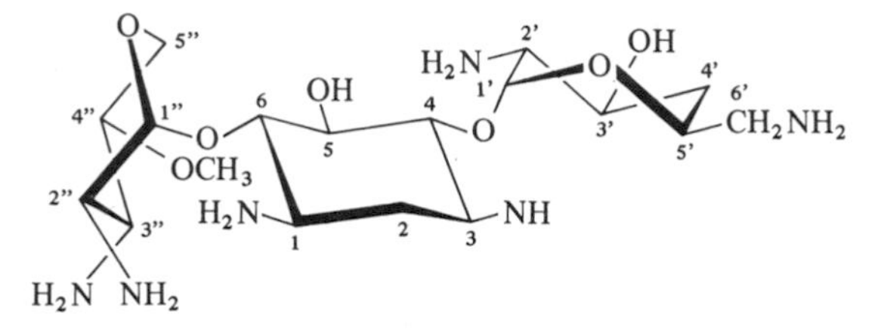

Fig. 12. Seldomycin factor 5

7. 3-Acetyltransferase [AAC(3)]

An enzyme found in the 105 S fraction of disrupted cells of *P. aeruginosa* 99 acetylated gentamicin C components (MITSUHASHI et al. 1971). A similar enzyme was found on *P. aeruginosa* 130 and 209, and the structure of gentamicin C_{1a} acetylated by this enzyme was determined to be the 3-acetate (BRZEZINSKA et al. 1972). The AAC(3) was specific for gentamicin C components.

The enzyme AAC(3) was divided into 4 groups (DAVIES and SMITH 1978): AAC(3)-I acetylated gentamicin C components and sisomicin, but did not acetylate, or very slowly acetylated, tobramycin, and kanamycins; AAC(3)-II isolated from *E. coli* K 12 harboring an R plasmid of *Klebsiella* origin was similar to AAC(3)-I in substrate profile but different in isoelectric point (LEGOFFIC et al. 1974); AAC(3)-III produced by *P. aeruginosa* PST 1 acetylated gentamicins, sisomicin, netilmicin, kanamycins, tobramycin, neomycins, and paromomycins; AAC(3)-IV produced by *E. coli* JR 225 had the broadest substrate range, acetylating all of the substrates of AAC(3)-III and apramycin (DAVIES and O'CONNOR 1978).

The AAC(3)-I was also found in *E. coli* K 12 C 600 R 135 which is resistant to gentamicin C components but not kanamycins (H. UMEZAWA et al. 1973 b). The strain was obtained by transduction of R factor in a clinically isolated *Enterobacter* with phage PIKc (WITCHITZ 1972). The AAC(3)-I from *E. coli* K 12 carrying an R plasmid of *K. pneumoniae* origin was purified by affinity chromatography on Indubiose–gentamicin C_1 and Indubiose–Kanamycin A columns (LEGOFFIC and

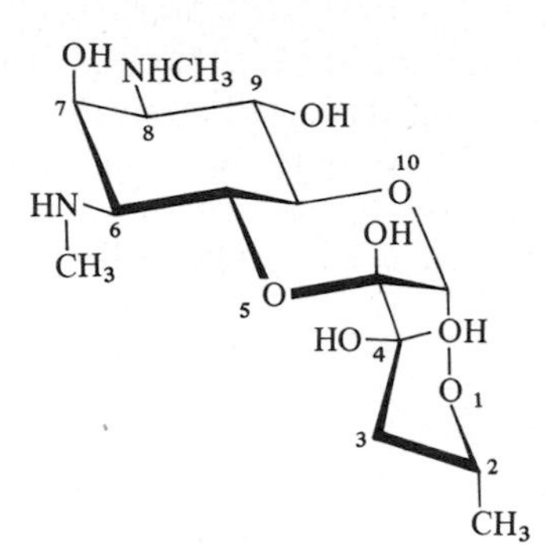

Fig. 13. Spectinomycin

MOREAU 1973). WILLIAMS and NORTHROP purified and characterized in detail the AAC(3)-I from *E. coli* C 600 JR 88 (WILLIAMS and NORTHROP 1976, 1978 a, b). The AAC(3)-I is a tetrameric protein of 63,000 mol. wt. (WILLIAMS and NORTHROP 1976), and the *N*-terminal amino acid sequence of 21 residues has been determined (HSIANG et al. 1978).

The AAC(3)-I in *E. coli* KY 8348 also acetylated the 3-amino group of seldomycin factor 5 (SATO et al. 1977).

8. 2′-Acetyltransferase [AAC(2′)]

AAC(2′), which transfers the acetyl group from acetyl CoA to the 2′-amino group of sisomicin, was found in a clinical isolate of *Providencia* (CHEVEREAU et al. 1974). The structure of 2′-*N*-acetylsisomicin was confirmed by mass spectrometric analysis. The 3′-deoxyaminoglycosides, such as gentamicin C components, tobramycin, and dibekacin, were the most effective substrates, and butirosins, gentamicin B, and kanamycin C were also substrates for AAC(2′). However, kanamycin B and neomycin were less effective substrates than kanamycin C and paromomycin, respectively. AAC(2′) was also found in other *Providencia* strains (YAMAGUCHI et al. 1974). Strains carrying this enzyme were resistant to lividomycin A and gentamicin C components, but sensitive to kanamycin A.

III. Resistance to Streptomycins

1. 3″-Adenylyltransferase [AAD(3″)]

H. UMEZAWA et al. (1968 a) first reported the mechanism of resistance to streptomycin involving AAD(3″). This enzyme was found in *E. coli* K 12 ML 1629 which also produced APH(3′) as described above, and the structure of the reaction product was determined by chemical methods to be streptomycin 3″-adenylate (H. UMEZAWA et al. 1968 a; TAKASAWA et al. 1968). YAMADA et al. also found enzymatic inactivation of streptomycin by AAD(3″) in *E. coli* (YAMADA et al. 1968). The AAD(3″) also adenylylated spectinomycin and its aminocyclitol moiety, actinamine. The position of adenylylation was suggested to be the 9-hydroxyl group from the similar *trans*-relation of the vicinal hydroxyl and methylamino groups in the actinamine moiety of spectinomycin and in the *N*-methyl-L-glucosamine moiety of streptomycin (BENVENISTE et al. 1970). Biochemical and genetic studies of AAD(3″) indicated that adenylylation of streptomycin, dihydrostreptomycin, bluensomycin, actinamine, spectinomycin, and dihydrospectinomycin was catalyzed by a single enzyme (SMITH et al. 1970).

An enzyme from *S. aureus* also adenylylated dihydrostreptomycin (KAWABE and MITSUHASHI 1971).

2. 3″-Phosphotransferase [APH(3″)]

OZANNE et al. found APH(3″) in *E. coli* JR 35, which is resistant to streptomycin but not to spectinomycin. The structure of streptomycin 3″-phosphate was confirmed chemically (OZANNE et al. 1969). The APH(3″) was also found in *E. coli* JR 66/W 677 (H. UMEZAWA et al. 1974) and *P. aeruginosa* TI-13, 99, 137, 138, 351, 10,126, and Cape 18 (KOBAYASHI et al. 1972). The structure of dihydrostreptomycin 3″-phosphate was clearly determined by ^{1}H NMR analysis (NAGANAWA et al. 1971 a).

Recently, resistance to streptomycin of phytopathogenic bacteria has been increasing. *Pseudomonas lachrymans* is known to be a plant pathogen which causes cucumber angular leaf spot and which is resistant to streptomycin because of APH(3″) (YANO et al. 1978; KAWABE et al. 1979). *Erwinia carotovora* from diseased plants also produces APH(3″) (FUKASAWA et al. 1980).

3. 6-Adenylyltransferase [AAD(6)] and 6-Phosphotransferase [APH(6)]

The enzymes AAD(6), found in *S. aureus* (SUZUKI et al. 1975), and APH(6), found in *P. aeruginosa* (KIDA et al. 1975), are also involved in resistance to streptomycin.

IV. Resistance to Fortimicins

The fortimicin group antibiotics which have been found in culture filtrates of *Micromonospora*, *Saccharopolyspora*, *Dactylosporangium*, and *Streptomyces* are interesting aminoglycosides. Fortimicin A, C, and D (NARA et al. 1977; EGAN et al. 1977; IIDA et al. 1979), SF-2052 or dactimicin (INOUYE et al. 1979), sporaricin A (DEUSHI et al. 1979 a, b), istamycin A (sannamycin A), and instamycin B (OKAMI et al. 1979; DEUSHI et al. 1979 c; WATANABE et al. 1979) exhibit good activity in inhibiting the growth of staphylococci and gram-negative bacteria, except *P. aeruginosa*. Strains producing AAC(3)-I are resistant to fortimicin group antibiotics, but other resistant strains are sensitive. The AAC(3)-I in *E. coli* acetylated the 1-amino group of fortimicin A (SATO et al. 1977).

V. Immobilization of Enzymes

As described above, the enzymes involved in resistance to aminoglycoside antibiotics are obtained in the 100 S fraction of disrupted cells of resistant bacteria. These enzymes can be extracted by conventional methods for enzyme extraction and purification, but more efficiently by using affinity columns with bound substrate antibiotics and their derivatives as ligands. The affinity column is made by linking

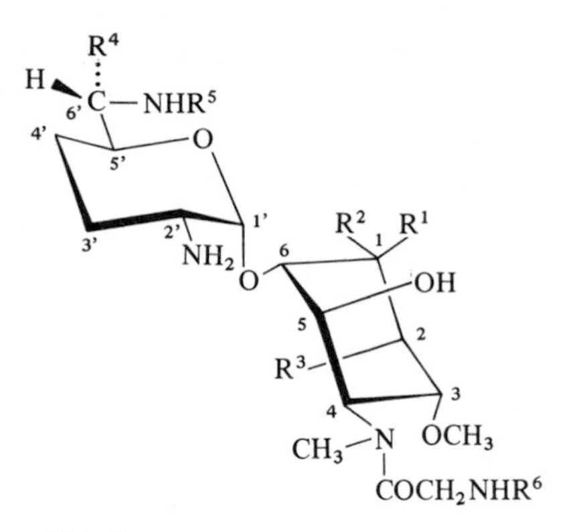

Fig. 14. Fortimicin group antibiotics

	R^1	R^2	R^3	R^4	R^5	R^6
Fortimicin A	NH_2	H	OH	CH_3	H	H
Fortimicin C	NH_2	H	OH	CH_3	H	$CONH_2$
Fortimicin D	NH_2	H	OH	H	H	H
Sporaricin A	H	NH_2	H	CH_3	H	H
Istamycin A	NH_2	H	H	H	CH_3	H
Istamycin B	H	NH_2	H	H	CH_3	H
Dactimicin	NH_2	H	OH	CH_3	H	$CH{=}NH$

the ligand to the solid matrix support by a covalent bond. Cyanogen bromide-activated Sepharose 4 B (Pharmacia Fine Chemicals, Uppsala) is commercially available and is convenient for the preparation of affinity columns.

These enzymes involved in resistance can also be immobilized on solid matrix supports. Then, reactions can be carried out with the immobilized enzymes and the reaction products can be easily isolated (H. UMEZAWA et al. 1974).

Growing cells of *E. coli* carrying R plasmid or *P. aeruginosa* were disrupted and the 100 S fraction was dialyzed against 20 m*M* phosphate buffer at pH 7.2. The enzymes in the dialyzed solution were coupled with cyanogen bromide-activated Sepharose 4 B under gentle stirring at 4 °C for 16 h. The supports with enzymes were treated with 1.0 *M* monoethanolamine, and washed with 0.1 *M* acetate buffer (pH 4.0) in 1.0 *M* sodium chloride and with 0.1 *M* borate buffer (pH 8.0) in 1.0 *M* sodium chloride, successively. When the enzyme in 1 ml of the 100 S fraction was coupled with 125 mg cyanogen bromide-activated Sepharose 4 B, the activity of the immobilized APH(3')-I prepared from *E. coli* K 12 J 5 R 11-2 was 4.18 µmol kanamycin A/wet g/h and 9.09 µmol lividomycin A/wet g/h. If the 100 S fraction contains more than one enzyme, all the enzymes are immobilized. The immobilized enzyme prepared from *E. coli* JR 66/W 677 showed APH(3')-II activity (33 µmol butirosin A/wet g/h and 20 µmol kanamycin A/wet g/h) and APH(3'') activity (1.64 µmol streptomycin/wet g/h). Cyanogen bromide-activated cellulose was also used as a solid matrix support for the immobilization of enzymes.

Continuous enzyme reactions can be carried out on a column of immobilized enzyme. The APH(3')-II–Sepharose 4 B (22 µmol kanamycin A/wet g/h, 1 wet g) prepared from partially purified APH(3')-II from *E. coli* JR 66/W 677 was packed into a column (0.6 × 4.4 cm) and a 250-ml solution containing kanamycin B

(121 mg, 250 μmol), ATP-Na·$3H_2O$ (756 mg, 1 mmol), magnesium acetate (2.5 mmol), and potassium chloride (15 mmol) in 20 m*M* phosphate buffer (pH 7.8) was passed through the column at the rate of 4 ml/h at 37 °C. In this way, kanamycin B was completely phosphorylated and kanamycin B 3′-phosphate (115 mg) was isolated by a single column chromatography on Amberlite CG-50 resin (NH^+ form) which was eluted with 0.1 *M* ammonia. Dihydrostreptomycin 3″-phosphate was obtained as crystals by phosphorylation on an APH(3″)–Sepharose 4 B column followed by adsorption on a column of Amberlite CG-50 resin (NH^+:H^+, 7:3) and elution with 0.5 *M* ammonia.

The activity of the immobilized enzyme is dependent on the purity of the enzyme used for the preparation. The enzyme is much more stable in the immobilized state than in solution.

VI. Structural Elucidation of Modified Antibiotics by Spectrometry

In the early studies the structures of enzyme reaction products were elucidated by chemical methods, including synthesis. Recently, structures have been determined solely by spectrometric methods, that is, by ^1H and ^{13}C NMR spectroscopic methods and by mass spectrometry. The development of high-resolution NMR spectroscopy has made it possible to identify almost all the protons or ^{13}C-atoms of all aminoglycoside antibiotics.

The chemical shift of the proton on a carbon bound to a phosphoric ester group is about 0.5 ppm to lower field than that of the parent antibiotic. By irradiation of the signal of ^{31}P (40.49113 MHz), the coupling of the proton on a carbon bearing a phosphate group can be clearly observed and the stereochemistry confirmed. The P-O-C-H coupling constant is about 8 Hz (NAGANAWA et al. 1971 a; MAEDA et al. 1968). The chemical shift of the proton on a carbon bearing an amino group moves by 0.3–0.6 ppm to lower field upon *N*-acetylation (YAGISAWA et al. 1972 b; YAMAMOTO et al. 1972 c).

In ^{13}C NMR spectra, the chemical shift of the carbon bearing the phosphoric ester group shifts by 3–6 ppm to lower field and the signal shows P-C coupling of about 5 Hz (TODA et al. 1978). The β-shift measurements of ^{13}C NMR spectra are also useful for determination of the position of *N*-acetylation.

Mass spectrometry has been applied to the determination of the structures of 3-*N*-acetylgentamicin C_1 (BRZEZINSKA et al. 1972; H. UMEZAWA et al. 1973 b) and 4′-*O*-adenylyltobramycin (LEGOFFIC et al. 1976).

VII. Similarity to Enzymes Involved in Biosynthesis

If an enzyme involved in biosynthesis of an antibiotic is similar to an enzyme involved in plasmid-mediated resistance, the appearance of resistant strains after widespread use of the antibiotic is easily understood. Some aminoglycoside-modifying enzymes involved in biosynthesis have been found: APH(6) in streptomycin-producing strains (WALKER and SKORVAGA 1973), APH(3′) in a neomycin-producing strain (BENVENISTE and DAVIES 1973) and a butirosin-producing strain (MATSUHASHI et al. 1977; COURVALIN et al. 1977), and AAC(6′) in a kanamycin-producing strain (SATOH et al. 1975). Furthermore, 3-*N*-acetyl derivatives of neomycin

(RINEHART 1964), kanamycin B (MURASE et al. 1970), and ribostamycin (KOJIMA et al. 1975) were isolated from the fermentation broth of the antibiotic-producing strains. Although APH(3′) in a butirosin producer, *Bacillus circulans*, was the APH(3′)-II-type enzyme by substrate specificity, it did not cross-react with rabbit antiserum prepared against APH(3′)-II from *E. coli* JR 66/W 677 (MATSUHASHI et al. 1977).

On the other hand, purified DNAs from *B. circulans* and the plasmid ColEl-Ap^R were digested with *Eco*RI endonuclease and the resulting fragments covalently joined with polynucleotide ligase. The recombined DNA was used to transform *E. coli* and ampicillin–neomycin-resistant colonies were selected. The development of neomycin resistance in the *E. coli* transformants was due to the presence of the APH(3′) gene in *B. circulans* (COURVALIN et al. 1977). However, it is not yet certain whether a plasmid for biosynthesis of an antibiotic is related in its origin to a plasmid for biosynthesis of an enzyme involved in resistance.

C. Derivatives Active Against Resistant Strains

Based on the biochemical mechanisms of resistance to aminoglycoside antibiotics, a synthetic approach to derivatives that do not undergo the enzyme reactions and thus inhibit the growth of resistant bacteria was started by the UMEZAWA group. 3′-*O*-Methylkanamycin A (H. UMEZAWA et al. 1972b) and 3′-*O*-methylneamine (S. UMEZAWA et al. 1972a) had only weak antibacterial activity. The 3′-*O*-methyl group seems to hinder the binding of these antibiotics to bacterial ribosomes. However, deoxygenation of the 3′-hydroxyl group gave active compounds: 3′-deoxykanamycin A (S. UMEZAWA et al. 1971a), 3′-deoxykanamycin B (tobramycin) (TAKAGI et al. 1973), 3′-deoxykanamycin C (KONDO et al. 1977), 3′-deoxyribostamycin (IKEDA et al. 1973b), 3′-deoxybutirosin B (IKEDA et al. 1975), and 3′-deoxyneomycin B (WATANABE et al. 1973b). The 3′-deoxy compounds showed increased antibacterial activity compared with the parent antibiotics, and inhibited resistant bacteria producing APH(3′) enzymes. The 3′,4′-dideoxy compounds also showed good activity; 3′,4′-dideoxykanamycin A (TSUCHIYA et al. 1979), 3′,4′-dideoxykanamycin B (dibekacin) (H. UMEZAWA et al. 1971), 3′,4′-dideoxykanamycin C (KONDO et al. 1977), 3′,4′-dideoxyribostamycin (S. UMEZAWA et al. 1972b), 3′,4′-dideoxybutirosin B (IKEDA et al. 1973a), and 3′4′-dideoxyneamine (S. UMEZAWA et al. 1971b) were synthesized. Dibekacin was found to be a valuable chemotherapeutic agent effective not only against infections of resistant bacteria but also against pseudomonas infections, and was commercially available. Deoxygenation of the 4′-hydroxyl group did not increase antibacterial activity, but 4′-deoxykanamycin A (S. UMEZAWA et al. 1974; NAITO et al. 1974) and 4′-deoxykanamycin B (ABE et al. 1977) inhibited resistant bacteria producing APH(3′)-II. Recently, 4′-deoxyneomycin possessing the intrinsic activity of the parent antibiotic was also synthesized (HANESSIAN and VATELE 1980).

However, deoxygenation of the 5-hydroxyl group of ribose in lividomycins and ribostamycin markedly reduced antibacterial activity; 5″-deoxylividomycin A (YAMAMOTO et al. 1972b), 5″-deoxylividomycin B (S. UMEZAWA et al. 1972c), and 3′,4′,5″-trideoxyribostamycin (S. UMEZAWA et al. 1972b) were synthesized. The 5″-

Table 2. Minimum inhibitory concentrations (μg/ml) of the 1-*N*-AHB derivatives of dibekacin (DKB), 6′-*N*-methyldibekacin (6′-*N*-MeDKB), 6′(*R*)-*C*-methyldibekacin [6′(*R*)-*C*-MeDKB], and 6′(*S*)-*C*-methyldibekacin [6′(*S*)-*C*-MeDKB]

Test organism	AHB-DKB	AHB-6′-*N*-MeDKB	AHB-6′(*R*)-*C*-MeDKB	AHB-6′(*S*)-*C*-MeDKB
Staphylococcus aureus FDA 209P	0.39	0.39	0.78	1.56
S. aureus Ap01 [a]	0.78	1.56	0.78	1.56
Escherichia coli K-12	3.13	3.13	0.78	1.56
E. coli K-12 R5 [b]	100	6.25	100	6.25
E. coli K-12 ML1629 [c]	3.13	6.25	3.13	3.13
E. coli K-12 LA290 R55 [d]	6.25	6.25	3.13	3.13
E. coli JR66/W677 [d, e]	6.25	6.25	6.25	6.25
E. coli K-12 C600 R135 [f]	1.56	1.56	0.78	1.56
E. coli JR225 [f]	3.13	3.13	1.56	1.56
Serratia marcescens	50	25	25	50
Providencia sp. Pv16 [g]	25	50	50	12.5
Pseudomonas aeruginosa A3	3.13	6.25	3.13	6.25
P. aeruginosa H9 [e]	6.25	12.5	25	25
P. aeruginosa TI-13 [c]	3.13	25	25	25
P. aeruginosa GN315 [b]	6.25	25	50	50

[a] AAD(4′)
[b] AAC(6′)
[c] APH(3′)-I
[d] AAD(2″)
[e] APH(3′)-II
[f] AAC(3)
[g] AAC(2′)-producing strains

amination of these antibiotics restored antibacterial activity, but increased toxicity; 5″-amino-5″-deoxylividomycin A (YAMAMOTO et al. 1972b), 6′,5″,6‴-triamino-6′,5″,6‴-trideoxylividomycin A, 6′,5″-diamino-6′,5″-dideoxylividomycin B (KONDO et al. 1976), 5″-amino-5″-deoxyneomycin, 5″-amino-5″-deoxyparomomycin (HANESSIAN et al. 1977), 5″-amino-5″-deoxybutirosin (CULBERTSON et al. 1973), 5″-amino-3′,5″-dideoxybutirosin A (WATANABE et al. 1978), and 5″-amino-3′,4′,5″-trideoxybutirosin A (WOO et al. 1975) were synthesized.

As already described, butirosins which contain the (*S*)-4-amino-2-hydroxybutyryl (AHB) group on the 1-amino group, are not modified by APH(3′)-I. Based on this reasoning, 1-*N*-AHB-kanamycin A (amikacin) (KAWAGUCHI et al. 1972), 3′-deoxyamikacin, 3′,4′-dideoxyamikacin, 4′-deoxyamikacin (TSUCHIYA et al. 1979), 1-*N*-AHB-kanamycin B, 1-*N*-AHB-dibekacin (KONDO et al. 1973a, b), 1-*N*-AHB-kanamycin C, 1-*N*-AHB-3′-deoxykanamycin C, 1-*N*-AHB-3′,4′-dideoxykanamycin C (KONDO et al. 1977), 1-*N*-AHB-gentamicin B (NAGABHUSHAN et al. 1978b), 1-*N*-AHB-gentamicin C_{1a} (WRIGHT et al. 1976), 1-*N*-AHB-gentamicin C_1 (DANIELS et al. 1974b), 1-*N*-AHB-lividomycin A (WATANABE et al. 1973a), and 1-*N*-AHB-3′,4′-dideoxyneamine (S. UMEZAWA et al. 1973) were synthesized. The modification of the 1-amino group gives derivatives which are active not only against resistant strains containing APH(3′)-I but also against resistant strains producing AAD(2″). It is easily understood that modification of the 1-amino group by the AHB group causes steric hindrance against AAD(2″). Amikacin has been

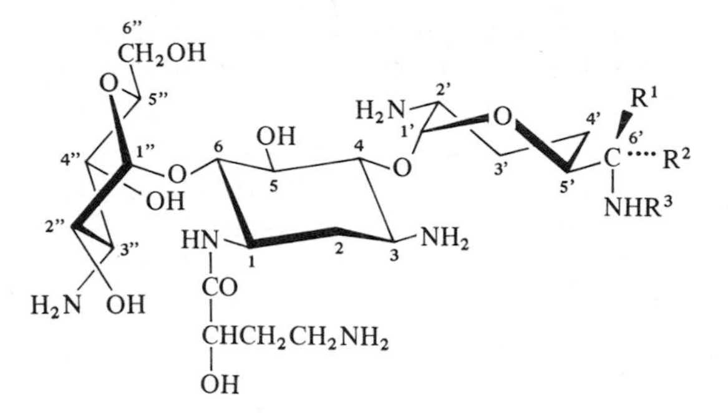

Fig. 15. Derivatives of dibekacin. 1-*N*-AHB-dibekacin: R^1, R^2, R^3=H; 1-*N*-AHB-6′-*N*-methyldibekacin: R^1, R^2=H, R^3=CH_3; 1-*N*-AHB-6′(*S*)-*C*-methyldibekacin: R^1, R^3=H, R^2=CH_3; 1-*N*-AHB-6′(*R*)-*C*-methyldibekacin: R^1=CH_3, R^2=H

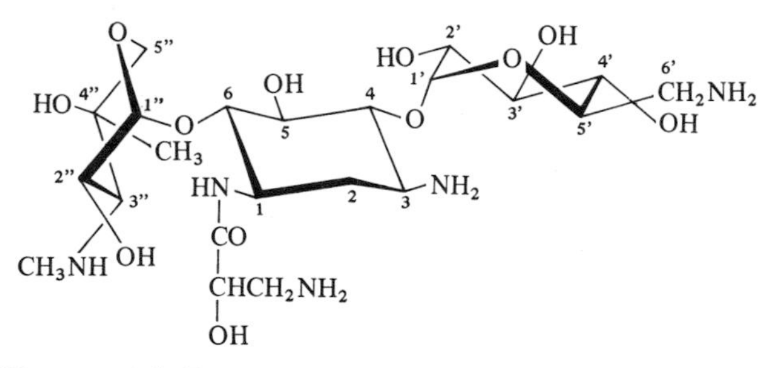

Fig. 16. 1-*N*-AHP-gentamicin B

widely used for infections of resistant bacteria. Furthermore, the 1-*N*-acylation of dibekacin with AHB (Table 2) and the 3′-deoxygenation of amikacin gave useful derivatives having a wide antibacterial spectrum against sensitive and resistant strains. These derivatives are expected to develop into valuable chemotherapeutic agents.

The isoseryl (3-amino-2-hydroxypropionyl, AHP) derivatives of the 1-amino group were also effective against resistant bacteria: 1-*N*-AHP-kanamycin A, 1-*N*-AHP-kanamycin B, 1-*N*-AHP-dibekacin (Kondo et al. 1974), 1-*N*-AHP-gentamicin C_1 (Daniels et al. 1974b), 1-*N*-AHP-gentamicin C_{1a} (Wright et al. 1976), 1-*N*-AHP-gentamicin B (Nagabhushan 1978b), and 1-*N*-AHP-sisomicin (Wright et al. 1976).

The 1-*N*-alkyl derivatives, 1-*N*-ethylsisomicin (netilmicin) (Wright 1976), 1-*N*-[(*S*)-4-amino-2-hydroxybutyl]kanamycin A (Richardson et al. 1977), and 1-*N*-(1,3-dihydroxy-2-propyl)kanamycin B (Richardson et al. 1979), were synthesized and showed interesting activity.

The 6′-*N*-alkyl derivatives of aminoglycoside antibiotics were synthesized to prevent reaction with AAC(6′); the 6′-*N*-methylation was not enough to inhibit the reaction of all AAC(6′) enzymes and the 6′-*N*-ethyl derivatives completely inhibited the reaction, but their activity was reduced to one-fourth or less than that of the parent antibiotics, 6′-*N*-Methylkanamycin A, 6′-*N*-methyldibekacin (H. Umezawa et al. 1972a), 6′-*N*-methylamikacin, 6′-*N*-ethylamikacin (H. Umezawa et al. 1975b), 4′-deoxy-6′-*N*-methylamikacin (NAITO et al. 1979), 1-*N*-AHP-6′-*N*-methyldibekacin, 1-*N*-AHB-6′-*N*-methyldibekacin (Table 2), 1-*N*-[(*S*)-5-amino-2-hydroxyvaleryl]-6′-*N*-methyldibekacin (H. UMEZAWA et al. 1975a), and 3′-deoxy-6′-*N*-methylneomycin B (WATANABE et al. 1973b) were synthesized.

The 6′-*C*-alkyl derivatives were synthesized through a 5′-deaminomethyl-5′-*C*-formyl derivative in good yield and two diastereomers, 6′(*S*)- and 6′(*R*)-*C*-alkyl derivatives, could be separated by column chromatography (IKEDA et al. 1979; H. UMEZAWA et al. 1979). The finding that 6′(*S*)-*C*-methyldibekacin, 6′(*S*)-*C*-methyltobramycin, 1-*N*-AHB-6′(*S*)-*C*-methyldibekacin, and 1-*N*-AHB-6′(*S*)-*C*-methyltobramycin are much more active than their *R* epimers against resistant bacteria producing AAC(6′)-1 is especially interesting (Table 2) (KONDO 1979).

It is also interesting that 5-deoxygenation of the 2-deoxystreptamine moiety gave active derivatives: 5-deoxykanamycin B (SUAMI et al. 1978), 5-deoxysisomicin (TESTA et al. 1974), and 5-deoxygentamicin C components (ROSSI et al. 1977). The 5-epimerization of sisomicin increased activity against *Pseudomonas*, *Providencia*, and *Proteus* spp. (WAITZ et al. 1978; FU and NEU 1978). Resistant strains possessing AAC(3)-I, AAD(2″), or AAC(2′) enzymes were much more sensitive to 5-*epi*-sisomicin and 5-*epi*-gentamicin B (VASTOLA et al. 1980). The 1-*N*-AHP-5-*epi*-sisomicin exhibited excellent activity but indicated a level of nephrotoxicity several times higher than that of sisomicin (DANIELS et al. 1979).

4″-*epi*-Tobramycin exhibited antibacterial activity similar to that of tobramycin (TANABE et al. 1977). 3′,4′,4″,6″-Tetradeoxyamikacin and 1-*N*-AHB-3′,4′,4″,6″-tetradeoxykanamycin B showed good activity against gram-negative and -positive bacteria, except against *Pseudomonas aeruginosa* (H. UMEZAWA 1979; MIYASAKA et al. 1980). However, it was reported that 4″-deoxygentamicin C_1 exhibited very weak antibacterial activity against some sensitive gram-positive bacteria and was otherwise inactive (MALLAMS et al. 1973).

Recently, 2′,3′-dideoxygentamicin B, 3′,4′-dideoxygentamicin B, and 2′-desaminosisomicin were synthesized, and their 1-*N*-acyl derivatives with AHP showed activity similar to that of amikacin (DANIELS et al. 1979). However, 2′,3′-epiminoribostamycin, 2′,3′-epiminokanamycin B, and 2″,3″-epiminokanamycin B showed little or no intrinsic activity (KUMAR et al. 1980).

2″-Deoxygentamicin C_2 showed good activity against resistant strains producing AAD(2″) but lower activity than the parent antibiotic against sensitive strains. 2″-*epi*-Gentamicin C_1 was without antibacterial activity in vitro at levels up to 25 μg/ml (DANIELS et al. 1974a).

The activity of the 3″-de-*N*-methyl derivatives of gentamicin C_2, gentamicin B, and sisomicin was similar to that of their parent antibiotics. The 3″-*N*-propyl, 3″-*N*-butyl, and 3″-*N*-(4‴-aminobutyl) derivatives of 3″-de-*N*-methylgentamicin C_2 were also active (NAGABHUSHAN et al. 1978a).

3″-Deoxydihydrostreptomycin was synthesized and found to inhibit resistant bacteria producing APH(3″) or AAD(3″) (SANO et al. 1976). However, many strains of *P. aeruginosa* were resistant to the compound. 1-Deamidino-, 3-deamidino-, and 1,3-di-(deamidino)-dihydrostreptomycins showed very weak activity, but the 3-guanidino group was more important than the 1-guanidino group for the antibacterial activity of dihydrostreptomycin. The 1-*N*-AHB-1-deamidino-dihydrostreptomycin and 1-*N*-[(*S*)-4-guanidino-2-hydroxybutyryl]-1-deamidinodihydrostreptomycin exhibited only weak activity, indicating that the successful modification of kanamycins by 1-*N*-acylation did not apply to the streptomycins (USUI et al. 1978).

D. Conclusion

The enzymatic mechanism of resistance to aminoglycoside antibiotics was clarified and the development of derivatives which are active against resistant organisms was successful. This study will continue parallel to the elucidation of new types of resistance mechanisms or to the discovery of new compounds.

Dibekacin is the first semisynthetic aminoglycoside antibiotic to be developed based on a knowledge of the enzymatic mechanism of resistance. This type of development will give more and more compounds which are useful in the treatment of resistant infections. On the other hand, the development of compounds which are active against resistant organisms with altered cell permeability must be sought in the near future.

References

Abe Y, Nakagawa S, Fujisawa K, Naito T, Kawaguchi H (1977) Aminoglycoside antibiotics. XI. Synthesis and activity of 4′-deoxykanamycin B. J Antibiot (Tokyo) 30:1004–1007

Akiba T, Koyama K, Isshiki Y, Kimura S, Fukushima T (1960) On the mechanism of the development of multiple drug resistance clones of *Shigella* (in Japanese). Nippon Iji Shimpo 1866:46–50

Benveniste R, Davies J (1971a) R-factor mediated gentamicin resistance: a new enzyme which modifies aminoglycoside antibiotics. FEBS Lett 14:293–296

Benveniste R, Davies J (1971b) Enzymatic acetylation of aminoglycoside antibiotics by *Escherichia coli* carrying an R-factor. Biochemistry 10:1787–1796

Benveniste R, Davies J (1973) Aminoglycoside antibiotic-inactivating enzymes in *Actinomycetes* similar to those present in clinical isolates of antibiotic-resistant bacteria. Proc Natl Acad Sci USA 70:2276–2280

Benveniste R, Yamada T, Davies J (1970) Enzymatic adenylylation of streptomycin and spectinomycin by R-factor-resistant *Escherichia coli.* Infect Immun 1:109–119

Brzezinska M, Davies J (1973) Two enzymes which phosphorylate neomycin and kanamycin in *Escherichia coli* strains carrying R factors. Antimicrob Agents Chemother 3:266–269

Brzezinska M, Benveniste R, Davies J, Daniels PJL, Weinstein J (1972) Gentamicin resistance in strains of *Pseudomonas aeruginosa* mediated by enzymatic N-acetylation of the deoxystreptamine moiety. Biochemistry 11:761–765

Chevereau M, Daniels PJL, Davies J, LeGoffic F (1974) Aminoglycoside resistance in bacteria mediated by gentamicin acetyltransferase II, an enzyme modifying the 2′-amino group of aminoglycoside antibiotics. Biochemistry 13:598–603

Cochran TG, Abraham DJ (1972) Stereochemistry and absolute configuration of the antibiotic spectinomycin: an X-ray diffraction study. J Chem Soc Chem Commun 494–495

Courvalin P, Weisblum B, Davies J (1977) Aminoglycoside-modifying enzyme of an antibiotic-producing bacterium acts as a determinant of antibiotic resistance in *Escherichia coli.* Proc Natl Acad Sci USA 74:999–1008

Culbertson TP, Watson DR, Haskell TH (1973) 5″-Amino-5″-deoxybutirosin, a new semisynthetic aminoglycoside antibiotic. J Antibiot (Tokyo) 26:790–793

Daniels PJL, Weinstein J, Tkach RW, Morton J (1974a) Gentamicin derivatives modified at the 2″-position. The preparation of 2″-*epi*-gentamicin C_1 and 2″-deoxygentamicin C_2. J Antibiot (Tokyo) 27:150–154

Daniels PJL, Weinstein J, Nagabhushan TL (1974b) The syntheses of 1-N-[(*S*)-4-amino-2-hydroxybutyryl]gentamicin C_1 and 1-N-[(*S*)-3-amino-2-hydroxypropionyl]gentamicin C_1. J Antibiot (Tokyo) 27:889–893
Daniels PJL, Cooper AB, McCombie SW, Nagabhushan TL (1979) Some recent advances in the chemistry of antibiotics of the gentamicin series. Jpn J Antibiot 32:S195–S204
Davies J, O'Connor S (1978) Enzymatic modification of aminoglycoside antibiotics: 3-N-acetyltransferase with broad specificity that determines resistance to the novel aminoglycoside apramycin. Antimicrob Agents Chemother 14:69–72
Davies J, Smith DI (1978) Plasmid-determined resistance to antimicrobial agents. Ann Rev Microbiol 32:469–518
Deushi T, Iwasaki A, Kamiya K, Kunieda T, Mizoguchi T, Nakayama M, Itoh H, Mori T, Oda T (1979a) A new broad-spectrum aminoglycoside antibiotic complex, sporaricin. I. Fermentation, isolation and characterization. J Antiobiot (Tokyo) 32:173–179
Deushi T, Nakayama M, Watanabe I, Mori T, Naganawa H, Umezawa H (1979b) A new broad-spectrum aminoglycoside antibiotic complex, sporaricin. III. The structures of sporaricins A and B. J Antibiot (Tokyo) 32:187–192
Deushi T, Iwasaki A, Kamiya K, Mizoguchi T, Nakayama M, Itoh H, Mori T (1979c) New aminoglycoside antibiotics, sannamycin. J Antibiot (Tokyo) 32:1061–1065
Doi O, Ogura M, Tanaka N, Umezawa H (1968a) Inactivation of kanamycin, neomycin, and streptomycin by enzymes obtained in cells of *Pseudomonas aeruginosa*. Appl Microbiol 16:1276–1281
Doi O, Miyamoto M, Tanaka N, Umezawa H (1968b) Inactivation and phosphorylation of kanamycin by drug-resistant *Staphylococcus aureus*. Appl Microbiol 16:1282–1284
Doi O, Kondo S, Tanaka N, Umezawa H (1969) Purification and properties of kanamycin-phosphorylating enzyme from *Pseudomonas aeruginosa*. J Antibiot (Tokyo) 22:273–282
Egan RS, Stanaszek RS, Cirovic M, Mueller SL, Tadanier J, Martin JR, Collum P, Goldstein AW, Devault RL, Sinclair AC, Fager EE, Mitscher LA (1977) Fortimicins A and B, new aminoglycoside antibiotics. III. Structural identification. J Antibiot (Tokyo) 30:552–563
Fu KP, Neu HC (1978) Activity of 5-episisomicin compared with that of other aminoglycosides. Antimicrob Agents Chemother 14:194–200
Fukasawa K, Sakurai H, Shimizu S, Naganawa H, Kondo S, Kawabe H, Mitsuhashi S (1980) 3″-Phosphoryldihydrostreptomycin produced by the inactivating enzyme of *Erwinia carotovora*. J Antibiot (Tokyo) 33:122–123
Haas M, Biddlecome S, Davies J, Luce CE, Daniels PJL (1976) Enzymatic modification of aminoglycoside antibiotics: a new 6′-*N*-acetylating enzyme from *Pseudomonas aeruginosa* isolate. Antimicrob Agents Chemother 9:945–950
Hanessian S, Vatele J (1980) Aminoglycoside antibiotics. 4′-Deoxyneomycin and 4′-deoxyparomamine. J Antibiot (Tokyo) 33:675–678
Hanessian S, Massé R, Capmeau M (1977) Aminoglycoside antibiotics: synthesis of 5″-amino-5″-deoxyneomycin and 5″-amino-5″-deoxyparomomycin. J Antibiot (Tokyo) 30:893–896
Hirayama N, Shirahata K, Ohashi Y, Sasada Y, Martin JR (1978) Structure of fortimicin B. Acta Crystallogr Sect B Struct Crystallogr Cryst Chem B34:2648–2650
Hsiang MW, White TJ, Davies JE (1978) NH_2-Terminal sequence of the aminoglycoside acetyltransferase (3)-I mediated by plasmid RIP135. FEBS Lett 92:97–99
Hori M, Umezawa H (1967) Miscoding activities of biologically inactivated kanamycins. J Antiobiot (Tokyo) A20:386–387
Iida T, Sato M, Matsubara I, Mori Y, Shirahata K (1979) The structures of fortimicins C, D, and KE. J Antibiot (Tokyo) 32:1273–1279
Ikeda D, Tsuchiya T, Umezawa S, Umezawa H, Hamada M (1973a) Synthesis of 3′,4′-dideoxybutirosin B. J Antibiot (Tokyo) 26:307–309
Ikeda D, Tsuchiya T, Umezawa S, Umezawa H (1973b) Synthesis of 3′-deoxyribostamycin. J Antibiot (Tokyo) 26:799–801
Ikeda D, Nagaki F, Umezawa S, Tsuchiya T, Umezawa H (1975) Synthesis of 3′-deoxybutirosin B. J Antibiot (Tokyo) 28:616–618

Ikeda D, Miyasaka T, Yoshida K, Iinuma K, Kondo S, Umezawa H (1979) The chemical conversion of gentamine C_{1a} into gentamine C_2 and its 6′-epimer. J Antibiot (Tokyo) 32:1357–1359

Inouye S, Ohba K, Shomura T, Kojima M, Tsuruoka T, Yoshida J, Kato N, Ito M, Amano S, Omoto S, Ezaki N, Ito T, Niida T, Watanabe K (1979) A novel aminoglycoside antibiotic, substance SF-2052. J Antibiot (Tokyo) 32:1354–1356

Kawabe H, Mitsuhashi S (1971) Inactivation of dihydrostreptomycin by *Staphylococcus aureus*. Jpn J Microbiol 15:545–548

Kawabe H, Kondo S, Umezawa H, Mitsuhashi S (1975) R factor-mediated aminoglycoside antibiotic resistance in *Pseudomonas aeruginosa:* a new aminoglycoside 6′-N-acetyltransferase. Antimicrob Agents Chemother 7:494–499

Kawabe H, Naganawa H, Kondo S, Umezawa H, Mitsuhashi S (1978) New plasmid-mediated phosphorylation of gentamicin C in *Staphylococcus aureus*. Microbiol Immunol 22:515–521

Kawabe H, Sakurai H, Fukasawa K, Shimizu S, Hasuda K, Iyobe S, Mitsuhashi S (1979) Phosphorylation and inactivation of streptomycin by plant pathogenic *Pseudomonas lachrymans*. J Antibiot (Tokyo) 32:425–426

Kawaguchi H, Naito T, Nakagawa S, Fujisawa K (1972) BB-K 8, a new semisynthetic aminoglycoside antibiotic. J Antibiot (Tokyo) 25:695–708

Kida M, Igarashi S, Okutani T, Asako T, Hiraga K, Mitsuhashi S (1974) Selective phosphorylation of the 5″-hydroxy group of ribostamycin by a new enzyme from *Pseudomonas aeruginosa*. Antimicrob Agents Chemother 5:92–94

Kida M, Asako T, Yoneda M, Mitsuhashi S (1975) Phosphorylation of dihydrostreptomycin by *Pseudomonas aeruginosa*. In: Mitsuhashi S (ed) Microbial drug resistance. University of Tokyo Press, Tokyo, pp 441–448

Kobayashi F, Yamaguchi M, Eda J, Higashi F, Mitsuhashi S (1971) Enzymatic inactivation of gentamicin C components by cell-free extract from *Klebsiella pneumoniae*. J Antibiot (Tokyo) 24:719–721

Kobayashi F, Yamaguchi M, Sato J, Mitsuhashi S (1972) Purification and properties of dihydrostreptomycin-phosphorylating enzyme from *Pseudomonas aeruginosa*. Jpn J Microbiol 16:15–19

Kobayashi F, Koshi T, Eda J, Yoshimura Y, Mitsuhashi S, (1973) Lividomycin resistance in staphylococci by enzymatic phosphorylation. Antimicrob Agents Chemother 4:1–5

Kojima M, Ezaki N, Amano S, Inouye S, Niida T (1975) Bioconversion of ribostamycin (SF-733). II. Isolation and structure of 3-N-acetylribostamycin, a microbiologically inactive product of ribostamycin produced by *Streptomyces ribosidificus*. J Antibiot (Tokyo) 28:42–47

Kondo S (1979) Some chemical modifications of aminoglycoside antibiotics. Jpn J Antibiot 32:S228–S236

Kondo S, Okanishi M, Utahara R, Maeda K, Umezawa H (1968) Isolation of kanamycin and paromamine inactivated by *E. coli* carrying R factor. J Antibiot (Tokyo) 21:22–29

Kondo S, Yamamoto H, Naganawa H, Umezawa H, Mitsuhashi S (1972) Isolation and characterization of lividomycin A inactivated by *Pseudomonas aeruginosa* and *Escherichia coli* carrying R factor. J Antibiot (Tokyo) 25:483–484

Kondo S, Iinuma K, Yamamoto H, Maeda K, Umezawa H (1973a) Synthesis of 1-*N*-[(*S*)-4-amino-2-hydroxybutyryl]-kanamycin B and 3′,4′-dideoxykanamycin B active against kanamycin-resistant bacteria. J Antibiot (Tokyo) 26:412–415

Kondo S, Iinuma K, Yamamoto H, Ikeda Y, Maeda K, Umezawa H (1973b) Syntheses of (*S*)-4-amino-2-hydroxybutyryl derivatives of 3′,4′-dideoxykanamycin B and their antibacterial activities. J Antibiot (Tokyo) 26:705–707

Kondo S, Iinuma K, Hamada M, Maeda K, Umezawa H (1974) Syntheses of isoseryl derivatives of kanamycins and their antibacterial activities. J Antibiot (Tokyo) 27:90–93

Kondo S, Yamamoto H, Iinuma K, Maeda K, Umezawa H (1976) Syntheses of 6′,5″,6‴-triamino-6′,5″,6‴-trideoxylividomycin A and 6′,5″-diamino-6′,5″-dideoxylividomycin B. J Antibiot (Tokyo) 29:1134–1136

Kondo S, Miyasaka T, Yoshida K, Iinuma K, Umezawa H (1977) Syntheses and properties of kanamycin C derivatives active against resistant bacteria. J Antibiot (Tokyo) 30:1150–1152
Koyama G, Iitaka Y, Maeda K, Umezawa H (1968) The crystal structure of kanamycin. Tetrahedron Lett 1875–1879
Kumar V, Jones GS, Blacksberg I, Remers WA, Misiek M, Pursiano TA (1980) Aminoglycoside antibiotics. 3. Epimino derivatives of neamine, ribostamycin, and kanamycin B. J Med Chem 23:42–49
LeGoffic F (1977) The resistance of *S. aureus* to aminoglycoside antibiotics and pristinamycins in France in 1976–1977. Jpn J Antibiot 30:S286–S291
LeGoffic F, Chevereau M (1972) L'adenyl-gentamycine C_1: un derive de la gentamycine inactivée par des bacteries proteuses d'un R-facteur. C R H S Acad Sci, Ser C 274:535–536
LeGoffic F, Martel A (1974) La résìstance aux aminosides provoquée par une isoenzyme la kanamycine acétyltransférase. Biochimie 56:893–987
LeGoffic F, Moreau N (1973) Purification by affinity chromatography of an enzyme involved in gentamicin inactivation. FEBS Lett 29:289–291
LeGoffic F, Martel A, Witchitz J (1974) 3-N Enzymatic acetylation of gentamicin, tobramycin and kanamycin by *Escherichia coli* carrying an R factor. Antimicrob Agents Chemother 6:680–684
LeGoffic F, Martel A, Capmau ML, Baca B, Goebel P, Chardon H, Soussy CJ, Duval J, Bouanchaud DH (1976) New plasmid-mediated nucleotidylation of aminoglycoside antibiotics in *Staphylococcus aureus*. Antimicrob Agents Chemother 10:258–264
LeGoffic F, Martel A, Moreau N, Capmau ML, Soussy CJ, Duval J (1977) 2″-O-Phosphorylation of gentamicin components by a *Staphylococcus aureus* strain carrying a plasmid. Antimicrob Agents Chemother 12:26–30
Maeda K, Kondo S, Okanishi M, Utahara R, Umezawa H (1968) Isolation of paromamine inactivated by *Pseudomonas aeruginosa*. J Antibiot (Tokyo) 21:458–459
Mallams AK, Vernay HF, Crowe DF, Detre G, Tanabe M, Yasuda DM (1973) The synthesis of 4″-deoxygentamicin C_1. J Antibiot (Tokyo) 26:782–783
Matsuhashi Y, Yagisawa M, Kondo S, Takeuchi T, Umezawa H (1975) Aminoglycoside 3′-phosphotransferases I and II in *Pseudomonas aeruginosa*. J Antibiot (Tokyo) 28:442–447
Matsuhashi Y, Sawa T, Takeuchi T, Umezawa H (1976a) Purification of aminoglycoside 3′-phosphotransferase II. J Antibiot (Tokyo) 29:204–207
Matsuhashi Y, Sawa T, Takeuchi T, Umezawa H (1976b) Immunological studies of aminoglycoside 3′-phosphotransferases. J Antibiot (Tokyo) 29:1127–1128
Matsuhashi Y, Sawa T, Takeuchi T, Umezawa H, Nagatsu I (1976c) Localization of aminoglycoside 3′-phosphotransferase II on a cellular surface of R factor resistant *Escherichia coli*. J Antibiot (Tokyo) 29:1129–1130
Matsuhashi Y, Sawa T, Kondo S, Takeuchi T (1977) Aminoglycoside 3′-phosphotransferase in *Bacillus circulans* producing butirosins. J Antibiot (Tokyo) 30:435–437
Mitsuhashi S (1975) Proposal for a rational nomenclature for phenotype, genotype, and aminoglycoside-aminocyclitol modifying enzyme. In: Mitsuhashi S (ed) Drug action and drug resistance in bacteria. 2. Aminoglycoside antibiotics. University of Tokyo Press, Tokyo, pp 269–275
Mitsuhashi S, Kobayashi F, Yamaguchi M (1971) Enzymatic inactivation of gentamicin C components by cell free extract from *Pseudomonas aeruginosa*. J Antibiot (Tokyo) 24:400–401
Miyamura S (1961) Dysentery bacilli and its relation to the resistance (in Japanese). Nippon Saikingaku Zasshi 16:115–119
Miyasaka T, Ikeda D, Kondo S, Umezawa H (1980) Syntheses and properties of the 6″-deoxy or 4″,6″-dideoxy derivatives of the kanamycin antibiotics. J Antibiot (Tokyo) 33:527–532
Murase M, Ito T, Fukatsu S, Umezawa H (1970) Studies on kanamycin related compounds produced during fermentation by mutants of *Streptomyces kanamyceticus*. Isolation and properties. Progr Antimicrob Anticancer Chemother 2:1098–1110

Murray BE, Moellering RC Jr (1979) Aminoglycoside-modifying enzymes among clinical isolates of *Acinetobacter calcoaceticus* subsp. *anitratus* (*Herellea vaginicola*): explanation for high-level aminoglycoside resistance. Antimicrob Agents Chemother 15:190–199

Nagabhushan TL, Wright JJ, Cooper AB, Turner WN, Miller GH (1978 a) Chemical modification of some gentamicins and sisomicin at the 3″-position. J Antibiot (Tokyo) 31:43–54

Nagabhushan TL, Cooper AB, Tsai H, Daniels PJL, Miller GH (1978 b) The syntheses and biological properties of 1-N-(*S*-4-amino-2-hydroxybutyryl)-gentamicin B and 1-N-(*S*-3-amino-2-hydroxypropionyl)-gentamicin B. J Antibiot (Tokyo) 31:681–687

Naganawa H, Kondo S, Maeda K, Umezawa H (1971 a) Structure determination of enzymatically phosphorylated products of aminoglycosidic antibiotics by proton magnetic resonance. J Antibiot (Tokyo) 24:823–829

Naganawa H, Yagisawa M, Kondo S, Takeuchi T, Umezawa H (1971 b) The structure determination of an enzymatic inactivation product of 3′,4′-dideoxykanamycin B. J Antibiot (Tokyo) 24:913–914

Naito T, Nakagawa S, Abe Y, Fujisawa K, Kawaguchi H (1974) Aminoglycoside antibiotics. VIII. Synthesis and activity of 4′-deoxykanamycin A. J Antibiot (Tokyo) 27:838–850

Naito T, Nakagawa S, Toda S, Fujisawa K, Kawaguchi H (1979) Aminoglycoside antibiotics. XIII. Synthesis and activity of 4′-deoxy-6′-N-methylamikacin and related compounds. J Antibiot (Tokyo) 32:659–664

Nara T, Yamamoto M, Kawamoto I, Takayama K, Okachi R, Takasawa S, Sato T, Sato S (1977) Fortimicins A and B, new aminoglycoside antibiotics. I. Producing organism, fermentation and biological properties of fortimicins. J Antibiot (Tokyo) 30:533–540

Neidle S, Rogers D, Hursthouse MB (1968) The crystal and molecular structure of streptomycin oxime selenate. Tetrahedron Lett 4725–4728

Ochiai K, Yamanaka T, Kimura K, Sawada O (1959) Transfer of resistance from resistant dysentery bacteria to *E. coli* and *vice versa* in their mixed culture (in Japanese). Nippon Iji Shimpo 1861:34–37

O'Connor S, Lam LKT, Jones ND, Chaney MO (1976) Apramycin, a unique aminocyclitol antibiotic. J Org Chem 41:2087–2092

Okami Y, Hotta K, Yoshida M, Ikeda D, Kondo S, Umezawa H (1979) New aminoglycoside antibiotics, istamycins A and B. J Antibiot (Tokyo) 32:964–966

Okamoto S, Suzuki Y (1965) Chloramphenicol-, dihydrostreptomycin- and kanamycin-inactivating enzymes from multiple drug-resistant *Escherichia coli* carrying episome "R". Nature 108:1301–1303

Okanishi M, Kondo S, Suzuki Y, Okamoto S, Umezawa H (1967) Studies on inactivation of kanamycin and resistances of *E. coli*. J Antibiot (Tokyo) A20:132–135

Okanishi M, Kondo S, Utahara R, Umezawa H (1968) Phosphorylation and inactivation of aminoglycosidic antibiotics by *E. coli* carrying R factor. J Antibiot (Tokyo) 21:13–21

Ozanne B, Benveniste R, Tipper D, Davies J (1969) Aminoglycoside antibiotics: inactivation by phosphorylation in *Escherichia coli* carrying R factors. J Bacteriol 100:1144–1146

Richardson K, Jevons S, Moore JW, Ross BC, Wright JR (1977) Synthesis and antibacterial activities of 1-N-[(*S*)-ω-amino-2-hydroxyalkyl]kanamycin A derivatives. J Antibiot (Tokyo) 30:843–846

Richardson K, Brammer KW, Jevons S, Plews RM, Wright JR (1979) Synthesis and antibacterial activity of 1-N-(1,3-dihydroxy-2-propyl)kanamycin B (UK-31,214). J Antibiot (Tokyo) 32:973–977

Rinehart KL Jr (1964) The neomycins and related antibiotics. John Wiley, New York London Sidney

Rossi D, Goss WA, Daum SJ (1977) Mutational biosynthesis by idiotrophs of *Micromonospora purpurea*. I. Conversion of aminocyclitols to new aminoglycoside antibiotics. J Antibiot (Tokyo) 30:88–97

Sano H, Tsuchiya T, Kobayashi S, Hamada M, Umezawa S, Umezawa H (1976) Synthesis of 3″-deoxydihydrostreptomycin active against resistant bacteria. J Antibiot (Tokyo) 29:978–980

Santanam P, Kayser FH (1976) Tobramycin adenylyltransferase: A new aminoglycoside-inactivating enzyme from *Staphylococcus epidermidis*. J Infect Dis 134:S33–S39
Sato S, Iida T, Okachi R, Shirahata K, Nara T (1977) Enzymatic acetylation of fortimicin A and seldomycin factor 5 by aminoglycoside 3-acetyltransferase I [AAC(3)-I] of *E. coli* KY 8348. J Antibiot (Tokyo) 30:1025–1027
Satoh A, Ogawa H, Satomura Y (1975) Effect of sclerin on production of the aminoglycoside antibiotics accompanied by salvage function in *Streptomyces*. Agric Biol Chem 39:1593–1598
Smith DH, Janjigian JA, Prescott N, Anderson PW (1970) Resistance factor-mediated spectinomycin resistance. Infect Immun 1:120–127
Suami T, Nishiyama S, Ishikawa Y, Umemura E (1978) Modification of aminocyclitol antibiotics. 6. Preparation of 5-deoxykanamycin B. Bull Chem Soc Jpn 51:2354–2357
Suzuki I, Takahashi N, Shirota S, Kawabe H, Mitsuhashi S (1975) Adenylylation of streptomycin by *Staphylococcus aureus:* a new streptomycin adenylyltransferase. In: Mitsuhashi S (ed) Microbial drug resistance. University of Tokyo Press, Tokyo, pp 463–471
Takagi Y, Miyake T, Tsuchiya T, Umezawa S, Umezawa H (1973) Synthesis of 3′-deoxykanamycin B. J Antibiot (Tokyo) 26:403–406
Takasawa S, Utahara R, Okanishi M, Maeda K, Umezawa H (1968) Studies on adenylylstreptomycin, a product of streptomycin inactivated by *E. coli* carrying the R factor. J Antibiot (Tokyo) 21:477–484
Tanabe M, Yasuda DM, Detre G (1977) Aminoglycoside antibiotics: synthesis of nebramine, tobramycin and 4″-*epi*-tobramycin. Tetrahedron Lett 3607–3610
Testa RT, Wagman GH, Daniels PJL, Weinstein MJ (1974) Mutamicins; biosynthetically created new sisomicin analogues. J Antibiot (Tokyo) 27:917–921
Toda S, Nakagawa S, Naito T, Kawaguchi H (1978) Structure determination of amikacin derivatives modified by enzymes from resistant *S. aureus* strains. Tetrahedron Lett 3917–3920
Tsuchiya T, Jikihara T, Miyake T, Umezawa S, Hamada M, Umezawa H (1979) 3′-Deoxyamikacin and 3′,4′-dideoxyamikacin and their antibacterial activities. J Antibiot (Tokyo) 32:1351–1353
Umezawa H (1970) Mechanism of inactivation of aminoglycosidic antibiotics by enzymes of resistant organisms of clinical origin. Progr Antimicrob Anticancer Chemother 2:567–571
Umezawa H (1974) Biochemical mechanism of resistance to aminoglycosidic antibiotics. Adv Carbohydr Chem Biochem 30:183–225
Umezawa H (1975) Biochemical mechanism of resistance to aminoglycosidic antibiotics. In: Mitsuhashi S (ed) Drug action and drug resistance in bacteria. 2. Aminoglycoside antibiotics. University of Tokyo Press, Tokyo, pp 211–248
Umezawa H (1979) Studies on aminoglycoside antibiotics: enzymic mechanism of resistance and genetics. Jpn J Antibiot 32:S1–S14
Umezawa H, Ueda M, Maeda K, Yagishita K, Kondo S, Okami Y, Utahara R, Osato Y, Nitta K, Takeuchi T (1957) Production and isolation of a new antibiotic, kanamycin. J Antibiot (Tokyo) A10:181–188
Umezawa H, Okanishi M, Utahara R, Maeda K, Kondo S (1967 a) Isolation and structure of kanamycin inactivated by a cell-free system of kanamycin-resistant *E. coli*. J Antibiot (Tokyo) A20:136–141
Umezawa H, Okanishi M, Kondo S, Hamana K, Utahara R, Maeda K, Mitsuhashi S (1967 b) Phosphorylative inactivation of aminoglycosidic antibiotics by *Escherichia coli* carrying R factor. Science 157:1559–1561
Umezawa H, Takasawa S, Okanishi M, Utahara R, (1968 a) Adenylylstreptomycin, a product of streptomycin inactivated by *E. coli* carrying R factor. J Antibiot (Tokyo) 21:81–82
Umezawa H, Doi O, Ogura M, Kondo S, Tanaka N (1968 b) Phosphorylation and inactivation of kanamycin by *Pseudomonas aeruginosa*. J Antibiot (Tokyo) 21:154–155
Umezawa H, Umezawa S, Tsuchiya T, Okazaki Y (1971) 3′,4′-Dideoxykanamycin B active against kanamycin-resistant *Escherichia coli* and *Pseudomonas aeruginosa*. J Antibiot (Tokyo) 24:485–487

Umezawa H, Nishimura Y, Tsuchiya T, Umezawa S (1972a) Syntheses of 6′-N-methylkanamycin and 3′,4′-dideoxy-6′-N-methylkanamycin B active against resistant strains having 6′-N-acetylating enzymes. J Antibiot (Tokyo) 25:743–745
Umezawa H, Tsuchiya T, Muto R, Umezawa S (1972b) Studies on amino sugars. XXIX. - The synthesis of 3′-O-methylkanamycin. Bull Chem Soc Jpn 45:2842–2847
Umezawa H, Yamamoto H, Yagisawa M, Kondo S, Takeuchi T, Chabbert YA (1973a) Kanamycin phosphotransferase I: mechanism of cross-resistance between kanamycin and lividomycin. J Antibiot (Tokyo) 26:407–411
Umezawa H, Yagisawa M, Matsuhashi Y, Naganawa H, Yamamoto H, Kondo S, Takeuchi T, Chabbert YA (1973b) Gentamicin acetyltransferase in *Escherichia coli* carrying R factor. J Antibiot (Tokyo) 26:612–614
Umezawa H, Matsuhashi Y, Yagisawa M, Yamamoto H, Kondo S, Takeuchi T (1974) Immobilization of phosphotransferases obtained from resistant bacteria. J Antibiot (Tokyo) 27:358–360
Umezawa H, Iinuma K, Kondo S, Hamada M, Maeda K (1975a) Synthesis of 1-N-acyl derivatives of 3′,4′-dideoxy-6′-N-methylkanamycin B and their antibacterial activities. J Antibiot (Tokyo) 28:340–343
Umezawa H, Iinuma K, Kondo S, Maeda K (1975b) Synthesis and antibacterial activity of 6′-N-alkyl derivatives of 1-N-[(*S*)-4-amino-2-hydroxybutyryl]kanamycin. J Antibiot (Tokyo) 28:483–485
Umezawa H, Ikeda D, Miyasaka T, Kondo S (1979) Syntheses and properties of the 6′-C-alkyl derivatives of 3′,4′-dideoxykanamycin B. J Antibiot (Tokyo) 32:1360–1364
Umezawa S, Tsuchiya T, Muto R, Nishimura Y, Umezawa H (1971a) Synthesis of 3′-deoxykanamycin effective against kanamycin-resistant *Escherichia coli* and *Pseudomonas aeruginosa*. J Antibiot (Tokyo) 24:274–275
Umezawa S, Tsuchiya T, Jikihara T, Umezawa H (1971b) Synthesis of 3′,4′-dideoxyneamine active against kanamycin-resistant *E. coli* and *P. aeruginosa*. J Antibiot (Tokyo) 24:711–712
Umezawa S, Jikihara T, Tsuchiya T, Umezawa H (1972a) Syntheses of 3′- and 4′-O-methylneamine. J Antibiot (Tokyo) 25:322–324
Umezawa S, Tsuchiya T, Ikeda D, Umezawa H (1972b) Syntheses of 3′,4′-dideoxy and 3′,4′,5″-trideoxyribostamycin active against kanamycin-resistant *E. coli* and *P. aeruginosa*. J Antibiot (Tokyo) 25:613–616
Umezawa S, Watanabe I, Tsuchiya T, Umezawa H, Hamada M (1972c) Synthesis of 5″-deoxylividomycin B. J Antibiot (Tokyo) 25:617–618
Umezawa S, Ikeda D, Tsuchiya T, Umezawa H (1973) Synthesis of 1-N-((*S*)-4-amino-2-hydroxybutyryl)-3′,4′-dideoxyneamine. J Antibiot (Tokyo) 26:304–306
Umezawa S, Nishimura Y, Hata Y, Tsuchiya T, Yagisawa M, Umezawa H (1974) Synthesis of 4′-deoxykanamycin and its resistance to kanamycin phosphotransferase II. J Antibiot (Tokyo) 27:722–725
Umezawa Y, Yagisawa M, Sawa T, Takeuchi T, Umezawa H, Matsumoto H, Tazaki T (1975) Aminoglycoside 3′-phosphotransferase III. A new phosphotransferase in resistance mechanism. J Antibiot (Tokyo) 28:845–853
Usui T, Tsuchiya T, Umezawa S (1978) 1- and 3-Deamidino derivatives of dihydrostreptomycin and some 1-N-acyl derivatives. J Antibiot (Tokyo) 31:991–996
Vastola AP, Altschaefl J, Harford S (1980) 5-*epi*-Sisomicin and 5-*epi*-gentamicin B: substrates for aminoglycoside-modifying enzymes that retain activity against aminoglycoside-resistant bacteria. Antimicrob Agents Chemother 17:798–802
Waitz JA, Miller GH, Moss E Jr, Chiu PJS (1978) Chemotherapeutic evaluation of 5-episisomicin (Sch 22591), a new semisynthetic aminoglycoside. Antimicrob Agents Chemother 13:41–48
Walker JB, Skorvaga M (1973) Phosphorylation of streptomycin and dihydrostreptomycin by *Streptomyces*. Enzymatic synthesis of different diphosphorylated derivatives. J Biol Chem 248:2435–2440
Watanabe I, Tsuchiya T, Umezawa S, Umezawa H (1973a) Synthesis of 1-N-((*S*)-4-amino-2-hydroxybutyryl)lividomycin A. J Antibiot (Tokyo) 26:310–312

Watanabe I, Tsuchiya T, Umezawa S, Umezawa H (1973 b) Syntheses of 6′-amino-6′-deoxylividomycin B and 6′-deoxy-6′-methylamino- and 6′-deoxy-6′-(2-hydroxyethylamino)-lividomycin B. J Antibiot (Tokyo) 26:802–804
Watanabe I, Tsuchiya T, Nakamura F, Hamada M, Umezawa S (1978) Synthesis of 5″-amino-3′,5″-dideoxybutirosin A. J Antibiot (Tokyo) 31:863–867
Watanabe I, Deushi T, Yamaguchi T, Kamiya K, Nakayama M, Mori T (1979) The structural elucidation of aminoglycoside antibiotics, sannamycins A and B. J Antibiot (Tokyo) 32:1066–1068
Williams JW, Northrop DB (1976) Purification and properties of gentamicin acetyltransferase I. Biochemistry 15:125–131
Williams JW, Northrop DB (1978 a) Kinetic mechanisms of gentamicin acetyltransferase I. Antibiotic-dependent shift from rapid to nonrapid equilibrium random mechanisms. J Biol Chem 253:5902–5907
Williams JW, Northrop DB (1978 b) Substrate specificity and structure-activity relationships of gentamicin acetyltransferase. I. Dependence of antibiotic resistance upon substrate Vmax/Km values. J Biol Chem 253:5908–5914
Witchitz JL (1972) Plasmid-mediated gentamicin resistance not associated with kanamycin resistance in *Enterobacteriaceae.* J Antibiot (Tokyo) 25:622–624
Woo PWK (1975) 5″-Amino-3′,4′,5″-trideoxybutirosin A, a new semi-synthetic aminoglycoside antibiotic. J Antibiot (Tokyo) 28:522–529
Wright JJ (1976) Synthesis of 1-N-ethylsisomicin: a broad-spectrum semisynthetic aminoglycoside antibiotic. J Chem Soc Chem Commun 206–208
Wright JJ, Cooper A, Daniels PJL, Nagabhushan TL, Rane D, Turner WN, Weinstein J (1976) Selective N-acylation of gentamicin antibiotics. Synthesis of 1-N-acyl derivatives. J Antibiot (Tokyo) 29:714–719
Yagisawa M, Naganawa H, Kondo S, Hamada M, Takeuchi T, Umezawa H (1971) Adenylyldideoxykanamycin B, a product of the inactivation of dideoxykanamycin B by *Escherichia coli* carrying R factor. J Antibiot (Tokyo) 24:911–912
Yagisawa M, Naganawa H, Kondo S, Takeuchi T, Umezawa H (1972 a) Inactivation of 3′,4′-dideoxykanamycin B by an enzyme solution of resistant *E. coli* and isolation of 3′,4′-dideoxykanamycin B 2″-guanylate and 2″-inosinate. J Antibiot (Tokyo) 25:492–494
Yagisawa M, Naganawa H, Kondo S, Takeuchi T, Umezawa H (1972 b) 6′-N-Acetylation of 3′,4′-dideoxykanamycin B by an enzyme in a resistant strain of *Pseudomonas aeruginosa.* J Antibiot (Tokyo) 25:495–496
Yagisawa M, Yamamoto H, Naganawa H, Kondo S, Takeuchi T, Umezawa H (1972 c) A new enzyme in *Escherichia coli* carrying R factor phosphorylating 3′-hydroxyl of butirosin A, kanamycin, neamine and ribostamycin. J Antibiot (Tokyo) 25:748–750
Yagisawa M, Kondo S, Takeuchi T, Umezawa H (1975) Aminoglycoside 6′-N-acetyltransferase of *Pseudomonas aeruginosa:* structural requirements of substrate. J Antibiot (Tokyo) 28:486–489
Yamada T, Tipper D, Davies J (1968) Enzymatic inactivation of streptomycin by R factor-resistant *Escherichia coli.* Nature 219:288–291
Yamaguchi M, Mitsuhashi S, Kobayashi F, Zenda H (1974) A 2′-N-acetylating enzyme of aminoglycosides. J Antibiot (Tokyo) 27:507–515
Yamamoto H, Kondo S, Maeda K, Umezawa H (1972 a) Synthesis of lividomycin A 5″-phosphate, an enzymatically inactivated lividomycin A. J Antibiot (Tokyo) 25:485–486
Yamamoto H, Kondo S, Maeda K, Umezawa H (1972 b) Synthesis of 5″-deoxylividomycin A and its amino derivatives. J Antibiot (Tokyo) 25:487–488
Yamamoto H, Yagisawa M, Naganawa H, Kondo S, Takeuchi T, Umezawa H (1972 c) Kanamycin 6′-acetate and ribostamycin 6′-acetate, enzymatically inactivated products by *Pseudomonas aeruginosa.* J Antibiot (Tokyo) 25:746–747
Yano H, Fujii H, Mukoo H, Shimura M, Watanabe T, Sekizawa Y (1978) On the enzymatic inactivation of dihydrostreptomycin by *Pseudomonas lachrymans,* cucumber angular leaf spot bacterium: isolation and structural resolution of the inactivated product. Ann Phytopathol Soc Jpn 44:413–419

CHAPTER 7

Toxicology and Pharmacology of Aminoglycoside Antibiotics

T. KOEDA, K. UMEMURA, and M. YOKOTA

A. Introduction

The major toxic effect of aminoglycosides is nephrotoxicity. In general, aminoglycosides are not metabolized in vivo, but are excreted by glomerular filtration. However, a portion can be reabsorbed via the proximal tubules and remain in the kidney, a process which may induce nephrotoxicity due to the damage of the tubules. Clinical pharmacologists have studied the detection of the early signs of nephrotoxicity and have searched for drugs which will alleviate nephrotoxicity.

Another side effect of the aminoglycosides is ototoxicity, although the rate of this effect is not always parallel with that of nephrotoxicity. Ototoxicity occurs in animals at a dose level which is much higher than the usual clinical dose. It is generally agreed that this side effect does not occur in clinical practice if the blood level is maintained within the generally accepted limits.

The ototoxicity of the commercially available aminoglycosides can be generally classified into two types: (1) Morphological changes in cochlear hair cells and (2) impairment of the vestibular functions. Damage to cochlear hair cells results in a decrease of auditory sensitivity at higher frequency corresponding to the intensity of morphological change in the cochlear hair cells as found by histologic examination. Damage to the vestibular function is characterized by loss of equilibrium, though it can be compensated with visual function in the earlier stages of the disorder. Extensive attempts have been made to determine the mechanism by which aminoglycosides cause ototoxixity, but without success. Nevertheless, it is presumed that a long residence time in the cochlear lymph is one of the factors leading to the development of ototoxicity.

Aminoglycosides are readily passed through the placental membrane into the fetus with minimal effects. There are reports that large doses of aminoglycosides given to the dam result in failure of the newborns to react to the caloric test or loss of the cochlear marginal cells, but there is considerable variation in these studies.

In general, the aminoglycosides show a curare-mimetic action on the neuromuscular junctions when they are administered in large doses to experimental animals. This is thought to be due to decreased release of acetylcholine from the residues in the postsynaptic membranes. Thus, it has been shown that the agonistic action of these antibiotics is synergistic with competitive neuromuscular blocking agents but is antagonized by calcium chloride ($CaCl_2$). This blocking action on the neuromuscular junctions by large doses of aminoglycosides results in relaxation of skeletal muscle or in respiratory paralysis if the blood concentration of the antibiotics reaches a certain level, regardless of the route of administration. This action is thought to be the main cause of acute lethal toxicity in mice or rats.

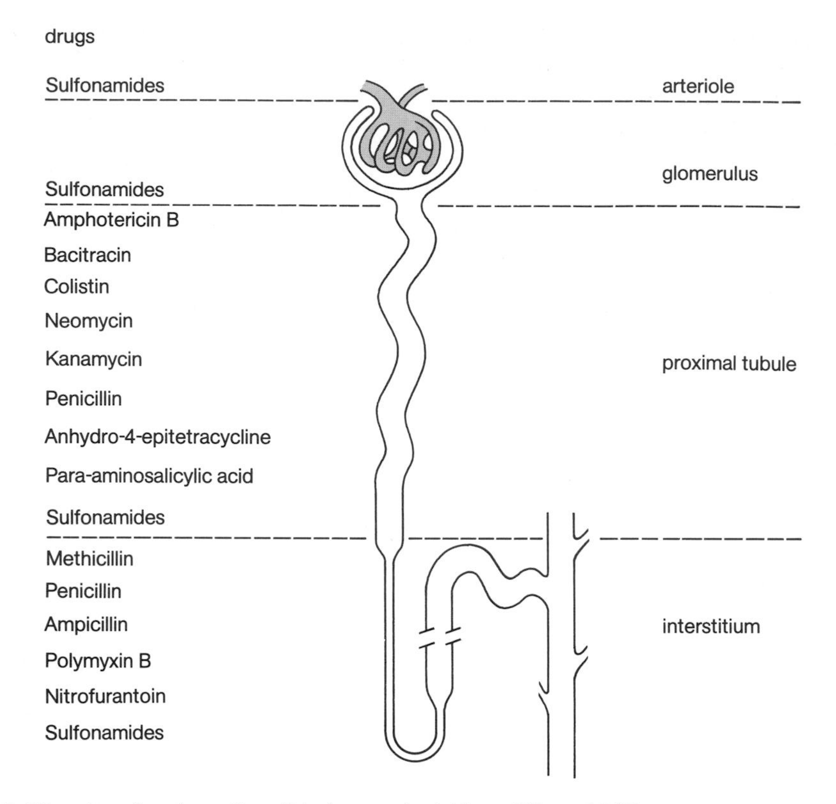

Fig. 1. The site of action of antibiotics on the kidney (UEDA 1969)

Clinically, the toxic effects of the aminoglycosides may be prevented by approriate control of the regimen, dose, and duration of administration. Recent advances in microquantitative assay methods for detection of these antibiotics, and a better understanding of their pharmacokinetics, make it possible to anticipate and prevent the appearance of toxic effects. This chapter will deal with the published animal and clinical data on the toxicology, pharmacology, and pharmacokinetics of the aminoglycosides.

B. Nephrotoxicity of Aminoglycosides

Many chemotherapeutic agents and antibiotics have nephrotoxic effects (WAITZ et al. 1971; WAKSMAN 1949; S. HAWKINS 1958; JACKSON and FINLAND 1969; GARROD et al. 1979; HARA et al. 1980; UEDA 1969; KOEDA et al. 1973a, b; MATSUZAKI et al. 1975a–d; KURAMOTO et al. 1975; KAJIMOTO and KURAMOTO 1967; HARADA et al. 1975; I. UMEZAWA et al. 1976a, b). Drugs are usually classified by sites of toxic effects in the kidney into three groups (UEDA 1969; Fig. 1): (1) those which damage the renal arteries and the glomeruli, (2) those which damage the interstitium, and (3) those which damage the proximal renal tubules. Aminoglycosides predominantly damage the proximal tubules when large doses are given. They are excreted from the glomerular capillaries into the urine by ultrafiltration and damage the epithelial cells lining the proximal tubules, leading to tubular necrosis. The renal function deteriorates as evidenced by changes in serum creatinine, creatinine clearance, and BUN values and by urinary findings such as proteinuria, casts, etc. Observations under a light microscope reveal hyaline droplets in the epithelium of the proximal tubules and calcification, degeneration, and necrosis of the epithelial cells. However, on the basis of the findings presented below, it can be concluded that all of these changes are reversible.

Sisomicin (New Drug Symposium of Japan Society of Chemotherapy, 1977) intramuscularly injected in beagle dogs for 3 months in daily doses ranging from 3 to 16 mg/kg causes degeneration, necrosis, and regeneration of the tubular epithelial cells, which recover within 3 months after discontinuance of the drug. When tobramycin (HARADA et al. 1975) is intramuscularly injected at a daily dose of 30 mg/kg, necrosis, desquamation, and regeneration of the epithelium in the proximal convoluted renal tubule and the distal convoluted renal tubule of the cortical tubules are observed on histologic examination. Desquamated epithelial cells are observed in the medullary proximal tubules and protein casts are also seen. Biochemical tests indicate increases in serum BUN, creatinine, and creatinine clearance. However, 1 month after tobramycin is discontinued, complete regeneration is observed in the most desquamated epithelium of the proximal tubules which have been damaged by the drug, and the only findings are a scattered hypertrophy of the basal membrane of the proximal convoluted renal tubule, slight cellular infiltration of the stroma, and a few protein casts in the medullary tubules. These findings indicate that the nephrotoxicity caused by aminoglycosides is reversible.

I. Nephrotoxicity of Individual Aminoglycosides

The nephrotoxicity of streptomycin is relatively mild, whereas that of neomycin is extremely potent (UEDA and NAKAMURA 1968; UEDA 1969). Proteinuria, hematuria, and urinary protein casts are usually observed after administration of therapeutic doses of neomycin. In some clinical cases the serum BUN is elevated, and histopathologic examination shows that neomycin causes abnormalities such as necrosed and obstructed tubules. The nephrotoxicity of kanamycin is intermediate between that of streptomycin and neomycin. Gentamicin (SAIRIO et al. 1978) causes turbid and edematous tubules and necrosed proximal tubules. Vacuolization and lysosomal myeloid bodies are observed on electon microscopic examination. Tobramycin, amikacin, sisomicin, and dibekacin (UEDA et al. 1975; YAMASAKU 1974) also cause the same abnormalities as those described above, and these are primarily localized in the proximal tubules (Fig. 2).

II. Intensification of Nephrotoxicity of Aminoglycosides by Concomitant Use with Other Drugs

The nephrotoxicity caused by the aminoglycosides may be intensified by the concomitant use of other antibiotics such as polypeptides and β-lactam antibiotics, or by plasma expanders such as sodium alginate (YAMASAKU 1974; OHTANI et al. 1977, 1978a, b; LAWSON 1972; HSU et al. 1974; MORI et al. 1972a). MOMOSE (1969) ob-

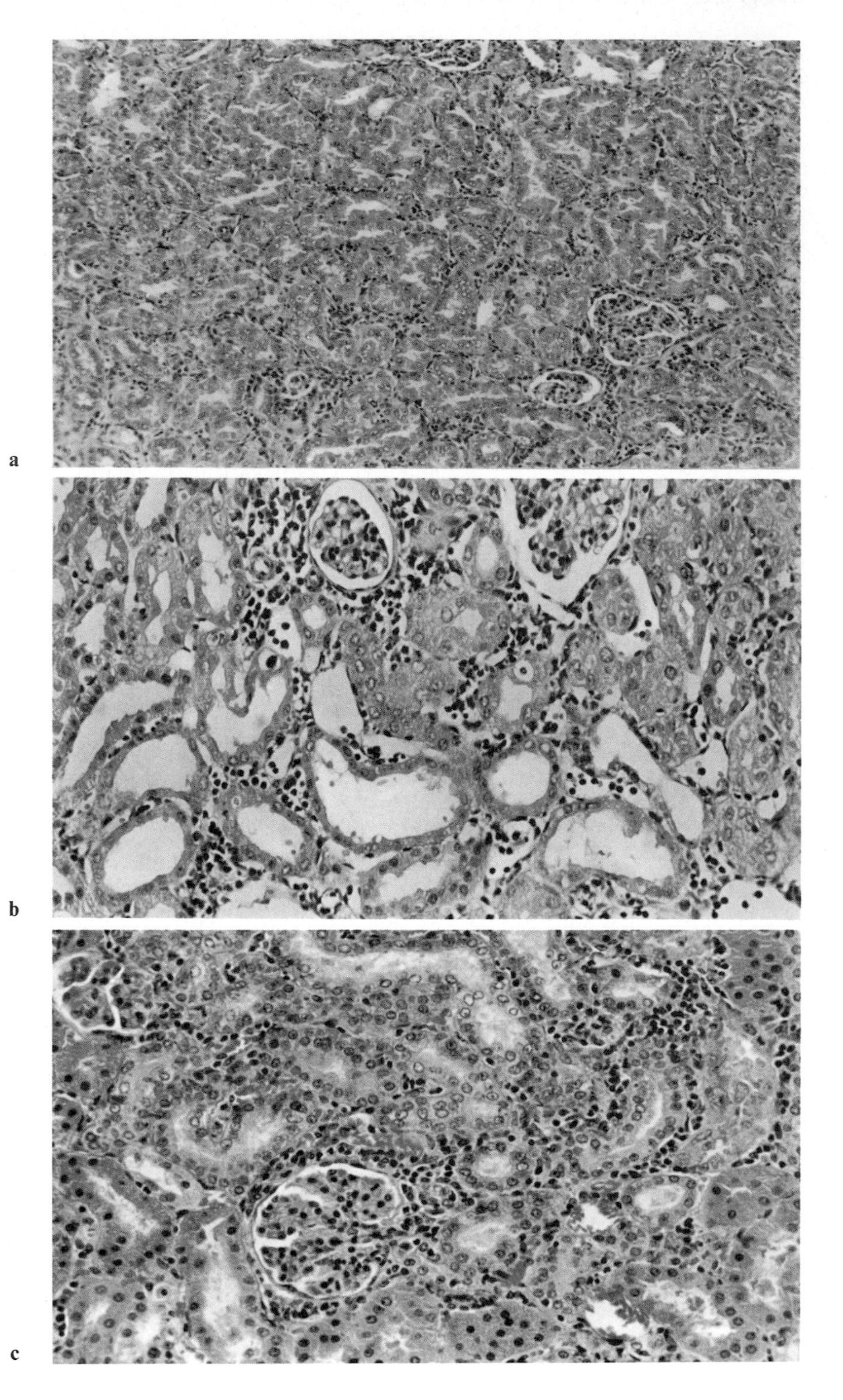
a
b
c

served that white, cloudy precipitates were produced when kanamycin and sodium alginate were mixed in vitro. Such a reaction can also occur in the renal tubules and may be the mechanism for the intensification of nephrotoxicity seen with the concomitant use of kanamycin and sodium alginate. The concomitant use of aminoglycosides and diuratics is also known to intensify nephrotoxicity. LAWSON (1972) has suggested that it involves renin–angiotensin, an allergic reaction, reduced blood flow, and increased antibiotic concentration in the serum. Furosemide, a diuretic agent, causes a decrease of oxygen consumption in the renal cells, which may cause an accumulation of aminoglycosides in the kidney owing to a decrease in antibiotic excretion. Other authors agree that renal toxocity may be aggravated by the above mechanism. In any case, it seems evident that nephrotoxicity is increased due to a decrease in renal excretion and an increase in aminoglycoside concentration in the kidney and serum when aninoglycosides are administered with diuretics.

III. Reduction of Nephrotoxicity of Aminoglycosides by Concomitant Use of Other Drugs

FURUNO et al. (1976a, b) reported that nephrotoxicity caused by kanamycin alone, or together with dextran, was reduced by simultaneous administration of D-glucurate to dehydrated rats. NIIZATO et al. (1976) also observed reduced nephrotoxicity by concomitant administration with D-glucaro-δ-lactam (Table 1).

IV. Experimental Methods for Investigating Nephrotoxicity

Since aminoglycosides can cause nephrotoxicity, it is important in clinical practice to detect nephrotoxicity at an early stage. In recent years, a variety of methods to do this have been developed and tried clinically.

1. Determination of Lysozyme

This method is based on the finding of UEDA et al. (1975) that urinary lysozyme increases when nephrotoxicity appears in the proximal tubules after administration of aminoglycosides. Intramuscular injection for 21 days of aminoglycosides in Wistar rats or rabbits at daily doses five to ten times higher than the usual therapeutic dose in patients caused nephrotoxicity which was most severe with kasugamycin and neomycin, and less severe with kanamycin, gentamicin, dibekacin, tobramycin, amikacin, and streptomycin. The toxicity was reflected in the increase in urinary lysozyme.

◄ **Fig. 2a–c.** Light microscopic findings in Wistar rat treated with dibekacin 200 mg/kg (i.m., **a**) and gentamicin 100 mg/kg (i.m., **b, c**) for 35 days. **a** Diffuse necrosis and regeneration of urinary tubuli. (×150, HE) **b** Atrophy, degeneration, necrosis, and regeneration of tubular epithelia with interstitial infiltration of round cells. (×300, HE) **c** Regeneration of urinary tubular epithelia. (×300, HE)

Table 1. Protective effect of D-glucaro-δ-lactam potassium salt (GL-K) on kanamycin (KM) or dibekacin (DKB). (NIIZATO et al. 1976)

Aminoglycoside	Compound	Dose (mg/kg)	Route	KER (%)	Urine		Antibiotic assay		BUN (mg/dl)	GOT (mU/ml)	InP (mg/dl)	LDH (mU/ml)	Mean score of morphological damage per rat[a]					
					Volume (ml)	pH	Serum (μg/ml)	Kidney (μg/g)					1	2	3	4	5	6
KM + dextran	GL-K	284	i.m.	1.09 ± 0.08	5.1	6.0	1	527	39 ± 14	239 ± 102	5.6 ± 0.4	749 ± 189	1.0		0	0.4	0	0
KM + dextran	–	–	–	1.39 ± 0.12	4.8	5.8	31	1,073	125 ± 33	267 ± 100	7.4 ± 2.5	696 ± 119	1.9		0.8	2.0	0.6	0.5
Control (dextran)	–	–	–	0.99 ± 0.09	3.4	6.0	0	0	22 ± 4	185 ± 47	5.1 ± 1.0	805 ± 216	1.1		0	0	0	0
DKB + dextran	GL-K	459	i.m.	0.92 ± 0.04	3.1	6.0	2	101	65 ± 34	342 ± 182	6.4 ± 1.0	598 ± 112	0.1	0.4	0	0.1		0
DKB + dextran	–	–	–	1.13 ± 0.12	1.3	6.0	30	198	132 ± 68	444 ± 308	12.0 ± 4.3	730 ± 325	1.6	2.3	0.6	1.4		1.0

Each group of 8 dehydrated rats weighing 200 g on an average was given KM (300 mg base/kg) or DKB (100 mg base/kg) and dextran (2 g/kg), with or without prior administration of GL-K. Renal damage was determined 24 h after antibiotic injection

[a] 1, Vacuolation of tubular epithelia cells; 2, hyaline droplet degeneration of tubular epithelial cells; 3, necrosis of tubular epithelial cells; 4, dilatation of tubular lumina; 5, cast in tubules; 6, abnormalities of collecting ducts

2. Determination of Alanine Aminopeptidase (AAP) Activity

MONDORF et al. (1978) published a method for determining renal toxicity by measuring the AAP activity which appears in the urine when the cell cycle of the brush border membrane in the proximal tubules is impaired. Urinary AAP activity is three to four times higher than that of the normal group (2,208.7 mU/24 h) after i.m. injection of amikacin (10 mg/kg, 3 times) to healthy subjects. Gentamicin, sisomicin, tobramycin, or netilmicin (3 mg/kg, 3 times) also cause a similar increase in the urinary AAP activity.

3. Determination of *N*-Acetyl-*β*-D-Glucosaminidase (NAG) Activity

HIROKAWA et al. (1979) reported a method for detection of nephrotoxicity by quantitative determination of the urinary para-nitrophenyl-*N*-acetyl-*β*-d-glucosaminidase activity. This method may be capable of detecting the early stages of nephrotoxicity. Urinary NAG activity was found to increase on the third or fourth day and finally reach values 20 times higher (10 mU/h) than normal (0.5 mU/h) on the seventh day in patients receiving gentamicin (120–240 mg/day). Urinary

NAG activity was found to be less than 2.5 mU/h in patients who received dibekacin (300 mg/man) for around 10 days. No abnormal findings were detectable with renal function tests and urinalysis.

4. Determination of β_2-Microglobulin

BERGGARD and BEARN (1968) reported that β_2-microglobulin is produced by nucleated cells and abundantly excreted in the urine when the renal tubules are damaged. Urinary β_2-microglobulin in patients who received aminoglycosides after a surgical operation was higher after treatment with gentamicin or amikacin than with tobramycin.

C. Ototoxicity of Aminoglycosides

The ototoxicity of aminoglycosides has been extensively investigated since the first report on streptomycin ototoxicity. Aminoglycosides can be classified into two groups according to the nature of the ototoxic symptoms: (1) those which primarily damage the cochlear hair cells, and (2) those which primarily impair vestibular function.

I. Effects on Cochlear Hair Cells

ENGSTRÖM and KOHONEN (1965) investigated the effect of kanamycin on cochlear hair cells of guinea pigs using a cochlear surface preparation and reported the following findings: (1) At the basal end of the first turn of the cochlea, the outer hair cells are damaged more quickly than the inner hair cells, and in the outer hair cells, the innermost layer of hair cells is apparently the most susceptible. (2) When the damage spreads in the cochlea, the outer hair cells disappear and damage also progresses from the first turn to the upper turns of the cochlea and, in the fourth turn, the inner hair cells often disappear much sooner than the outer hair cells. (3) If the damage progresses further, the nerve endings and nerve fibers frequently are atrophied and disappear after the disappearance of the hair cells.

Later, many other investigators (AKIYOSHI and SATO 1968, 1969a, 1971, 1973; AKIYOSHI et al. 1968, 1972, 1974a, 1975a, 1977; BROWN and FELDMAN 1978; LINDSEN et al. 1960; S. HAWKINS 1958; LANGE 1975; ENGSTRÖM and KOHONEN 1965; PARKER and JAMES 1978; HORI and KAWAMOTO 1972; TAMURA et al. 1972; REIFENSTEN et al. 1973; JACKSON and FINLAND 1969; YOKOTA 1977; YOKOTA et al. 1976, 1977; BRUMMETT 1972; LURIE and RAHWAY 1956; J. HAWKINS 1959; J. HAWKINS and ENGSTRÖM 1964; MORIYAMA 1959; J. HAWKINS and ARBOR 1976) studied the changes in the cochlear inner and outer hair cells after aminoglycoside treatment. At the present time, it has been confirmed that the outer hair cells regularly disappear from the first turn to the upper turns corresponding to the degree of damage and the decrease in auditory acuity (Fig. 3).

Functionally, the pinna reflex decreases or disappears with a decrease in auditory function. The threshold of auditory function decreases from 20,000 Hz to lower frequencies in guinea pigs receiving aminoglycosides. KANZAKI (1966) and AKIYOSHI and SATO (1969b) comparatively studied the pinna reflex and morphological changes in the cochlear hair cells of guinea pigs after i.m. injection of vari-

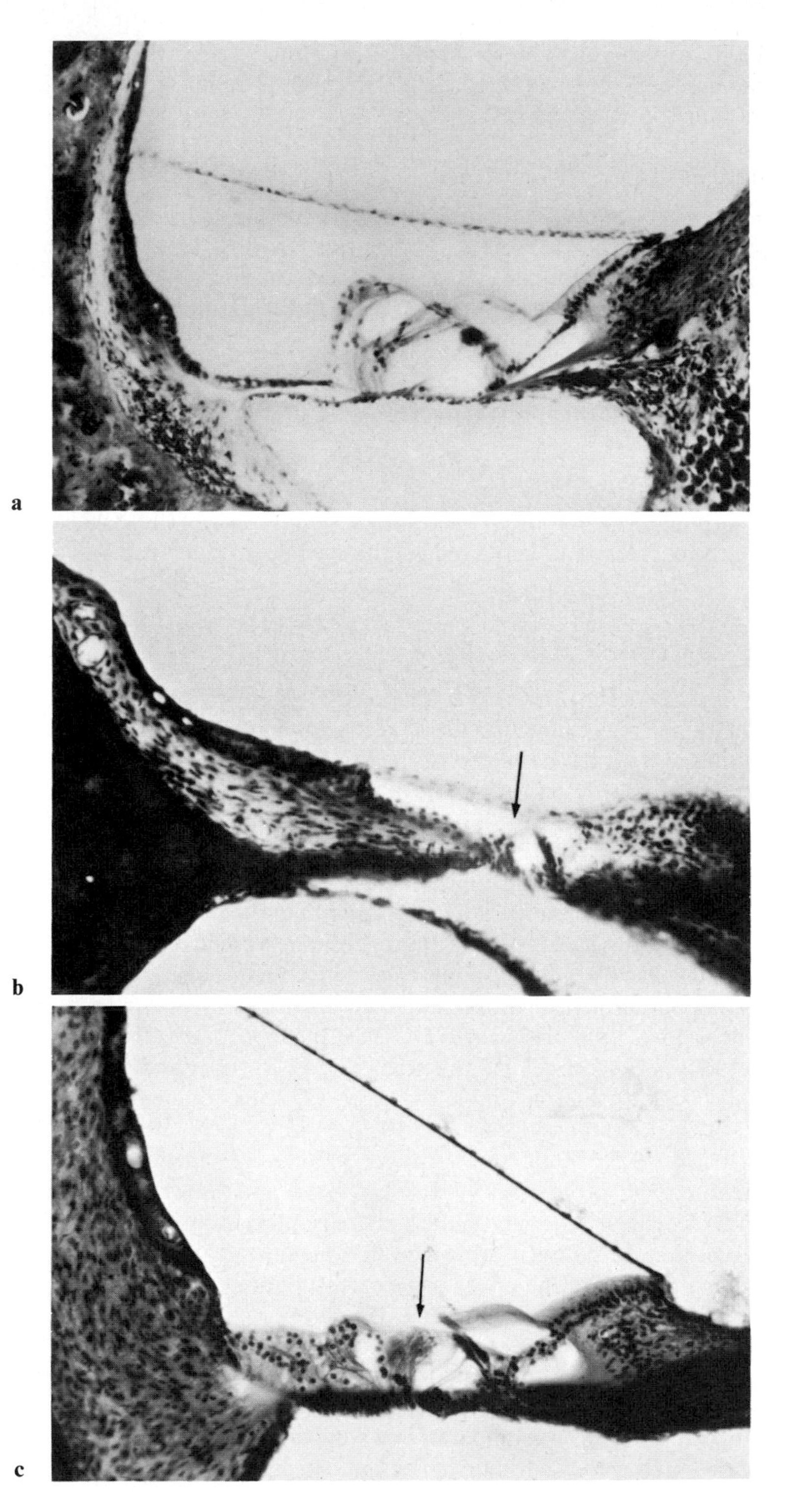
a
b
c

ous aminoglycosides in daily doses of 50–500 mg/kg for 4 weeks. They found ototoxicity in the following decreasing order: gentamicin, sisomicin, neomycin, tobramycin, dibekacin, kanamycin A, kanamycin B, fortimicin A, amikacin, butirosin, spectinomycin, and ribostamycin when compared at equal dose levels.

On administration of kanamycin A to guinea pigs at a daily dose of 200 mg/kg for 21 days, MOOTZ et al. (1972) observed with the electron microscope that structural damage of the mitochondria and intensive osmophile granules occured. In addition, NAKAI et al. (1972, 1974), SATO and HAMA (1979), and SATO et al. (1979) reported that fused, deformed, and missing outer hair cells from the innermost to the outermost row of the outer hair cells were observed in the cochlea of guinea pigs by the scanning electron microscope.

It is well established that there is a good correlation between the ototoxicity caused by administration of aminoglycosides and changes in the cochlear microphonics (CM) and in summational potentials (SP) among the electric phenomena in the cochlea (TASAKI et al. 1954; TANAKA et al. 1975; ASAKUMA et al. 1975; WATANUKI and GOTTESBERG 1971; BRUMMETT et al. 1975; WEFER and BRAY 1930; OHYAMA and YOSHIMURA 1975; SHIRAIWA 1966; MOOTZ et al. 1972; J. HAWKINS and ARBOR 1976). Cochlear microphonics and positive SP originate from the outer hair cells while negative SP originates from the inner hair cells. It is reported that CM decreases together with the disappearance of the outer hair cells following administration of streptomycin into the inner ear of guinea pigs.

OHTANI et al. (1979) treated rabbits with i.v. dibekacin or tobramycin in daily doses of 40 mg/kg for 30 days and investigated daily changes in the CM potentials with permanent electrodes placed on the round window of the ear. Cochlear microphonics decreased in one of four rabbits treated with dibekacin and in all four rabbits treated with tobramycin (Fig. 4). In addition, histopathologic studies showed a good correlation between the decrease in CM and the disappearance of the outer hair cells in these animals. They assumed that the decrease in CM and the loss of outer hair cells were more pronounced after administration of tobramycin than after dibekacin, because the former accumulated more in the inner ear than did the latter.

Studies on biochemical changes in ototoxicity (AKIYOSHI and SATO 1967a, b, 1968b; SPOENDLIN and GALOGH 1964; YAMASHITA 1972; OGAWA 1975) have been mainly oriented to the changes in succinic dehydrogenase (SDH) activity in the cochlear hair cells. AKIYOSHI and SATO (1967b) reported that SDH activity in the hair cells varies in the outer hair cells corresponding to changes in the threshold of the pinna reflex, and that it decreases parallel to the degree of induced damage of the cochlear cells when ototoxicity occurs after administration of aminoglycosides.

◀ **Fig. 3a–c.** Ototoxic effects of ribostamycin, kanamycin, and gentamicin on inner ear of adult guinea pigs. **a** Effects of ribostamycin 400 mg/kg (i.m., for 35 days) on the outer hair cells in Corti's organ, showing intact outer and inner hair cells. (×100) **b** Effects of kanamycin 400 mg/kg (i.m., for 35 days) on the outer hair cells in Corti's organ, showing loss of the outer hair cells (*arrow*) and the marginal cells. (×200) **c** Effects of gentamicin 80 mg/kg (i.m., for 35 days) on the outer hair cells in Corti's organ, showing loss of the outer hair cells from basal end to ¾ turn of cochlea (*arrow*). (×100)

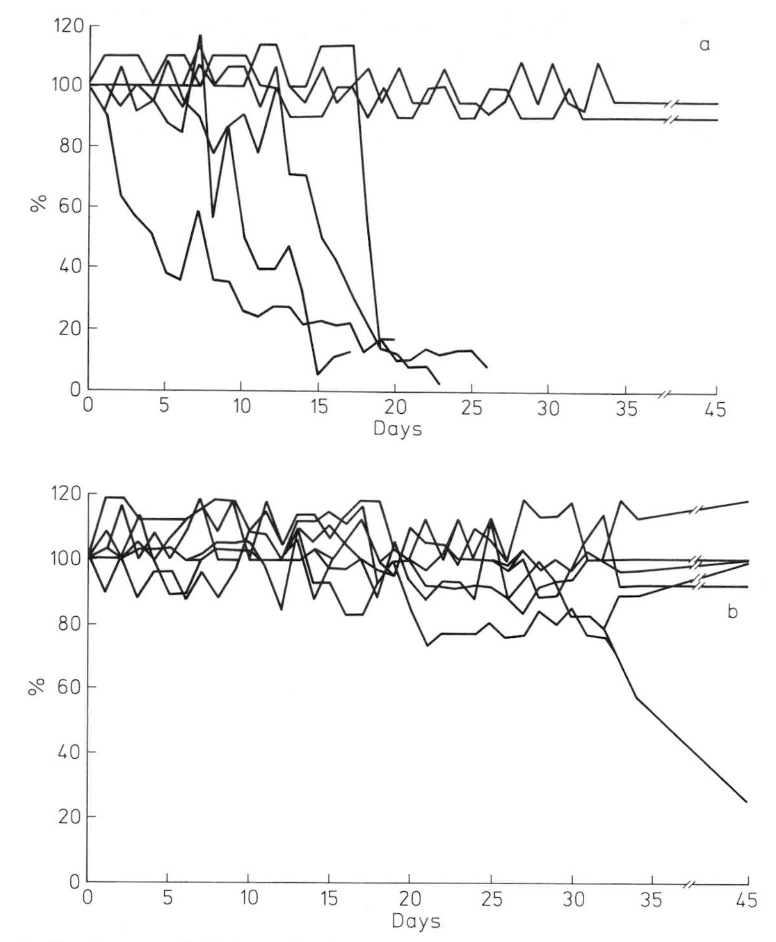

Fig. 4. a Daily changes of CM amplitude to a pure tone 15,000 Hz, 100 dB, represented as relative amplitude in rabbits administered tobramycin 40 mg/kg by i.v. infusion. **b** Daily changes of CM amplitude to a pure tone 15,000 Hz, 100 dB, represented as relative amplitude in rabbits administered dibekacin 40 mg/kg by i.v. infusion (OHTANI et al. 1979)

II. Effects on Vestibular Organs

BERG (1951) reported ataxia and nystagmus possibly due to the disturbance of vestibular organs and histopathologic changes in the crista ampullaris of the semicircular canals after administration of streptomycin to cats. However, dihydrostreptomycin (J. HAWKINS et al. 1956–1957), a derivative of streptomycin, has been confirmed to cause no vestibular disturbance, its pattern of toxicity being clearly different from that of streptomycin.

Summarizing the published data, vestibular dysfunction seems to be most associated with streptomycin and gentamicin, but less with other aminoglycosides such as kanamycin, amikacin, and tobramycin.

Many investigators have reported on the development of vestibular dysfunction (Fig. 5 shows the vestibular organ). According to OGAWA (1975), after admin-

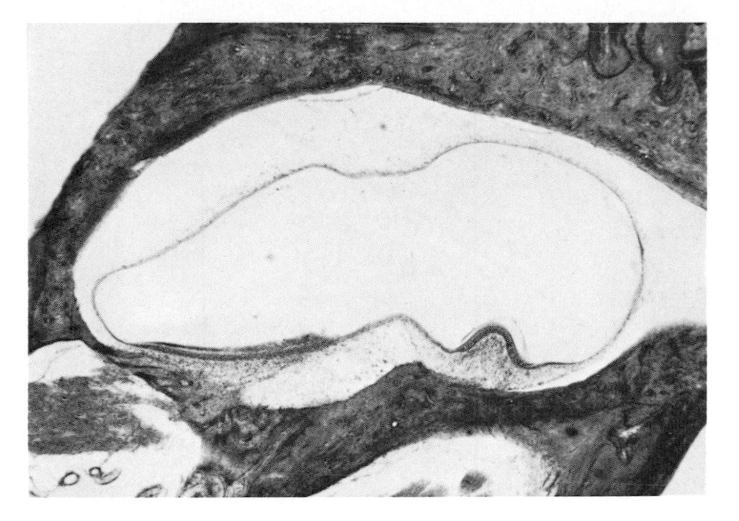

Fig. 5. Effects of ribostamycin 200 mg/kg (i.m., for 28 days) on the vestibular organ of adult guinea pigs, showing intact vestibular epithelium of crista ampullaris and utriculus and sacculus (OGAWA 1975)

istration of aminoglycosides to guinea pigs vestibular disturbance is found predominantly in the vestibular sensory cells from the crista ampullaris, being most severe in its center, to the utriculus and sacculus, being severest in the striola with type I sensory cells being affected more than type II sensory cells.

III. Ototoxicity by Concomitant Use of Aminoglycosides with Other Drugs

Ototoxicity caused by aminoglycosides is, like nephrotoxicity, intensified by combination with diuretics such as ethacrynic acid and furosemide (WEST and BRUMMETT 1973; NAKAI et al. 1975; BRUMMETT et al. 1975). Ethacrynic acid and furosemide, both loop diuretics, inhibit ATP-ase activity in the membrane of the cochlear outer hair cells, resulting in swelling of the cell bodies. Variations in the threshold of pinna reflex, degeneration of the outer hair cells, a decrease in cochlear electrical potential, and a marked decrease in reductive reaction with nitro blue tetrazolium in the in situ outer hair cells due to the temporary disturbance of metabolism appear after accumulation of aminoglycosides such as kanamycin in the cochlear lymph, when the aminoglycoside is given together with the diuretic.

IV. Correlation Between Renal Toxicity and Ototoxicity of Aminoglycosides

It is well known that different aminoglycosides induce nephrotoxicity, primarily in the proximal tubules, to different extents. The correlation between the nephrotoxicity and ototoxicity of individual aminoglycosides (SMITH et al. 1979) is not yet clear. However, OHTANI et al. (1977) reported that nephrotoxicity pro-

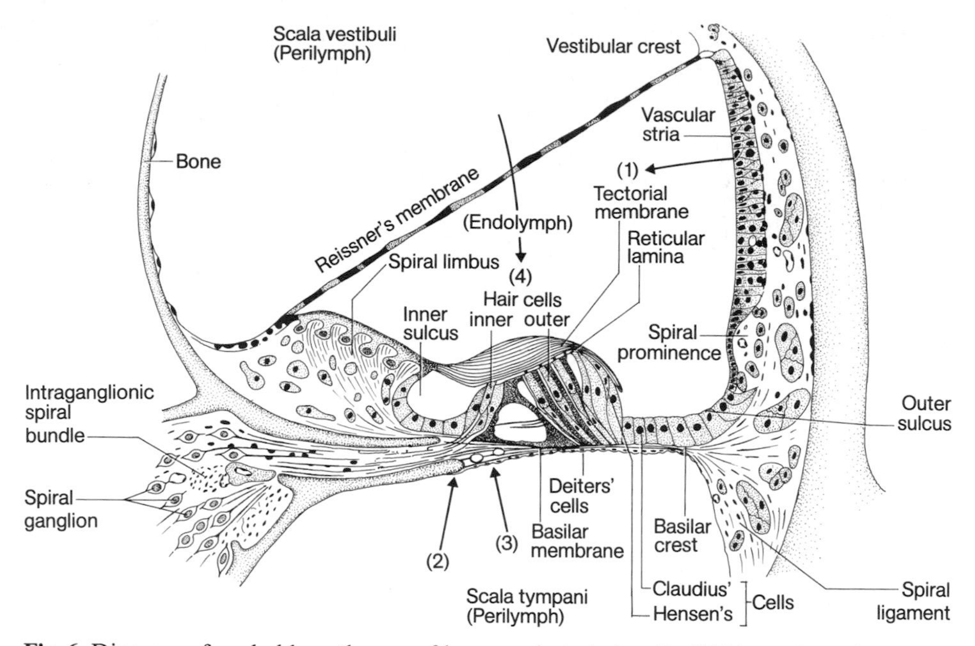

Fig. 6. Diagram of probable pathways of kanamycin to hair cells. (1) From the stria vascularis via endolymph. (2) From perilymph in the scala tympani through the basilar membrane. (3) Directly from the vas spirale. (4) From perilymph in the scala vestibuli via endolymph (WATANABE et al. 1971)

duced by the administration of aminoglycosides to experimental animals such as rabbits is accompanied by ototoxicity.

AKIYOSHI and SATO (1973) found that when kanamycin, lividomycin, and neomycin were intramusculary injected in guinea pigs and rats there was not always a correlation between the nephrotoxicity and ototoxicity. The following results were obtained: (1) Nephrotoxicity and ototoxicity were both mild, (2) nephrotoxicity and ototoxicity were both severe, (3) nephrotoxicity was mild but ototoxicity was severe, and (4) nephrotoxicity was severe but ototoxicity was mild.

V. Transfer Routes of Aminoglycosides into the Inner Ear Fluids

In general, there may be four different transfer routes of chemical compounds into the inner ear fluids (WATANABE et al. 1971; KELLERHALS 1979; ISRAEL et al. 1976; KANEKO et al. 1970): (1) direct transfer into the hair cells through the endolymph, (2) direct transfer from the vas spirale, (3) transfer from the tympanic endolymph into the hair cells through the pores of the basal membrane, and (4) transfer from the vestibular perilymph into the hair cells through Reissner's membrane and the endolymph (Fig. 6).

AKIYOSHI (1979) proposed that aminoglycosides transfer into the lymph of the inner ear from the bloodstream finally distributed around the outer hair cells after removing through the capillary vessels to the endolymph, passing through the

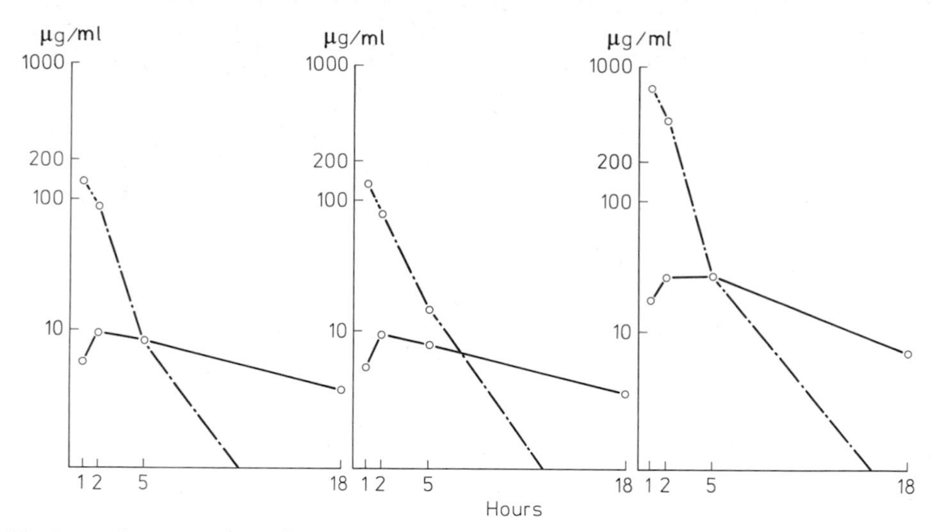

Fig. 7 a–c. Concentration of **a** gentamicin, **b** tobramycin, and **c** amikacin in serum and perilymph of guinea pigs after a single s.c. injection of 50 mg/kg antibiotic. ———, perilymph; ·—·—, serum (AKIYOSHI 1979)

basal membrane, and reaching the cochlear lymph (Fig. 7), while there may be little passage of aminoglycosides from the endolymph to the cochlear lymph because of the obstacle of the inner hair cells surrounded with supporting cells.

The rate of transfer of aminoglycosides into the hearing organs is considered to be the most important factor affecting the induction of ototoxicity.

VI. Fetal Ototoxicity of Aminoglycosides

Since ROBINSON and CAMBON (1964) reported from clinical experience on ototoxicity in a newborn delivered from a dam which received aminoglycosides during pregnancy, numerous publications on this problem have apeared (OTORI 1967; FUKUSHIMA and FUJITA 1970; MORI et al. 1972b, 1973; KOEDA and MORIGUCHI 1973; HASEGAWA et al. 1975; MATSUZAKI et al. 1975b, c; ALLEVA and BALZAS 1978; AKIYOSHI et al. 1974b, 1975a, b). However, there may be great individual differences in fetal ototoxicity; for example, ROBINSON and CAMBON (1964) reported that a newborn from a mother which received 1 g streptomycin during the 6th to the 14th week of pregnancy showed a high degree of deafness and a loss of reaction to caloric test in both ears, while WATSON and STOW (1948) reported that a newborn delivered from a mother which received streptomycin from the fourth month of pregnancy did not show any ototoxicity. AKIYOSHI et al. (1974b) found degeneration in the inner ear of newborn guinea pigs derived from dams which were given kanamycin and gentamicin (Fig. 8).

D. Acute Lethal Toxicity of Aminoglycosides

The LD_{50} values of the aminoglycosides obtained with rats and mice are shown in Tables 2–5. It is difficult to compare these data directly since conditions such

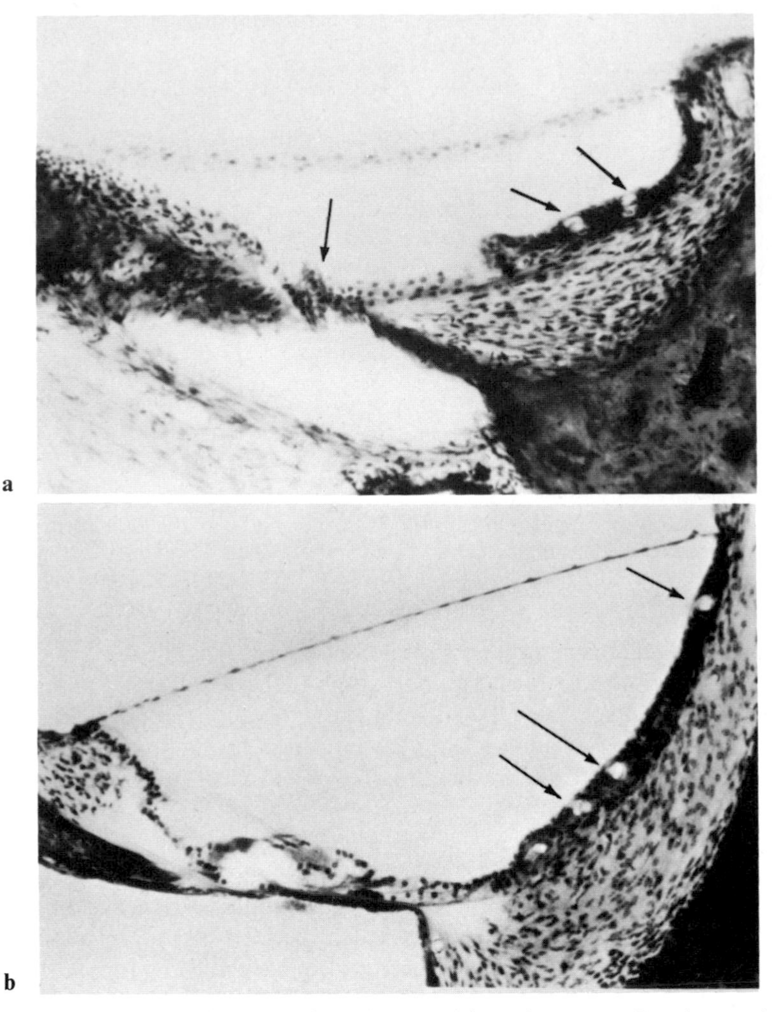

Fig. 8 a, b. Ototoxic effect of kanamycin and gentamicin on inner ear of newborn guinea pigs. **a** Effect of kanamycin 200 mg/kg (i.m., for 35 days) on the outer hair cells in Corti's organ in a newborn baby derived from the kanamycin-medicated pregnant guinea pig, showing loss of the outer hair cells (*left arrow*) and marginal cells (*right two arrows*) in Corti's organ. (×100) **b** Effect of gentamicin 40 mg/kg (i.m.) on the outer hair cells in Corti's organ in a newborn baby derived from the gentamicin-medicated pregnant guinea pig, showing loss of marginal cells (*arrows*) in Corti's organ at the first turn of the cochlea. (×100)

as administration route and speed, animal species, age, drug concentration, pH, and others were not always standardized. The LD_{50} values increase in the order of intravenous, intramuscular, subcutaneous, intraperitoneal, and oral administration.

A large dose of aminoglycosides causes respiratory paralysis and death in rats and mice. In general, aminoglycosides have a neuromuscular blocking action on the isolated diaphragm–phrenic nerve preparation of the rat with a very narrow safety margin between the noneffective dose and complete blocking dose. The on-

Table 2. Acute toxicity of aminoglycosides in male mice

Drugs	Strain	LD_{50} (mg/kg)					Calculation formula
		i.v.	i.p.	s.c.	i.m.	p.o.	
Amikacin	DDB	340 (250–375)[b]	2,930 (2,000–3,500)	3,250 (2,000–4,000)	3,250 (2,000–4,000)	> 6,000	Litchfield–Wilcoxon
Butirosin	CF-1 (Carworth)	650		4,070			
Dibekacin	ICR-JCL	72 (67–78)	605 (517–707)	528 (486–575)	431 (407–457)	> 6,950	Litchfield–Wilcoxon
Destomycin A[a]	ICL-ICR		13 (12–15)	460 (422–501)		120 (98–148)	Litchfield–Wilcoxon
Fortimicin		380		400			
Gentamicin	ICR-JCL	65 (60–71)	375 (336–418)		252 (210–302)		Litchfield–Wilcoxon
Kanamycin A	ICR-JCL	240 (221–261)	1,860 (1,699–2,036)	2,020 (1,788–2,283)	1,320 (1,266–1,377)	18,700 (17,251–20,271)	Litchfield–Wilcoxon
Kanamycin B	ddM	125 (115–136)	800 (742–862)	750 (669–842)	700 (620–791)	> 10,000	Litchfield–Wilcoxon
Kasugamycin		4,570	7,500	11,750		20,900	
Lividomycin A	ICR-JCL	246 (233–258)		1,249 (1,207–1,293)	1,348 (1,282–1,418)	> 10,000	Van der Wärden
Neomycin		15–53	116–133	265–358		> 7,200	
Paromomycin				1,062 (954–1,182)		17,800 (15,700–20,200)	
Netilmicin	ICR-JCL	23 (21–26)		69 (66–72)	65 (62–69)		Litchfield–Wilcoxon
Ribostamycin	ICR-JCL	300 (267–335)	2,900 (2,636–3,190)	3,350 (2,926–3,836)	2,230 (2,000–2,486)	> 10,000	Litchfield–Wilcoxon
Sisomicin	ICR-JCL.	37 (34–40)		280 (255–308)	280 (252–310)		Litchfield–Wilcoxon
Spectinomycin	ddY		2,440 (2,313–2,574)	8,400	> 5,000	> 10,000	Litchfield–Wilcoxon
Streptomycin		200		900		> 9,000	
Tobramycin	ICR-JCL	70 (64–78)			456 (416–500)	> 11,500	Van der Wärden

The observation period was 7 days [a] Observation period of 14 days [b] Figures in ( ) have a 95% confidence limit

Table 3. Acute toxicity of aminoglycosides in female mice

Drugs	Strain	LD_{50} (mg/kg)					Calculation formula
		i.v.	i.p.	s.c.	i.m.	p.o.	
Amikacin	DDB	350 (275–400) [a]	3,000 (2,000–4,000)	3,450 (2,000–4,500)	3,450 (2,000–4,500)	>6,000	Litchfield–Wilcoxon
Dibekacin	ICR-JCL	63 (59–66)	431 (365–509)	521 (474–573)	396 (354–444)	>6,950	Litchfield–Wilcoxon
Gentamicin	ICR-JCL				175 (164–186)		Litchfield–Wilcoxon
Kanamycin A	ICR-JCL	245 (229–262)	1,980 (1,854–2,115)	1,970 (1,743–2,226)	1,190 (1,119–1,265)	17,500 (16,417–18,655)	Litchfield–Wilcoxon
Kanamycin B	ddM	112 (103–121)	760 (691–836)	740 (661–828)	628 (561–730)	>10,000	Litchfield–Wilcoxon
Lividomycin A	ICR-JCL	225 (214–237)		1,249 (1,217–1,282)	1,400 (1,340–1,462)	>10,000	Van der Wärden
Netilmicin	ICR-JCL	22 (20–24)		69 (66–73)	63 (60–66)		Litchfield–Wilcoxon
Ribostamycin	ICL-JCL	320 (297–345)	2,830 (2,527–3,170)	3,490 (3,173–3,879)	2,300 (2,018–2,622)	>10,000	Litchfield–Wilcoxon
Sisomicin	ICR-JCL	38 (35–42)		272 (252–294)	296 (285–308)		Litchfield–Wilcoxon
Spectinomycin	ddY		2,350 (2,210–2,499)	8,600	>5,000	>10,000	Litchfield–Wilcoxon
Tobramycin	ICR-JCL	70 (63–78)			465 (423–510)	>11,500	Van der Wärden

The observation period was 7 days
[a] Figures in ( ) have a 95% confidence limit

Table 4. Acute toxicity of aminoglycosides in male rats

Drugs	Strain	LD_{50} (mg/kg)					Calculation formula
		i.v.	i.p.	s.c.	i.m.	p.o.	
Amikacin	Wistar	460 (375–550)[b]		>4,000	>4,000	>4,000	Litchfield–Wilcoxon
Dibekacin	Wistar	177 (166–190)	799 (727–879)	1,668 (1,273–2,185)	560 (513–610)	>6,950	Litchfield–Wilcoxon
Gentamicin	Wistar	108 (100–117)	630 (583–680)		360 (340–381)		Litchfield–Wilcoxon
Kanamycin A	Wistar	225 (150–350)	3,200 (2,500–4,000)	3,200 (2,500–4,000)	>4,000	>4,000	Litchfield–Wilcoxon
Kanamycin B[a]	Wistar	150 (121–186)	1,590 (1,440–1,755)	1,970 (1,812–2,141)	1,600 (1,404–1,824)	>10,000	Litchfield–Wilcoxon
Kasugamycin		5,200	12,000	17,000			
Lividomycin A	SD-JCL	379 (362–397)		1,819 (1,696–1,950)	1,750 (1,654–1,850)	>10,000	Van der Wärden
Paromomycin					1,200 (1,150–1,240)	21,620 (20,510–22,780)	
Netilmicin	SD-JCL	41 (38–44)	273 (246–303)	203 (186–221)	200 (185–216)	>10,000	Litchfield–Wilcoxon
Ribostamycin	Wistar	535 (493–580)	4,850 (4,429–5,311)	>8,000	2,900 (2,544–3,306)	>10,000	Litchfield–Wilcoxon
Sisomicin	Wistar	58 (52–65)		560 (530–590)	450 (417–484)		Litchfield–Wilcoxon
Spectinomycin	Wistar		2,340 (2,235–2,450)	>5,000	>2,500	>5,000	Litchfield–Wilcoxon
Tobramycin	Wistar	116 (106–126)			946 (883–1,015)	>7,500	Van der Wärden

The observation period was 7 days
[a] Observation period of 14 days
[b] Figures in ( ) have a 95% confidence limit

Table 5. Acute toxicity of aminoglycosides in female rats

Drugs	Strain	LD_{50} value (mg/kg)					Calculation formula
		i.v.	i.p.	s.c.	i.m.	p.o.	
Amikacin	Wistar	455 (350–550) [b]		>4,000	>4,000	>4,000	Litchfield–Wilcoxon
Dibekacin	Wistar	140 (123–160)	1,015 (894–1,152)	1,376 (1,280–1,479)	577 (524–635)	>6,950	Litchfield–Wilcoxon
Gentamicin	SD-JCL				472 (429–519)		Litchfield–Wilcoxon
Kanamycin A	Wistar	245 (150–375)	3,350 (2,500–4,000)	>4,000	4,000	>4,000	Litchfield–Wilcoxon
Kanamycin B [a]	Wistar	141 (127–157)	1,400 (1,244–1,575)	1,900 (1,664–2,170)	1,420 (1,279–1,576)	>10,000	Litchfield–Wilcoxon
Lividomycin A	SD-JCL	365 (346–384)		1,888 (1,750–2,038)	1,767 (1,661–1,879)	>10,000	Van der Wärden
Netilmicin	SD-JCL	43 (40–47)	230 (207–255)	168 (159–177)	168 (155–182)	>10,000	Litchfield–Wilcoxon
Ribostamycin	Wistar	565 (533–599)	4,400 (3,764–4,884)	>8,000	3,900 (3,171–4,197)	>10,000	Litchfield–Wilcoxon
Sisomicin	Wistar	49 (44–55)		500 (470–530)	404 (385–424)		Litchfield–Wilcoxon
Spectinomycin	Wistar		2,020 (1,908–2,139)	>5,000	>2,500	>5,000	Litchfield–Wilcoxon
Tobramycin	Wistar	122 (112–134)			929 (849–1,017)	>7,500	Litchfield–Wilcoxon

The observation period was 7 days
[a] Observation period of 14 days
[b] Figures in ( ) have a 95% confidence limit

Table 6. Serum concentration of dibekacin determined immediately after the death of mice given almost the same dose as LD_{100}. (KOMIYA et al. 1981 b)

Route of administration	Dose (mg/kg)	Serum concentration (µg/ml) mean ± SE
Infusion [a]	280–330	880 ± 76 (n = 9)
i.v.	75	825 ± 79 (n = 8)
i.m.	700	934 ± 66 (n = 6)
i.p.	700	850 ± 78 (n = 5)

[a] Infusion period = 8–9 min

Table 7. Reduction of lethal toxicity in mice of gentamicin by combination with calcium chloride. (WAGMAN et al. 1966)

Dose (mg/mouse)	No. of living animals/No. of experimental animals		
	Hydrochloride	Sulfate	Calcium chloride
60			2/15
45			9/15
30			9/15
25			10/15
22			15/15
20			15/15
11		0/15	
10		8/15	
9	0/15		
8	1/15	9/15	
7	5/15	14/15	
6	10/15	15/15	
5	15/15	15/15	
4	15/15		

set of action is rapid once a certain concentration in serum is achieved. KOMIYA et al. (1981 b) reported that no death occurred in mice receiving dibekacin until the serum concentration reached a certain level, irrespective of the route of administration and the dosage (Table 6).

There is a good correlation between the acute toxicity and the speed of injection of aminoglycosides; that is, an i.v. drip infusion results in lower toxocity than a i.v. bolus injection.

As will be discussed later in Sect. F, the blocking action of aminoglycosides on the neuromuscular junction is antagonized by $CaCl_2$. Furthermore, there are several reports concerning the concomitant use of aminoglycosides and $CaCl_2$ to reduce the acute toxicity of aminoglycosides. For example, WAGMAN et al. (1966) clearly observed reduction of the acute toxicity of gentamicin when it was injected at a dose of 12.5 mg in combination with $CaCl_2$ in doses ranging from 4 to 16 mg in male mice (Table 7). Moreover, CHILD et al. (1956–1957), KELLER et al. (1955), and WEITNAUER et al. (1957) reported similar findings on the reduction of the acute toxicity of streptomycin and dihydrostreptomycin by combination with $CaCl_2$.

In summary, it is possible to conclude that the acute toxicity of aminoglycosides is induced by neuromuscular blocking action and subsequent respiratory paralysis after the serum concentration has reached a critical level. The blockade of the isolated rat diaphragm–phrenic nerve preparation after application of aminoglycosides is antagonized by posttreatment with $CaCl_2$. The acute toxicity of aminoglycosides is also reduced by concomitant use of $CaCl_2$ in vivo.

E. Correlation Between Chemical Structure and LD_{50} Values of Aminoglycosides

H. UMEZAWA (1964), FUJISAWA et al. (1974), ITO (1962a, b, 1963), and INOUE (1972) pointed out that there is a correlation between the structure and LD_{50} of aminoglycosides. Most of the aminoglycosides treated in this review contain the 2-deoxystreptamine (DOS) moiety as a common structural unit, to which various aminosugars are attached by glycosidic linkage. On the basis of their chemical structure, these aminoglycosides can be classified into: (1) kanamycin group, (2) gentamicin group, (3) neomycin group, and (4) ribostamycin group (Table 8). The correlation between the chemical structures of these antibiotics and their LD_{50} values when administered to mice by i.v. injection is discussed here.

I. Kanamycin Group

This group includes kanamycin A, B, and C, amikacin, dibekacin, tobramycin, etc. We will discuss kanamycin B which is considered to be representative of this group. Kanamycin B has 2,6-diamino-2,6-dideoxy-α-D-glucose (2,6-AG) bound at the 4 position of DOS, and 3-amino-3-deoxy-α-D-glucose (3-AG) bound at the 6 position of DOS. Tobramycin is deoxygenated at the 3 position of 2,6-AG of kanamycin B. Dibekacin is dideoxygenated both at the 3 and 4 positions of 2,6-AG of kanamycin B. The LD_{50} values of the latter two aminoglycosides are about one-half that of kanamycin B.

Kanamycin A has a hydroxyl group in place of the amino group at the C-2 position of the 2,6-AG moiety of kanamycin B. Its LD_{50} value is higher than that of kanamycin B. Amikacin is produced by acylation of the C-1 amino group of kanamycin A with L-γ-amino-α-hydroxybutyric acid (AHB). Its LD_{50} value is higher than that of kanamycin A.

Kanamycin C has a hydroxyl group in place of the amino group at C-6 of the 2,6-AG of kanamycin B. Its LD_{50} value is twice that of kanamycin B.

II. Gentamicin Group

Gentamicin consists of a mixture of gentamicin C_1, C_{1a}, and C_2. Gentamicin C_{1a} has purpurosamine (2,6-diamino-2,3,4,6-tetradeoxy-α-D-glucose) at the 4 position of DOS, and garosamine at the 6 position of DOS. The LD_{50} of this compound is about one-half that of kanamycin B. Sisomicin has a double bond at the 4 and 5 positions (purpurosamine) of gentamicin C_{1a}. Its LD_{50} is about one-half that of gentamicin C_{1a}. Netilmicin is produced by *N*-ethylation of the C-1 amino group of sisomicin. Its LD_{50} is about one-third that of gentamicin.

Table 8. Correlation between chemical structure and LD_{50} of aminoglycosides

Group	Drug	LD_{50} values (mg/kg)	Chemical structure					
			R_1	R_2	R_3	R_4	R_5	R_6
Neomycin	Neomycin B	24	OH	NH_2	OH	CH_2NH_2	H	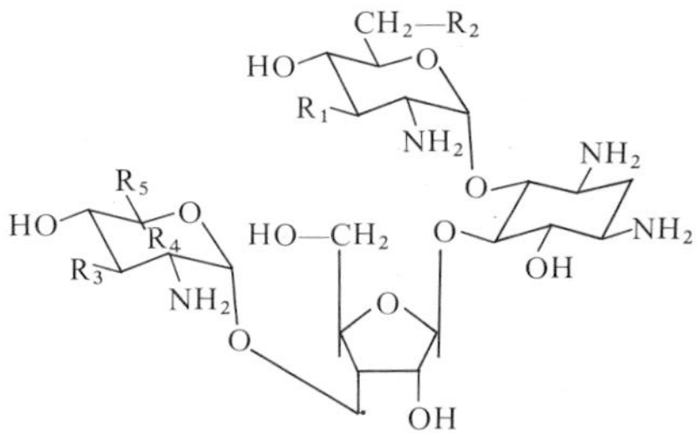 –
	Neomycin C	44	OH	NH_2	OH	H	CH_2NH_2	–
	Paromomycin I	160	OH	OH	OH	CH_2NH_2	H	–
	Lividomycin A	140	H	OH	MAN [a]	CH_2NH_2	H	–
Kanamycin	Kanamycin A	240	H	OH	OH	OH	CH_2NH_2	3Ag [b] 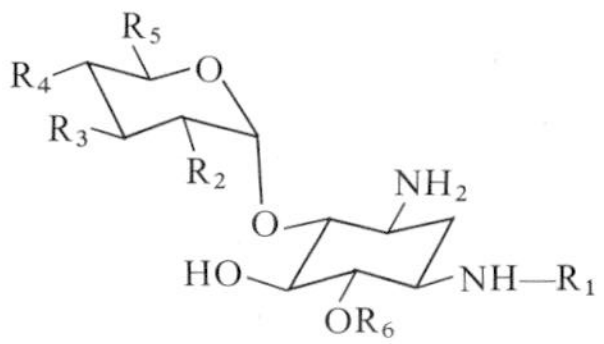
	Kanamycin B	125	H	NH_2	OH	OH	CH_2NH_2	3Ag [b]
	Kanamycin C	225	H	NH_2	OH	OH	CH_2OH_2	3Ag [b]
	Amikacin	340	AHB	OH	OH	OH	CH_2NH_2	3Ag [b]
	Tobramycin		H	NH_2	OH	OH	CH_2NH_2	3Ag [b]
	Dibekacin	300	H	NH_2	H	H	CH_2NH_2	3Ag [b]
Gentamicin	Gentamicin (C_{1a})	70	H	NH_2	H	H	CH_2NH_2	GAR [c]
	Sisomicin	37	H	NH_2	H	C=C		GAR [c]
	Netilmicin	23	C_2H_5	NH_2	H	C=C		GAR [c]
Ribostamycin	Ribostamycin	300	H	OH	NH_2	H	OH	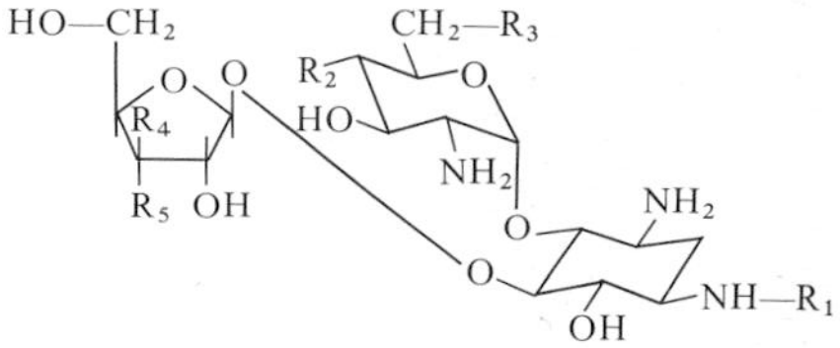 –
	Xylostasin	280	H	OH	NH_2	OH	H	–
	Butirosin	650	AHB	OH	NH_2	OH	H	–

[a] D-mannosyl
[b] 3-Amino-3-deoxy-D-glucosyl residue
[c] Garosaminyl residue

III. Neomycin Group

This group includes neomycin B and C, paromomycin I, and Lividomycin A and B.

Neomycin B has 2,6-AG at the 4 position of DOS, and neobiosamine B (2,6-diamino-α-L-idosyl-β-D-ribose) at the 5 position of DOS; neomycin C contains 2,6-AG and an epimer of neobiosamine B (2,6-diamino-α-D-glucosyl-β-D-ribose). Its LD_{50} is about twice that of neomycin B.

Paromomycin I has a hydroxyl group substituted for the amino group at the 6 position of the 2,6-AG moiety of neomycin B. Its LD_{50} is about four times greater than that of neomycin B. Lividomycin B is deoxygenated at the C-3 position of paromomycin I. Lividomycin A has an α-D-mannose moiety at the C-3 position of neobiosamine B of lividomycin B. Both LD_{50} values are significantly higher than those of paromomycin I and neomycin B.

IV. Ribostamycin Group

Ribostamycin has a 2,6-AG residue at the C-4 position of DOS and a β-D-ribose at the C-5 position. Its LD_{50} is about one and a half times that of kanamycin A. Butirosin B is *N*-acylated with AHB at the C-1 amino group of ribostamycin. Xylostasin has a xylose moiety in place of the ribose of ribostamycin. Its LD_{50} is nearly the same as that of ribostamycin. Butirosin A is a derivative of xylostasin containing AHB at the C-1 amino group and has a higher LD_{50} than ribostamycin.

From the comparison of LD_{50} values described above, there seems to exist a correlation between the chemical structure and LD_{50} value of aminoglycosides. In our overall judgment, however, any simple correlation is difficult to make though the LD_{50} values of aminoglycosides seem to be shifted regularly by modification or removal of functional groups. Further study on these aspects may make it possible to establish such a correlation between the chemical structure and acute toxicity of the aminoglycosides.

F. General Pharmacology of Aminoglycosides

This section deals with the general pharmacologic effects of aminoglycosides (OSHITA 1959; KOEDA et al. 1970a, b, 1973c; BENZI et al. 1972; ARATANI et al. 1968; ADAMS et al. 1974; TAKEDA et al. 1975; MATSUZAKI et al. 1975e; HASHIMOTO et al. 1977) on the skeletal muscle, smooth muscle, cardiovascular system, and central nervous system.

I. Effect on Neuromuscular Junctions

The aminoglycosides exert a blocking action on the neuromuscular junction (BRAZIL and CORRADO 1957; BRAZIL and PRADO-FRANCESCHI 1969; ALBIERO et al. 1978; PARADELIS et al. 1974, 1977; ADAMS 1973; MOLGÓ et al. 1979; STANLEY et al. 1969; CRAWFORD and BOWEN 1971; SINGH et al. 1978; GERGIS et al. 1971; WEINSTEIN 1970). Aminoglycosides have a curare-mimetic action on the isolated rat diaphragm–phrenic nerve preparation, as indirect electric stimulation may be in-

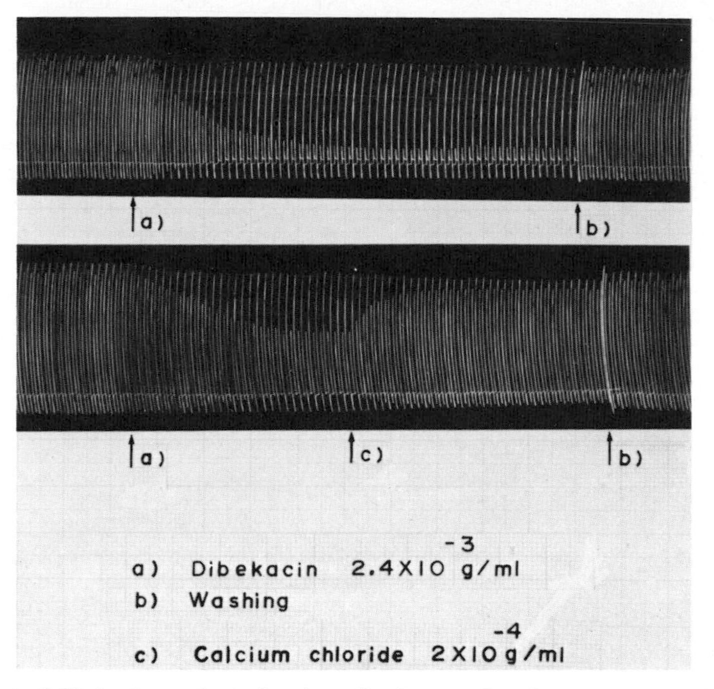

Fig. 9. Effect of dibekacin on the isolated rat diaphragm–phrenic nerve preparation. *a*, Dibekacin 2.4×10^{-3} g/ml; *b*, washing; *c*, calcium chloride 2×10^{-4} g/ml

hibited or disappear with time after application of aminoglycosides to the preparation.

This blocking action differs in intensity from compound to compound and depends on the drug concentration. The range between the noneffective dose and the complete blocking dose is very narrow. However, blockade is reversed by posttreatment with calcium chloride (Fig. 9), but is enhanced by concomitant use of magnesium chloride or d-tubocurarine. The neuromuscular blocking action of d-tubocurarine is reversed by posttreatment with physostigmine but is not affected by calcium chloride. These findings indicate that aminoglycosides have a different mechanism of neuromuscular blocking action from that of d-tubocurarine.

Dibekacin at concentrations of less than 0.01% has no influence on the isolated rat diaphragm–phrenic nerve preparation, but exhibits a blocking action at concentrations of more than 0.01%. A 0.3% concentration of dibekacin results in about 50% of maximal action. The blocking action by dibekacin disappears after treatment with 0.02% calcium chloride.

According to PARADELIS et al. (1974), gentamicin exhibits a blocking action at concentrations of more than 0.02% with complete blocking action at a 0.05% concentration on the isolated rat diaphragm–phrenic nerve preparation. The combined application of noneffective dose levels of gentamicin and d-tubocurarine causes a blocking action. The action of gentamicin alone is reversed by treatment with calcium chloride, but not by neostigmine. Other aminoglycosides such as amikacin, kanamycin, ribostamycin, sisomicin, and tobramycin have an action similar

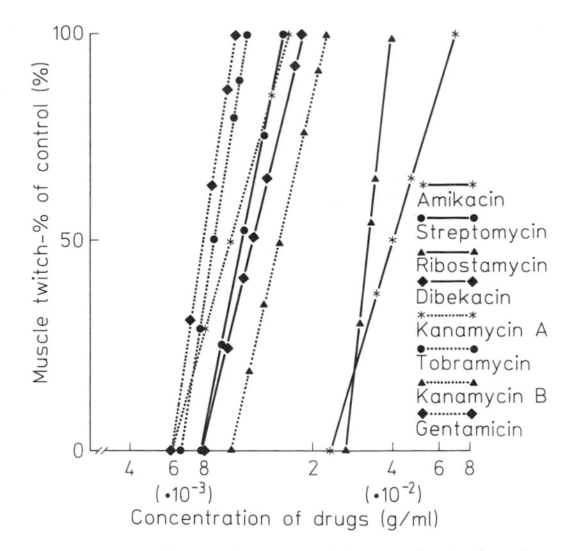

Fig. 10. Dose response curves for aminoglycosides on the isolated rat diaphragm–phrenic nerve preparation

to the above aminoglycosides. Concerning the mechanism of blocking action of aminoglycosides, BRAZIL and PRADO-FRANCESCHI (1969) suggested that aminoglycosides might competitively inhibit the binding of acetylcholine to acetylcholine receptors and thus block impulses from the motor nerve endings to the receptors in the nerve and plates.

They also reported that release of acetylcholine from the nerve endings markedly decreased after application of neomycin and gentamicin to the rat diaphragm–phrenic nerve preparation suspended in Tyrode's solution.

In summary, it is concluded that aminoglycosides exhibit a neuromuscular blocking action (Fig. 10) by a competitive antagonism towards calcium ion on the presynptic membranes of the neuromuscular junction, and then inhibit release of acetylcholine from the nerve endings (GERGIS et al. 1971).

II. General Pharmacologic Actions, Especially on Smooth Muscle and Cardiovascular System

Table 9 presents a summary of the general pharmacology of amikacin (MATSUZAKI et al. 1975e). Usually, aminoglycosides do not show any specific pharmacologic effects at therapeutic dose levels. Some compounds may show an antihypertensive action at higher dose levels (YAMAMOTO et al. 1975). This action of decreasing blood pressure is not reduced by pretreatment with atropine, tetraethylammonium, antihistamines, propranolol, and sodium nitrate, and also is not affected by vagotomy and spinalectomy. This action is accompanied by fluctuation of respiration, a decrease in the heart rate, and a decrease in the cardiac motility and dilation of peripheral blood vessels.

Aminoglycosides inhibit smooth muscle activity and decrease the tonus and amplitude of the isolated rabbit and guinea pig intestine and uterus, antagonizing the contractive action of acetylcholine, histamine, barium chloride, serotonin, and nicotine (Table 9).

Tobramycin was reported to have monosynaptic effects on the spinal reflex potentials of decerebrated animals; this may not be a central effect because the mode of action is different from that of mephenesin, a central muscle relaxant. In general, it is believed that aminoglycosides are not transferred across the blood–brain barrier to exert an action on the central nervous system.

G. Pharmacokinetics

I. Recent Progress in Assay Methods for Aminoglycosides in Serum and Other Body Fluids

Microbiologic assay is the most widely used method for determining the concentration of an antibiotic. This is reasonable since the effectiveness of an antibiotic depends on its antimicrobial activity. However, the microbiologic assay method lacks accuracy and speed. Body fluid may affect the antimicrobial activity and it is difficult to assay two or more antibiotics given simultaneously.

Recent progress in the field of analytic chemistry has resulted in new assay methods to accurately determine trace amounts of drug in biologic fluids. Of these new methods, the radioimmunoassay and high-performance liquid chromatography methods are the most widely used. In addition, an enzymatic assay method based on biochemical and radioisotope techniques is being employed in some laboratories. The microbiologic assay method has not been forgotten but continues to be improved.

1. Microbiologic Assay

The antimicrobial activity of aminoglycosides is affected by the culture medium pH, and the kind and concentration of coexisting ions. LAMB et al. (1972) carried out a study on the effects of these factors in the determination of tobramycin. To avoid the effects of interfering substances in body fluids, LAMB et al. (1972) adsorbed the antibiotic from the body fluid onto a paper disk, extracted it, and then assayed the antibiotic.

Tobramycin and dibekacin are administered in smaller doses than streptomycin and kanamycin, ordinarily only one-fifth to one-tenth the dose of the older drugs. Their concentration in the body fluids is accordingly considerably lower and the sensitivity of assay organisms is not great enough to permit easy assay of these antibiotics in trace amounts in body fluids. SIMON and YIN (1970), DAVIS and STOUT (1971), and YOSHIDA et al. (1975) have studied the application of microdetermination methods such as the paper disk method and the agar well method.

With two or more antibiotics present, it was necessary to separate them and carry out individual assays. LUND et al. (1973) developed a method to assay gentamicin mixed with other antibiotics, using a *Klebsiella pneumoniae* strain resistant to all the antibiotics present, except gentamicin. STEVENS and YOUNG (1977) have made use of the selective binding ability of cellulose phosphate powder for aminoglycosides; in this method only the aminoglycoside is extracted from the test serum and then assayed.

Table 9. General pharmacology of amikacin. (MATSUZAKI et al. 1975e)

Subjects (species)	Dose	Effects
Blood pressure (rabbit)	20 mg/kg i.v.	Decreased, 8 mm Hg
urethane anesthesia	80 mg/kg i.v.	Decreased, 10 mm Hg
Heart rate (cat)		
phenobarbital-Na anesthesia	40 mg/kg i.v.	Decreased, 205→175/min
	80 mg/kg i.v.	Decreased, 205→160/min
ECG, unanesthesia rabbit	100 mg/kg i.v.	No effect
Respiration (rabbit)		
urethane anesthesia	80 mg/kg i.v.	No effect
Respiration (cat)		
phenobarbital-Na anesthesia	80 mg/kg i.v.	Increased amplitude
Heart isolated (guinea pig)	1 mg/0.5 ml	Decreased amplitude
Atria isolated (guinea pig)	10^{-3} g/ml	Decreased amplitude and beats
Peripheral vessel		
Ear vessel (rabbit)	2×10^{-1} g/ml	No effect
Hind limb vessel (rat)	2×10^{-3} g/ml	Vasoconstriction
Intestine isolated (rabbit)		
Duodenum, jejunum, and ileum	2×10^{-3} g/ml	Inhibition
Ileum (mouse, rat)	5×10^{-4} g/ml	Inhibition
Trachea muscle isolated (guinea pig)	5×10^{-4} g/ml	Inhibition
Stomach isolated (rat)	5×10^{-4} g/ml	Inhibition
Uterus isolated (rat)	10^{-5} g/ml	Inhibition
Seminal vesicle isolated (rat)		
anti-Adr	10^{-3} g/ml	No inhibition
Aorta isolated (rabbit)		
anti-Adr	10^{-3} g/ml	No inhibition
Ileum isolated (guinea pig)		
anti-Ach	3×10^{-3} g/ml	Inhibition
anti-His	10^{-3} g/ml	Inhibition
anti-$BaCl_2$, anti-5-HT	5×10^{-4} g/ml	Inhibition
anti-Nicotine	10^{-3} g/ml	Inhibition
Stomach in vivo (rabbit)	80 mg/kg i.v.	No effect
Intestine in vivo (rabbit)	80 mg/kg i.v.	No effect
Uterus in vivo (rat)	40 mg/kg i.v.	No effect
Urinary bladder (rabbit)	80 mg/kg i.v.	Inhibition
Gastrointestinal propulsion (mouse)	400 mg/kg i.p.	No effect
Phrenic-diaphragm (rat)	10^{-3} g/ml	No effect
Anticonvulsant effect (mouse)		
Strychnine, picrotoxin, pentetrazol	400 mg/kg i.p.	No effect
Hexobarbital-sleeping (mouse)	400 mg/kg i.p.	No effect
Spontaneous movement (mouse)	200 mg/kg i.p.	No effect
Analgesic effect (mouse)		
Hot plate and D'Amour-Smith method	400 mg/kg i.p.	No effect
Writing method, acetic acid	400 mg/kg i.p.	Inhibition
Muscle relaxant (mouse)		
Traction and inclined test	400 mg/kg i.p.	No effect
Surface anesthesia (guinea pig)	20% Insitil	No anesthesia
Infiltration anesthesia (guinea pig)	10% i.c.	No anesthesia
Gastric secretion (Schild rat)	40 mg/kg i.v.	No effect
Bile secretion (rat, rabbit)	40 mg/kg, 200 mg/kg i.v.	No effect
Local irritation test		
Capillary permeability (rabbit)	40 mg/ml i.c.	No effect
Pleural effusion (rat)	80 mg/ml intrapleurally	No effect
Muscular irritation (rabbit)	250 mg/ml i.m.	No effect

Table 10. Tobramycin specificity.[a] (BROUGHTON et al. 1976a)

Drug	Concentration for 50% B/B_0 (ng/ml)	Cross-reactivity (%)
Tobramycin	28	100.0
Kanamycin	350	8.0
Gentamicin	1,900	1.5
Amikacin	3,500	0.8
Sisomicin	3,500	0.8

[a] The concentration for 50% B/B_0 was the concentration of drug necessary to reduce binding of [^{123}I]-tobramycin by 50%. The percentage of cross-reactivity was the relative efficiency of competition by the other aminoglycoside drugs compared to tobramycin

2. Radioimmunoassay

In recent years it has become increasingly common for aminoglycosides to be administered by continuous i.v. infusion. To monitor blood levels an assay method is needed with small blood samples. Radioimmunoassay meets these requirements. There are many reports concerning the radioimmunoassay of aminoglycosides, but the following methods can be considered as representative of the most commonly used techniques. The aminoglycoside is conjugated with bovine serum albumin through reaction with a bonding agent such as 1-ethyl-3-(3-dimethylaminopropyl)-corbodiimide. This conjugate is then emulsified in Freund's complete adjuvant and injected subsutaneously to rabbits to stimulate antibody formation. These antibodies bind specifically with the aminoglycoside which was used to make the antigen, and to the same aminoglycoside labeled with ^{125}I. When both the aminoglycoside and the ^{125}I-aminoglycoside are present, the binding reaction with the antibody fraction becomes competitive. It is then possible to carry out radioimmunoassay by making use of that competitive reaction. Radioimmunoassay methods have been reported for gentamicin by LEWIS et al. (1972), for tobramycin by BROUGHTON et al. (1976a), for amikacin by LEWIS et al. (1975), and for sisomicin by BROUGHTON et al. (1976b). In addition, NOONE et al. (1974) employed radioimmunoassay to monitor the serum concentration of gentamicin during clinical treatment.

Radioimmunoassay employs the specificity of the antibody–antigen reaction. Nevertheless, it is possible that cross-reaction may occur between the antigen and a compound which is very similar in chemical structure to the antibody-inducing antigen. Table 10 presents data of BROUGHTON et al. (1976a) on the cross-reactivity between tobramycin and other aminoglycosides. In clinical therapy, it is quite rare for two or more aminoglycosides having similar chemical structures to be administered concurrently, so this capacity for cross-reactivity does not present a very great practical problem. Radioimmunoassay kits, consisting of the antibody, the labeled antibiotic, and the standard antibiotic, have become commercially available in recent years.

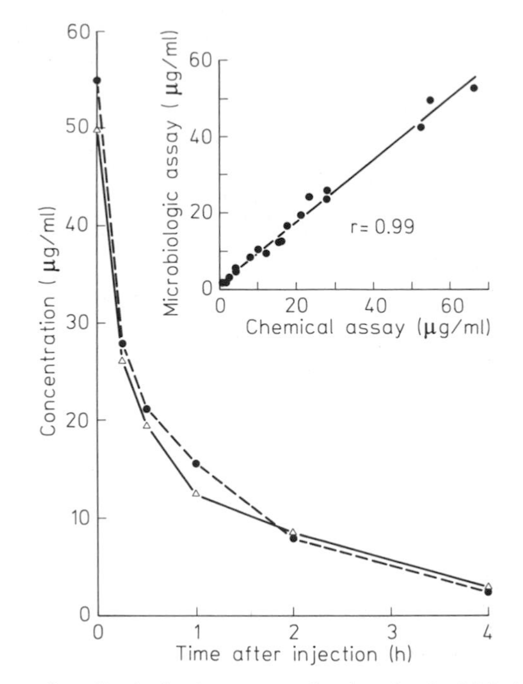

Fig. 11. Correlations of amikacin in the serum of a dog (male, 30 kg) after i.v. injection of 225 mg amikacin. ●, HPLC assay, 7.5-min peak was used; △, microbiologic assay. *Insert*, linear regression analysis of amikacin concentration in three dogs determined by HPLC and microbiologic assay; r is the correlation coefficient and the line is represented by the equation $y=0.823 \times +1.32$ (MAITRA et al. 1978)

3. High-Performance Liquid Chromatography (HPLC)

High-performance liquid chromatography has been used for serum assays of aminoglycosides. Chromatography is usually utilized in situations demanding a high degree of sensitivity. With aminoglycosides, the technique usually uses fluorescence produced by the reaction of the amino groups of the antibiotic reagents such as *o*-phthalaldehyde. Since aminoglycosides contain amino group, this detection method can be applied to nearly all of these drugs if the reaction conditions used to form the fluorescing derivative are properly chosen. The application of HLPC to the assay of aminoglycosides has been reported by MAYS et al. (1976) for kanamycin, ANHALT (1977) for gentamicin, MAITRA et al. (1978) for amikacin, and PENANG et al. (1977) for netilmicin.

When assaying aminoglycosides by the HPLC method, it is possible to separate two or more of these antibiotics from a mixture and then quantify them. It is also posible to determine the amounts of the various components contained in a drug such as gentamicin, and even the minor component kanamycin B that is contained in kanamycin. Amikacin consists of only one component; the HPLC assay of this drug (MAITRA et al. 1978) is presented in Fig. 11. It can be seen that these assay results agree well with the results obtained by the microbiologic assay method.

Generally, the sample is passed through the chromatography column, then through the reactor, and finally detected in the form of its fluorescing derivative.

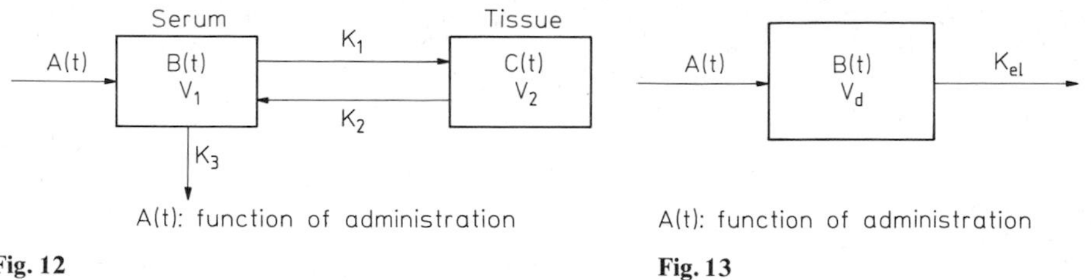

Fig. 12

Fig. 13

Fig. 12. Two-component model. A(t), function of administration

Fig. 13. One-compartment model. A(t), function of administration

An alternative procedure is to first carry out the reaction between the antibiotic and the reagent, and then pass the fluorescing derivative through the column.

4. Enzymatic Assay

In this method, the amino groups of the aminoglycosides are acetylated through the use of acetyltransferase and ^{14}C-labeled acetylcoenzyme A. The amount of antibiotic is assayed by determining the radioactivity of the sample. Most of the work on this method has used gentamicin or related antibiotics, as reported by BROUGHALL and REEVES (1975a, b), HAAS and DAVIS (1973), amd HOLMES and SANFORD (1974). The acetyltransferase most commonly employed in this technique is obtained from *Escherichia coli*. The specificity of this technique depends upon a specific enzyme reaction with the amino group of deoxystreptamine. Therefore, it is possible to employ this method only with those aminoglycoside antibiotics that contain the deoxystreptamine structural unit and which are acetylated by this enzyme.

II. Pharmacokinetics of Aminoglycosides

1. Compartment Models for Pharmacokinetic Analysis and Calculation of Parameters

The one-compartment model and the two-compartment model, shown in Figs. 12 and 13, are both commonly used to carry out the pharmacokinetic analysis of aminoglycosides.

As will be discussed later, aminoglycosides are not metabolized in the body and the main route of elimination of the drug from the body is urinary excretion. In addition, these antibiotics are usually administered by i.m. or i.v. injection. For these reasons, the fate of these drugs in the body is pharmacokinetically simple. Accordingly these two basic models are sufficient for carrying out the analysis of the serum concentrations of aminoglycosides.

The serum drug concentration can be expressed as B(t), as a function of time t. It is then possible to derive the following equations using the two-compartment model in relation to each route of administration.

a) Intramuscular Administration

The function of administration, A(t), is expressed by the Eq. (1):

$$A(t) = W \cdot K_a \cdot \exp(-K_a \cdot t), \quad (1)$$

where
W = the dose of the drug
K_a = rate constant of drug transport from site of administration to serum.

Using the one-compartment model,

$$B(t) = W \cdot K_a / \{V_d(K_a - K_{el})\} \cdot \{\exp(-K_{el} \cdot t) - \exp(-K_a \cdot t)\} \quad (2)$$

can be derived. In Eq. (2),
V_d = volume of distribution
K_{el} = elimination rate constant from serum.

Using the two-compartment model, Eq. (3) is obtained:

$$\begin{aligned} B(t) = W \cdot K_a / \{V_1(\alpha - \beta)\} \cdot \{&(K_2 - K_a)(\alpha - \beta) \cdot \exp(-K_a \cdot t) \\ &+ (K_2 - \alpha)(\beta - K_a) \cdot \exp(-\alpha t) \\ &+ (\beta - K_2)(\alpha - K_a) \cdot \exp(-\beta t)\} / \{(K_a - \alpha)(K_a - \beta)\}, \end{aligned} \quad (3)$$

where
V_1 = volume of serum compartment
V_2 = volume of tissue compartment
K_1 = rate constant of drug transport from serum compartment to tissue compartment
K_2 = rate constant of drug transport from tissue compartment to serum compartment
K_3 = elimination rate constant from serum compartment
and where α and β represent the constants that satisfy the following conditions:

$$\alpha + \beta = K_1 + K_2 + K_3$$

$$\alpha\beta = K_2 K_3$$

$$\alpha > \beta .$$

Here, constant β is the apparent elimination rate constant for the drug from the serum compartment when the concentration of the drug in the tissue compartment and its concentration in the serum compartment have reached a state of quasi-equilibrium; this has the same meaning as K_{el} in the one-compartment model.

b) Bolus Intravenous Injection

When the drug is rapidly injected intravenously, A(t) takes on the definition given in Eq. (4):

$$A(t) = W\delta(t), \quad (4)$$

where $\delta(t)$ is a unit impulse function (delta function).

The serum concentration, B(t), is given in Eq. (5) and (6) for the one- and two-compartment models, respectively.

With the one-compartment model,

$$B(t)=W/V_d \cdot \exp(-K_{el} \cdot t)\,. \tag{5}$$

With the two-compartment model,

$$B(t)=W/\{V_1(\alpha-\beta)\} \cdot \{(\alpha-K_2) \cdot \exp(-\alpha t)+(K_2-\beta) \cdot \exp(-\beta t)\}\,. \tag{6}$$

c) Constant-Rate Intravenous Infusion

When the dose of the drug, W, is administered to the patient intravenously at a constant rate over the time period from $t=0$ to $t=T$, the equation for A(t) becomes as given in Eqs. (7) and (8) below.

When $t \leqq T$,

$$A(t)=W/T\,. \tag{7}$$

When $t>T$,

$$A(t)=0\,. \tag{8}$$

Hence, using the one-compartment model, when $t \leqq T$,

$$B(t)=W/(TV_d \cdot K_{el}) \cdot \{1-\exp(-K_{el} \cdot t)\}\,. \tag{9}$$

When $t>T$,

$$B(t)=W/(TV_d \cdot K_{el}) \cdot \{1-\exp(-K_{el} \cdot T)\} \cdot \exp\{-K_{el}(t-T)\}\,. \tag{10}$$

And, using the two-compartment model, when $t \leqq T$,

$$B(t)=W/\{TV_1(\alpha-\beta)\} \cdot [(\alpha-K_2)\{1-\exp(-\alpha t)\}/\alpha+(K_2-\beta)\{1-\exp(-\beta t)\}/\beta]\,. \tag{11}$$

When $>T$,

$$B(t)=W/\{TV_1(\alpha-\beta)\} \cdot [(\alpha-K_2)\{1-\exp(-\alpha T)\}/\alpha \cdot \exp\{-\alpha(t-T\} \\ +(K_2-\beta)\{1-\exp(-\beta T)\}/\beta \cdot \exp\{-\beta(t-T)\}]\,. \tag{12}$$

d) Calculation of Pharmacokinetic Parameters

The data obtained for the value of the serum concentration of a drug, B(t), are substituted into the above equations. Then, by applying the method of least squares, it is possible to calculate the various parameters in the models, that is, V_d, K_a, V_1, V_2, K_1, K_2, K_3, α, β, etc.

In addition, Eq. (13) can be used to calculate the value of area under curve (AUC), which is an index of the drug availability.

$$AUC=\int_0^\infty B(t)dt\,. \tag{13}$$

Once these parameters have been calculated, it is possible to employ Eqs. (14)–(17) to calculate the biologic half-life, $T_{1/2}$, of the drug and the body or serum clearance, C_b, thereof in the case of each model.

Using the one-compartment model,

$$T_{1/2} = \ln 2/K_{el} = 0.693/K_{el}, \quad (14)$$

$$C_b = W/AUC = V_d K_{el}. \quad (15)$$

Using the two-compartment model,

$$T_{1/2} = \ln 2/\beta = 0.693/\beta, \quad (16)$$

$$C_b = W/AUC = V_1 K_3. \quad (17)$$

It is clear that K_{el} in the one-compartment model and β in the two-compartment model have the same meaning. Substitution of β for K_{el} and making use of the relationship between Eqs. (15) and (17) results in Eq. (18) giving the relationship between V_1 and V_d:

$$V_d = V_1 K_3/\beta. \quad (18)$$

The cumulative renal excretion of the drug can be measured and expressed as a function of time t: E(t). Then the renal clearance, C_r, can be calculated using Eq. (19):

$$C_r = E(t)/\int_0^t B(t)dt. \quad (19)$$

Equation (19) has been applied to the administration of dibekacin by UMEMURA et al. (1977), and to tobramycin by TAKIMOTO et al. (1976) in order to calculate the value of C_r.

2. Pharmacokinetic Parameters in Normal Animals

There are many reports on the administration of aminoglycosides to experimental animals and the calculation of the pharmacokinetic parameters based on the serum concentration of the drug. Data for the biologic half-life, $T_{1/2}$, and the volume of distribution, V_d, taken from various publications are compiled in Table 11.

Although discrepancies do exist in these data obtained by various research groups, the differences are not as great as those seen for other drug groups. The differences between the aminoglycosides are also small, and the method and route of administration of the drugs did not have much of an effect on the results.

It is seen that the value for $T_{1/2}$ in dogs and rabbits ranges from 70 to 100 min, while this value is 20 to 50 min in rats and 20 min in mice. The value for V_d falls within a range of 230 to 338 ml/kg in dogs and rabbits. Accordingly, in the case of i.m. administration using a dose of 10 mg/kg, the actual maximum serum concentration is 40 μg/ml or less.

3. Pharmacokinetic Parameters in Human with Normal Renal Function

Data on the pharmacokinetic parameters calculated for aminoglycosides administered to healthy humans or adult human patients with normal renal function are compiled in Table 12.

Table 11. Pharmacokinetic parameters of aminoglycosides in normal animals

Antibiotics	Animals	Administration	Biologic half-life $T_{1/2}$ (min)	Volume of distribution V_d (ml)	Reference
Kanamycin	Dog	i.m.	99.6	–	MURATA et al. (1971)
	Dog	i.v.	42.0	230/kg	CABANA and TAGGART (1973)
	Dog	i.m.	55.8–61.8	–	CABANA and TAGGART (1973)
Ribostamycin	Dog	i.m.	72.6	–	MURATA et al. (1971)
	Rat	i.m.	26.0	–	MURATA et al. (1971)
	Rat	i.v.	29.2	–	MURATA et al. (1971)
	Rat	i.p.	57.1	–	MURATA et al. (1971)
Gentamicin	Rat	i.v.	21.0	48.9/rat	TRONOVEC (1978)
	Rat	i. tracheal	23.1	–	TRONOVEC (1978)
	Rat	i.m.	46 ± 6	–	MIRHIJ et al. (1978)
	Rat	i.m.	22.4	–	IKEDA et al. (1979)
	Mice	s.c.	18.5	–	IKEDA et al. (1979)
	Dog	i.m.	69.66–70.5	262–312/kg	FUJITA et al. (1973)
	Dog	i.m.	73.0	–	IKEDA et al. (1979)
Tobramycin	Rat	i.v.	30	–	YAMADA et al. (1975)
	Rat	i.m.	25–30	–	YAMADA et al. (1975)
Dibekacin	Dog	i.m.	88.6–100.6	264–338/kg	FUJITA et al. (1973)
	Dog	i.v. infusion	66.8 ± 4.28	96.6 ± 7.4/kg	KOMIYA et al. (1981a)
	Rabbit	i.v.	80.64	–	FUJITA et al. (1973)
	Rabbit	i.m.	83.34	324/kg	FUJITA et al. (1973)
	Rabbit	i.v. infusion	67.26 ± 6.42	94.7 ± 7.9/kg	KOMIYA et al. (1981a)
Amikacin	Rat	i.m.	47 ± 15	–	TRONOVEC (1978)
	Dog	i.v.	51	250/kg	CABANA and TAGGART (1973)
	Dog	i.m.	55.8–61.8	–	CABANA and TAGGART (1973)
Sisomicin	Mice	s.c.	19.4	–	IKEDA et al. (1979)
	Rat	i.m.	23.5	–	IKEDA et al. (1979)
	Dog	i.m.	75.6	–	IKEDA et al. (1979)

As has already been noted for animal models, there was little difference between the various antibiotics tested, and differences between individual patients were also relatively small.

In most of the reported cases, the value of $T_{1/2}$ fell within the range of 120 ± 30 min, while V_d was found to be 250 ± 50 ml/kg in most cases. Accordingly, after administration of an aminoglycoside at a dose of 10 mg/kg by the i.m. route, the maximum serum concentration of the drug should be within the range of 30 to 50 μg/ml.

When an aminoglycoside is administered intramuscularly, the rate constant for the transport of the drug from the site of injection to the serum, K_a, is generally very large, falling within the range of 0.02 to 0.08 min^{-1} in most cases. This means that by 10–30 min after the injection of the drug, about one-half of the administered dose has already been transported from the site of administration to the serum. This indicates that aminoglycoside are extremely well dispersed from an i.m. injection site.

Table 12. Pharmacokinetic parameters of aminoglycosides in man with normal renal function

Antibiotics	Administration	Biologic half-life $T_{1/2}$ (min)	Volume of distribution V_d (ml)	Reference
Kanamycin	i.m.	126 –138	217 – 236/kg	CABANA and TAGGART (1973)
Ribostamycin	i.m. 500 mg/man	97.62 ± 37.26	14,760 ± 4,050/man	YAMASAKU et al. (1980)
	i.m. 1,000 mg/man	96.36 ± 12.9	16,480 ± 3,800/man	YAMASAKU et al. (1980)
	i.m. 1,500 mg/man	107.04 ± 23.58	18,670 ± 4,010/man	YAMASAKU et al. (1980)
	Constant-rate i.v.	94.2 ± 24	10,440 ± 2,010/man	YAMASAKU et al. (1980)
Gentamicin	i.m.	÷120	–	LOCKWOOD and Bower (1973)
	Constant-rate i.v.	103.8 ± 8.4	–	SIMON et al. (1973)
	i.v.	127.8 ± 42	140 ± 50/kg	WALKER et al. (1979)
	i.m.	146.4 ± 24.6	–	REVERT et al. (1978)
	i.v.	126 ± 78	200/kg	SAWCHAK and ZASKE (1976)
	i.m.	129 ± 19.2	–	THUILLIER et al. (1977)
Tobramycin	i.m. 40 mg/man	97.8 ± 4.2	–	SIMON et al. (1973)
	i.m. 80 mg/man	128.4 ± 3.6	–	SIMON et al. (1973)
	Constant-rate i.v.	95.4 ± 4.8	–	SIMON et al. (1973)
	i.m.	÷120	–	LOCKWOOD and BOWER (1973)
	i.m.	÷120	–	OKSENHENDLER et al. (1977)
	i.v., i.m.	55 – 82	123/kg	PECHÉRE et al. (1976a)
Dibekacin	i.m.	105.6 –241.8	153 – 199/kg	SAITO et al. (1978)
	i.m. 1 mg/kg	106.8 ± 22.8	192.2 ± 33.1/kg	UMEMURA et al. (1977)
	i.m. 1.5 mg/kg	121.8 ± 13.8	226 ± 13.8/kg	UMEMURA et al. (1977)
	i.m. 2 mg/kg	112.8 ± 11.4	218 ± 19.9/kg	UMEMURA et al. (1977)
Amikacin	i.m.	132 –144	222 – 225/kg	CABANA and TAGGART (1973)
	i.m.	168	–	BODEY et al. (1974)
	Constant-rate i.v.	114 –120	–	BODEY et al. (1974)
	i.v.	118 ± 15.6	170 ± 80/kg	WALKER et al. (1979)
	i.m.	102 ± 18	350 ± 51/kg	VOGELSTEIN et al. (1977a)
Sisomicin	i.m.	210	201/kg	ROTH et al. (1976)
	i.m.	103	–	SAITO et al. (1978)
Netilmicin	i.m., i.v.	124.4 –173.3	66 – 108/kg	PECHÉRE and DUGAL (1978), PECHÉRE et al. (1978a, b)
	i.m.	÷ Sisomicin	–	MEYERS et al. (1977)
	i.m., i.v.	126	250/kg	SCHROGIE et al. (1977)

ICHIKAWA et al. (1973) and SAITO et al. (1978) have pointed out that the value of K_a differs as a function of the conditions at the time of administration, even in the same individual.

Table 13 presents a summary of pharmacokinetic parameters obtained from the administration of aminoglycoside antibiotics to infants and children. These data are from a number of reports by pediatricians, and patients had normal renal function. Compared with the results for adults, it is seen that these young patients' data for $T_{1/2}$ and V_d show a large degree of variance. Perhaps the reason for this is that pediatric patients are in the growth stage, with large differences between the subjects in terms of body size and age.

TAKIMOTO et al. (1976) administered tobramycin to newborn infants and analyzed the serum concentration of the drug. Their data showed that the value of $T_{1/2}$ was between 360 and 420 min on the first day after birth, but became shorter with

Table 13. Pharmacokinetic parameters of aminoglycosides in infants and children

Antibiotics	Age	Administration	Biologic half-life $T_{1/2}$ (min)	Volume of distribution V_d (ml)	Reference
Tobramycin	2–18 yr	Constant rate i.v.	97 (52–137)	420±38/kg	Hoecker (1978)
	Newborn 0–7 days	i.m.	$\left[\frac{8.69}{x+1.29}+1.21\right]\cdot 60$ x = postnatal age (days) when x = 7, $T_{1/2}$ = 170	–	Takimoto et al. (1976)
Dibekacin	20 days	i.m.	118.8– 22.8	130–134/kg	Nakazawa et al. (1973)
	3–4 yr	i.m.	76.2– 98.4	93–141/kg	
	7–14 yr	i.m.	117.6–147.6	142–360/kg	
	4–16 yr	i.v.	96	320/kg	Vogelstein et al. (1977b)
Amikacin	10 yr	i.m.	63	221.9/kg	Yoshioka et al. (1974)
	7 yr	i.m.	80.4	295/kg	

the passage of time, reaching 120 min on the seventh day. These results can be interpreted as indicating that renal function develops rapidly within a short period of time following birth.

4. Relationship Between Serum Level, Acute Toxicity, and Mode of Administration in Experimental Animals

As was noted previously, the acute lethal activity of aminoglycosides occurs as a result of a neuromuscular blocking action that is dependent on the serum concentration of the drug.

When an aminoglycoside is administered intramuscularly and the one-compartment model is used, the maximum serum concentration will be reached at the time T_{max}, which can be calculated using Eq. (2). The maximum concentration can then be calculated by substituting T_{max} for t in Eq. (2).

$$T_{max} = \ln(K_a - K_{el})/(K_a - K_{el}) . \tag{20}$$

In addition, when the drug is administered rapidly by the i.v. route, the maximum serum concentration occurs immediately after the administration is completed. That concentration can be calculated by substituting $t=0$ into Eqs. (5) and (6).

Using the one-compartment model,

$$B(T_{max}) = B(0) = W/V_d . \tag{21}$$

Using the two-compartment model,

$$B(T_{max}) = B(0) = W/V_1 . \tag{22}$$

Since, in these cases, the aminoglycoside is being administered very rapidly into the bloodstream, during the initial period following administration is must be considered that no equilibrium of the drug between the serum and the tissues has yet been reached. For this reason, the one-compartment model is not very suitable for calculation of the maximum serum concentration, $B(T_{max})$, and Eq. (22) given above for the two-compartment model provides data that coincide well with the actual situation.

In the case of i.v. infusion of an aminoglycoside antibiotic at a constant rate, T_{max} is the same as the time T when the infusion has been completed. The value of the drug serum concentration at that time, $B(T_{max})$, is the same as B(T), and this value can be calculated by substituting T for t in Eqs. (9) and (11). When T is a relatively large number, e.g., >15–20 min, the actual determined values for the concentration and those calculated using the one-compartment model nearly coincide.

Figure 14 presents a concentration curve for ribostamycin in human serum when the drug is administered by constant-rate i.v. infusion; this was prepared by YAMASAKU et al. (1980) using the technique of computer simulation. It is clear from this graph that the maximum serum concentration of the drug is less as the value of T becomes larger (that is, as the administration rate becomes slower).

The acute lethal toxicity of aminoglycosides depends on the serum concentration of the drug. As has been seen above, the maximum serum concentration of

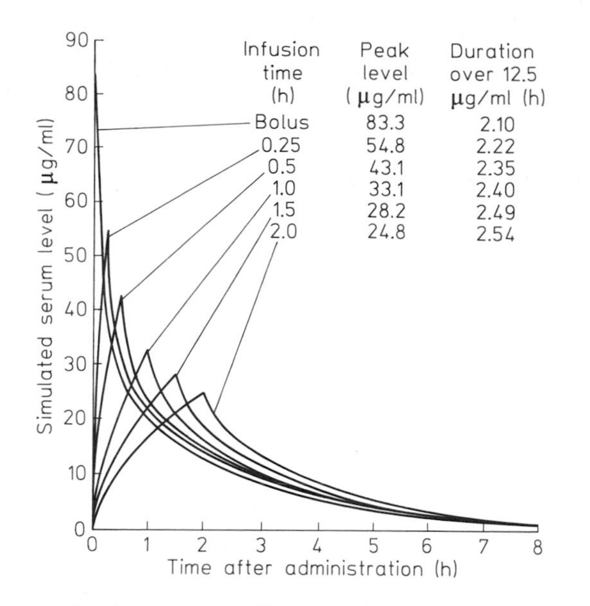

Fig. 14. Simulated serum levels when 0.5 g ribostamycin was intravenously infused over different periods of time (YAMASAKU et al. 1980)

a drug can be controlled by means of the administration method, the route, and the dose. Accordingly, when aminoglycosides are administered clinically, it is essential that the physician carefully selects the dose, the route, and the administration conditions so that the serum concentration does not exceed a safe level.

III. Metabolism and Excretion

1. Metabolism

There have been no reports to date that aminoglycosides are metabolized in the body, but there have been many reports that aminoglycosides are not subject to in vivo metabolic processes.

MURATA et al. (1971) administered ^{3}H-labeled ribostamycin to rats, and KOMIYA et al. (1973) carried out similar experiments in rats with labeled dibekacin. Both of these groups found close agreement between the microbiologic assay of the drug in the serum or in the urine, and the radioactivity values obtained for the same body fluids. Figure 15 shows the thin-layer chromatography analysis of dibekacin excreted in the urine of rats; these results indicate that the radioactive material excreted in the urine consisted completely of dibekacin.

YAMADA et al. (1975) have published similar results for tobramycin, while IKEDA et al. (1979) have performed similar studies on sisomicin and again obtained similar results.

These results indicate that aminoglycosides are not metabolized in the body but are excreted unchanged in the urine.

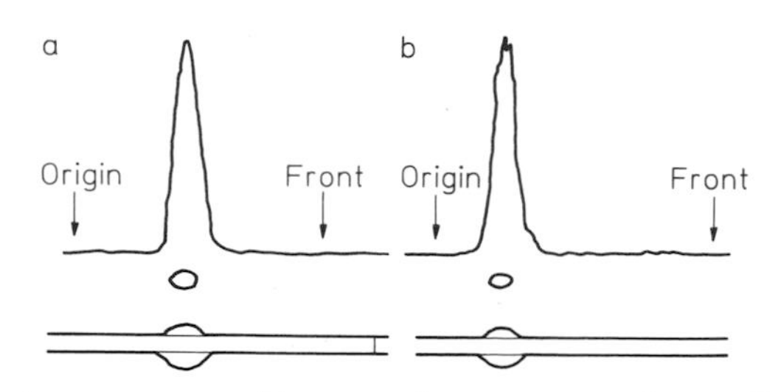

Fig. 15. Thin-layer chromatograms (Eastman chromatogram sheet, n-BuOH-EtOH-$CHCl_3$-17%-NH_4OH=4:5:2:5) of urine of rats after ion exchange fractionation with Amberlite CG-50 type I. *A*, ^{3}H-dibekacin dissolved in urine of rats; *B*, urine of rats administered ^{3}H-dibekacin 20 mg/kg i.m.

2. Excretion

Researchers have administered aminoglycosides to normal animals and then determined the amount of the drug excreted in the urine. In all cases, the urinary recovery of the antibiotic is 80%–100% of the administered dose within the first 24 h following administration.

The urinary recovery of the drugs has also been determined in humans with normal renal function. Various groups have carried out studies using the various aminoglycosides available. The following is a list of several such reports: CABANA and TAGGART (1973), kanamycin; YAMASAKU et al. (1980), ribostamycin; LOCKWOOD and BOWER (1973), SIMON et al. (1973), WALKER et al. (1979), REVERT et al. (1978), SAWCHUK and ZASKE (1976), THUILLIER et al. (1977), gentamicin; SIMON et al. (1973), LOCKWOOD and BOWER (1973), OKSENHENDLER et al. (1977), PECHÉRE and DUGAL (1976), PECHÉRE et al. (1976a, b), tobramycin; SAITO et al. (1978), UMEMURA et al. (1977), dibekacin; CABANA and TAGGART (1973), BODEY et al. (1974), WALKER et al. (1979), BERNARD et al. (1977), VOGELSTEIN et al. (1977a), KENDALL et al. (1978), amikacin; ROTH et al. (1976), SAITO et al. (1978), sisomicin; PECHÉRE et al. (1978a, b), MEYERS et al. (1977), SCHROGIE et al. (1977), netilmicin.

The results of all of these research groups are in agreement: within 4 h after drug administration, 50%–60% of the administered dose is recovered in the urine, 60%–70% is recovered within 6 h, and 70%–90% of the drug has been excreted in the urine by 20 h after administration.

In addition, UMEMURA et al. (1977) reported that the body clearance (C_b) and renal clearance (C_r) of dibekacin in humans are practically the same. This finding indicates that the elimination of dibekacin from the body is by renal excretion.

These data from animals and humans show that the main route of excretion of aminoglycosides is via the urine. Concerning the mechanism of renal excretion, it is generally considered that there are three aspects involved: glomerular filtration, active and passive secretion by the renal tubules, and active and passive reabsorption.

BOGER and GAVIN (1958–1959) administered streptomycin and kanamycin to human subjects and concurrently administered probenecid, a drug that inhibits active secretion. They reported that this drug had no effect on the serum concentration of the two aminoglycosides, and that the renal clearance of kanamycin was 83%–88% of the creatinine clearance. Furthermore, YAMASAKU et al. (1980) re-

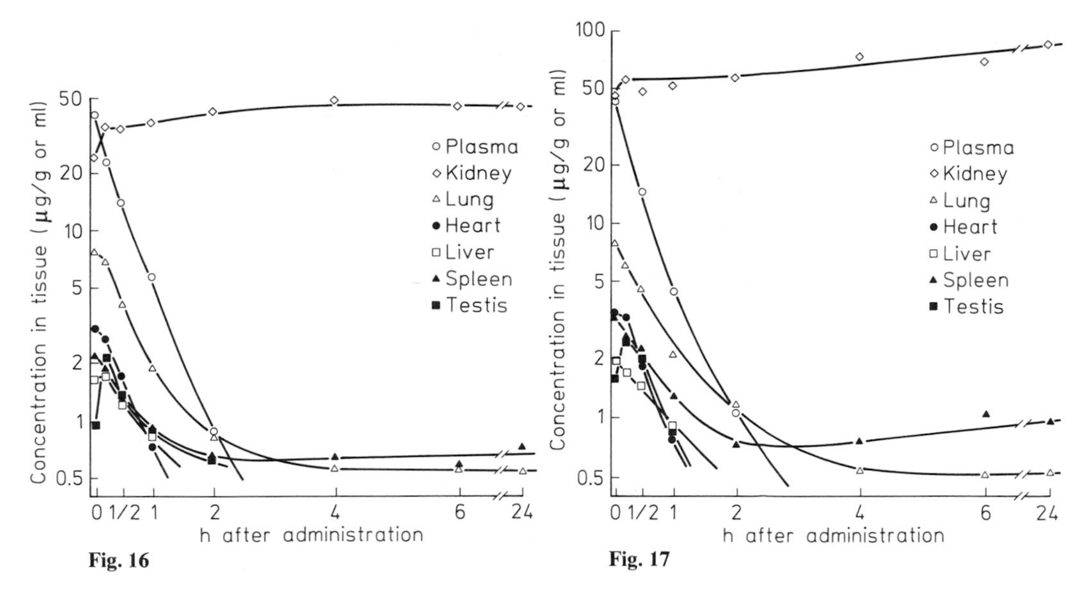

Fig. 16. Distribution of gentamicin after i.m. injection of 10 mg/kg into rats (IKEDA et al. 1979)

Fig. 17. Distribution of sisomicin after i.m. injection of 10 mg/kg into rats (IKEDA et al. 1979)

ported that the body clearance of ribostamycin administered to humans and the creatinine clearance were practically the same. CHIU et al. (1976) reported that gentamicin administered to rats showed a renal clearance which was about 80% of the renal clearance of inulin, a compound that is excreted from the kidneys only by glomerular filtration. They suggested that the remaining 20% of gentamicin was reabsorbed by the kidneys. CHIU et al. (1977) also reported that in separate experiments using rats, the 24-h urinary recovery of administered gentamicin and netilmicin reached 71%–90% of the administered dose, regardless of the volume of urine excreted. In another study using rats, CHIU and LONG (1978) noted that when furosemide was administered to the animals to reduce the level of glomerular filtration, the excretion rate of administered gentamicin decreased in a corresponding fashion.

Summarizing these experimental findings, it appears that the urinary excretion of aminoglycosides occurs primarily by glomerular filtration. Active secretion, on the other hand, is negligible, while a small amount of the drug is reabsorbed by the kidneys.

IV. Tissue Distribution

1. Tissue Distribution in Animals

Many reports have been published concerning the tissue distribution of aminoglycosides in animals. Figures 16 and 17 present data obtained by IKEDA et al. (1979) in relation to the tissue distribution of gentamicin and sisomicin in rats. Each of these drugs was administered by i.m. injection, and the concentration of the drug

Table 14. Distribution of ^{3}H-dibekacin in various tissues of rats. Time after injection = 24 h; dose = 2.5 mg/kg i.m. (KOMIYA et al. 1973)

Tissue	Percentage of dose			L-value [a]		
	Maximum	Minimum	Mean	Maximum	Minimum	Mean
Blood				0.0424	0.0081	0.0252
Lymph node	0.0049	0.0029	0.0059	0.0794	0.0607	0.0700
Site of administration (muscles)	0.5364	0.2778	0.4071	0.7165	0.2202	0.4683
Brain	0.0025	0.0010	0.0018	0.0046	0.0019	0.0033
Eyeball	0.0005	0.0001	0.0003	0.0055	0.0033	0.0044
Thyroid	0.0003	0.0001	0.0002	0.0387	0.0219	0.0303
Thymus	0.0036	0.0024	0.0030	0.0289	0.0196	0.0243
Heart	0.0058	0.0026	0.0042	0.0161	0.0031	0.0121
Lung	0.0192	0.0127	0.0159	0.0456	0.0368	0.0412
Liver	0.2934	0.2526	0.2730	0.0901	0.0773	0.0837
Spleen	0.0124	0.0099	0.0111	0.0804	0.0569	0.0686
Pancreas	0.0034	0.0024	0.0029	0.0179	0.0147	0.0163
Adrenal	0.0005	0.0005	0.0005	0.0399	0.0337	0.0368
Kidney	12.3639	10.4942	11.4291	15.8652	15.1431	15.5042
Testis	0.0084	0.0053	0.0069	0.0100	0.0072	0.0036
Seminal vesicle	0.0035	0.0015	0.0025	0.0141	0.0100	0.0121
Prostate	0.0014	0.0011	0.0013	0.0129	0.0086	0.0108
Bladder			0.0014			0.0405
Stomach	0.0081	0.0060	0.0071	0.0184	0.0166	0.0175
Small intestine	0.0398	0.0265	0.0331	0.0270	0.0235	0.0252
Caecum	0.0106	0.0086	0.0096	0.0416	0.0414	0.0415
Large intestine	0.0104	0.0089	0.0096	0.0293	0.0254	0.0276
Contents of stomach	0.0010	0.0006	0.0008	0.0111	0.0082	0.0097
Contents of small intestine	0.0188	0.0108	0.0148	0.0176	0.0142	0.0159
Contents of caecum	0.0299	0.0262	0.0281	0.0603	0.0301	0.0452
Contents of large intestine	0.0028	0.0018	0.0023	0.0539	0.0211	0.0375
Faeces	0.1939	0.1133	0.1536	0.8881	0.0909	0.4895
Urine	86.5090	83.2196	84.8643			

[a] L-value is a parameter indicating the localization of drug and calculated by the following equation: L = radioactivity in g tissue/(administered radioactivity/body weight)

in the tissues was determined by microbiologic assay. Except for the kidneys, the concentration of these antibiotics in the various body tissues increased rapidly in response to an elevation of the plasma level, while a decrease in the plasma concentration resulted in a gradual drop in concentration in the tissues. Only the kidney maintained a concentration that was equal to or greater than the maximum plasma concentration, and this drug level had hardly dropped at 24 h postadministration.

Table 14 shows the results of experiments carried out by KOMIYA et al. (1973) in rats. They administered ^{3}H-dibekacin and then monitored the tissue distribution of the radioactivity for 24 h. Since dibekacin is not metabolized in vivo, the distribution of the radioactivity represents the distribution of the administered dibekacin. As had been found for gentamicin and sisomicin, 10% or more of the administered dose of dibekacin was retained in the kidneys, at a high concentration. Similar results have been reported for other aminoglycosides in experiments in other animal species. For example, MURATA et al. (1971) reported on the tissue distribution of ribostamycin in rats, KORNGUTH and KUNIN (1971) dealt with the tissue distribution of gentamicin and amikacin in rabbits, YAMADA et al. (1975) studied the tissue distribution of tobramycin in rats, and FUJITA et al. (1973) reported on sisomicin's distribution in mice. TAKABATAKE et al. (1978a, b) used pregnant rabbits and investigated the distribution of administered dibekacin in the uterus, oviducts, ovaries, fetus, placenta, and amniotic fluid. They reported that the concentration of the antibiotic in these tissues increased in response to an elevation of the serum level of the drug. TOYODA and TACHIBANA (1978) found that the transfer of administered kanamycin to the kidneys and perilymph in guinea pigs was rapid, but the elimination from those tissues and fluid was slow; this resulted in accumulation of kanamycin in those tissues.

Tissues consist of the tissue cage and the interstitial fluid. RAUWS and VAN KLINGEREN (1978) carried out experiments on gentamicin using rat tissue. They found that the concentration of the antibiotic in the interstitial fluid shifted in almost the same manner as the concentration in the serum, while the gentamicin concentration in the tissue cage changed more slowly. SZWED et al. (1974) employed gentamicin and tobramycin and studied the transfer of these drugs to the lymph of dogs. Their results indicated that the lymph concentration of these antibiotics was almost the same as their concentration in the serum.

Research has also been performed in relation to the uptake of aminoglycosides by tissues which have been isolated from an animal and incubated in vitro. For example, TULKENS and TROUET (1978) carried out studies using incubated fibroblasts that were isolated from trypsinized rat embryo carcasses. They reported that the relative rate of uptake of various aminoglycosides was as follows: gentamicin = amikacin > kanamycin = streptomycin. In addition, GOODMAN (1978) used incubated smooth muscle isolated from rabbits and determined the uptake of gentamicin. He found that the uptake of gentamicin was reduced by the presence of calcium ions. This finding is interesting in view of the fact that Ca^{2+} is known to generally reduce the toxicity of aminoglycosides.

2. Tissue Distribution in Humans

Research on the tissue distribution of aminoglycosides is considerably more difficult to carry out in humans than in animals. Nevertheless, our knowledge of this aspect of antibiotic therapy is increasing since studies are being performed using postmortem and surgically excised tissues. Drug concentrations are determined in those tissues, together with the interstitial fluid, and the serum. These data are analyzed using the previously mentioned two-compartment model, and the concentration of the drug in the tissue compartment is calculated.

SCHENTAG (1977) administered gentamicin to 47 patients by either i.v. or i.m. injection, and then carried out a pharmacokinetic analysis of the fate of the drug in the body. They calculated the volume of distribution and then estimated the tissue distribution. During the course of therapy, 6 of those patients died due to the basic disease conditions. It was found that, except for the bones, the concentration of gentamicin in all of the tissues was higher than the final serum concentration, and the concentration of the drug in the kidneys was the highest.

DASCHNER et al. (1977) administered amikacin to children at a dosage level of 7.5 mg/kg and then performed surgery. They determined the concentration of amikacin in the excised tissues and reported that an amikacin concentration of 1 μg/g or more was maintained in the muscles for 3 h or more postadministration and in the fat for more than 4 h. TAN and SALSTROM (1977) administered gentamicin, tobramycin, and amikacin to healthy humans, sampled the interstitial fluid, and then compared the concentration of the drug in that fluid with the concentration in serum obtained at the same time. Their results showed that the ratio of the interstitial fluid concentration to the serum concentration was larger with gentamicin and tobramycin than with amikacin. This finding indicates that gentamicin and tobramycin are more readily transferred to the interstitial fluid than is amikacin. In addition, SCHENTAG et al. (1978a–c) administered gentamicin and tobramycin to patients and then analyzed the serum drug concentration using the two-compartment model. It was inferred on the basis of this analysis that gentamicin attains a higher concentration than tobramycin in the tissue compartment.

V. Accumulation in Kidneys

As was mentioned previously, when aminoglycosides are administered to animals, the concentration of the drug in the various tissues rises and falls in direct response to the change in the serum concentration of the antibiotics. However, only in the kidney tissue does the concentration of these drugs attain a very high level and maintain that level for periods of as long as 24 h postadministration. And even when it is no longer possible to detect the drug in the serum, the concentration in the kidney tissue is still high.

Accordingly, when aminoglycoside therapy is carried out, it is possible that the drug will accumulate in the kidney tissue. It is thought that this accumulation is related to the development of renal impairment, a side effect shared by all the aminoglycosides. For this reason, much research has been performed in relation to the renal accumulation of these drugs and the mechanism thereof.

1. Renal Accumulation in Animals

Figure 18 presents data from the experiments of LUFT and KLEIT (1974). They determined the elimination of a single dose of aminoglycosides from the kidneys of rats. It is known that the various aminoglycosides disappear almost completely from the serum within 24 h postadministration. It is thus clear that the elimination of these drugs from the kidney tissue is very slow in comparison with their elimination from the serum. Of the aminoglycosides, only streptomycin is eliminated quickly from the kidney tissue.

EZER et al. (1976) administered ^{3}H-labeled tobramycin, gentamicin, and amikacin to rats and reported that these aminoglycosides accumulated in the kidney tissue at concentrations 100 times higher than in other organs. They also found that the site of the drug accumulation in the kidney tissue was primarily the cortex, with the ratio of the concentration in the cortex and the medulla being 50:1. NURAZYAN (1976) administered neomycin to rabbits and found that a high concentration of this drug remained in the cortex and the medulla, even at 6 days postadministra-

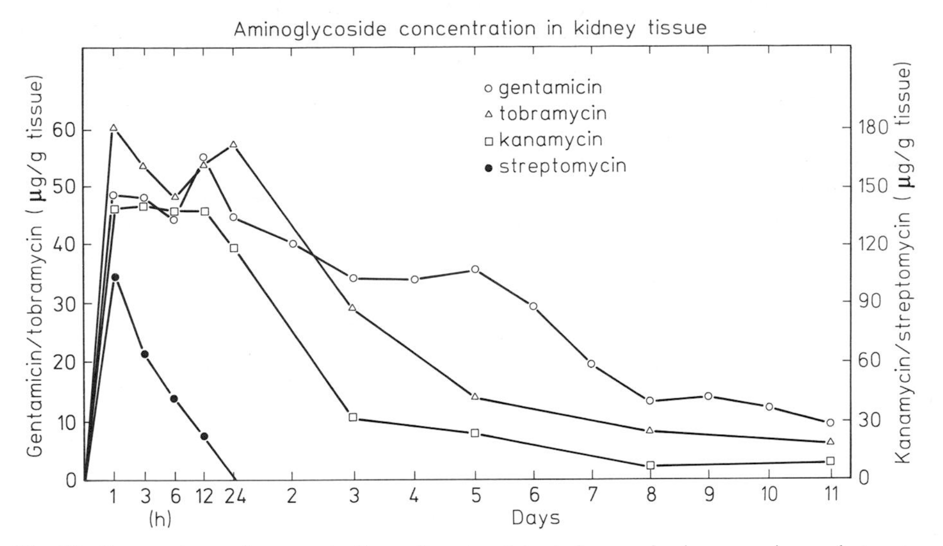

Fig. 18. Comparison of concentration of gentamicin, tobramycin, kanamycin, and streptomycin in renal tissue of rats after a single s.c. injection of 10 mg/kg gentamicin or tobramycin or of 150 mg/kg kanamycin or streptomycin (LUFT and KLEIT 1974)

tion. NIEMINEN et al. (1978) administered gentamicin, tobramycin, and amikacin to rats and investigated the state of these drugs in the kidney tissue. They reported that the aminoglycoside molecules existed in the kidneys in both the free and bound state, and that the ratio of the amount in these two states was constant, independent of the administered dosage. They also found that the total concentration of the free and bound forms of the drug was 200 µg/g or less, and that there was no evidence of histologic damage to the kidneys.

CHAUVIN et al. (1978) and RUDHARDT et al. (1978) both administered gentamicin to rats for 21 days at a dosage of 4 mg/kg/day. They reported that gentamicin could be detected in the kidney tissue at a level of 50 µg/g 2 weeks after the termination of dosing and at 15 µg/g after as long as 15 weeks. WHELTON et al. (1975) employed gentamicin in dogs and found that the concentration of the drug in the cortex of the kidney was 20 times as high as the concentration in the serum. The concentration in the medulla was also 4 times higher than the serum gentamicin concentration. They also reported that hydration did not exert any great effect on the renal accumulation of gentamicin by these animals. BEGERON and TROTTIER (1979) administered multipledoses of gentamicin and netilmicin to rats. They reported that the concentration of these antibiotics in the renal cortex rose to levels of 53–719 µg/g, and that the accumulation increased as the frequency of drug administrations increased. JERAULD and SILVERBLATT (1978) administered ^{14}C-gentamicin to rats that had already been administered *N*-methyl-nicotinamide. It was found that the renal clearance of the gentamicin was greater than in the control animals, and the concentration of the antibiotic in the renal tissue was lower. They interpreted these findings as indicating that the transfer of gentamicin to the kidneys at high concentrations is due to reabsorption by the kidneys. In addition, KLUWE and HOOK (1978) proposed that the nephrotoxicity of gentamicin is due to its renal accumulation, which is in turn the result of selective uptake of the drug by the renal tissue.

The above-mentioned findings are in agreement with the idea that renal accumulation of aminoglycosides is due to the transfer of a high concentration of the drugs to the cortex of the kidney. However, KUHAR et al. (1979) have detected the binding and accumulation of gentamicin in the portions of the renal tubules that contain mucopolysaccharide-rich microvilli. This evidence was obtained as a result of administration of ^{3}H-gentamicin to mice, followed by microautoradiography. There are also reports that the renal accumulation of aminoglycosides can be suppressed by concurrent administration of other drugs. For example, FURUNO et al. (1976b, 1977) studied the concomitant use of D-glucarate with kanamycin while DELLINGER et al. (1976) experimented with joint administration of cephalothin and gentamicin. The results obtained by both of these groups indicated that concurrent administration suppressed the accumulation of the aminoglycosides in the kidneys of the rats.

In vitro experiments have been carried out using isolated tissues in an attempt to determine the mechanism by which renal accumulation of aminoglycosides occurs. HSU et al. (1977), for example, employed rat cortex slices and reported that active transport resulted in the uptake of ^{3}H-gentamicin. LUTZ (1978) used a similar experimental system with ^{3}H-gentamicin and discovered that biologic energy is required for the uptake of the drug to occur. They also reported that the gentamicin which was taken up was strongly bound to the cortex tissue. They proposed that this binding of aminoglycosides to the renal tissue has a closer relationship to the expression of nephrotoxicity by these drugs than does simple uptake. In addition, MITCHELL et al. (1977) perfused rat kidneys with gentamicin and neomycin. COLLIER et al. (1978) experimented with the incubation of renal tubules in gentamicin solutions. The results obtained by both of these groups indicated that these aminoglycoside antibiotics, and especially neomycin, are readily taken up by the renal tissues.

2. Renal Accumulation in Humans

The accumulation of aminoglycosides by the human kidney has been studied in the organs of patients who have died in the course of therapy. LUFT et al. (1975) used biopsy to obtain samples of renal tissue from patients who were being treated with gentamicin. They found that, as with animal studies, the concentration of gentamicin was high in human kidney tissue, with the concentration 3 to 4 times higher in the cortex than in the medulla. EDWARDS et al. (1976) excised kidney tissues from 10 patients who had died in the course of therapy which included the administration of gentamicin or amikacin. They then determined the concentration of those antibiotics in the extirpated tissues. Gentamicin was present in the cortex at levels ranging from 140 to 540 μg/g and in the medulla from 128 to 230 μg/g, while amikacin was detected in the cortex at concentrations between 365 and 1,030 μg/g and in the medulla between 270 and 718 μg/g. They also reported that the level of renal accumulation of these antibiotics had no correlation with the renal function of the patients prior to death. SCHENTAG et al. (1978a) reported that in patients in whom the administration of gentamicin had been terminated, the concentration of gentamicin in the kidneys was gradually decreased over a period of days after termination of drug administration.

Summarizing the above experiments in relation to the renal accumulation of aminoglycosides in animals and humans yields the following principles:

(1) The renal accumulation of aminoglycosides in animals and in humans is very similar.

(2) Aminoglycosides are taken up by the renal tissues as a result of active transport from the urine, and the concentration of these drugs in the renal tissues is much higher than the concentration in other tissues of the body.

(3) The concentration attained by aminoglycosides in the renal cortex tissue is several times higher than the concentration in the medulla.

(4) The elimination of aminoglycosides from the renal tissues is much slower than the elimination from other body tissues. In spite of many reports concerning the slow elimination of aminoglycosides from the renal tissues, there is still almost nothing known about the mechanism of this phenomenon. In fact, it can be said that the accumulation of drugs in the body tissues is due more to slow elimination than to exceptional uptake of the drug by those tissues. Accordingly, it is hoped that in the coming years research will shed light on this aspect of elimination. It is thought that this will require elucidation of the mechanism by which aminoglycosides are bound to the renal tissues.

VI. Binding to Biopolymers

1. Binding to Heparin

Heparin is an acid mucopolysaccharide and is therefore able to bind electrostatically to aminoglycosides, which are basic substances. Raab and Windisch (1973) reported that the antimicrobial activity of neomycin against *Staphylococcus aureus* was decreased by the addition of heparin, and postulated that this reduction in activity was due to electrostatic binding with heparin. Moreover, it is also reported that the s.c. injection of neomycin can result in the appearance of biologically active amines such as histamine that had been inactivated by heparin in the skin; thus a cutaneous reaction from free amines occurs as the result of neomycin injection.

There are occasions when the physician must administer heparin to a patient in order to prevent clot formation. If an aminoglycoside is then administered to such a heparin-treated patient, a reduction in the antimicrobial activity of the antibiotic should occur due to binding between it and the heparin. Regamey et al. (1972) administered heparin to patients, followed by gentamicin. Microbiologic assay of gentamicin in the serum showed a lower than expected level of the drug. They also reported that the addition of heparin to blood samples so that coagulation would not occur prior to determination of gentamicin resulted in low values for the antibiotic. The extent to which the activity of the drug was lowered differed as a function of the ratio of the gentamicin and the heparin and of their concentration. As can be seen from the data presented in Table 15, when dilution lowered the concentration, keeping the ratio of the heparin and gentamicin constant, the measured values for gentamicin activity were close to the theoretically expected values. These results indicate that the bond between gentamicin and heparin can be broken by dilution, and that their binding is a reversible reaction.

Table 15. Reversibility by dilution of the inhibitory effect of heparin on the assayable concentration of gentamicin. (REGAMEY et al. 1972)

Heparin concentration (units/ml)	Gentamicin (μg/ml)	
	Concentration present	Concentration measured by assay
500	16	8.6 (54%)[a]
250	8	5.7 (71%)
125	4	3.35 (84%)
62	2	1.78 (89%)
31	1	0.9 (90%)

[a] Percentage of expected value

Table 16. Serum protein binding of five aminoglycoside antibiotics as determined by ultrafiltration. (GORDON et al. 1972)

Antibiotic	Concentration in serum (μg/ml)	No. of ultrafiltrations	Mean binding ± SE	p[a] (%)
Gentamicin	5	9	− 2.0 (± 2.0)	>0.3
Tobramycin	5	8	− 2.1 (± 1.9)	>0.3
Kanamycin	5	12	+ 2.8 (± 6.4)	>0.5
Kanamycin	15	6	− 0.7 (± 4.4)	>0.7
Streptomycin	15	6	+35.4 (± 0.9)	<0.001

[a] For tobramycin, gentamicin, and kanamycin, the mean binding percentages do not differ significantly from zero as determined by the t test.

2. Binding to Serum Proteins

In general, the binding of drugs and serum proteins is important because it affects the pharmacokinetic behavior of the drug and can influence its pharmacologic activity and effectiveness.

Table 16 presents data prepared by GORDON et al. (1972) in relation to the binding of aminoglycosides to serum proteins. The determinations were carried out by means of ultrafiltration. The results indicate that, except for streptomycin, aminoglycosides do not bind to serum proteins to a great extent. ZIV and SULMAN (1972) employed the sera of cows and ewes and measured the protein binding of streptomycin. When the equilibrium dialysis method was employed in the case of the ewe sera, it was found that 9.6% ± 2.2% of the streptomycin had become bound to the serum proteins, while a value of 13.6% ± 3.5% was obtained when the measurements were carried out by ultrafiltration. In the case of the cow sera, equilibrium dialysis was used to make the determinations; there was considerable variation between individual cows, and the range of binding of the streptomycin was calculated to be 5.8%–11%. These data show that the measured binding of streptomycin to serum proteins differs with the origin of the serum and with the method of determination.

Table 17. Binding of aminoglycosides to human serum determined by equilibrium dialysis.[a] (RAMIREZ-RONDA et al. 1975)

Aminoglycoside	Concentration (μg/ml)[b]		Percentage bound
	Free	Bound (corr)	
Gentamicin	1.05	2.72	72
Gentamicin C_1	0.88	4.11	82
Gentamicin C_{1a}	0.89	3.44	79
Gentamicin C_2	0.86	3.87	82
Tobramycin	0.76	2.31	75
Sisomicin	0.56	3.33	85
Kanamycin	7.20	8.60	54
Amikacin (BB-K8)	6.00	13.28	69

[a] In 0.05 *M*, pH 7.4, Tris-Cl buffer. Data represent average of experiments performed in triplicate. Assays were performed by enzymatic methods

[b] The initial concentration of antibiotic in the dialysis buffers was approximately 1 μg/ml for gentamicin, gentamicin C_1, C_{1a}, and C_2, tobramycin, and sisomicin, and 7 μg/ml for kanamycin and amikacin

RAMIREZ-RONDA et al. (1975) reported that divalent cations such as Ca^{2+} and Mg^{2+} greatly influence the serum binding of aminoglycoside antibiotics. Table 17 presents data on the degree of binding of aminoglycosides to human serum proteins in the absence of divalent cations. It is seen that the measured values are very high, i.e., 54%–85% of the antibiotics are bound under these conditions. Table 18, on the other hand, shows gentamicin binding to human serum proteins in the presence of various concentrations of Ca^{2+} and Mg^{2+}. The addition of these divalent cations results in a striking reduction in the degree of human serum protein binding of gentamicin. In fact, at a concentration of 1.0 m*M* Mg^{2+} and 2.5 m*M* Ca^{2+}, gentamicin was not bound at all. Under physiologic conditions, human serum normally contains a Mg^{2+} concentration of 0.71 m*M* and a Ca^{2+} concentration of 2.33 m*M*, which are very close to the concentrations at which no binding occurred in the in vitro experiments reported above. This leads to the conclusion that probably very little binding of aminoglycoside antibiotics to serum proteins takes place in humans under clinical conditions.

The binding of gentamicin to microbial cells was investigated using ^3H-labeled gentamicin compound. With *Pseudomonas aeruginosa* cells, it was found that divalent cations had a very large effect on the binding, with a high level of binding of gentamicin to cells when such cations were absent. In the case of *Escherichia coli*, however, divalent cations did not exert much influence on gentamicin binding.

VII. Relationship Between Renal Function and Pharmacokinetics: Clinical Applications

As was discussed in the preceding sections, aminoglycosides are not metabolized when they are administered to humans and animals. Most of the administered dose

Table 18. Effect of Ca^{2+} and Mg^{2+} concentration on the binding of gentamicin to human serum. (RAMIREZ-RONDA et al. 1975)

Divalent cations[a] (m*M*)		Gentamicin (µg/ml)		Percentage bound[b]
Mg^{2+}	Ca^{2+}	Free	Bound (corr)	
1.0	2.5	5.03	0	0
1.0	0	5.21	0.03	6
0.5	0	5.06	0.79	14
0.25	0	4.58	7.44	62
0	2.5	4.69	1.59	25
0	1.25	4.98	3.85	44
0	0.675	4.53	4.30	48
0	0	4.22	8.53	67
0.5	2.5	4.87	2.70	35
0.25	2.5	4.17	11.00	72
1.0	1.25	5.56	1.57	22
1.0	0.675	5.99	0.14	2.3

[a] In 0.05 *M*, pH 7.4, Tris-Cl buffer containing 0.15 *M* NaCl
[b] The concentration of gentamicin added to each buffer before dialysis was approximately 5.1 µg/ml. Assays were performed by the enzymatic method. Data represent averages from experiments performed in triplicate. Experiments were performed by equilibrium dialysis as described in the text

of these drugs is excreted unchanged in the urine. Accordingly, the pharmacokinetic behavior of these antibiotics is decisively influenced by renal function. The renal excretion of aminoglycosides occurs mainly as the result of glomerular filtration. Therefore, much research has been carried out with regard to the relationship between the pharmacokinetics of these drugs and parameters, such as the glomerular filtration rate and creatinine clearance, that give an indication of the level of renal function.

YAMASAKU et al. (1980) divided human subjects into four groups on the basis of creatinine clearance values, administered ribostamycin to them, and then studied the pharmacokinetic behavior of the antibiotic. Figure 19 shows the serum concentration curves which were simulated for ribostamycin on the basis of the average values for the pharmacokinetic parameters for each group. It is evident from these curves that the three groups whose members showed below-normal creatinine clearance values show simulated ribostamycin serum concentrations that are higher and are maintained at high levels for longer periods of time than in the case of group I, whose members had normal creatinine clearance values. This pattern is true not only for ribostamycin, but also for the other aminoglycosides; for example, LOCKWOOD and BOWER (1973) reported similar findings with tobramycin and gentamicin, and YAMASAKU and KABASAWA (1976) obtained similar results with dibekacin.

Figure 20 presents a graph prepared by SCHENTAG et al. (1978b) showing the linear relationship between the body clearance of tobramycin and the creatinine clearance in humans. YAMASAKU and KABASAWA (1976) and YAMASAKU et al. (1980) published similar linear relationship curves on the basis of their data con-

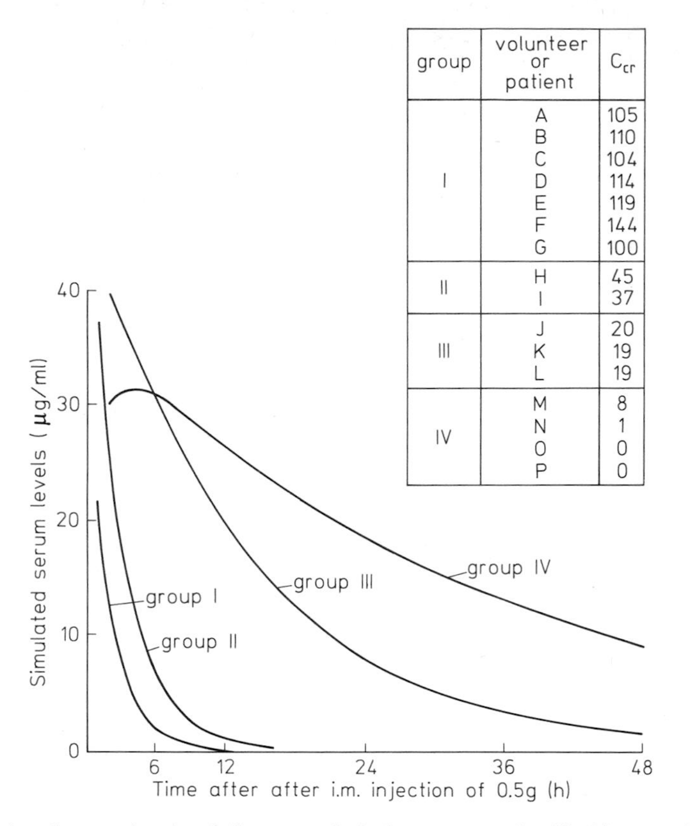

group	volunteer or patient	C_{cr}
I	A	105
	B	110
	C	104
	D	114
	E	119
	F	144
	G	100
II	H	45
	I	37
III	J	20
	K	19
	L	19
IV	M	8
	N	1
	O	0
	P	0

Fig. 19. Simulated serum levels of ribostamycin in four groups classified by creatinine clearance (YAMASAKU et al. 1980)

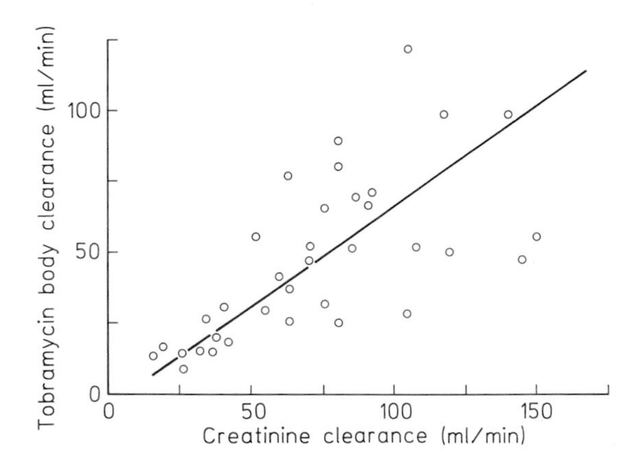

Fig. 20. Relation between tobramycin body clearance (Cln) and Ccr is described by the regression equation Cln = 0.71 (Ccr) − 4.1; $r = 0.65$; $P < 0.01$. If the regression line is placed through the origin, the regression equation describing this relationship is Cln = 0.66 (Ccr); $r = 0.66$; $P < 0.01$ (SCHENTAG et al. 1978b)

Table 19. First-order equation expressing linear correlation between the elimination constants K_{el} of aminoglycosides and creatinine clearance c_{cr}
$X = C_{cr}$ ml/min
$Y = K_{el}$%/hr $\quad Y = AX + B$

Aminoglycoside	A	B	Reference
Ribostamycin	0.3853	4.5651	YAMASAKU et al. (1980)
Amikacin	0.331	−0.42	MCHENRY et al. (1976b)
Dibekacin	0.43	0.4	YAMASAKU and KABASAWA (1976)
Sisomicin	0.312	3.16	PECHÉRE et al. (1976b)

cerning the body clearance of dibekacin and ribostamycin. The body clearance of these drugs was calculated using the previously presented Eq. (15). Since the elimination of aminoglycoside antibiotics from the bloodstream is primarily dependent upon renal glomerular excretion, the linear relationship between the body clearance of the drug and the creatinine clearance is exactly as expected.

In Eq. (15), assuming that there is little individual variation in the volume of distribution V_d, the body clearance C_b and the elimination constant K_{el} become proportional. Accordingly, the relationship between K_{el} and the creatinine clearance should also take on a linear form. Various research groups have actually reported a high degree of correlation between these two values for several aminoglycosides. Table 19 presents the first order equation obtained on the basis of data from YAMASAKU and KABASAWA (1976), YAMASAKU et al. (1980), MCHENRY et al. (1976b), and PECHÉRE et al. (1976b).

If we ignore reabsorption which may occur during the process of the renal excretion of aminoglycosides, the value of A in Table 19 should be equal to $6/V_d$(L). Then, if we assume a body weight of 75 kg and calculate on the basis of V_d being 20% of the body weight, as shown in Table 19, A = 0.4. This value is very close to the values shown in Table 19. Also, if V_d is small, the value of A will become large. In this connection, we should note that in Table 19 the relatively large values for A were obtained by YAMASAKU et al. (1980) and YAMASAKU and KABASAWA (1976) when using ribostamycin nd dibekacin in Oriental patients, who have relatively small physiques. The other two groups of subjects were Westerners and were therefore relatively large in physical build, and the values of A obtained for those groups were smaller. Therefore, it is not possible to claim that differences in the value of A as seen in Table 19 always arise as a result of differences between the aminoglycosides being investigated. Reports on the correlation between the drug elimination constant K_{el} and the creatinine clearance have also been made by MCHENRY et al. (1976a, b) for amikacin and by PECHÉRE et al. (1978a, b) for netilmicin.

As is evident from Eq. (14), since K_{el} and the biological half-life $T_{1/2}$ have an inversely proportional relationship, there should be a linear correlation between the reciprocal of $T_{1/2}$ and the creatinine clearance or the glomerular filtration rate. HOEFFLER et al. (1976) and PIJCK et al. (1976) have demonstrated this correlation with amikacin.

Often aminoglycosides must be administered to patients out of therapeutic necessity, even though the patients are known to have abnormal renal function. In such cases, to avoid side effects of the aminoglycoside the concentration of the drug in the patient's bloodstream must be regulated. To this end, the first step is to ascertain the level of the renal function of the patient and then apply those results and the above-mentioned correlation so that pharmacokinetic parameters such as $T_{1/2}$ and K_{el} can be estimated. Then the serum concentration of the drug corresponding to various administration protocols should be calculated. Finally, the drug administration program most suited to the needs of the patient must be worked out.

For example, let us consider the case where an aminoglycoside must be administered to a patient at time interval T_i. If we administer the same dosage of the drug to a patient having abnormal kidney function as would be given to a patient with normal renal function, we can expect that the serum concentration of the antibiotic will be higher than desired, and there will be a risk of side effects developing. In this case, it is essential to control the administered dose at the proper level so that the serum concentration of the aminoglycoside will be the same as it would be with normal kidney function. DETTLI (1971) studied the problem of finding an administration program calling for the periodic administration of dose D at intervals of time T_i for patients with abnormal renal function. They proposed that the following equations be used for the calculation of the initial dose, $\hat{D}_*$, and the maintenance dose, $\hat{D}$.

$$\hat{D} = D \cdot \hat{K}/K_N, \tag{23}$$

$$\hat{D}_* = \hat{D}/\{1 - \exp(-\hat{K}T_i)\}. \tag{24}$$

In these equations, K_N is the elimination constant, K_{el}, for patients with normal renal function, while $\hat{K}$ represents that value in the case of the patients with abnormal renal function.

The most convenient parameter to assess renal function is creatinine clearance. However, in order to calculate the creatinine clearance, it is necessary to determine both serum and urinary creatinine. This determination is faced with the problem of manpower needed to carry out both the serum and urinary creatinine determinations, and also the fact that in patients with poor renal function the amount of urine excreted is often very small and may be insufficient to determine the creatinine content. In such cases, it is necessary to estimate the pharmacokinetic parameters from data obtained by blood analysis, for example, BUN, the serum creatinine concentration, the hematocrit value, etc.

If we assume that the production rate of creatinine in the body is a constant, with no individual differences, the serum creatinine concentration and the creatinine clearance should take on an inversely proportional relationship. Then, on the basis of the previously mentioned correlation, the serum creatinine concentration and the biologic half-life of aminoglycosides should have a linear relationship. MCHENRY et al. (1976a, b) and LEVY and KLASTERSKY (1975) reported that on the basis of this assumption, it was possible to estimate the K_{el} and the biologic half-life of amikacin from the serum creatinine concentration.

BARZA et al. (1974), on the other hand, reported that they found a degree of correlation between the serum creatinine concentration and the biologic half-life of gentamicin, but that this correlation was not exact enough to permit clinical application of the biologic half-life value. In fact, they claimed that there was a better correlation between the biologic half-life and the value of the serum creatinine concentration divided by the hematocrit. How well the pharmacokinetic parameters estimated using this technique coincide with reality depends on the degree to which the above assumptions fit the actual situation in the body. BARZA et al. (1975) maintain that the serum concentration of gentamicin should be monitored for safety with patients having poor renal function, because there is a tendency in such patients for the serum concentration of the drug to become too high. Thus, while the drug is being administered according to the program formulated from the estimated pharmacokinetic parameters, monitoring of the serum concentration of the antibiotic can serve as a valuable safeguard against inadvertent overdosing.

BARZA et al. (1974) also reported that there is no correlation between the volume of distribution of gentamicin and the renal function of the patient.

SCHENTAG et al. (1976), PECHÉRE and DUGAL (1976), PECHÉRE et al. (1976a, b), and YAMASAKU et al. (1980) have actually carried out the formulation of aminoglycoside administered protocols through the application of calculations based on the renal function of patients. RITSCHEL et al. (1977), meanwhile, have developed a computer program whereby it is possible to enter data relating to renal function, and obtain an administration protocol for kanamycin. This program may also be applicable to amikacin administration without any alteration, since KIRBY et al. (1976) have reported that the pharmacokinetic parameters of kanamycin and amikacin are the same.

There is concern that the administration of aminoglycosides to patients who already have impairment of renal function may result in increased impairment. WHELTON et al. (1976) administered gentamicin to 12 patients who required renal surgery. They then determined the concentration of gentamicin in the cortex of the kidneys that were removed during surgery. The gentamicin concentration in impaired kidney cortex was much lower than the concentration in the cortex of normal kidneys.

Aminoglycosides are often used concurrently with penicillins. The amino group of aminoglycosides is able to react chemically with the β-lactam group of penicillins. This reaction does not occur in patients having normal renal function because the rate of the reaction in vivo is much slower than the rate of clearance of these drugs from the bloodstream. However, in patients in whom renal function is greatly reduced, the clearance rate of these antibiotics from the serum is decreased and their concentration in the blood is not reduced as quickly as in the normal patient. Thus, when an aminoglycoside is administered to such a patient concomitantly with a penicillin-type drug, serum concentrations remain high enough so that they are able to react, and the antibiotics are inactivated. The decrease in the serum level of the aminoglycoside is accordingly considerably more rapid than when it is administered alone, i.e., not concomitantly with a penicillin.

This situation has been reported as actually occurring by ERVIN et al. (1976). They administered gentamicin alone, or together with ticarcillin or carbenicillin, to patients having renal impairment and found that the disappearance of gentamicin activity from the serum was accelerated when the penicillin drugs were given concurrently. These results are presented in Fig. 21. This chemical reaction resulting in the inactivation of gentamicin is a common feature of all aminoglycosides

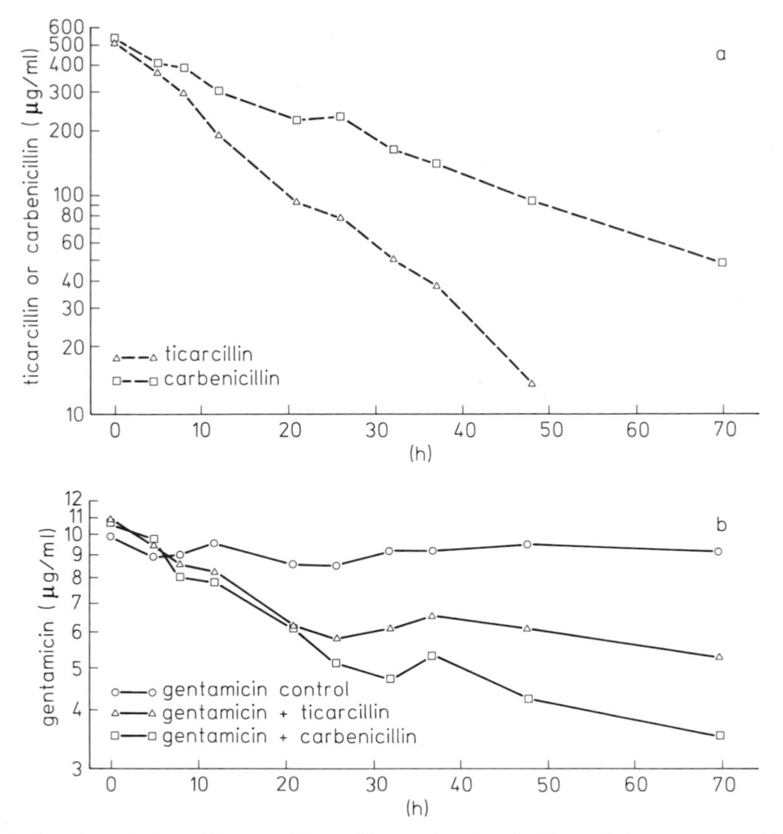

Fig. 21 a, b. In vitro study. **a** Decay of ticarcillin and carbenicillin activity in serum at 37 °C. **b** Decay curves of gentamicin activity in the presence of ticarcillin or carbenicillin. Penicillin concentration at each interval as depicted in **a** (ERVIN et al. 1976)

and may occur with any aminoglycoside administered with a penicillin to patients with reduced renal function.

In the case of patients suffering from severe renal dysfunction, it is often necessary to carry out hemodialysis or peritoneal dialysis in order to eliminate metabolic products from the body. If these dialysis procedures are performed on a patient receiving an aminoglycoside, the antibiotic will be eliminated from the body together with the metabolic products. Increasing the rate at which dialysis is performed will accelerate the desired reduction in the serum creatinine and blood urea concentrations. At the same time, however, rapid dialysis will shorten the biologic half-life of an administered aminoglycoside. Figures 22 and 23 present data obtained by REGEUR et al. (1977) and show the correlation between the biologic half-life of amikacin and the decrease in serum creatinine and blood urea when dialysis is performed. Similar results have been obtained by LETOURNEAU SASEB et al. (1977) and DANISH et al. (1974) with gentamicin, by DANISH et al. (1974) with kanamycin, by MALACOFF et al. (1975) and JAFFE et al. (1974) with tobramycin, and by MADHAVAN et al. (1976) with amikacin.

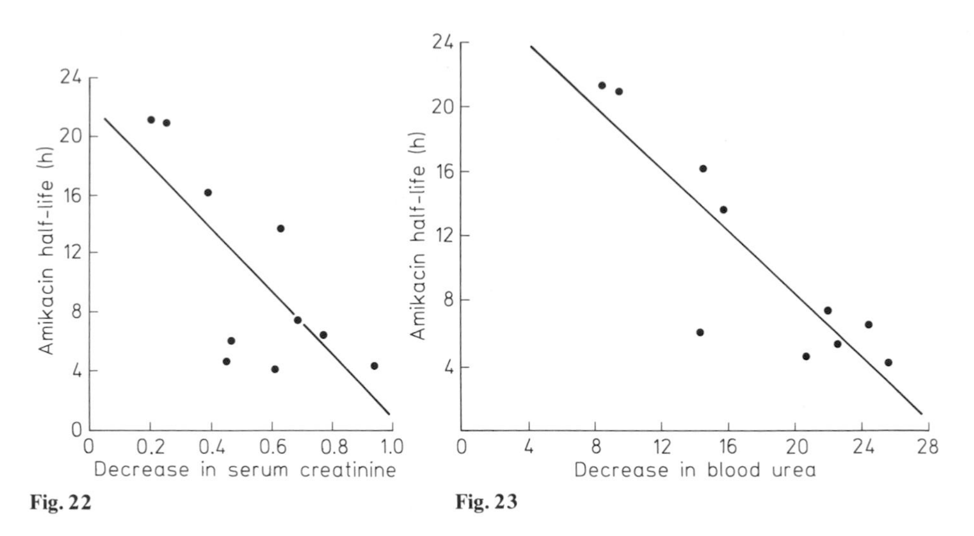

Fig. 22 **Fig. 23**

Fig. 22. Correlation between the half-life of amikacin and the decrease in serum creatinine during hemodialysis and peritoneal dialysis. $r = -0.71$; $P < 0.05$ (REGEUR et al. 1977)

Fig. 23. Correlation between the half-life of amikacin and the decrease in blood urea during hemodialysis and peritoneal dialysis. $r = -0.66$; $P < 0.05$ (REGEUR et al. 1977)

References

Adams HR (1973) Neuromuscular blocking effect of aminoglycoside antibiotic in nonhuman primate. J Am Vet Med Assoc 163:613–616

Adams HR, Goodman FR, Weiss GB (1974) Alteration of contractile function and calcium ion movements in vascular smooth muscle by gentamicin and other aminoglycoside antibiotics. Antimicrob Agents Chemother 5:640–646

Akiyoshi M (1979) Inner ear damage, its evaluation and safety administration of ototoxic aminoglycoside antibiotics, innermost row of the outer hair cells. Clin Bacteriol 6:353–361

Akiyoshi M, Sato K (1967a) Histopathological and enzyme histochemical studies on ototoxicity due to gentamicin and kanamycin in guinea pigs. Chemotherapy (Tokyo) 15:501–512

Akiyoshi M, Sato K (1967b) Histochemical demonstration of succinic dehydrogenase activity of the hair cells by means of intravital perfusion of the cochlea. Audiology Jpn 10:48–56

Akiyoshi M, Sato K (1968) Functional, histopathological and histochemical studies on the ototoxicity in guinea pigs due to aminosidine. Chemotherapy (Tokyo) 16:134–138

Akiyoshi M, Sato K (1969a) Experimental study on the ototoxicity of aminodeoxykanamycin in guinea pig, pinna reflex and histopathologic findings. Chemotherapy (Tokyo) 17:1656–1663

Akiyoshi M, Sato K (1969b) Reevaluation of the pinna reflex test as screening for ototoxicity of antibiotics. Prog Antimicrob Anticancer Chemother. University of Tokyo Press, vol 1, pp 621–627

Akiyoshi M, Sato K (1971) Ototoxicity of vistamycin. Audiology Jpn 14:189–201

Akiyoshi M, Sato K (1973) Histochemical study of reduction potency of ubiquinone of hair cells of the spiral organ in guinea pigs. Acta Histochem Cytochem 233–247

Akiyoshi M, Sato K, Sugahiro K, Shoji T (1968) Functional, histochemical and histopathological studies on ototoxicity of enduracidin in guinea pigs. Chemotherapy (Tokyo) 16:511–520

Akiyoshi M, Sato K, Tamura H (1972) Ototoxicity of liviodomycin. Audiology Jpn 15:220–223

Akiyoshi M, Sato K, Nakada H, Tojima T (1974a) Audiometrical and histopathological evaluation of ototoxicity of 3′,4′-dideoxykanamycin B (DKB), a new semisynthetic aminoglycoside antibiotic in guinea pigs. Jpn J Antibiot 27:15–26

Akiyoshi M, Sato K, Shoji T, Sugahiro K, Tajima T, Koeda T, Odaki M, Yokata M (1974b) Ototoxic effect of 3′,4′-dideoxykanamycin B on the inner ear in the intrauterine guinea pigs. Jpn J Antibiot 27:735–745

Akiyoshi M, Sato K, Nakada H, Nara T, Tajima T, Sasaki K, Ogawa M (1975a) Ototoxicity of tobramycin in guinea pigs. Chemotherapy (Tokyo) 23:1522–1543

Akiyoshi M, Sato K, Nakada H, Tajima T, Suzuki K, Kishimoto K (1975b) Evaluation of ototoxicity of amikacin (BB-K 8) by animal test. Jpn J Antibiot 28:288–304

Akiyoshi M, Iwazawa T, Yano S, Shoji T, Tajima T, Hara T, Shimizu M (1977) Animal test for evaluation of ototoxicity and safety of KW-1062. Chemotherapy (Tokyo) 25:1892–1914

Albiero L, Ongini E, Parravicini L (1978) The neuromuscular blocking activity of a new aminoglycoside antibiotic netilmicin sulphate. Eur J Pharmacol 50:1–7

Alleva FR, Balzas T (1978) Toxic effects of potential administration of streptomycin sulfate to rats. Toxicol Appl Pharmacol 45:855–859

Anhalt JP (1977) Assay of gentamicin in serum by highpressure liquid chromatography. Antimicrob Agents Chemother 11:651–655

Aratani H, Yamanaka Y, Onishi R, Kono S, Hashimoto T, Hirozane T (1968) Pharmacological studies on amidosidine. Chemotherapy (Tokyo) 6:114–120

Asakuma S, Shida S, Suzuki M, Abe N (1975) Experimental study on the mutual relation between endocochlea DC potential and cochlear microphonics. Audiology Jpn 18:246–254

Barza M, Brown RB, Shen D, Gibaldi M, Weinstein L (1974) Predictability of blood levels of gentamicin in man. Clin Res 22:687A

Boger WP, Gavin JJ (1958–1959) Kanamycin: its cerebrospinal fluid diffusion, renal clearance and comparison with streptomycin. Antibiot Annu 676–677

Brazil OV, Corrado AP (1957) The curariform action of streptomycin. J Pharmacol Exp Ther 120:452–459

Brazil OV, Prado-Franceschi J (1969) The neuromuscular blocking action of gentamicin. Arch Int Pharmacodyn Ther 179:65–76

Broughall JM, Reeves DS (1975a) Properties of the gentamicin acetyltransferase enzyme and application to the assay of aminoglycoside antibiotics. Antimicrob Agents Chemother 8:222–223

Broughall JM, Reeves DS (1975b) The acetyltransferase enzyme method for the assay of serum gentamicin concentrations and a comparison with other methods. J Clin Pathol 28:140–145

Broughton A, Strong JE, Pickering LK, Bodey GP (1976a) Radioimmunoassay of iodinated tobramycin. Antimicrob Agents Chemother 10:652–656

Broughton A, Strong JE, Bodey GP (1976b) Radioimmunoassay of sisomicin. Antimicrob Agents Chemother 9:247–250

Brown RD, Feldman AM (1978) Pharmacology of hearing and ototoxicity. Annu Rev Pharmacol Toxicol 18:233–252

Barza M, Brown RB, Shen D, Gibaldi M, Weinstein L (1975) Predictability of blood levels of gentamicin in man. J Infect Dis 132:165–174

Benzi G, Arrigoni E, Pancer P, Berte F (1972) Action on gentamicin, aminosidine, and ampicillin on uterine tone and motility. Jpn J Pharmacol 22:571–576

Berg K (1951) The toxic effect of streptomycin on the vestibular and cochlear apparatus. Acta Otolaryngo [Suppl] (Stockh) 97:1–47

Bergeron MG, Trottier S (1979) Influence of single or multiple doses of gentamicin and netilmicin on their cortical, medullary and papillary distribution. Antimicrob Agents Chemother 15:635–641

Berggärd I, Bearn AG (1968) Isolation and properties of low molecular weight β^2-microglobulin occurring in human biological fluids. J Biol Chem 243:4095–4103

Bernard B, Abate M, Thielen PF, Attar H, Ballard CA, Wehrle PF (1977) Maternal-fetal pharmacological activity of amikacin. J Infect Dis 135:925–932
Bodey GP, Valdivieso M, Feld R, Rodriguez V (1974) Pharmacology of amikacin in humans. Antimicrob Agents Chemother 5:508–512
Brummett RE (1972) A comparative study of the ototoxicity of tobramycin and gentamicin. Arch Otolaryngol 96:505–512
Brummett RE, Traynor J, Brown R, Himes D (1975) Cochlear damage resulting from kanamycin and furosomide. Acta Otolaryngol (Stockh) 80:86–92
Cabana BE, Taggart JG (1973) Comparative pharmacokinetics of BB-K8 and kanamycin in dogs and humans. Antimicrob Agents Chemother 3:478–483
Chauvin JM, Rudhardt M, Bluauchard P, Gaillard R, Fabre J (1978) Le compartment de la gentamicine dans le parenckyme renal. Schweiz Med Wochenschr 108:1020–1025
Child KJ, Davis B, Sharpe HM, Tomich EG (1956–1957) Toxicologic studies on the sulfate and pantothenates of streptomycin and dihydrostreptomycin. Antibiot Annu 574–580
Chiu PJS, Long JF (1978) Effects of hydration on gentamicin excretion and renal accumulation in furosemide-treated rats. Antimicrob Agents Chemother 14:214–217
Chiu PJS, Brown A, Miller G, Long JF (1976) Renal extraction of gentamicin in anesthetized dogs. Antimicrob Agents Chemother 10:277–282
Chiu PJS, Miller GH, Brown AD, Long JF, Waitz JA (1977) Renal pharmacology of netilimicin. Antimicrob Agents Chemother 11:821–825
Collier VU, Mitch WE, Lietman PS (1978) Tubular uptake of gentamicin by the intact kidney. Clin Res 26:288A
Crawford LM, Bowen JM (1971) Calcium binding as a property of kanamycin. Am J Vet Res 32:357–359
Danish M, Schultz R, Jusco J (1974) Pharmacokinetics of gentamicin and kanamycin during hemodialysis. Antimicrob Agents Chemother 6:841–847
Daschner F, Reiss E, Engert J (1977) Distribution of amikacin in serum, muscle and fat in children after a single intramuscular injection. Antimicrob Agents Chemother 11:1081–1083
Davis WW, Stout TR (1971) Disk plate method of microbiological antibiotic assay II, novel procedure offering improved accuracy. Appl Microbiol 22:666–670
Dellinger P, Murphy T, Barza M, Pinn V, Weinstein L (1976) Effect of cephalothin on renal cortical concentration of gentamicin in rats. Antimicrob Agents Chemother 9:587–588
Dettli L (1971) Multiple dose kinetics and drug dosage in patients with kidney disease. Acta Pharmacol Toxicol 29:211
Edwards CQ, Smith CR, Baugman KL, Rogers JF, Lietman PS (1976) Concentration of gentamicin and amikacin in human kidneys. Antimicrob Agents Chemother 9:925–927
Engström H, Kohonen A (1965) Cochlear damage from ototoxic antibiotics. Acta Otolaryngol (Stockh) 59:171–178
Ervin FR, Bullock WE Jr, Nuttal CE (1976) Inactivation of gentamicin by penicillins in patients with renal failure. Antimicrob Agents Chemother 9:1004–1011
Ezer J, Mahon WA, Inaba T (1976) Tissue distribution and selective kidney uptake of tritiated aminoglycosides in the rats. Pharmacologist 18:206
Fujisawa K, Hoshiya T, Kawaguchi H (1974) Aminoglycoside antibiotics. VII. Acute toxicity of aminoglycoside antibiotics. J Antibiot (Tokyo) 27:677–681
Fujita M, Fukushima K, Abe M, Tomono N, Umemura K (1973) Experimental studies on absorption, excretion, distribution, and metabolism of 3′,4′-dideoxykanamycin B. II. Absorption, excretion, and distribution in rabbits and dogs. Jpn J Antibiot 26:55–60
Fukushima K, Fujita M (1970) Teratological study of vistamicin. Clin Rep 4:52–61
Furuno K, Andoh K, Suzuki S (1976a) Effect of D-glucarates on basic antibiotic-induced renal damage in rats. J Antibiot (Tokyo) 29:187–194
Furuno K, Matsubara S, Andoh K, Suzuki S (1976b) Preventive effect of D-glucarate against renal damage induced by kanamycin. J Antibiot (Tokyo) 29:950–953
Furuno K, Suzuki S, Hirata K (1977) Influence of dehydration and D-glucarate on distribution and excretion of kanamycin in rats. Jpn J Pharmacol 27:371–378
Garrod LP, Gruenwaldt G, Marget W, Wellta H (1979) New aspects of aminoglycoside therapy, sisomicin. Infection 7:294–300

Gergis SD, Dretchen KL, Sokoll MD, Long JP (1971) The effects of neuromuscular blocking agents on acetylcholine release. Proc Soc Exp Biol Med 38:693–695
Goodman FR (1978) Distribution of gentamicin in vascular smooth muscle. Pharmacology 16:17–25
Gordon RC, Regamey C, Kirby WMM (1972) Serum protein binding of the aminoglycoside antibiotics. Antimicrob Agents Chemother 2:214–216
Haas MJ, Davis J (1973) Enzymatic acetylation as a means of determining serum aminoglycoside concentrations. Antimicrob Agents Chemother 4:497–499
Hara T, Nishikawa S, Miyazaki H, Ohguro Y (1980) Studies on the safety of KW-1062 (Fifth report), a comparative study on the renal toxicity of KW-1062 and gentamicin in rats by light and electron microscopies. Jpn J Antibiot 33:1–9
Harada Y, Mori S, Teshima K, Ino M, Nakatani Y, Hirota K, Ishikawa M, Toyota H, Kawase M, Matsumura S, Kimoto S, Uno O, Nakao T (1975) Subacute toxicologic studies with tobramycin and its recovery studies in beagle dogs. Chemotherapy 23:1494–1521
Hasegawa Y, Yoshida T, Kozen T, Yamagata H, Sakaguchi I, Okamoto A, Ohara T, Kozen T (1975) Teratological studies on tobramycin in mice and rats. Chemotherapy 23:1544–1553
Hashimoto T, Ichikawa S, Kojima T (1977) The general pharmacological action of KW-1062, a new aminoglycoside antibiotics. Jpn J Antibiot 30:362–385
Hawkins JE Jr (1959) The ototoxicity of kanamycin. Ann Otol Rhinol Laryngol 68:698–715
Hawkins JE Jr, Arbor A (1976) Drug ototoxicity. In: Kiedel WD, Neff WD (eds) Auditory system. Clinical and special topics. Springer, Berlin Heidelberg New York (Handbook of sensory physiology, vol 5/3, pp 707–748)
Hawkins JE Jr, Engström H (1964) Effects of kanamycin on cochlear cytoarchitecture. Acta Otol Laryngol [Suppl] (Stockh) 188:100–107
Hawkins JE Jr, Wolcott H, O'Skanny WJ (1956–1957) Ototoxic effects of streptomycin and dihydrostreptomycin pantothenates in the cat. Antibiot Annu 554–563
Hawkins S (1958) Pharmacology of neomycin. In: Waksman SA (ed) Neomycin, its nature and practical application. Williams & Wilkins, Baltimore, pp 130–146
Hirokawa N, Haruyama A, Oike S, Naruse T (1979) Clinical evaluation of *N*-acetyl-β-D-glucosaminidase activity in 60 patients treated with aminoglycosides. Curr Chemother Infect Dis 1:626–627
Hoecker JL (1978) Clinical pharmacology of tobramycin in children. J Infect Dis 137:592–596
Hoeffler D, Koeppe P, Demers HG (1976) Pharmacokinetics of amikacin for treatment of urinary tract infections in patients with reduced renal function. J Infect Dis 134:S369–373
Holmes RK, Sanford JP (1974) Enzymatic assay for gentamicin and related aminoglycoside antibiotics. J Infect Dis 129:519–527
Hori K, Kawamoto K (1972) The experimental study of the side effect of lividomycin on the inner ear. Audiology Jpn 15:212–219
Hsu CH, Kurtz TW, Easterling RE, Weller JM (1974) Potentiation of gentamicin nephrotoxicity by metabolic acidosis (38212). Proceedings of the Society for Experimental Biology and Medicine 146:894–897
Hsu CH, Kurtz TW, Weller JM (1977) In vitro uptake of gentamicin by rat renal cortical tissue. Antimicrob Agents Chemother 13:192–194
Ichikawa T, Nakano I, Hirokawa I, Okada K, Abe M, Umemura K (1973) Experimental studies on absorption, excretion, distribution, and metabolism of 3′-4′-dideoxykanamycin B. III. Pharmacokinetic analysis in man. Jpn J Antibiot 26:262–266
Ikeda C, Tachibana A, Yano K (1979) Absorption, distribution, metabolism, and excretion of sisomicin in mice, rats, and dogs. Jpn J Antibiot 32:312–322
Inoue S (1972) Recent progress in the aminosugar antibiotics. Sci Rep Meiji Seika Kaisha 12:1–55
Israel KS, Welles JS, Black HR (1976) Aspects of the pharmacology and toxicology of tobramycin in animals and humans. J Infect Dis [Suppl] 134:97–103
Ito Y (1962a) Chemistry of basic oligosaccharide antibiotics (1). Pharm Month 34:1–35
Ito Y (1962b) Chemistra of basic oligosaccharide antibiotics (2). Pharm Month 34:74–99

Ito Y (1963) Recent advances in the chemistry of basic oligosaccharide antibiotics. Pharm Month 34:293–315

Jackson GG, Finland M (1969) International symposium on gentamicin, a new aminoglycoside antibiotic. J Infect Dis 119:4–5

Jaffe G, Meyers BR, Hirschman SZ (1974) Pharmacokinetics of tobramycin in patients with stable renal impairment, patients, undergoing peritoneal dialysis, and patients on chronic hemodialysis. Antimicrob Agents Chemother 5:611–616

Jerauld R, Silverblatt FJ (1978) Effect of *N*-methylnicotinamide on the renal accumulation and reabsorption of gentamicin in rats. Antimicrob Agents Chemother 13:893–894

Kajimoto Y, Kuramoto M (1967) Toxicity of gentamicin. Chemotherapy (Tokyo) 15:490–496

Kaneko Y, Nakagawa T, Tanaka K (1970) Reissner's membrane after kanamycin administration. Arch Otolaryngol 92:457–462

Kanzaki J (1966) The Preyer's reflex of the guinea pig as the hearing index. Audiology Jpn 60:940–948

Keller H, Krupe W, Sous H, Muckter H (1955) The reduction of the toxicity of basic streptomyces antibiotics. I. Streptomycin and dihydrostreptomycin. Arzneim Forsch 5:170–176

Kellerhals B (1979) Perilymph production and cochlear blood flow. Acta Otolaryngol (Stockh) 187:370–374

Kendall MJ, Wisc R, Andrews JM, Bedford KA (1978) A pharmacological study of VK-18892 and amikacin. Antimicrob Agents Chemother 4:459–463

Kirby WMM, Clarke JT, Libke RD, Regamey C (1976) Clinical pharmacology of amikacin and kanamycin. J Infect Dis 134:S312–315

Kluwe WM, Hook JB (1978) Functional nephrotoxicity of gentamicin in the rat. Toxicol Appl Pharmacol 45:163–175

Koeda T, Moriguchi M (1973) Teratological studies of 3′,4′-dideoxykanamycin B in rats and mice. Jpn J Antibiot 26:40–48

Koeda T, Odaki M, Niizato T, Watanabe H (1970a) Toxicological studies of vistamycin. Clin Rep 4:14–37

Koeda T, Shibata U, Nakazawa T, Asaoka H, Yamagami K (1970b) Pharmacological studies on vistamycin. Clin Rep 4:39–51

Koeda T, Odaki M, Hisamatsu T, Sasaki H, Yokota M, Niizato T, Uchida S (1973a) Studies on subacute toxicity of 3′,4′-dideoxykanamycin B (DKB). Jpn J Antibiot 26:228–246

Koeda T, Odaki M, Hisamatsu T, Sasaki H, Yokota M, Niizato T, Uchida S (1973b) Studies on chronic toxicity of 3′,4′-dideoxykanamycin B. Jpn J Antibiot 26:247–261

Koeda T, Shibata U, Asaoka H, Kabata Y, Yamaki Y (1973c) Pharmacological studies on 3′,4′-dideoxykanamycin B (DKB). Jpn J Antibiot 26:28–39

Komiya I, Hayasaka Y, Murata S, Komai T, Umemura K (1973) Experimental studies on absorption, excretion, distribution, and metabolism of 3′,4′-dideoxykanamycin B. I. Absorption, excretion, distribution, and metabolism in rats. Jpn J Antibiot 26:49–54

Komiya I, Murata S, Umemura K, Tomono N, Kikai S, Fujita M (1981a) Pharmacokinetics of dibekacin in rabbits and dogs. J Pharm Dyn, vol 4, pp 362–373

Komiya I, Murata S, Umemura K, Tomono N, Kikai S, Fujita M (1981b) Acute toxicity and pharmacokinetics of dibekacin in mice. J Pharm Dyn, vol 4, pp 356–361

Kornguth ML, Kunin CM (1977) Distribution of gentamicin and amikacin in rabbit tissues. Antimicrob Agents Chemother 11:974–977

Kuhar MJ, Mak LL, Lietman P (1979) Autoradiographic localization of [3H] gentamicin in the proximal renal tubules of mice. Antimicrob Agents Chemother 15:131–133

Kuramoto M, Okubo T, Lee S, Ishimura Y, Morimoto J (1975) Toxicological studies of tobramycin in mice and rats. Chemotherapy (Tokyo) 23:1470–1493

Lamb JW, Mann JM, Simmons RJ (1972) Factors influencing the microbiological assay of tobramycin. Antimicrob Agents Chemother 1:323–328

Lange G (1975) Das Verhalten der Labyrinth-Funktionen des Affen (Macacus rhesus) unter Streptomycin-Belastung. Arch Otorhinolaryngol 211:35–41

Lawson DH (1972) Effects of furosemide on antibiotic-induced renal damage in rats. J Infect Dis 126:593–600

Letourneau Saseb L, Lapierre L, Daigneault R, Homme MP, St Lous G, Sirois G (1977) Gentamicin pharmacokinetics during hemodialysis in patients suffering from chronic renal failure. Int J Clin Pharmacol Biopharm 15:116–120

Levy J, Klastersky J (1975) Correlation of serum creatinine concentration and amikacin half-life. J Clin Pharmacol 15:705–707

Lewis JE, Nelson JS, Elder HA (1972) Radioimmunoassay of an antibiotic gentamicin. Nature New Biol 239:214–215

Lewis JE, Nelson JC, Elder HA (1975) Amikacin; a rapid and sensitive radioimmunoassay. Antimicrob Agents Chemother 7:42–45

Lindsen JR, Proctor LR, Work WP (1960) Histopathologic inner ear changes in deafness due to neomycin in a human. Laryngoscope 70:382–392

Lockwood WR, Bower JD (1973) Tobramycin and gentamicin concentrations in the serum of normal and anephric patients. Antimicrob Agents Chemother 3:125–129

Luft FC, Kleit SA (1974) Renal parenchymal accumulation of aminoglycoside antibiotics in rats. J Infect Dis 130:656–659

Luft FC, Walker PD, Yum MN, Kleit SA (1975) Gentamicin concentration in human kidney cortex. Clin Res 23:477A

Lund ME, Blazevic DJ, Matsen JM (1973) Rapid gentamicin bioassay using a multiple-antibiotic-resistant strain of *Klebsiella pneumoniae*. Antimicrob Agents Chemother 4:569–573

Lurie MH, Rahway NJ (1956) The ototoxicity of dihydrostreptomycin and neomycin in the cat. Ann Otol Rhinol Laryngol 62:1128–1148

Lutz MD (1978) Characteristic of gentamicin accumulation by proximal straight renal tubules in vitro. Clin Res 26:140A

Madhavan T, Yaremchuk K, Levin N, Pohlod D, Burch K, Fisher E, Cox F, Quinn EL (1976) Effect of renal failure and dialysis on the serum concentration of the aminoglycoside, amikacin. Antimicrob Agents Chemother 10:464–466

Maitra SK, Yoshikawa TT, Steyn CM, Guze LB, Schotz MC (1978) Amikacin assay in serum by high-performance liquid chromatography. Antimicrob Agents Chemother 14:880–885

Malacoff RE, Finkelstein FO, Andriole VT (1975) Effect of peritoneal dialysis on serum levels of tobramycin and clindamycin. Antimicrob Agents Chemother 8:574–580

Matsuzaki M, Nakamura K, Akutsu S, Sekino M, Hirata A, Asano M, Kishimoto K, Fukushima M (1975a) Studies on the toxicity of amikacin (BB-K8), I. Acute toxicity and subacute toxicity in rats. Jpn J Antibiot 28:415–433

Matsuzaki M, Nakamura Y, Yoshida A, Sekine M, Iisue K, Asano M, Onodera K, Watanabe K (1975b) Studies on the toxicity of amikacin (BB-K8). II. Chronic toxicity in rats. Jpn J Antibiot 28:434–457

Matsuzaki M, Akutsu S, Yoshida A, Onodera A, Sekine M, Tsuchida M, Asano M (1975c) Studies on the toxicity of amikacin (BB-K8). III. Subacute toxicity of amikacin (BB-K8) in dogs. Jpn J Antibiot 28:458–484

Matsuzaki M, Yoshida A, Akutsu S, Nakamura K, Sekino M, Okuyama D, Asano M (1975d) Studies on the toxicity of amikacin (BB-K8). IV. Chronic toxocity in dogs. Jpn J Antibiot 28:485–523

Matsuzaki M, Onodera K, Okazaki I, Nakajima A, Akima T, Koshino M, Kishimoto K (1975e) Pharmacological studies of amikacin (BB-K8). Jpn J Antibiot 28:385–400

Mays DL, VanApeldoorn RJ, Lauback RG (1976) High-performance liquid chromatographic determination of kanamycin. J Chromatogr 120:93–102

McHenry MC, Wagner JG, Hall PM, Vidt DG, Gavan TL (1976a) Amikacin in renal failure. Clin Pharmacol Ther 19:112a

McHenry MC, Wagner JG, Hall PM, Vidt DG, Gavan TL (1976b) Pharmacokinetics of amikacin in patients with impaired renal function. J Infect Dis 134:S343–354

Meyers BR, Hirschman SZ, Warmser G, Siegel D (1977) Pharmacokinetic study of netilmicin. Antimicrob Agents Chemother 12:122–123

Mirhij NJ, Roberts RJ, Myers MG (1978) Effect of hypoxemia upon aminoglycosides serum pharmacokinetics in animals. Antimicrob Agents Chemother 14:344–347

Mitchell CJ, Bullock S, Ross BD (1977) Renal handling of gentamicin and other antibiotics by the isolated rat kidney. Antimicrob Agents Chemother 3:593–600
Molgó J, Lameignan M, Uchiyama T, Lechat P (1979) Inhibitory effect of kanamycin on evoked transmitter release. Reversal by 3′,4′-diaminopyridine. Eur J Pharmacol 57:93–97
Momose S (1969) A new approach to the pathogenesis of acute tubular necrosis: with special reference to tubular damages occurred from coincidental administration of aminoglycoside antibiotics and sodium alginate. Jpn J Urol 60:823–833
Mondorf AW, Breider J, Hendus J, Scherberich JE, Mackenrodt G, Shah PM, Stille W, Schoeppe W (1978) Effect of aminoglycosides on proximal tubular membranes of the human kidney. Eur J Clin Pharmacol 13:133–142
Mootz W, Schöndorf J, Werner G (1972) Elektronenmikroskopische Untersuchungen am Plexus cochlearis nach Kanamycinintoxikation. Acta Otolaryngol (Stockh) 73:38–43
Mori H, Koga T, Kawahara T, Tamura H, Nakamura T (1972a) The safety test of lividomycin (1). Acute, subacute and chronic toxicity test of lividomycin. Pharmacometrics 6:787–812
Mori H, Kakishita T, Katoh Y (1972b) The safety test of lividomycin (2). Effect of lividomycin on development of fetuses and newborns' mouse. Pharmacomedia 6:813–820
Mori H, Saitoh N, Katoh Y (1973) The safety test of liviodomycin (5). Effect of lividomycin on development of fetuses and newborn of rabbits. Pharmacomedia 7:1241–1250
Moriyama S (1959) Studies on streptomycin deafness in its early stage. Jpn Otolaryngol 62:107–118
Murata S, Kadosawa H, Shomura T, Umemura K (1971) Distribution, metabolism and excretion of ribostamycin. Yakuzaigaku 3:1–7
Nakai Y, Yamamoto K, Iwamoto T (1972) Electromicroscopic study of kanendomycin and vistamycin ototoxicity. Audiology Jpn 15:202–210
Nakai Y, Yamamoto K, Zushi K, Fujimoto A (1974) The influence of amikacin (BB-K8) upon the cochlea. An electron microscopical study. Jpn J Antibiot 27:212–217
Nakai Y, Fujimoto A, Yamamoto K (1975) Combined effect of aminoglycoside antibiotics and potent diuretics on the cochlea. Audiology Jpn 18:290–298
Nakazawa S, Satoh H, Watanabe O, Sadaoka K, Fujii N, Abe M, Umemura K (1973) Experimental studies on absorption, excretion, distribution, and metabolism of 3′,4′-dideoxykanamycin B. IV. Pharmacokinetic analysis in pediatric field. Jpn J Antibiot 26:454–458
Nieminen L, Kasaun A, Kangas L, Sairio E, Anttila M (1978) Renal accumulation of amikacin, tobramycin, and gentamicin in the rat. Experientia 34:1335–1336
Niizato T, Koeda T, Tsuruoka T, Inoue S, Niida T (1976) Protective effects of D-glucaro-δ-lactam against aminoglycoside-induced nephrotoxicity in rats. J Antibiot (Tokyo) 29:833–840
Noone P, Pasaons TMC, Pattison JR, Slack RCB, Garfield-Davis D, Hughes K (1974) Experience in monitoring gentamicin therapy during treatment of serious gram-negative sepsis. Br Med J 1:477–481
Nurazyan AG (1976) Absorption, distribution, and retention of neomycin in gravid rabbits and fetus. Antibiotiki 21:625–630
Ogawa A (1975) The effects of ototoxic antibiotics on the sensory epithelia of the inner ear; a functional and histochemical study. Audiology Jpn 18:1–19
Ohtani I, Ohtsuki K, Omata T, Ouchi J, Saito T (1977) Potentiation of cochlear and renal damage resulting from furosemide and aminoglycoside antibiotics. Chemotherapy (Tokyo) 25:2348–2360
Ohtani I, Ohtsuki K, Omata T, Ouchi J (1978a) Interaction of bumetanide and kanamycin. Audiology Jpn 81:554–561
Ohtani I, Ohtsuki K, Omata T, Ouchi J, Saito T (1978b) Potentiation and its mechanism of cochlear damage resulting from furosemide and aminoglycoside antibiotics. ORL 40:53–63
Ohtani I, Ohtsuki K, Aikawa T, Ouchi J, Nakayoshi T (1979) A comparative study on the ototoxicity of dibekacin and tobramycin administered by intravenous infusion. Jpn J Antibiot 32:990–997

Ohyama S, Yoshimura M (1975) The role and behavior of the endocochlear potential in the inner ear. Audiology Jpn 18:255–260

Oksenhendler G, Leroy A, Humbert G, Fillastre JP, Winkler C (1977) Pharmacocinetique des nouveaux antibiotiques du groupe des aminosides: tobramycine, lividomycine, amikacine, sisomycine chez le sujet a function renale normale et chez l'insuffisant renal regles de posologie. Anesth Analg (Paris) 34:93–110

Oshita K (1959) Pharmacological studies on kanamycin. Med J Hiroshima Univ 7:1029–1062

Otori H (1967) Influence of gentamicin on the fetuses of Wistar rats and KR-JCK mice. Chemotherapy (Tokyo) 15:497–500

Paradelis AG, Triantaphyllidis C, Fidani V, Logaras G (1974) The action of the aminoglycosidic antibiotic gentamicin on isolated rat diaphragm. Arzneim Forsch (Drug Res) 24:1774–1779

Paradelis AG, Triantaphyllidis C, Markomichelakis JM, Logaras G (1977) The neuromuscular blocking activity of aminodeoxykanamycin as compared with that of other aminoglycoside antibiotics. Arzneim Forsch 27:141–143

Parker FL, James WL (1978) The effect of various topical antibiotic and antibacterial agents on the middle and inner ear of the guinea pig. J Pharm Pharmacol 30:236–239

Pechére JC, Dugal R (1976) Pharmacokinetics of intravenously administered tobramycin in normal volunteers and renal impaired and hemodialyzed patients. J Infect Dis 134:S118–124

Pechére JC, Roy B, Dugal R (1976a) Distribution and elimination kinetics of intravenously and intramuscularly administered tobramycin in man. Int J Clin Pharmacol Biopharm 14:313–318

Pechére JC, Pechére M-M, Dugal R (1976b) Clinical pharmacokinetics of sisomicin: dosage schedules in renal impaired patients. Antimicrob Agents Chemother 9:761–765

Pechére JC, Dugal R, Pechére MM (1978a) Kinetics of netilmicin in man. Clin Pharmacol Ther 23:677–684

Pechére JC, Dugal R, Pechére MM (1978b) Pharmacokinetics of netilmicin in renal insufficiency and hemodialysis. Clin Pharmacokinet 3:395–506

Penang GW, Jackson GG, Chion WK (1977) High-pressure liquid chromatographic assay of netilmicin in plasma. Antimicrob Agents Chemother 12:707–709

Pijck J, Hallynck T, Soep H, Baert L, Daneels R, Baelaert J (1976) Pharmacokinetics of amikacin in patients with renal insufficiency: relation of half-life and creatinine clearance. J Infect Dis 134:5331–5341

Raab WP, Windisch J (1973) Antagonism of neomycin by heparin. Arzneim Forsch 23:1326–1328

Ramirez-Ronda CH, Holms RK, Sanford JP (1975) Effect of divalent cations on binding of aminoglycoside antibiotics to human serum proteins and to bacteria. Antimicrob Agents Chemother 7:239–245

Rauws AG, VanKlingeren B (1978) Estimation of antibiotic levels in interstitial fluid from whole tissue levels. Scand J Infect Dis [Suppl] 14:186–188

Regamey C, Schaberg D, Kirby WMM (1972) Inhibitory effect of heparin on gentamicin concentrations in blood. Antimicrob Agents Chemother 1:329–332

Regeur L, Golding H, Jensen H, Kampman JP (1977) Pharmacokinetics of amikacin during hemodialysis and peritoneal dialysis. Antimicrob Agents Chemother 11:214–218

Reiffensten JC, Holmes SW, Hottendorf GH, Bierwagen MF (1973) Ototoxicity studies with BB-K8, a new semisynthetic aminoglycoside antibiotic. J Antibiot (Tokyo) 26:94–100

Revert C, Fillastre JP, Godin M, Leroy A (1978) Pharmacocinetique de la gentamicine; administration intramusculare de trois doses differentes chez des sujets ayant une fonction renale normale. Therapie 33:713–722

Ritschel WA, Banarer M, Lau Chang EF (1977) Computer-calculated kanamycin dosage regimen and monitoring. Int J Clin Pharmacol Biopharm 15:121–125

Robinson GC, Cambon KG (1964) Hearing loss in infants of tuberculous methods treated with streptomycin during pregnancy. N Engl J Med 271(18):949–951

Roth S, Naber K, Scheer M, Gruenwaldt G, Lange H (1976) Pharmacokinetics of sisomicin in patients with normal and impaired renal functions. Eur J Clin Pharmacol 10:357–365
Rudhardt M, Blauchard P, Fabre J (1978) Accumulation et persistance de aminosides dans le parenchyme renal. Nouv Presse Med 7:3819–3823
Sairio E, Kasanen A, Kangas L, Nieminen AL, Nieminen L (1978) The nephrotoxicity of renal accumulation of amikacin, tobramycin and gentamicin in rats, rabbits and guinea pigs. Exp Pathol (Jena) 15:370–375
Saito A, Katoh Y, Ishikawa K, Uemura H, Tomizawa M, Nakayama I, Satoh K (1978) Studies on sisomicin. Chemotherapy (Tokyo) 26:99–106
Sato K, Hama K (1979) Scanning electron microscopic observations of the under-surface of the tectorial membrane. J Electron Microsc (Tokyo) 28:36–42
Sato K, Koeda T, Yokota M (1979) Histopathological study on the vestibular toxicity of dibekacin and other aminoglycoside antibiotics. J Kanazawa Med Univ 4:172–175
Sawchuk RJ, Zaske DE (1976) Pharmacokinetics of dosing regimes which utilize multiple intravenous infusions; gentamicin in burn patients. J Pharmacokinet Biopharm 4:183–195
Schentag JJ (1977) Gentamicin disposition and tissue accumulation on multiple dosing. J Pharmacokinet Biopharm 5:559–577
Schentag JJ, Abrutyn E, Jusca WJ (1976) Pharmacokinetic characterization of gentamicin accumulation in man. Clin Pharmacol Ther 19:114
Schentag JJ, Cumbo TJ, Jusco WJ, Plaut ME (1978 a) Gentamicin tissue accumulation and nephrotoxic reactions. J Am Med Assoc 240:1067–2069
Schentag JJ, Lasezkay G, Cumbo TJ, Plaut ME, Jusco WJ (1978 b) Accumulation pharmacokinetics of tobramycin. Antimicrob Agents Chemother 13:649–656
Schentag JJ, Lasezkay G, Plaut ME, Jusco WJ, Cumbo TJ (1978 c) Comparative tissue accumulation of gentamicin and tobramycin in patients. J Antimicrob Chemother 4:23–30
Schrogie JJ, Costello R, Hensley MM (1977) Pharmacokinetics of netilmicin in healthy volunteers. Clin Pharmacol Ther 21:116–117
Shiraiwa M (1966) Studies on permanent electrodes implanted on the round window of rabbits. Audiology Jpn 69:631–660
Simon HJ, Yin EJ (1970) Microbioassay of antimicrobial agents. Appl Microbiol 19:573–579
Simon VK, Mösinger EU, Malerczy V (1973) Pharmacokinetic studies of tobramycin and gentamicin. Antimicrob Agents Chemother 3:445–450
Singh YN, Marshall IG, Harrey AL (1978) Some effects of the aminoglycoside antibiotic amikacin on neuromuscular and autonomic transmission. Br J Anaesth 50:109–117
Smith CR, Lipsky JJ, Lietman PS (1979) Relationship between aminoglycoside-induced nephrotoxicity and auditory toxicity. Antimicrob Agents Chemother 15:780–782
Spoendlin H, Galogh K (1964) Licht- und elektronenmikroskopische Darstellung von Dehydrogenasen in der Schuche nach Intravitalinkubation. OPL 26:159
Stanley VF, Giesecke AH, Jenkins MT (1969) Neomycin – curare, neuromuscular block and reversal in cats. Anesthesiology 31:228–232
Stevens P, Young LS (1977) Simple method for elimination of aminoglycosides from serum to permit bioassay of other antimicrobial agents. Antimicrob Agents Chemother 12:286–287
Szwed JJ, Luft FC, Black HR, Elliot RA, Stuart A (1974) Comparison of the distribution of tobramycin and gentamicin in body fluids of dogs. Antimicrob Agents Chemother 5:444–446
Takabatake H, Oda T, Shiina M, Satoh Y, Ohno T (1978 a) Studies on diffusion of chemotherapeutic agent into blood, uterine, oviduct, and ovary of rabbits and urinary recovery, of dibekacin and ampicillin. Jpn J Antibiot 31:303–306
Takabatake H, Oda T, Shiina M, Satoh Y, Ohno T (1978 b) Studies on diffusion of chemotherapeutic agents in uterine muscle, fetus, placenta, amnion, and amniotic fluid of pregnant rabbits, of dibekacin and ampicillin. Jpn J Antibiot 31:307–309
Takeda H, Nakanishi H, Matumura S, Matsuda S, Kawakami M, Otani K, Uno O, Kaneshiro A (1975) Pharmacological studies on tobramycin, effects of tobramycin on cardiovascular, respiratory, muscular, and urinary excretory systems. Chemotherapy (Tokyo) 23:1440–1459

Takimoto M, Fujita K, Maruyama S, Yoshida H (1976) Safety test of lividomycin. III. Experimental study of the cochlear damage induced by lividomycin. Pharmacometrics 6:845–855

Tamura H, Fukakusa Y, Ogawa Y, Ouchi J (1972) The pharmacokinetics of tobramycin following intramuscular administration in new born infants. Chemotherapy (Tokyo) 24:1268–1271

Tan JS, Salstrom SJ (1977) Levels of carbenicillin, ticarcillin, cephalothin, cefazolin, cefamandole, gentamicin, tobramycin, and amikacin in human serum and interstitial fluid. Antimicrob Agents Chemother 11:698–700

Tanaka Y, Asanuma A, Yanagisawa K, Katsuki Y (1975) Microphonic and D.C. potentials in the organ of corti and tectrial membrane. Audiology Jpn 18:241–245

Tasaki I, Davis H, Eldredge DH (1954) Exploration of cochlear potentials in guinea pigs with microelectrode. J Acoust Soc Am 26:765–773

Thuillier C, Fillastre JP, Godin M (1977) Pharmacokinetic data on single dose of 280 mg gentamicin i.m. J Antimicrob Chemother 3:527–528

Toyoda Y, Tachibana M (1978) Tissue levels of kanamycin in correlation with oto- and nephrotoxicity. Acta Otolaryngol (Stockh) 86:9–14

Tronovec T (1978) Pharmacokinetics of gentamicin administered intratrancheally to rats. Antimicrob Agents Chemother 14:165–167

Tulkens P, Trouet A (1978) The uptake and intracellular accumulation of aminoglycoside antibiotics in lysosomes of cultures rat fibroblasts. Biochem Pharmacol 27:415–424

Ueda Y (1969) Nephrotoxicity of antibiotics. Chemotherapy (Tokyo) 17

Ueda Y, Nakamura N (1968) Nephrotoxicity of antibiotics. Farumashia 4:179–183

Ueda Y, Saitoh A, Uchiura G (1975) Nephrotoxicity of antibiotics. Gekkan Yakuji 17:35–39

Umemura K, Komiya I, Nakadori S, Sien-Yao Chow (1977) Pharmacokinetics of dibekacin after intramuscular administration in man. Jpn J Antibiot 30:650–656

Umezawa H (1964) Aminoglycoside antibiotics. In: Umezawa H (ed) Recent advances in chemistry and biochemistry of antibiotics. Nissin Tosho Insatsu, Tokyo, pp 67–84

Umezawa I, Ogawa H, Kawakubo Y, Morino T, Nishiyama Y (1976a) Studies on acute and subacute toxicity of spectinomycin dihydrocloride pentahydrate. J Antibiot (Tokyo) 29:43–54

Umezawa I, Ogawa H, Komiyama K, Kawakubo Y, Morino T, Nishiyama Y (1976b) Studies on chronic toxicity of spectinomycin dihydrochloride pentahydrate. Jpn J Antibiot 29:55–60

Vogelstein B, Kowarski AA, Lietman PS (1977a) Continuous sampling as a pharmacokinetic tool. Clin Pharmacol Ther 22:131–139

Vogelstein B, Kowarski AA, Lietman PS (1977b) The pharmacokinetics of amikacin in children. J Pediat 91:333–339

Wagman GH, Oden EM, Weinstein MJ, Irwin S (1967) Effect of calcium on the toxicity of gentamicin. Antimicrob Agents Chemother 1966:175–181

Waitz JA, Moss EL Jr, Weinstein MJ (1971) Aspects of the chronic toxicity of gentamicin sulfate in cats. J Infect Dis 124:125–129

Waksman SA (1949) Clinical use of streptomycin. Streptomycin, nature and practical application. Williams & Wilkins, Baltimore, pp 279–560

Walker JM, Wise R, Mitchard M (1979) The pharmacokinetics of amikacin and gentamicin in volunteers: a comparison of individual differences. J Antimicrob Chemother 5:95–99

Watanabe Y, Nakajima R, Oda R, Uno M, Naitoh T (1971) Experimental study on the transfer of kanamycin to the inner ear fluids. Med J Osaka Univ 21:257–263

Watanuki K, Gottesberg AM (1971) Toxic effects of streptomycin and kanamycin upon the sensory epithelium of the *crista ampullaris*. Acta Otolaryngol (Stockh) 72:59–67

Watson EH, Stow RM (1948) Streptomycin therapy, effects on fetus. J Am Med Assoc 137:1599–1600

Wefer G, Bray C (1930) The nature of acoustic response. J Exp Physiol 13:373

Weinstein L (1970) Chemotherapy of microbial disease. In: Goodman LS; Gilman A (eds) The pharmacological basis of therapeutics. Macmillan, New York Toronto London, pp 1090–1247

Weitnauer G, Mattei A, Sinoncini F (1957) Acute and chronic toxicity of some complex salts of streptomycin and dihydrostreptomycin. Farmaco [Sci] 12:899–927
Whelton A, Carter GG, Walker WG (1975) Gentamicin concentrations in healthy and diseased kidneys. Clin Rev 23:225A
Whelton A, Carter GG, Bryant HH, Fox L, Walker WG (1976) Therapeutic implications of gentamicin accumulation in severely diseased kidneys. Arch Intern Med 136:172–176
West BA, Brummett RE (1973) Interaction of kanamycin and ethacrynic acid. Arch Otolaryngol 98:32–37
Yamada H, Yoshida T, Hirano K, Kimura Y, Ichihashi T, Doi M, Konaka J, Katagiri K (1975) Absorption, excretion, distribution and metabolism of tobramycin. Chemotherapy (Tokyo) 23:894–899
Yamamoto K, Yoshimura K, Hirono S, Inoue Y, Sakamori M, Matsumura S, Morishige E (1975) The effects of tobramycin on the central nervous system. Chemotherapy (Tokyo) 23:1460–1469
Yamasaku F (1974) Nephrotoxicity. Chemotherapy (Tokyo) 22:210–213
Yamasaku F, Kabasawa T (1976) Serum levels of dibekacin in normal subjects and uremic patients following intramuscular injections. Chemotherapy (Tokyo) 24:1515–1520
Yamasaku F, Suzuki Y, Umemura K (1980) Pharmacokinetics of ribostamycin in healthy volunteers and patients with impaired renal function. Jpn J Antibiot 33:1318–1331
Yamashita T (1972) Histochemical studies on the effects of oxygen deprivation in the hair cells of the cortis organ. Otol Fukuoka 65:591–613
Yokota M (1977) Ototoxic effects of some aminoglycoside antibiotics on the inner ear in guinea pigs. J Showa Medical 37:535–544
Yokota M, Odaki M, Koeda T, Sato K, Akiyoshi M (1976) The safety evaluation of fradiomycin-gramicidin-S troches "Meiji". Jpn J Antibiot 29:841–849
Yokota M, Odaki M, Koeda T, Sato K (1977) Ototoxic effects of some aminoglycoside antibiotics on the inner ear in the spontaneously hypertensive rats (SHR). Jpn J Antibiot 30:738–743
Yoshida M, Kimura Y, Doi M, Katagiri K (1975) Micromethod for microbiological assay of tobramycin concentrations in body fluids. Chemotherapy (Tokyo) 23:886–893
Yoshioka H, Takimoto M, Nakatsugawa T, Maeda T, Tasaka Y (1974) Pharmacokinetics and clinical evaluation of BB-K8 in children. Jpn J Antibiot 27:382–388
Ziv G, Sulman FG (1972) Binding of antibiotics to bovine and ovine serum. Antimicrob Agents Chemother 2:206–213

Subject Index

Handbook of Experimental Pharmacology

Continuation of "Handbuch der experimentellen Pharmakologie"

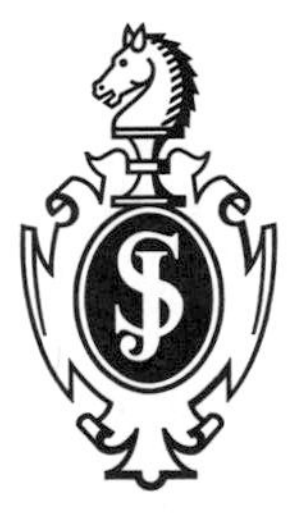

Springer-Verlag
Berlin
Heidelberg
New York

Volume 18
Histamine and Anti-Histaminics

Part 1
Histamine. Its Chemistry, Metabolism and Physiological and Pharmacological Actions

Part 2
Histamine II and Anti-Histaminics

Volume 19
5-Hydrocytryptamine and Related Indolealkylamines

Volume 20: Part 1
Pharmacology of Fluorides I

Part 2
Pharmacology of Fluorides II

Volume 21
Beryllium

Volume 22: Part 1
Die Gestagene I

Part 2
Die Gestagene II

Volume 23
Neurohypophysial Hormones and Similar Polypeptides

Volume 24
Diuretica

Volume 25
Bradykinin, Kallidin and Kallikrein

Volume 26
Vergleichende Pharmakologie von Überträgersubstanzen in tiersystematischer Darstellung

Volume 27
Anticoagulantien

Volume 28: Part 1
Concepts in Biochemical Pharmacology I

Part 3
Concepts in Biochemical Pharmacology III

Volume 29
Oral wirksame Antidiabetika

Volume 30
Modern Inhalation Anesthetics

Volume 32: Part 2
Insulin II

Volume 34
Secretin, Cholecystokinin, Pancreozymin and Gastrin

Volume 35: Part 1
Androgene I

Part 2
Androgens II and Antiandrogens/Androgene II und Antiandrogene

Volume 36
Uranium - Plutonium - Transplutonic Elements

Volume 37
Angiotensin

Volume 38: Part 1
Antineoplastic and Immunosuppressive Agents I

Part 2
Antineoplastic and Immunosuppressive Agents II

Handbook of Experimental Pharmacology

Continuation of "Handbuch der experimentellen Pharmakologie"

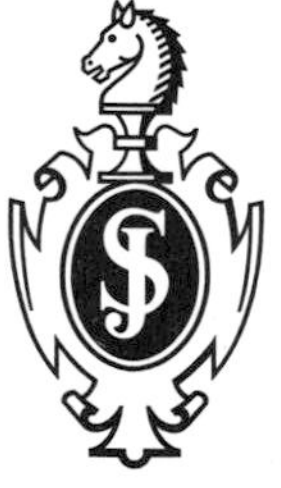

Springer-Verlag
Berlin
Heidelberg
New York

Volume 39
Antihypertensive Agents

Volume 40
Organic Nitrates

Volume 41
Hypolipidemic Agents

Volume 42
Neuromuscular Junction

Volume 43
Anabolic-Androgenic Steroids

Volume 44
Heme and Hemoproteins

Volume 45: Part 1
Drug Addiction I

Part 2
Drug Addiction II

Volume 46
Fibrinolytics and Antifibrinolytics

Volume 47
Kinetics of Drug Action

Volume 48
Arthropod Venoms

Volume 49
Ergot Alkaloids and Related Compounds

Volume 50: Part 1
Inflammation

Part 2
Anti-Inflammatory Drugs

Volume 51
Uric Acid

Volume 52
Snake Venoms

Volume 53
Pharmacology of Ganglionic Transmission

Volume 54: Part 1
Adrenergic Activators and Inhibitors I

Part 2
Adrenergic Activators and Inhibitors II

Volume 55: Part 1
Antipsychotics and Antidepressants I

Part 2
Antpsychotics and Antidepressants II

Part 3
Alcohol and Psychotomimetics, Psychotropic Effects of Central Acting Drugs

Volume 56, Part 1 + 2
Cardiac Glycosides

Volume 57
Tissue Growth Factors

Volume 58
Cyclic Nucleotides
Part 1: **Biochemistry**
Part 2: **Physiology and Pharmacology**

Volume 59
Mediators and Drugs in Gastrointestinal Motility
Part 1: **Morphological Basis and Neurophysiological Control**
Part 2: **Endogenis and Exogenis Agents**

Volume 60
Pyretics and Antipyretics

Volume 61
Chemotherapy of Viral Infections